Medical Armageddon

UPDATE 2000

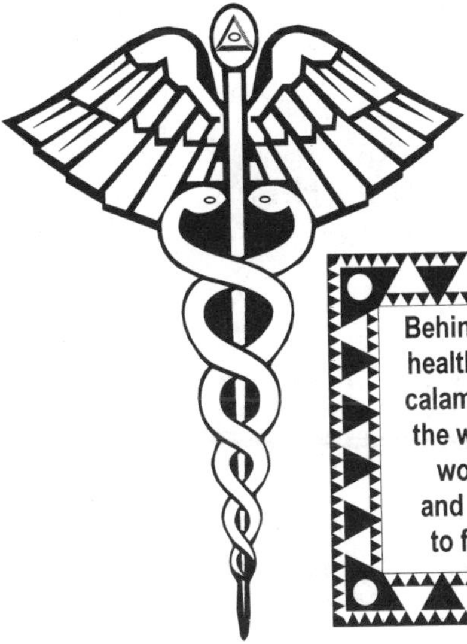

Behind the healthcare calamity of the whole world and how to fix it

Michael L. Culbert DSc

C AND C COMMUNICATIONS
San Diego, California

First Printing: Fall 1997

LIBRARY OF CONGRESS CATALOGUE CARD NUMBER 97-069817

ISBN: 0-9636487-5-6

MADE IN CANADA

Dedicated to the memory of
Gylah Bess Culbert

1910-1995

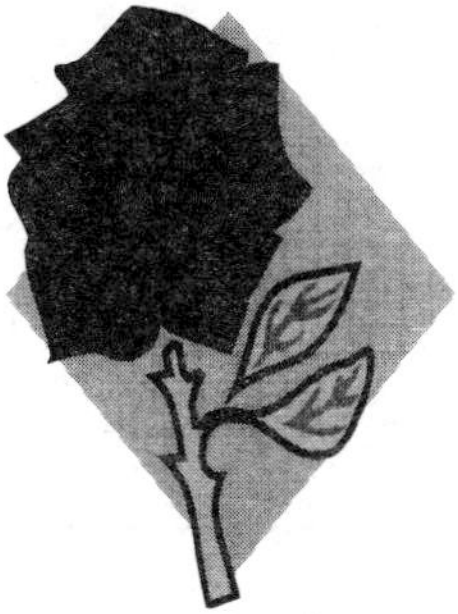

". . . and behold, a pale horse, and its rider's name was Death, and Hades followed him; and they were given power over a fourth of the earth, to kill with sword and with famine and with pestilence . . ."

REVELATION 6:8

". . . for thy merchants were the great men of the earth, and all nations were deceived by thy sorcery . . ."

REVELATION 18:23

TABLE OF CONTENTS

AUTHOR'S PREFATORY NOTE

This book was edited and readied for publication at about the same time a new dimension in medical terror was developing — the increasing likelihood that biological warfare-derived "weaponized" microbes, for which the Persian Gulf War of 1991 may have been a kind of dress rehearsal, were spreading throughout both the military and civilian populations of many countries. (See Chapter XIV)

The appearance of microscopic structures almost certainly manufactured as "stealth" weapons presents a new concern to a world population already threatened with virtually uncontrolled metabolic/immunological chronic conditions and antibiotic-resistant "old" bacteria.

These combined threats, some coming simply from Mother Nature, others from the expanding human civilization on this planet, still others from what mankind is consciously doing to *mankind, present the world's population with the most serious of challenges as a new millennium begins.*

There is now a greater need than ever before for a thorough alteration of the Western-led medical paradigm which "guides" so much of therapy and for the continual presence of openmindedness in dealing with new theories and approaches.

It is my hope that this book is a contribution to both.

Michael L. Culbert DSc PhD (Hon.)
San Diego, California
Fall 1997

ACKNOWLEDGMENTS

While the author cannot possibly list all the individuals and organizations who and which have played some role in helping bring *Medical Armageddon* to fruition, he feels impelled to mention the following:

- Dr. Robert Bradford, Bradford Research Institute/American Biologics, an innovative medical thinker with whom the author has long been associated.
- Rodrigo Rodriguez MD, medical director, and the staff of the American Biologics-Mexico SA Medical Center, Tijuana, Mexico, with whom he has also been associated since the beginning.
- Dr. Anton Jayasuriya, Sri Lanka, whose worldwide Medicina Alternativa organization has helped provide a sounding board for new ideas concerning, and new directions for, world medicine.
- Attorney William Moore Jr. who originated some of the conceptual phrases referred to in this book.
- Bruce Halstead MD, whose lifelong dedication to new ideas in medicine and medical thought has been a continuing inspiration to so many.
- California biochemical researcher Henry W. Allen, who for years has been of invaluable assistance in explaining complicated issues in an understandable way.
- The late Ernst T. Krebs Jr. DSc and Dean Burk PhD, of laetrile fame, who often served as mentors and intellectual stimulants to a frequently doubting journalist.

He is also indebted to Bernardino S. Juat Jr. for proofreading. Of course the constantly-altered manuscript would never have been ready for publication without the dedicated PC input of his colleague and companion Dante I. Camino.

INTRODUCTION:
The birth of a paradigm

"To every action there is an equal and opposite reaction."
— Newton's Third Law of Motion

Dawn breaks in Virginia

These were truly historic moments:

Never before had standard medical practitioners (allopaths), homeopaths, naturopaths, chiropractors, acupuncturists, herbalists, Native American healers, experts in meditation, dietitians, physical therapists and self-styled medical eclecticists converged in one place at one time.

But it occurred in Virginia in 1992, after an earlier meeting had also taken place in the Old Dominion to set the stage for this one:

The "working group on unconventional medical practices" was established by the federal National Institutes of Health (NIH) as an ad hoc gathering of 110 proponents of what the American medical establishment was variously calling "unproven," "unorthodox," "unconventional," and "alternative" medicine.

The tone was easily perceptible: American medicine is losing the war against chronic diseases — and millions of citizens are turning to "alternative" treatments for everything from persistent back pain (the number-one medical complaint in the Western world) to cancer. Perhaps varying schools of medicine might learn from each other.

I was on the ad hoc group, and I inhaled with deep satisfaction the atmosphere of a paradigm shift, however slight:

The mere fact that ideological and vested-interest adversaries could be gathered together under the banner of the NIH was itself a tremendous propaganda victory for the concept of the need for a new paradigm in medicine. That it had been stimulated into creation because former Congressman Berkley Bedell (D-Iowa) and sitting Senator Tom Harkin (D-Iowa) had had positive experiences with "alternatives" was icing on the cake.

I was among the minority of ad hoc committee members arguing for three central ideas: that the new paradigm in medicine ought to be called *integrative* rather than "alternative" (since the latter word suggests that somehow "standard" treatments are still preferred and are the criterion against which any other treatments should be measured), that the only rational assessment of multifactorial, essentially nutritional therapies should be *end results*, and that only a restoration of a decentralized free market in medicine and medical ideas could or should be the sociopolitical filter through which the new paradigm was presented.(1)

In 1993 two landmark events followed these earlier meetings:

First, the Office of Alternative Medicine (OAM) within the NIH maze became a working unit, an outgrowth of the Virginia meetings, invested with a small budget and a tiny staff; and, perhaps of equal or more importance, a startling national poll published in the strictly orthodox *New England Journal of Medicine* sent shock waves reverberating through what we are calling throughout this book the Allopathic Industrial Complex (AIC) — that is, the governmental-pharmaceutical-medical "establishment".

A random survey of 1,539 adults had found(2) that in 1990 *one out of three* Americans had used or were using "alternative" treatments of one kind or another — and, more stunning from the AIC's eye-on-the-bottom-line perspective — they had paid $13.7 billion for such services (chiropractic and herbs topping the list), with $10.3 billion paid out-of-pocket (as opposed to $12.8 billion spent out-of-pocket for all hospitalizations in 1990). Of almost equal weight, the *NEJM* survey found that American patients had made 425 million visits to "alternative" healthcare professionals in 1990, or substantially more than the 388 million visits to "standard" family doctors and internists.

Putting it conservatively, Dr. David Eisenberg, Harvard Medical School, told *USA Today*: "The scope is far larger than anticipated."[3]

Quite so.

The national poll was only the most recent tidal wave invading the littoral of the AIC: as we note elsewhere in this account, by 1993 it was an accepted fact that Americans were spending $4 billion per year on vitamin and other nutritional supplements, that a half or more of adult Americans were consuming them occasionally and some 60 million were doing so daily and that Americans in record numbers were seeking solutions to their chronic disease problems *outside* the United States — usually Mexico.

While earlier research had essentially dispelled the myth that Americans who seek "alternative" cancer treatments are somehow undereducated, misinformed dolts, the *NJEM* and other research looked at the even broader field of seekers of "alternatives" in general:

They were, said the authors, well-educated and among the more affluent of the population.

The extreme "quackbuster" phalanx of the AIC had little to say about the poll itself, since the figures spoke for themselves, but it did have rhetoric to hurl at the new OAM office as "a waste of time and money."

The same oft-quoted, court case-appearing "quackbusters" intoning such standard claptrap were often the same individuals who, unable to explain away a vast increase in consumption by the American public of vitamin pills, attempted to dismiss the whole effort as one leading only to "more expensive urine."

But the dinosaurian pro-drug industry "quackbusters" and the embattled party ideologues of allopathy may or may not have had any understanding of what was really happening — a paradigm shift and a grass-roots movement far vaster in scope and concept than the scattered elements of outright health fraud, gouging and profiteering which also went with them.

The nutritional supplements/"healthfoods"/herbal industries have become explosive elements in the domestic economy:

—By 1994 supplements/herbs were bringing in $7 billion a year, a market growing by 20 percent per year, according to 1996 figures.[4] By 1996, the total market in "natural products" had zoomed to $9.17 billion.[5] One estimate placed the "nutrition industry" at $17 billion that year with projected annual increments of 14 to 16 percent, with an estimate of $30 billion-plus by 2000.[6] These figures still trail the gargantuan synthetic drug industry (*see VII*) but the latter is clearly feeling the heat and has belatedly "discovered" how nutrient sales can inflate the bottom line, as we shall see.

Within four years of pivotal 1993, it became clear to many, including some in the AIC (if not to its sociopath minority wing), that a revolution — a shift in thought-constructs or paradigms — regarding medicine was in the works, and that it reached deep into the American (and Western) psyche.

At the political level, and borrowing a page from the state-by-state "decriminalization" movement for laetrile in the late 1970s/early 1980s, various freedom-of-medical-choice organizations began lobbying for and passing legislation at the state level.

At the time of this update (1997) eight states had written into law legislation which either generally protected "alternative" medicine or some particular aspect of it, and bills to do the same were incubating in more than a dozen others.

At the federal level, sweeping medical freedom legislation had been offered in both Houses but, as expected by numerous activists, had not gotten very far since the combined lobbying clout of the AIC is massive and ubiquitous at that level.

Perhaps of even more significance, "alternative" medicine had become an area of legitimate medical study at major American universities. By mid-decade, divisions of, courses in, or even departments devoted to, "alternative" medicine were in place at some 30 percent of teaching hospitals and/or universities including those of the University of Arizona, Boston, Case Western Reserve,

Cincinnati, City University of New York, Columbia, Georgetown, George Washington, Harvard, Indiana, Johns Hopkins, Louisville, Maryland, Medical College of Philadelphia, Miami, Michigan State, Minnesota, Mount Sinai School of Medicine, Pennsylvania State, Rochester, Rush Medical College, Southern Illinois, Stanford, Temple, Tufts, UCLA, Uniformed Services University of Health Sciences, University of California-San Francisco, Virginia, Wayne State and Yale.[(7)]

By 1997, naturopathy had secured licensing or relicensing in twelve states, and was available in one form or another in more than two dozen others. Rapidly resurging homeopathy, while long "legal" in the US but cold-shouldered by the AIC (and its major turf competitor in the 19th century — *see V*), was covered by specific "practice acts" in only three states but interest in its *pharmacopeia,* an authorized medical document in the US since 1938 though elements of it are over a century old, was blossoming practically everywhere.

The number of homeopathic practitioners exploded toward the end of the century in the USA — from an estimated 200 in 1970 to some 2,000 in 1995.[(8)]

Chiropractic, this century's major challenge to medical orthodoxy, was a licensed profession in all 50 states.

And acupuncture was regulated by "practice acts" in 26 states as of 1995[(9)] with some 3,000 physicians nationwide using the ancient technique.[(10)]

Indeed, if acupuncture is lumped in with "oriental medicine," as of 1996 practitioners of the latter were licensed or registered in 24 states with licensure under the supervision of a "physician" (allopath) available in three others and oriental medicine without licensure available in at least five other states. All told, as of that year some 7,200 individuals were involved in the practice of oriental medicine, 6,500 of whom were licensed.[(11)]

A Health Policy Institute of the Medical College of Wisconsin survey in 1996 projected that the supply of "alternative" medical clinicians (definable as chiropractors, naturopaths, and practitioners of oriental medicine) would grow by 88 percent between 1994 and 2010, while the "physician" (that is, allopath) supply would grow only by 16 percent.[12]

The Wisconsin survey set the number of "alternative" physicians (again, as narrowly defined) in 1994 at 59,000, or "equivalent to 10 percent of the number of patient care physicians (including osteopaths) in that year."[13]

It added that as of 1994 there were 16 chiropractic colleges, 29 colleges of oriental medicine and three naturopathic colleges, with a fourth expected by 1997.

This was before the announcement of the first student year at the new Capital University of Integrative Medicine in Washington DC, an accredited institution offering degrees in both "integrative" and "physiatric" medicine for health professionals already holding other degrees.

While at this time chiropractic remains quantitatively the major form of "alternative" medicine, the growth of "oriental medicine" is projected to be more impressive between now and 2010 (a 230 percent increase.[14]).

Harking back to the most ancient form of medicine (touch — *see IV*), some 24 states had licensed "massage therapists" by 1996 — another manifestation of upwardly spiralling interest in non-pharmaceutical therapy.[15]

As tepid moves toward integrating medical practices began to be seen, a 1996 report[16] indicated that numerous allopathic physicians were using acupuncture, herbal therapy and other "alternative" approaches in their practices, while the American Academy of Family Physicians was recommending continuing medical education (CME) credits for courses in spinal manipulation[17] and many allopathic doctors, especially those in "primary" care, were referring patients to "alternative" clinicians.[18] In a ground-breaking event for government-based medicine, in 1995 a "natural medicine clinic" was approved as a part of the King County (WA) Department of Health, to be managed by the accredited naturopathic Bastyr University.

Incredibly, in 1996 the National Institutes of Health (NIH) recommended that medical and nursing students learn about "alternative" medicine — on the heels of a University of Maryland survey that showed that 70 percent of doctors wanted to learn more about the subject since 40 percent of their patients wanted such treatments.[19]

Even the *New York Times* was forced to admit editorially in 1996 that "alternative medical treatments have grown into a big business and a powerful force in modern medicine."[20]

Breaking at least in part with the AIC, by 1997 at least 18 major insurance companies, several small ones and a growing number of HMOs were at least timidly beginning to cover — or soon planned to cover[21] — certain "alternative" medical practices in several states, if only on an experimental basis.

This was in response not only to the merits of "natural therapies" but to the drives for "cost containment" and "managed care" — since "alternative medicine" usually costs less.

Behind the paradigm shift

Several currents were converging in the stream racing toward medical change:

— The ever-more-visible failure of "standard" (that is, allopathic) medicine, as enshrined in the AIC, to stave off chronic, systemic, metabolic diseases and immunological challenges, whose numbers, both in incidence and fatality, had been growing with rapidity during the prior decades. Cancer and AIDS were the more notable of these, but the population was also adrift in a polluted sea of arthritis (at ever younger ages), diabetes and prediabetic conditions; the full spectrum of maladies lumped together as "heart disease"; increases in such "incurable" disorders as multiple sclerosis (MS), lupus, osteoporosis, rheumatoid arthritis, Parkinson's and Alzheimer's; the rapidly-growing Chronic Fatigue Syndrome (CFS) and Gulf War Illness (GWI) and a veritable plague of immunological disorders and environmental poisonings of all kinds; weirdly named syndromes rare or unheard of a century before; and a growing list of geriatric and pediatric conditions.

And, by the mid-1990s, the accelerated presence of antibiotic-resistant bacteria and of "emerging" new viral diseases, all seemingly incurable, greatly enhanced public concern. Both failure in curbing these civilization-threateners, and the high economic and social costs of such failure, could no longer be hidden or easily explained away.

— The dietary/nutritional revolution was blossoming, an outgrowth of several currents in American society. The connection between dietary excesses and deficiencies and health and disease was being joined by an ever-greater national debate over the nature of food processing itself and the chemicalization of the food supply. In the "heart disease" sector, it was being demonstrated on all sides that more balanced eating programs, reducing fats while increasing fruits, vegetables and grains, and encouraging physical exercise, clearly correlated to lower fatalities and fewer cardiac problems. "Food faddism," or the popularization of dietary plans promoted to enhance good health, and ranging from the demonstrably useful to the absurdly eccentric, became hallmark "counterculture" activities of the 1960s which reached the mainstream in the 1970s and 1980s.

— The advent of meditative/mind-body techniques from the East and their virtual "Americanization" as a part of a generally "holistic" paradigm developing primarily within the 1960s and enhanced by political forces (America's "opening to China" and the spread of communism in Asia, which indirectly stimulated a flow of Asian religion-centered practices toward the West.) Some of these were championed by entertainers and other famous personages; some were continuations of the Eastern occult tradition which had intermittently entered the West earlier in the 20th century and throughout the 19th. The Western need to quantify results and subject such practices to "scientific" scrutiny has led to an avalanche of information on what we call the "X factor" and its relationship to health and disease (*see XVII.*)

— The political success of the laetrile movement in the 1970s/1980s had been a prime catalyst. As we examine elsewhere (*XII*), the promotion, distribution and use of an apricot kernel derivative against cancer posed the greatest challenge to the AIC since its struggle with homeopathy in the 19th century and was of even greater impact than its war in the twentieth with chiropractic. That 24 states representing more than half the American population would either "decriminalize" or "legalize" an unpatentable plant-derived nutritional factor for use against cancer while the totality of the AIC (and most of the administrative/statutory and media apparatus which it controls or strongly influences) and the enormous marriage of vested industrial and research interests we have called Cancer Inc. (*XI*) vehemently opposed it, was a reality of historic, sociological and political significance. More than any other element (though the battle for the vindication of Vitamin C against disease was not far behind), laetrile drew attention to the realities that nutrition plays giant roles in the induction and control of chronic diseases and that dietary change alone provides at least a partial barrier to the development of such disorders.

The laetrile movement was also parallel to, and at times part of, a general antiestablishment mindset which particularly flourished in the 1960s/1970s, the decades which straddled sociopolitical concern over civil rights and America's involvement in an intensely unpopular war. The movement to secure "freedom of choice in cancer therapy" for laetrile, in which this writer was intimately involved, became part of the larger movement to secure "freedom of choice in medicine" for physician and patient "with informed consent" — and it stood as a major adversary to entrenched bureaucracy, assumed authority, and the virtual religiosity with which the AIC presented itself to the masses as the arbiter, dispenser, controller and ideological policeman of all things medical in the United States.

— And, last but not least, biochemical research was raising the tantalizing possibility that the human lifespan could be lengthened — in good health — with a constellation of nutrients, hormones, drugs and lifestyle changes. The herd instinct not only to survive but thrive was demanding a review of basic medical wisdom.

'Quackbusters' attack

The arbiters and gatekeepers of American medicine simply do not like to be challenged in any way. This writer was directly assailed in 1993 in one of the final numbers of the *New York State Medical Journal* by one of the more rational "quackbusters," who attempted to link my stated dissent from the AIC's "line" on AIDS (its causation by a single "new" virus, primarily) with a "rightwing conspiracy theory" involving black nationalists and *left*-leaning journalists. The author made a major point that "suspicion of authority is a national characteristic of Americans, and is easily aroused," as if this were some sort of inherited disorder.[22]

The laetrile movement, and all that flowed from it, did in fact arouse — with very good reason — a "suspicion of authority," one in alignment (I argued) with the arousal in 1775-1776 which gave birth to the Republic. But the notion that the Allopathic Industrial Complex somehow is the single defender of revealed truth in medicine, and that all dissidents thereto are either deranged or charlatans, remains the self-defeating defense mechanism of that very AIC.

For, even as the notion of *integrative medicine* — joining the best of all worlds of medical practice into a united concept of healing — began to rise at the conceptual and intellectual levels, the policing powers of the AIC remained intact, and as vicious as ever.

Even so, it was all akin to a Greek drama: the bemused American public (and increasingly that of Western civilization) was televisionally treated to case after case of "unorthodox" practitioners arrested, led off in handcuffs and irons, and of violent raids on their clinics by uniformed goons. Each new police action had the effect of setting off a thousand new FAXes and inspiring E-mail activists to send messages of protest to state or national capitals or to load the rapidly advancing — and as yet uncontrolled — cyberspace of the Internet with damning information.

Every AIC action, then, was producing an equal and opposite reaction, confirming Newton.

As we indicate later in this account, "quackbusting" is international, and very much at the behest of international pharmaceutical food and energy concerns which (correctly) see in the surge of interest in vitamins, minerals/metals, herbs and all manner of "non-nutritive food factors" and "phytochemicals" natural and mostly *unpatentable* challenges to the empire of synthetic chemicals and the medical model which ideologically nurtures it.

As the millennium approaches, no small portion of the political questions relating to human liberty *vis-a-vis* the incubating New World Order revolves around international efforts to squelch medical free choice in the interests of monopoly over drugs, foods, seeds and even genes, and to use both regional and international law to do so (*see VIII and XV*).

From my own world tours of 1996 and 1997 (Philippines, Thailand, Malaysia, New Zealand, Spain, Italy, Sri Lanka) I found a planet in medical-freedom ferment with millions of people beginning to be aware of the all-out struggle between the forces of free choice and liberty and those which seek to impose total control, including total *health* control, over the whole world.

These tours, and the onrush of new information — some frightening, some heartening — caused me to update and re-release as a single large study *Medical Armageddon*, whose first two volumes appeared in late 1994 and the subsequent two in 1995.

The war is on. We dare not lose it.

San Diego, California
Fall, 1997

REFERENCES

1. Committee for Freedom of Choice in Medicine Inc. statement to National Institutes of Health (NIH), June 2, 1992.
2. Eisenberg, DM, *et al.*, "Unconventional medicine in the United States; prevalence, costs and patterns of use." *New Eng. J. Med.*, Jan. 28, 1993.
3. *The Choice*, XIX:1, 1993.
4. *Newsweek*, May 6, 1996.
5. Emerich, Monica, *Natural Foods Merchandiser,* June 1996.
6. "Revenge of the witch doctor." Multnomah OR: *Oregon Business*, December 1996.
7. *Alternative Medicine*, March 1995.
8. *Alt. Med. Digest* 13, 1996.
9. *Overview of Legislative Developments Concerning Alternative Health Care in the United States,* Fetzer Institute, 1995.
10. Appleby, Julie, "Cultures and cures." Pleasanton CA *Valley Times*, Dec. 8, 1996.
11. Cooper, RA, and SJ Stoflet, "Trends in the education and practice of alternative medicine clinicians." *Health Affairs* XV: 3, Fall 1996.
12. *Ibid.*
13. *Ibid.*
14. *Ibid.*
15. Cohen, MH, "Holistic health care: including alternative and complementary medicine in insurance and regulatory schemes." *Arizona Law Rev.* 38:1, Spring 1996.
16. Cooper, *op. cit.*
17. Page, L, "Manipulative therapy gains interest; DOs seek more study." *Am. Med. News,* June 26, 1995.
18. Borkan, J, *et al.*, "Referrals for alternative therapies." *J. Fam. Prac.* 39: 6, 1994.
19. Kritz, Fran, "Doctors, nurses need alternative medicine training." *Medical Tribune*, July 18, 1996.
20. Cited in *Alt. Med. Digest.* 13, 1996.
21. Pelletier, KR, presentation to Medical Board of California Alternative Medicine Colloquium, University of California-San Diego, Aug. 22, 1997.

22 Sampson, WI, "AIDS: frauds, finances and fringes." *NY State Med. J.*, February 1993.

I
FEDSTAPO:
The incredible story of health-freedoms suppression in America

"I'm naive. I believe everybody wants to be well, and to have the freedom to make medical decisions concerning their health."

— Indiana osteopath Dr. Cal Streeter after a 30-man FDA raid on his clinic, 1996

". . . A female employee's apartment was raided by eight officials. One official knocked on the door, refusing to identify himself. She looked through the peephole, did not know the person, went into her bedroom to call 911. They then broke the door down with guns drawn, forcing her to the floor with a gun to her temple . . . In another example . . . agents broke into a Southern California home while a mother was breast-feeding her infant. The mother was handcuffed for eleven hours while the agents ransacked her home."

— Life Extension Foundation, 1993

"These people are quacks . . . We had to play a little rough to send a message to the whole industry . . . When you get these kinds of off-balance people combined with a patient population that is more than a little crazy, then you would want to have plenty of firepower too when you raided one of these so-called clinics."

— FDA spokesman "explaining" the Wright clinic raid in Washington State, 1992

"Former employees received subpoenas for depositions. I was placed under surveillance and followed. Members of my family were followed. Telephones were tapped . . . My home was ransacked, with nothing stolen. Days and weeks later, various business documents could not be found. An 'insider' in the police department let it slip that they were under orders to release no information about the investigation of the break-in. . ."

— Imprisoned chiropractor Lawrence Hall DC, Florida, 1991

". . . I was still chained to the bed. Two guards were assigned to me on 8-hour shifts. When I went to the bathroom, both ankles were chained together and a woman guard went to the bathroom with me. The only more secure measures are taken with prisoners on Death Row."

— FDA veterinary vitamin products prisoner Sissy Harrington-McGill, 1990

In an American Gulag

In fall 1990, Gertrude (Sissy) Harrington-McGill, 57, of El Cajon CA, found herself in a maximum-security federal prison in San Diego, surrounded by federal felons — drug runners, traffickers in illegal immigrants, embezzlers, perpetrators of bank frauds, and assorted other women who in one form or another had run afoul of federal laws and statutes (and of federal judges, who are all-powerful in the "American judicial system.")

The self-described member of the California Teachers Assn. (CTA) and the National Education Assn. (NEA), though asthmatic, had been assigned to "vacuuming" duties at the Metropolitan Correctional Center — a "hard time" maximum security detention facility.

Ms. Harrington-McGill could only move "off the floor" while shackled at the wrists, ankles and waist. She slept horizontally on rusty, antediluvian beds while wrapped up in castoff Navy fatigues to protect herself against the nightly cold.

Once she was placed in the prison hospital for severe hypertension. Later she was rushed as an emergency case of possible stroke to a San Diego hospital, where she was taken to the neuro-surgery intensive care unit.

She recalled:

> On my left side was a monitor with white wires and a pulse meter attached to it. On my right side were brown wires and an automatic blood pressure cuff that inflated every few minutes. I was still chained to the bed. Two guards were assigned to me on 8-hour shifts. When I went to the bathroom, both ankles were chained together and a woman guard went to the bathroom with me. The only more secure measures are taken with prisoners on Death Row.(1)

It was finally determined she had not had a stroke but had in fact undergone severe anxiety and stress. She was put on a heavy regimen of tranquilizers and returned to prison — where, a few days later, she suffered another "occurrence" in which she temporarily had severe pains in her head, right arm and right leg.

Younger women took a liking to the woman they called "Miss Harrington" and warned her to be careful of all the pills the prison was prescribing. Even when she gave in and took "one little yellow pill" instead of the four she had been prescribed she slept 24 hours one day and 22 the next.

At one point, virtually comatose, she was awakened by her alarmed cellmates who brought her to her feet and walked with her to keep her awake. She was told by prison officials she had had "an unexpected reaction" to the medication.

In her mostly coherent moments, Ms. Harrington-McGill made some mental notes. One of her prison companions was in "max" for 40 days for smuggling illegal aliens. Another had drawn 90 days for writing $10,000 worth of bad checks on a government base (with no restitution necessary). Another woman was doing four months for a $168,000 embezzlement, and yet another four months for $150,000 in bank fraud.

Sissy Harrington-McGill did 114 days' "hard time" (just shy of four months).

Her crime? Americans who believe ours is "the land of the free and the home of the brave" should steel themselves for the answer:

"Criminal contempt of court" in a tangled federal legal brawl growing out of a 12-year running battle with the Food and Drug Administration (FDA) over labels and "health claims" made on 13 health foods and supplements for . . .

Dogs, cats and horses.

For a good deal of her professional life, Sissy Harrington-McGill has owned and operated Solid Gold, a veterinarian-oriented company providing dietary supplements and healthfood products for animals — and serving some of the better-known names in Western civilization, including presidents and royal families.

It is instructive to note that only a community newspaper and our own The Choice *magazine (national organ of the Committee for Freedom of Choice in Medicine, Inc.) made much of a fuss about the incredible story.*

In the American Gulag, this well-educated, otherwise non-criminal, taxpaying, responsible American citizen simply ceased to exist for 114 days.

Assuming, if necessary, that she was somehow guilty of the "crime," that she had had poor prior legal advice, that she could have cut deals — which prosecutors and lawyers love to do — and could have avoided her nightmare experience by paying a $500 fine, the question that nettled everyone, that is, everyone, *who knew of her case was uniformly the same:*

So what?

How could this woman be placed into extreme peril and crypto-human incarcerative conditions because of "health claims" — beginning with "veterinarian brewer's yeast" products for dogs and horses? How, indeed . . .

The Choice *gave both the federal judge as well as the FDA a chance to answer the question. The beyond-public-access jurist declined. An FDA bureaucrat, a "consumer safety officer, division of compliance, center for veterinary medicine" (yes, there is such a bureaucrat and there is such an office within the tax-sapping FDA) did in fact respond.*

He sent along several documents, all in order, including a "complaint for injunction" (1988) which "summarizes the government's allegations that Ms. McGill violated the law by promoting and distributing unapproved new animal drugs"; a "consent degree of permanent injunction" (when Harrington-McGill "did not comply" with the court order, the FDA brought "contempt proceedings" against her and Solid Gold) — and the "information" document on which the proceedings were based.[2]

So much for the icily correct bureaucratic response.

Not one to keep her head down, the operator of Solid Gold began a long, protracted legal battle with the Feds, and had scored one mini-victory by 1993. She claimed to be far from finished. "Major media" ignored the story.

The great B-vitamin bust

The "major media," however, could not overlook what happened May 6, 1992, in Kent WA, simply because a cool-headed employee had the gumption to alert the media to the outrage and videotape footage captured part of it.

On that date, reported the Seattle WA *Post-Intelligencer*:

> *Dozens of state and federal law enforcement officers broke down the doors of a Kent medical clinic. . .*
>
> *They burst through the back door with guns drawn. "They came in with their guns pointing at us and told us to freeze," said Julie Gallegos, a medical assistant at the clinic.*
>
> *Receptionist Marge Murphy said FDA agents wearing flak vests "broke through the main door yelling" and one of them pointed a gun in her face. "He told me, 'Get your hands up where I can see them,'" Murphy said.*
>
> *Clinic manager Pennie Morehead said agents yanked telephone lines out of walls after one employee tried to make a call.*[3]

The *P-I* reported that one employee had suffered a mild heart "irregulation" during the action and that officers carted off equipment, business records and other documents while also raiding a pharmacy in the same complex where the target facility, the Tahoma Clinic, was located.

Luckily, an employee who was hiding behind a column was able to make telephone contact with the outside world before the clinic's two dozen employees were corraled into a "holding area" by the raiders.

This police action, led by the FDA, is typical of operations by the *DEA* directed at suspected purveyors of dangerous drugs and devices. What were the dangerous drugs and devices which the Feds and the Kent police found being dispensed at Dr. Jonathan Wright's Tahoma Clinic?

They were — among other essentially harmless things — German brands of injectable Vitamin B complex, folic acid, and

Vitamin B12, injectable adrenal cortical extract, injectable licorice extract, the naturally occurring substance adenosine monophosphate, and a machine widely used in Europe for the detection of allergies. Which is to say, only by the FDA's broadest stretch of the word "drugs," particularly anything injected, and implied lack of approval of certain substances or devices used medically, were there "illegal" items on the premises.

The Kent WA police, used by the FDA in the raid, indicated in various ways that they had been "had." An FDA-watching newsletter quoted a Kent policeman who had participated in the goon squad-like assault:

> *"FDA officials asked for our help . . . We looked at the search warrant and saw it had been signed by a federal magistrate. We made a critical mistake in not reading the search warrant. The FDA guys were all pumped up. It pumped us up. We were told to break down the doors. We didn't have any idea who we would encounter. We knew that illegal drugs were involved. But FDA didn't tell us it was for old ladies with allergies.*
>
> *"The whole incident has been extremely embarrassing. We look and feel like class A idiots. The next time those jerks ask us for some help, we'll let them find some other patsies. It would be pretty funny unless you saw the terror on the faces of those people."*[(4)]

The same newsletter wrested from an FDA official this intriguing response to the question as to why such force had been used in the confiscation of a U-Haul truckful of records, equipment and natural substances (none of them truly synthetic drugs in the liberal definition thereof):

> *"These people are quacks. They mislead innocent people into believing they can be cured of all kinds of illness just with vitamin shots. We had to play a little rough to send a message to the whole industry . . .*
>
> *"And these people are slippery, if you think you can let them get away with anything. When you get these kinds of*

off-balance people combined with a patient population that is more than a little crazy, then you would want to have plenty of firepower too when you raided one of these so-called clinics."[5]

And, then, what of Jonathan Wright MD himself? A career hoodlum? A known quack? A clear and present social danger?

In fact, the creative and medically progressive Dr. Wright — a maverick, an original thinker, an individualist in an American Medical Association (AMA) sea of toe-the-line obeisance — was a Harvard-and-University of Michigan-educated physician who had been practicing what some call "holistic" or "complementary" medicine for 20 years, who had never undergone disciplinary action, and none of whose patient population of about 1,200 had complained against him. Far from it: they took to the print and electronic media *in defense* of their doctor.

At a time when FDA-approved modalities were/are killing at least 100,000 Americans per year (*IX*), and while not a single substance of those which were seized, confiscated or placed under surveillance by the FDA/Kent raiders had been known to maim, let alone kill, anybody, we were constrained to wonder just what *had* Jonathan Wright done? Since he was not the only well credentialed medic who believed in and used various vitamin products (whatever their technical legality might be), was there some other murky specter lurking in his medical closet?

And, sure enough, there was:

The FDA had already swung into enthusiastic high gear over the L-tryptophan scandal: the appearance in the USA of a production-contaminated version of an amino acid which thousands of doctors had administered to hundreds of thousands (possibly millions) of patients over many years as a kind of natural, non-drug, non-addictive tranquilizer/sedative. Because there had been scattered cases of actual deaths and poisonings attributable to the foreign version of the product, the FDA — waiting for almost 20 years to re-assert itself in the vitamin supplements industry, a growing competitor to the far more profitable synthetic drug business — had seen in the L-tryptophan case an excuse to move against the entire supplements area, with drug companies applauding from the sidelines. (*IX*)

Hence, FDA raiders had been going around confiscating contaminated L-tryptophan — possibly a worthwhile endeavor. They of course did not stop there: they nabbed *any* L-tryptophan they could get their bureaucratic hands on. Then, unlike actions against the friendlier food and drug industries (recent examples had included the Tylenol capsule and imported grape tampering cases) the product in general (that is, *all* L-tryptophan in oral form) remained banned, contaminated or not.

The FDA had seized Dr. Wright's uncontaminated L-tryptophan — a mainstay not only of his practice but of that of numerous "holistic" doctors. But Jonathan Wright had had the brassbound gall to sue the federal agency for its return.

The imperious — and, as we shall see, multiply corrupted and often thug-like — federal agency, even though allegedly existing at the will of "the people," does not like to be sued. When suits occur, it fights back, and will use a battery of attorneys good to the taxpayers' last dollar in efforts to rid the landscape of dissidents.

As Citizens for Health detailed it in a publication for holistic and other independent-minded physicians:

> *Dr. Wright's attorney has informed us that the lawsuit filed against the FDA by Dr. Wright to have uncontaminated L-tryptophan returned from a pharmacy and his clinic was filed in August 1991. According to the FDA's affidavit attempting to justify their armed raid on May 6, 1992, they began their investigation of his clinic . . . on Sept. 23, 1991.*
>
> *On that date they began searching the business complex's trash dumpster for any evidence that might be used as probable cause to raid his clinic. The dumpster serves a sandwich shop, computer software accounting company, a pharmacy, a laboratory, the clinic, and other*

businesses. The dumpster was checked periodically from late September 1991 through March 19, 1992.[6]

The time frame thus suggests to the minimally IQ-efficient a revenge attack on an outspoken, popular holistic/integrative physician who had had the temerity to fight Big Brother.

This had been going on for a long time, of course — FDA, state and local SWAT teams breaking down doors, arresting doctors, harassing nurses, terrifying patients, confiscating records, intimidating witnesses and in general behaving as Gestapoid-Communist thugs was well-known to practitioners and patients of "alternative" medicine in "the land of the free, the home of the brave."

It was simply that this time part of the government's vicious and criminal behavior was captured on videotape. The Wright case became a *cause celebre*, and generated so many FAXes, telephone calls and telegrams to the federal government in such numbers that a special "hot line" FAX was set up at the White House to deal with them.

The pressure paid off: in 1995 the US Justice Department ordered an end to the Wright probe and also mandated the FDA to return the $100,000 worth of medical materials it had wrongfully seized during the 1992 raid. The 1992-1995 Tahoma Clinic raid and followup constituted a pivotal turning point in the battle for health freedoms in America and graphically demonstrated that — until the Constitution is revoked — an outraged and informed citizenry still has the power to successfully oppose governmental tyranny.

Heavy-handedness at Highland Labs

At an overflow hearing of the King County (WA) Council's Law and Justice Committee after the Kent raid, an employee of another recently raided facility, Highland Laboratories in Oregon, was on hand to report on just what had gone on there. The employee had reportedly made the trip because the FDA, in a statement to the county council's chairman, had denied the federal agency was involved in a general campaign of suppression of alternative/nutritional medicine and products.

In 1991, some two dozen federal and state officers showed up to raid Highland Laboratories, Mount Angel OR, over supposed labelling violations first brought to Highland's attention in 1989, when the FDA had originally "visited" the highly respected supplements manufacturer.

The combination federal-state operations — which startled residents of the small town, some of whom wondered just what dangerous activity might be going on at Highland — resulted in the confiscation of 14 products, office and personnel records, and printing plates for the 200 products Highland was manufacturing.

At issue was the nature of "labelling" (FDA has always had an interesting view of what "labelling" is — it has often been construed to mean a book or pamphlet about a natural supplement in a healthfood store located apparently within *any* proximity to a bottle, box or other container that may have a supply of the natural supplement). The implied message of the action at Highland seemed to have been: "When the FDA says change labels we *mean* it" (witness Sissy Harrington-McGill).

The campaign of the FDA against Highland was what a company spokesman called a pattern of harassment which

> *. . . involves (1) the force used by FDA to conduct a simple regulatory proceeding, (2) the tactics used by the FDA to discredit Highland with clients and state granting agencies before judicial proceedings began, (3) the clear intent of FDA to run Highland out of business, and (4) FDA's campaign to usurp business rights to free speech and individuals' free choice of medical and nutritional care.*[7]

The Highland raid, ultimately resulting in hefty legal fees (more than six figures by 1992) for defense (a primary weapon used by the government against presumed violators, since the government itself has the endless treasure trove of American tax dollars with which to pay for wave after wave of Justice

Department attorneys in grinding down the victim), was one of 1991's major negative news items from the FDA compliance world.

Double trouble at Century Clinic

In 1990, another example of government muscle flexed for the murkiest of reasons took place at the Century Clinic, Reno NV.

On two separate occasions, Sept. 6 and Oct. 25, FDA and state agents raided a clinic run by Yiwen Tang MD and his wife — the first "visit" lasting an estimated 16 hours, the other 13. Patients were denied the right to leave the premises for most of those hours, The Choice *was told.*

The raiders seized 72 patient records, various natural supplement products, homeopathic medical equipment and, said Mrs. Tang, acted like "Nazis."

She told me:

> They came in with an open warrant. They've been here twice. They said they were looking for Wobe-Mugos enzymes [*a European-produced line of protein-digesting natural enzymes*]. They were also looking for things we don't have and never heard of. I can't imagine this happening; I'm ready to leave the country. They even took homeopathic medicines. Those are supposed to be legal in Nevada. We can't figure out what we did wrong. What kind of country is this?[(8)]

What kind, indeed.

I contacted the FDA about this particular raid and was told by a spokeswoman: "We went in twice for search and seizure, with a warrant to seize a number of products, including Nieper drugs and medical devices."

"Nieper drugs" apparently referred to any number of the innovative nutritional supplements developed by Hans Nieper MD of Hanover, Germany, one of Europe's most famous integrative practitioners. The FDA had been routinely seizing and confiscating some of these from US recipients for years, usually arguing

that they were "illegal new drugs" (typically, anything used even vaguely for medical purposes which had not gone through the labyrinthine FDA approval process, an apparatus designed for synthetic drugs.)

The FDA apparently was also interested in an electro-diagnostic machine called the Dermatron, favored by many homeopaths and naturopaths but which, particularly when of foreign manufacture, ran afoul of FDA control over "medical devices" — anything, in fact, which even remotely could be construed as being involved in the practice of medicine. The FDA had also seized Dermatrons and similar equipment in offices in Florida and Washington.

ITEM: None of the products or devices referred to had been known to have killed or injured anybody.

In a sinister parallel to the Century raids, the mother of a former patient at the clinic told The Choice *she had been visited by a self-identified FDA officer at her home.*

According to the mother, the agent intimidated her with threats of a subpoena, particularly after she spoke in favor of the treatment her 8-year-old daughter had received there. The mother added that the agent had told her "I could be in trouble" for sending the child to the clinic in the first place.[9]

Century Clinic patients rallied around their treatment center. By 1994 the clinic was working out its differences with the FDA, but the memory of the events remained etched in many patients' minds, and whatever the federal agency had hoped to accomplish with the high-profile tactics had faded from media interest.

American storm troopers

In 1991, a particularly active year for high-profile, thuggish activity by the FDA, agency-led raids were carried out in Washington, Oregon and Utah at various sites and offices from which Vitacel-7 nutritional products were sold or records concerning which were kept. They apparently were part of an ongoing effort to crush Gerovital (procaine hydrochloride, a vitamin-like substance), or GH3, both names for the "anti-aging" compound developed by the late gerontologist Ana Aslan of Rumania, and similar products.

Biochemist Robert Koch DSc, also developer of some of these procaine-based products, told *The Choice* that a lengthy investigation of them by US postal authorities had failed to turn up any complaints against them.

Koch said that on May 21, 1991:

— FDA and postal authorities, accompanied by armed police and federal marshals, entered an Oregon mail forwarding agency contracted by a British West Indies manufacturer and began seizing company mail.

— Agents entered the Seattle Computer Center and seized a computer, data discs, records, and whatever was related to the products.

— In South Jordan UT, "agents, police and federal marshals wearing bulletproof vests and brandishing guns surrounded and entered [my] home, scaring [my] daughter and granddaughter. They seized all of [my] research records, personal and business records, computer, computer discs and software printers, etc., and [my] bank account."[10]

An employee who exclaimed, "What about our rights?" was said to have been shoved into a chair and told, "You don't have any rights!"

It is instructive to note that this gun-toting multi-agency, multi-state raid on business locations was not directed at cocaine trafficking, heroin, uppers, downers, illicit gold bullion, or smuggled arms or aliens but against vitamin-like supplements used by thousands of people and which somehow, some way, may indeed have violated some statute or presumed statute of state or federal law.

Gerovital was also a focus of aggressive federal activity in 1993 in both California and New Mexico.

In the former, observers reported that eight FDA and

Customs agents surrounded and raided a home in Fresno whose occupant was being investigated for the alleged illegal importation and distribution of the compound. His father had already been jailed on similar charges. In the Fresno raid the man's 8-months-pregnant wife and 83-year-old grandmother were allegedly held at gunpoint for 10 hours.

In Albuquerque NM, raiders also swung into action against Rodger Sless' Tierra Marketing, approximating the same kind of gun-wielding incursions as in California.

Fighting back, Sless let it be known by all who would listen just what the ironies of the crackdown on Gerovital were:

The drug is "vitaminic" in that it breaks down to the B-vitamin PABA and the related substances choline and acetylcholine, among other things, and was legally available in the State of Nevada and in an estimated 40 foreign countries.

Defenders of GH3 or Gerovital have also noted that an FDA consumer affairs officer was already on record as stating it was not illegal to possess GH3 for personal use and another FDA officer had stated there was no safety problem with it.

If in fact this essentially harmless compound had been illegally imported, the question remained unanswered: why so much federal muscle to stop the smuggling?

In June 1994 it was Sless — not the FDA — who prevailed in court, as he was acquitted on 11 of 15 charges and no decision was reached on 4 others.[11]

Beating the Feds in court — example one

Throughout part of the 1990s, nutritional supplements purveyors or proponents Life Extension International/Life Extension Foundation were continually harassed by the FDA. After FDA-incited embargoes of Life Extension's products in Arizona were lifted by the Arizona state attorney general, FDA seemed all the more eager to keep LE under surveillance.

In October 1991, Life Extension won an important victory: US District Court Judge James C. Paine ordered the FDA to return to the Foundation and its officers property — supplements and documents — which the federal agency had illegally seized on Feb. 26, 1987.

In a lawsuit, Life Extension officers Saul Kent and William Faloon said they had taken action "because the FDA has been spending millions of taxpayer dollars on a criminal 'investigation' to stop plaintiffs from criticizing FDA policies and practices" through publishing articles, brochures, and advertisements and by providing press and congressional information on the FDA's misadventures. They added:

> The FDA has been trying to silence the Foundation with threats of indictment and jailing of its leaders, even though the FDA has yet to present a shred of evidence that the Foundation has ever harmed anyone![12]

By 1993, Life Extension, as a continuing thorn in the side of the FDA, had won another sweet victory: a federal judge forced the FDA to pay attorneys' fees in the amount of $4,392.22 in the lawsuit over the FDA's holding "without just cause" company property for more than four years.[13]

This was evidence that persistence enough, and enough legal fees, could at least keep the Feds at bay. In fact, the record is that if a company has enough money and patience it may win in the end.

Beating the Feds in court — example two

By 1992, biochemist Stephen Levine, operator of Nutricology/Allergy Research Group in Northern California, reported he had spent $300,000 in a year's time to defend his companies against FDA claims of mail fraud and selling "unapproved new drugs" or "unsafe food additives" — that is, nutritional supplements.

By 1994, the feisty Dr. Levine had been in and out of court enough times to become something of an expert in FDA law, and had won against Big Brother at least five times. At several of the hearings and legal chess moves, a US federal judge repeatedly admonished the federal agency for its behavior.

The FDA had been monitoring Allergy Research Group since 1982, intermittently informing Levine that the agency considered various natural supplements (among others, flaxseed oil, coenzyme Q10, organic germanium, borage oil, an extract of hen egg yolks, and several natural antioxidants) to be "unlicensed new drugs."

Claiming Levine and associates had not sufficiently cooperated with the agency, a dozen agents and US marshals had finally raided and shut down the company's operations for two days while they made copies of files and records — and, Dr. Levine told me, "scared the employees, took down their license plate numbers, and videotaped them."[14]

Intimidating employees through name-taking and videotaping is part of federal/state tactics designed to create the illusion the victims are involved in organized crime — just as going through trash and garbage to secure evidence ("garbage duty," in police enforcement parlance) and sticking presumed violators with as many charges at the *state* level as possible (the "porcupine tactic," in attorney talk) — is part of the investigative prosecutory process.

But Dr. Levine marshalled copious documentation on all the nutrients under FDA surveillance and inserted into the record research by major investigators, as well as 60 affidavits from doctors and nutritionists who expressed their positive opinions on the products' efficacy and safety.

In the first of several victories for judicial reason over the FDA's Gestapery, Judge Lowell Jensen rebuffed FDA arguments that Levine and associates had engaged in "misrepresentation" let alone "mail and wire fraud" on grounds of "insufficient evidence." Moreover, ruled Judge Jensen:

> *The government has brought forward no direct evidence that the products at issue here have caused any harm whatsoever to the consumer public. . .*
>
> *Because an apparently substantial percentage of*

defendants' products are used by patients upon the advice of their physicians, there is no significant threat of plaintiff's perceived danger of consumers opting in favor of defendants' products over alternative and arguably more efficacious methods of care.[15]

On Sept. 23, 1993, Judge Jensen again ruled against the FDA's attempt to stop Levine's companies from selling 14 of its nutrient products, which primarily were being distributed through doctors.

He denied the federal agency's motion for summary judgment, granted Nutricology's motion to eliminate the FDA's charges of "wire fraud" and "mail fraud" and even granted Nutricology's motion to throw out the FDA's demand that the company pay financial restitution for "improprieties" to the government.[16]

It appeared that all Levine was truly guilty of was fighting back — at enormous personal expense — against his initial harassment by the FDA. The FDA, as its long and shoddy history reveals (*IX*), does not like to be sued in return after it raids, confiscates and tramples on civil liberties. That a single purveyor of highly regarded nutritional supplements could be left standing following attack after attack by the FDA over several years was something of a record itself.

Nightmare for a 'chiro'

In February 1992 chiropractor Lawrence Hall DC entered Eglin Air Force Base, Florida, to begin five years of federal detention following conviction on various Medicare "mail fraud" counts after years of harassment of his successful chiropractic clinics across Florida — a harassment which may have begun, he believes, when he contributed to a defense fund for a fellow doctor facing similar charges earlier.

The Hall case was occurring just as chiropractors were winning their decade-old legal battle with the AMA and associates over conspiracy, restraint of trade and related matters (see VII) *and as chiropractic was enjoying a considerable surge in popularity by removing tens of thousands of Americans from drug-based allopathic medicine and hence posing the most severe challenge to "establishment" medicine (and the immense global pharmaceutical hydra which has nurtured it) since its 19th-century battle with homeopathy.*

By the end of 1991 the popular Dr. Hall said he had spent some $7 million over a five-year period while the federal government ground him down in every way possible, ultimately hitting him with 32 counts of various illegal activities. As he told The Choice,[17] *the basis of his hounding by Big Brother had to do with his preference for chiropractic and musculoskeletal adjustment therapies (even when used together with "standard" medicine) at five successful clinics in the state.*

Following five years of problems, audits and attorney games, Dr. Hall on Jan. 23, 1991, found himself placed in handcuffs and irons in front of a clinic full of his patients in Winter Haven, then whisked 60 miles to a courthouse jail in Tampa for appearance before a federal magistrate.

Information Dr. Hall turned up through a private investigator led to the discovery that Medicare had established a "hit list" of doctors to be put out of business and that Medicare field investigators had been told to do "whatever it takes" to close the listed clinics.

"The clinics were getting sick and hurting people well by the hundreds," he told me.

Claiming he had never been told in five years of investigation just what his supposed crimes were, Dr. Hall described months and years of hounding and nerve-wracking surveillance by the Feds, while virtually all his funds went into attorneys' fees and endless legal maneuvers.

Among the harassments:

> Former employees received subpoenas for depositions. I was placed under personal surveillance and followed. Members of my family were followed. Telephones were

tapped . . . My home was ransacked, with nothing stolen. Days and weeks later, various business documents could not be found. An 'insider' in the police department let it slip that they were under orders to release no information about the investigation of the break-in . . .[18]

It should be noted that this kind of policing/surveillance is normally used for investigating distributors of dangerous drugs — a job the federal side has seemed to do very badly — and other serious criminal enterprises. Whether Dr. Hall was totally innocent or made mistakes or not during the operation of a successful chiropractic practice again raised the question: So what? Did his professional life and reputation need to be junked by an investigation which over the span of years cost American taxpayers dearly — and just what kind of menace did he really *represent to society even if* any *or* all *of the counts against him had any validity?*

The ordeal of Jimmy Keller

On March 18, 1991 — as it was argued by his attorneys — noted "metabolic therapy" healer Jimmy Keller, an American beloved by many cancer patients who had sought out his Saint Jude Clinic in Tijuana, Mexico, was actually escorted across the international border from Mexico by *US federal agents* and immediately jailed. No deportation proceedings had taken place and the act, as his lawyers described it, might have violated Mexican-US treaties; at the very least it made a mockery of Mexican sovereignty.[19]

It should be pointed out that Keller, a long-time recovered "terminal" melanoma cancer patient who had healed himself through various natural methods, was not a doctor and did not claim to be one — nor had he broken any of the various layers of laws in the Republic of Mexico.

Through a combination of maneuvers involving one Mexican policing agency and an individual suspected of helping to set him up, Keller was grabbed by Americans on the strength of a "wire fraud" and "cancer quackery" indictment issued in 1984. At that time, he had operated a cancer treatment clinic in Matamoros, Mexico, on the other side of the country from Tijuana.

The 1984 indictment was largely an argument that Keller used a telephone to inform American cancer patients about treatments in Matamoros — on the face of it, a Constitutionally protected activity. The federal side argued that in essence the soft-spoken Louisianan had lured the ill-informed into the bowels of "cancer quackery" and promised to "cure" them. He claimed he had never promised any such thing (and this writer, who knew him for years, never heard him claim to cure anybody of anything). Even so, he had become a popular exponent of "alternative" therapies and, worse, seems to have infuriated at least one federal officer. One doesn't infuriate one of these "public servants" and get away with it.

Keller spent months in federal detention before his trial in Brownsville TX federal court. There, scores of Keller's patients were on hand not to denounce the "cancer quack" but to claim he had helped them.

A major government complaint against Keller (though, had this been an honest proceeding, it should have been Mexicans complaining, not Americans) was that he used radionics and L-arginine against cancer.

To the amazement of some reporters, and possibly even the federal judge, who could have doled out 55 years to Keller, it was learned that radionics, however seemingly bizarre (energy healing projected at a distance [*see XVII*]), is a legitimate form of therapy in several countries, with most of its early work having been done in the USA; and L-arginine, an amino acid, is known to have certain anti-cancer properties.

Neither, of course, is an "FDA-approved" remedy — though neither is specifically banned in Mexico, which normally views medicine and medical freedom other than the way "the Colossus of the North" does.

Despite widespread support for Keller, he drew two years in

federal prison for his "wire fraud" and defense of radionics, L-arginine and other non-toxic therapies in a friendly foreign country. Another "social menace" had been removed, thanks to America's ever-vigilant federals.

The major media did not see fit to make much of the Keller case. It remained, however, a legal abomination hatched in the Land of the Free, the Home of the Brave.

Grim humor from the FDA?

Possibly interested in occasional comic relief, the tax-supported FDA in 1991 brought its guns to bear down on a product of a Utah company called Pets Smell-Free (PSF).

The product was designed to stop odors from urine, feces, gas and bad breath in animals. But — and this may have been the crux of the absurdity — it also contained an antibiotic, enough for underworked federal FDA "compliance" officers to claim the product was an "unapproved new drug."

Luckily, a rational judge granted Pets Smell-Free a summary judgment against the FDA from destroying a quantity of the product it had (actually) seized and voiding an injunction against it.

The federal judge agreed with PSF's producer that an item designed to remove an offensive odor is not the treatment of a disease.[20] *Since it also was neither a food nor a cosmetic there were questions galore raised about just why the FDA — unless it was taking a needed respite from raiding healthfood stores or terrifying matronly recipients of foreign B-vitamins — even believed it* had *jurisdiction in this patently asinine case, whose prosecutory elements were paid for, of course, by US taxpayers.*

Burzynski battles to victory

By 1997, Polish-born emigre physician-biochemist Stanislaw Burzynski MD PhD, operating the Burzynski Research Institute (BRI) in Houston TX, had spent some 14 years learning about "the American way" of medical freedom, and wondering just what the differences were between it and the Polish Communist system he had left behind:

On the one hand, the FDA had long since raided the BRI and carted off so many medical records and other documents that many Burzynski patients — recipients of his experimental "antineoplaston" cancer treatment — were literally left twisting in the wind. While he fought off the FDA raiders, the compliant state of Texas, and even insurance companies which tried to avoid reimbursing his patients, the full weight of American medical orthodoxy, oncological subdivision, came down heavily on the very well-credentialed — and very brave — doctor.

On the other hand, the federal National Cancer Institute (NCI), conduit of federal funds for cancer research, had thought enough of Dr. Burzynski's extensive documentation from US and foreign sources on the theory and practice of antineoplastons against cancer that it had begun clinical (human) trials on the compounds, though one study was "truncated" when the NCI and the doctor could not come to terms.

While more and more patients claimed results, some of them spectacular, from antineoplastons at the medical researcher's Houston facility, the American war on cancer continued to be a heavily financed failure and the machinery of the allopathic orthodoxy and the state instruments at its disposal continued to smash every last vestige of freedom of choice in cancer therapies lest another laetrile headache (just winding down as the antineoplaston matter was coming to the fore) throb to the forefront.

The trouble with Burzynski is that he did not intimidate well and had the foreigner-fresh-to-our-shores point of view that the strength of America (at least once upon a time) lay in rugged individualism rather than in supine compliance to the state.

He had begun his investigation in Europe of antineoplastons. He described them as naturally occurring peptides and amino acid derivatives which (he argued) are components of a biochemical defense system which parallels the human immune system(s). The antineoplaston apparatus, he has long maintained, "normalizes" defective cells.

Aside from the laetrile wars of the 1970s and early 1980s, no "alternative" cancer therapy had arisen within the United States in recent memory with the good credentials and "anecdotal" evidence of antineoplastons. As we shall see (*XII*), what we style "Cancer Inc." does not like competitors, particularly upstart ones with good credentials, novel new theories and their own products, which are not derived from the pharmaceutical/research interlock of "Cancer Inc."

Hence, Burzynski and his loyal patients revolved in and out of court for more than a decade. By 1996, a federal grand jury (incredibly, the *fourth* grand jury empaneled to probe "Dr. B") had indicted him on 75 counts even while several of his patients had won significant settlements against medical insurance companies which had balked at paying for antineoplaston therapy, no matter how successful the outcome.[21]

And a key federal legislator had announced plans for a full Congressional investigation of the ongoing harassment of the physician/researcher.[22] As cancer was killing at least 1,500 Americans per day there was no way to estimate just how many millions of dollars American and Texas taxpayers had been clipped by their "public servants" to help put this maverick out of business.

A signal victory occurred March 3, 1997, when a US District Court jury in Houston deadlocked 6-6 on the latest Burzynski charges and the judge declared a mistrial and dismissed the meat of the cases — 34 counts of "mail fraud." He was acquitted on the other charges in May — a stellar victory after 14 years of harassment. While it was not clear the prosecution would let up on the physician, something else had happened:

The lap-dog national media (electronic and print), which usually faithfully parrot the position of the Allopathic Industrial Complex (AIC) against the challengers (usually derided as "quacks," predators, deceivers of the infirm and elderly, etc.) had

Burzynski and his patients in the public eye for so long that the affable physician/scientist was beginning to come off as a hero and a lovable father figure rather than the monster painted by the FDA and Department of Justice.

The fact that dozens of Burzynski patients and/or their relatives were paraded before cameras and interviewed by the press while it was hard to find anyone with a command of the facts willing to speak against him was not lost on the American public.

"Bad press" — a continuing tactic of Cancer Inc. and the AIC against dissenters — had boomeranged into "good press," clear evidence that American journalism is not beyond rescue, either.

Neutralizing a naturopath

On Nov. 2, 1993, naturopathic physician Dr. Joan Vera Allison, one of Nevada's most famed and beloved "alternative" practitioners, returned to her Reno clinic from lunch, just in time for an FDA-led, 12-man federal/local police raid.

Dr. Allison was handcuffed and arrested as she attempted a telephone consultation with her attorney while patients looked on.

The raiders seized all patient, financial and medical records, office and medical equipment, nutritional supplies, published literature and even all of Dr. Allison's certificates, diplomas and licenses.

Ultimately, the Nevada healer whose experience with "alternatives" dated back to the earlier laetrile days — she had been a nurse of the late Ernst T. Krebs Sr. MD, pioneer of the controversial treatment, and probably had more experience in treating cancer patients with laetrile than any living exponent of the compound — was charged with felony counts of "practicing medicine without a license," "furnishing a dangerous drug without a prescription" and "possession of a dangerous drug."

The "dangerous drugs" listed in the State of Nevada criminal complaint against the healer, who had only recently been elected president of the Nevada Naturopathic Medical Assn.

(NNMA), were the synthetic hormone progesterone, thyroid extract, the normal medical solution heparin, human growth hormone, and a brand of the chelating agent EDTA. There was no suggestion any of these things — part of a total nutritional practice against chronic disease — had killed anybody, though allegedly one person had had an allergic reaction to the perfectly-legal drug progesterone.

An eyewitness to the raid and investigation told The Choice: *"The FDA guy bragged about shutting down other naturopaths" in the Pacific Northwest.*[23]

While the Allison raid had the odor of intrastate Nevada politics it was also clear that the federal level (including the Drug Enforcement Administration, DEA) would do just about anything or find any technicality to put a high-visibility practitioner of "alternative" therapies out of business.

Before Dr. Allison agreed to plead guilty to one count simply to be able to survive economically, many patients in Nevada were suddenly without the services of a doctor who had treated patients from around the world — many of whom let their feelings about the weird raid be known to the Nevada media. Dr. Allison died in 1995. "They just broke her," said a friend.

How to crush a dissident

In 1992, Zane R. Gard MD, California, was admittedly near total financial ruin from some seven years of litigation with state authorities while trying to protect his license. An expert in environmental medicine and long-time proponent of metabolic therapies, he had argued that state officials were involved in "a conspiracy . . . to violate the civil rights of non-allopathic physicians in the State of California."

Among many elements which he said reflected the nature of the conspiracy of the State of California was the following conversation contained in a "pretrial conference" hearing:

> *Hearing officer to deputy attorney general: "How many complaints do you have against Dr. Gard?"*

Deputy attorney general: "One."

Hearing officer: "Why are you bringing charges against Dr. Gard with only one complaint?"

Deputy attorney general: "Dr. Gard believes that chemicals may harm man. He practices environmental medicine, and he has a detox program. We intend to stop this type of practice within the United States."[24]

In part of his lengthy and expensive defense against waves of litigatory harassment from Sacramento, Dr. Gard argued:

The medical establishment has been conducting campaigns against non-allopathic physicians or alternatives for over 50 years. The most recent and costly campaign has been against alternatives, but the difference between this campaign and others that have gone before it is that this [one] is being directly paid for by the pharmaceutical industry.

In this current campaign, the targets are many different alternative entities . . . The one thing that every single target . . . has is simple: They are basically non-pharmaceutical (or drugless) remedies. This makes the stimulating motivation for this campaign to be simply economics. *The pharmaceutical industry is dumping tens of millions of dollars into this campaign in order to knock out of existence their competition . . .*

In my case, there is clear evidence that the California Board of Medicine is involved in a general conspiracy and as part of this conspiracy this action was filed against me. Because of the nature of my practice . . . I was frequently called upon as an expert witness in toxic tort cases for my patients which brought me [into] direct conflict with those who manufactured, distributed, or handled toxic materials.[25]

Star chamber for a maverick

By 1992, California physician Valentine G. Birds MD,

veteran champion of metabolic, nutritional and non-toxic therapies, said he had spent more than $80,000 unsuccessfully attempting to protect his medical license — suspended by the California Medical Board — while he fought charges of dispensing an "illegal AIDS medication."

While Dr. Birds favored various nutritional therapies and even the controversial (and anecdotally successful) typhoid vaccine approach to AIDS, he denied that he had ever dispensed the suspect drug in question.

How was Dr. Birds' license lifted in the sovereign State of California?

He told The Choice *that the suspension occurred*

> when my wife and I left for New York. On that day, a deputy attorney general representing the Medical Board of California called my office . . . [and] told a member of my staff that a hearing to suspend my medical license was to be held the very next day in San Diego. There was no advance notification in writing and no chance for appeal or for postponement.
>
> At the hearing, my attorney was given 20 minutes to review more than 300 pages of information bearing on the case. Within an hour it was over. Without adequate opportunity to review the charges, let alone to answer them, my license to practice was suspended.[26]

Dr. Birds had indeed been brought to the star-chamber proceedings on a technicality — "dispensing an AIDS medication not approved by the FDA" — even when he had not dispensed the medication in question (though patients of his had requested he be in contact with the doctor who was *using it).*

But the North Hollywood medic had every reason to feel he was on the "hit list" anyway because he was a long-time proponent of "alternative" non-drug therapies, and had become well-known in the AIDS community for using them.

The treatment of AIDS is, as is the treatment of cancer, a virtual red flag for the Allopathic Industrial Complex (AIC).

High-visibility practitioners of non-drug (that is, non-allopathic) medicine can always expect to get into trouble, as Dr. Birds did.

It seemed not to matter one whit to California authorities that when Dr. Birds was on the way to the kangaroo-court proceeding that a full decade of AIDS research and treatments had occurred without the medical establishment having produced one single case of a cure.

'Get Halstead' was the order

By 1997, Committee for Freedom of Choice in Medicine Inc. Vice President Bruce Halstead MD, Colton CA, had been waiting *for several years* for imprisonment in a long, involved, expensive — and ultimately silly — conviction of using a Japanese herbal tea in the immunological management of cancer. And he finally *was* jailed for several months.

Dr. Halstead, however, was fully aware (*VII*) that the Oct. 25, 1983, *25*-man early-morning raid by the Los Angeles County District Attorney's office, the California Food and Drug Administration, the San Bernardino Sheriff's Department and the Colton Police Department was hardly in response to Japanese herbal tea (denounced by the state as "fecal matter and water"):

A widely respected world-class researcher (and World Health Organization consultant) in marine biology, biotoxicology, herbs and other specialties, he had long been a visible, high-profile exponent of and defender of EDTA chelation therapy, laetrile, DMSO, nutritional therapies and herbal medicine. He had known that the AIC would go to any lengths to "get" him, that all it needed was an excuse, no matter how slim.

In a February 1991 letter to a probation officer, the dauntless Dr. Halstead wrote:

> *They broke into my home, met me in the hall, and burst into our bedroom where my wife was still in bed . . . At the clinic, the doors were barricaded, most of the patients were prevented from coming in for treatment even though some of them had driven hundreds of miles to get here, telephone*

calls from pharmacies for medication were blocked, and the rights of the patients for treatment and medical care that day were seriously interrupted.[27]

He also told the officer:

While I was waiting in the hallway of the municipal court one day . . . the chief investigator for the prosecution . . . informed me that I had been targeted by "Sacramento" for prosecution.

He informed me that "Sacramento" told them to "get Halstead" no matter what . . .

I attempted to introduce witnesses concerning my selective prosecution, but the judge wouldn't let me put any of them on the stand. The trial was a farce. I would have done just as well in Iran or Libya.[28]

While Halstead was convicted on the Japanese herbal tea charge, he waited for orders for incarceration and exhausted the appeals process.

Incredibly, on Feb. 5, 1997, almost *14 years* after the well-muscled raid, Dr. Halstead, now 77 and diabetic, was led off to county jail, where he remained several months. Early efforts to release him on his "own recognizance" failed. While multi-million-dollar drug profiteers, murderers and white-collar swindlers, embezzlers and assorted other criminals were "OR'd" to roam the streets at will, a purveyor of Japanese herbal tea as an adjuvant therapy in cancer languished in jail. Justice in America?

Tyranny in the Empire State

While California's medical establishment has usually topped the list of most repressive state agencies in the brutal suppression of medical freedom of thought in the USA (since the medical lobby is normally the number-one legislative influence-peddler in the Golden State, whose major industry remains agriculture), New York for a long time kept fighting to jump from second to first place:

Empire State taxpayers have been taken for millions of

dollars by their own medical fascisti to prosecute such high-profile "alternative" physicians as Warren Levin MD, Robert Atkins MD and the brilliant centenarian physician/scientist Emanuel Revici MD as well as to make it very difficult for others to "step out of line" by advocating nutritional and metabolic therapies.

Dr. Levin in 1995 savored among the most succulent of victories over the state: not only was he finally cleared — after 14 years — of all charges brought against him for using 20 treatments and 18 diagnostic/monitoring techniques said to be "unproven" or "questionable" — but in the midst of it all he developed and overcame kidney cancer with some of those very modalities.

Warren Levin noted he had spent more than a half-million dollars in legal fees over the long period of state harassment. When all was said and done, the state had only one alleged "expert witness" — an ever-quoted "quackbuster" with a seeming obsession to do in all those who do not agree with him medically — against Levin, whose own expert witnesses included a who's-who of leaders in the "alternative" movement."[29]

The same professional "quackbuster" who failed to bring down Levin also misfired in the state's long-running battle with Dr. Revici, the gifted physician/biochemist who turned 100 in 1996 and to whom thousands of people around the world believe they owe their lives.

*Dr. Revici had won totally by 1991 and out of the tangled legal case came a landmark US Appeals Court decision (*Schneider vs. Revici*) that patients have a right to obtain "unconventional" medical treatment and that the patient could assume the risk of such therapy.*[30]

In 1993, one week after it was issued, a New York State Health Department "summary suspension" of the medical license of famed "complementary" physician (and best-selling author) Robert Atkins MD was vacated by a New York State Supreme Court judge.

In a case primarily involving Dr. Atkins' defense of ozone treatment, Judge Edward I. Greenfield said the state's license suspension of the Manhattan doctor had been "arbitrary, capricious, and overbroad." Thousands of telephone calls had been logged by Atkins supporters to Governor Mario Cuomo and New York Mayor David Dinkins over the unwarranted Atkins prosecution.[31]

Without question, New York's heavy-handed assault on medical freedom in these major cases helped spur citizen support of efforts to move that state into the victory column for freedom-of-choice proponents: it passed landmark free-choice legislation in 1994 which has at least ameliorated the political situation there.

The high crimes and misdemeanors of Albany are conceivably worse than those of the Sacramento sanitary sanhedrin since there are proportionally more sick people in NY — chronic disease-plagued New Yorkers are inhabiting the most atmospherically toxic confines of the USA outside the intermittently unhealthier Los Angeles Basin and are folks who really need *all the "alternatives" they can find.*

In the Land of the Free . . .

In May 1993, federal and local raiders hit 37 sites — including homes and healthfood stores — in seven states, executing warrants growing out of an international investigation (US/Mexico) pinpointing the alleged illegal distribution in the United States of products (many, but not all, natural supplements) allegedly made abroad and illegally brought into the US.

While the health-freedoms movement in general was not defending acts which might truly have been illegal, it was, as *The Choice* recounted, amazed at the excess amount of compliance and police force used against what was, by any measure, far from being a major international dangerous drug operation.

Both the Life Extension Foundation (LEF), itself a constant target of FDA "compliance," and eyewitnesses reported to the Committee for Freedom of Choice in Medicine Inc. on the obscene amount of police muscle used.

The LEF reported that

In San Diego, a female employee's apartment was raided by eight officials. One official knocked on the door, refusing to identify himself. She looked through the peephole, did not know the person, and went into her bedroom to call 911. They then broke the door down with guns drawn, forcing her to the floor with a gun to her temple. They confiscated a computer, a box of brochures and the woman's personal belongings.

In another example of terrorist tactics, agents broke into a Southern California home while a mother was breast-feeding her infant. The mother was handcuffed for eleven hours while the agents ransacked her home.[32]

A month later, the FDA raided three natural products companies in Nevada operated by G.S. Oden. The raiders seized $300,000 worth of products, particularly herbs and substances developed by the aforementioned metabolic pioneer Hans Nieper MD in Germany. An FDA spokeswoman said the Nieper products, particularly orotates, were both illegal and misleading because they "promote specific disease prevention but are not FDA approved."

And, naturally, that is simply not to be allowed in our liberty-loving republic.

The Las Vegas NV *Review-Journal/Sun* reported how Larry and Catherine Carpenter felt about their "protection" by the FDA:

Orthodox medicine had told Catherine Carpenter, 38, of Las Vegas, that there was no effective treatment for her brain cancer. So she had turned to "alternative" medicine, particularly herbs and "Nieper products" which actually seemed to help her condition.

The newspaper quoted husband Larry, a private investigator: "Orthodox medicine had told us nothing can be done; they tell us chemotherapy will not work." Since the raid, the FDA "might as well put a gun to her head and pull the trigger."[33]

The Carpenters had been cheered to note that following such "unapproved," "unproven," "unorthodox," "unscientific" therapies a tumor on Catherine's left shoulder had been reduced — and that scans had shown there were no more brain tumors.

Remembering the Laetrile War

As we shall see (*XII*), the war between the Allopathic Industrial Complex (AIC) and laetrile involved the greatest medical controversy in this century. It also led to many federal- and state-level legal harassments of the ever-growing numbers of physicians who openly admitted using the apricot seed derivative.

Among the persistent targets — and eventual winners — in the seemingly endless battle was California physician James Privitera MD, whose sheer persistence became a lesson for all:

In 1991 the state's medical board agreed to dismiss "with prejudice" its accusation and "petition to revoke probation" growing out of Dr. Privitera's conviction in 1975 of a felony conspiracy to sell laetrile, a processed form of amygdalin from apricot kernels.

In the up-and-down Privitera affair, the felony conviction had been reversed by a state appeals court but had been reinstated in 1979. A national outcry had been raised against the short-term imprisonment of the popular medic and it led to his official pardon by Governor Edmund G. Brown Jr.

Between 1982 and 1987, he told me, he had been subjected to endless harassment by the medical board and had even been arrested in 1989 on an allegation of suspicion of "a written threat to extort" after he held a press conference.

Perceptively, a state superior court judge ruled that there was no such crime and that the physician/biochemist had every right to hold press conferences to continue to denounce his oppressors.

Throughout, Dr. Privitera believed he would eventually win and told all who would listen that persistence, openness and tenacity pay off against the forces of institutional darkness. Said he to other victims:

"Go public, go to the people, involve the press."[34]

The word is 'genocide'

The victimization of patients by "their" government is of course old news. We had already reported extensively on the kidnappings — either by state and local agents claiming to be acting in the "best interests" of the patients, or by parents trying to snatch their progeny out of the hands of the same — of child cancer victims.[35]

The plight of parents who wished their (usually) cancer-afflicted children to be treated by some other way than the cruelly debilitating cut-burn-poison approach of orthodoxy has made intermittent news since the 1970s. In some cases, there may have been validity to the arguments that certain couples were irresponsible parents for keeping their children out of the medical loop. In others, as in cases of harassment against Jehovah's Witnesses (whose religious teachings forbid blood transfusions), parents were hounded by the government for practicing their religion — many fleeing state to state before appearing in Mexico where they could find a hospital or clinic willing to treat their children without blood products.

In June 1984 the Committee for Freedom of Choice in Medicine Inc. included some of the child-kidnapping cases within a 70-page document filed with the United Nations Center for Human Rights, Geneva, and entitled A Complaint Against Medical Tyranny as Practiced in the United States of America: American Medical Genocide.[36]

This "complaint," a detailed account of health-freedoms suppression in the United States, while sent to every member of the United Nations, and submitted with the authority of Committee leaders, physicians and researchers in five countries, received responses (but not action from) only the Vatican, Cuba, Uganda, Zaire and Finland. It did not seem, in 1984, that the world was highly concerned about the deprivation of American medical liberties by its own establishment. After all, the USA is a "free country," isn't it?

The supreme irony in this "free country" is that neither

medicine nor medical choices are free, that optional health modalities have been vigorously suppressed on the one hand while being quietly co-opted on the other, that medical pioneers whose primary interest has been allegiance to the Hippocratic Oath are dragged out of their offices in handcuffs, and that an ostensibly well-informed public in the main has no idea that there are scores of rational health choices in existence which have nothing to do with surgery, radiation and chemotherapy ("cut, burn and poison.")

Only a minority of Americans is aware that the notion of freedom of choice in medicine is a guiding part of the spirit of international agreements — and that the United States is a signatory to the Declaration of Helsinki, adopted in Finland in 1964 by the 18th Medical Assembly.

Were the United States in the slightest loyal to the spirit, let alone the letter, of the Declaration of Helsinki, its Section II, Article 1 would be printed on a sheepskin hanging in the office of every medical practitioner, every state or federal medical bureaucrat and every office within the FDA:

> "In the treatment of the sick person, the doctor must be free to use a new therapeutic measure, if in his judgment it offers hope of saving life, re-establishing health, or alleviating suffering."

Fedstapo still at it

By mid-decade, the FDA and similars were still at it:

Life Extension Foundation reported[37] on a 1995 "visitation" by two FDA "enforcement" agents to the Maryland apartment of a US Navy computer software expert.

The agents told him it was a "serious" matter that he had attempted to import from abroad the procaine-based product KH3 — which has improved the health of many people over several decades — because the same had not been "approved" by the FDA.

The LEF noted that the man

was terrorized for 30 minutes by these government agents into thinking he was going to be arrested for importing a medication from Europe for his own personal use. The agents threatened to jail him if he attempted to import medications not approved by the FDA for his own personal use.

The spectacle of federal thugs appearing at private homes to threaten citizens into not buying something for their own use is simply one more scenario which gives the lie to the myth that the FDA and other federal bureaus somehow protect "the people."

Washington state cancer patients — and those from many places — were apoplectic in 1996 when the state's Medical Quality Assurance Commission revoked the license of board-certified oncologist Glenn Warner MD, one of the Pacific Northwest's best-known innovative cancer experts.

As long-time cancer writer and CANHELP director Patrick M. McGrady Jr. put it:

> "*Probably no other cancer doctor in the Seattle community can claim to match Dr. Warner's one thousand-plus surviving patients . . . Clearly, the Commission has engaged in a most vicious vendetta against a holistic physician, knowledgeable in both conventional and alternative evidence. This, despite all the evidence showing excellent results from his distinctive, compassionate approach.*"[38]

What particularly upset McGrady and other observers of the Warner witch hunt was that of 20,000 patients treated by the highly respected medic over 40 years there had been exactly six complaints, the most recent over eight years old! They also were piqued that the state commission's attorney claimed that cancer patients are "incapable" and "unqualified" to know whether they are receving appropriate care or not.[39]

Dr. Warner's real crime, of course, was that he was a high-profile proponent of "unconventional" therapies which pose a solid economic challenge to the $200-billion-per-year business of

Cancer Inc. (*XI*).

On July 31, 1996, according to the victimized doctor himself, more than 30 federal agents with the help of local police raided the office of Dr. Wilbert Calvin (Cal) Streeter, an osteopath who is one of Indiana's — and the nation's — best-known exponents of "alternative" therapy.

Dr. Streeter reported that they proceeded

> *"to interrogate all my employees, to confiscate all so-called 'non-approved' (FDA) health potions and medications [and] also loaded three thousand charts with the file cabinets into a semi-truck and took the hard drives out of all my computers and carted them off to the FDA office in Chicago.*
>
> *"They had a court order signed by a federal judge allowing them to search and seize at will whatever they deemed 'illegal' or FDA-unapproved substances."*[40]

A Streeter cancer patient from Florida left little doubt about his understanding of the sudden crackdown on the veteran doctor:

> *"Maybe he had done something wrong. That's not the issue. The issue is I went to him, and I'm still here. He didn't make any promises, and he said he'd do his best.*
>
> *"In my opinion, they are trying to stop Dr. Streeter as part of the pattern of suppression, the silencing of the modalities to treat cancer that threaten the status quo. If you do the things that prevent cancer, you control cancer. There's no money in prevention."*[41]

Noting that he assumed the raid — following which no charges had been filed at this book's time of publication (Fall 1997) — was an effort by the medical establishment to "get my license and shut me down," Dr. Streeter added:

> *"I'm naive. I believe everybody wants to be well, and to have the freedom to make decisions concerning their*

health."[42]

A challenge for us all

A 57-year-old veterinarian vitamin products manufacturer doing 114 days' hard time in a federal detention center in San Diego?

Physicians and vitamin products manufacturers spending themselves into financial oblivion for protection against wave after wave of federal or state or county or city litigation growing out of vague charges construing natural supplements as "illegal drugs"?

SWAT-type teams of up to two dozen or more police raiders from various jurisdictions breaking down doors, brandishing revolvers and terrorizing patients as they receive intravenous vitamin infusions?

US federal officers violating the sovereignty of a foreign country to nab an American who had broken no laws in the foreign country — and whose "crimes" in this one primarily involved the use of a telephone?

Children kidnapped by the state because their parents wished to protect them from chemotherapy and radiation in cases of cancer where there were no guaranteed "cures"?

An enormous display of federal, state and local police "compliance" against vitamin pills, "unapproved" diagnostic devices and "alternative" non-drug therapies while the United States is literally awash in a crime-drenched deluge of cocaine, heroin, stimulants, amphetamines, hallucinogens and a host of other illegal dangerous drugs?

Honest men and women in the medical profession hounded, humiliated, persecuted and prosecuted, treated as quacks, charlatans and criminals for attempting to help their patients while the American public dies in record numbers of cancer, AIDS, and "heart disease" or suffers from immunological disorders unknown just a few decades ago? A Food and Drug Administration (FDA) viciously and ruthlessly suppressing "alternatives" in medicine and therapeutics, most of which have killed or maimed no one while its own approved nostrums, medications and devices kill at least 100,000 Americans a year?

How can all of this be — and what can be done about it?

The answer to these questions is the purpose of this study.

References

1. *The Choice* XVII: 1, 1991.
2. Baker, DE, in *The Choice*, XVII: 2, 1991.
3. Seattle WA *Post-Intelligencer*, May 7, 1992.
4. *FDA Insider*, cited in The Choice, XVIII: 2, 1992.
5. *Ibid.*
6. *Townsend Letter For Doctors*, July 1992.
7. *The Choice*, XVII: 1, 1991.
8. *The Choice*, XVI: 4, 1990.
9. *The Choice*, XVII: 1, 1991.
10. *The Choice*, XVII: 3,4, 1991.
11. *The Choice*, XX: 1, 1994.
12. *The Choice*, XVII: 3,4, 1991.
13. *The Choice*, XIX: 2, 1993.
14. *The Choice*, XVII: 2, 1991.
15. *Ibid.*
16. *The Choice*, XIX: 3-4, 1993.
17. *The Choice*, XVII: 3,4, 1991.
18. *Ibid.*
19. Moore, WJ Jr. Esq., "Argument to arrest judgment" in *USA vs. Keller*, 1991, cited in *The Choice*, XVII: 3,4, 1991.
20. *The Choice*, XVIII: 2, 1992.
21. *The Choice*, XVIII: 2, 1992. (also XVIII: 1, 1992)
22. *Alt. Med. Digest*, #9, 1995.
23. *The Choice*, XVIII: 3, 1992.
24. *The Choice*, XVII: 3,4, 1991.
25. *Ibid.*
26. *The Choice*, XVII: 3,4, 1991.
27. *The Choice*, XVII: 3,4, 1991.
28. *Ibid.*
29. *The Choice*, XXI: 1, 1995.
30. *The Choice*, XVII: 1, 1991.
31. *The Choice*, XIX: 2, 1993.
32. *The Choice*, XIX: 2, 1993.
33. Las Vegas NV *Review-Journal Sun*, June 25, 1993.
34. *The Choice*, XVII: 3-4, 1991.
35. Culbert, ML, *What The Medical Establishment Won't Tell You that Could Save Your Life*. Norfolk VA: Donning, 1993.
36. *A Complaint Against Medical Tyranny as Practiced in the United States of America: American Medical Genocide*. San Francisco CA: The Committee for Freedom of Choice in Medicine Inc., 1984.
37. *The Choice*, XXI:2, 1995.
38. McGrady, PM, "The revocation of Dr. Glenn Warner's license is unjust and cruel." *Townsend Letter for Doctors and Patients*. Aug./Sept. 1996.
39. *Ibid.*
40. "Indiana chelation physician raided." *Townsend Letter for Doctors and Patients*, Feb/March 1997.
41. *Ibid.*
42. *Ibid.*

II
AN AMERICAN CHAMBER OF HORRORS:
Modern medicine as a threat to our health

"I would like the doctor to have to stand up, face the East, and say to the patient, 'I'm a greedy son-of-a-bitch and I'm sending you to a facility where you're going to be charged an outrageous sum for a procedure which is probably not necessary, may be harmful to your health, and I will pocket a large bunch of money for risking your health and come very close to doing things I promised not to do when I took the Hippocratic Oath.'"

— **Rep. Fortney H. Stark (D-CA) to *Medicare Compliance Alert* on how he thought doctors should disclose their ownership interests to patients (1990)**

"A physician is naturally reluctant to think that his treatment contributes to a patient's disability. It is easier to attribute new symptoms to an extension of an underlying disease than to obvious or occult drug toxicity . . . Too frequently, laboratory data or new symptoms that do not 'fit' into the anticipated course of a disease are ignored."

— **Kenneth L. Melmon MD**

"Medical technology and the system built upon it have now themselves become an increasingly important cause of disease and disability, both because of the inherent dangers of powerful diagnostic and therapeutic methods and because of their misuse by incompetent and venal personnel and institutions."

— **V.M. Sidel and R. Sidel (*A Healthy State*)**

"The fact that most individuals unhesitatingly entrust their bodies and lives to doctors about whom they know nothing is a remarkable testimony to the power of social conventions and etiquette."

— **Marcia Millman (*The Unkindest Cut*)**

". . . The greatest danger to your health is the doctor who practices Modern Medicine."

— **Robert S. Mendelsohn MD (*Confessions of a Medical Heretic*)**

An American medical nightmare

Multiple sclerosis patient Al Fine, then 61, was both happy and enraged:

— Happy that he was among the most dramatic responders to a form of "alternative" therapy for MS in Mexico — and not allowed, of course, in the United States — to the point where he had graduated from wheelchair to cane to walking without the need for the latter.

— And enraged that his American insurance company, which had paid for an initial round of the "experimental" therapy, would pay for no more such treatments (none approved by the Food and Drug Administration) even though the company had picked up the considerable tab for the earlier "recognized" if mostly useless treatments for MS, primarily steroids.

It was 1988, or 10 years after the former stockbroker had been diagnosed with the crippling neurological autoimmune disorder and confined, originally, to a wheelchair.

That same year, Fine told fellow patients and doctors at the "experimental" or "alternative" treatment center in Tijuana, where he had returned for "booster" treatments:

"Just look at me!" He added that "for years, those SOBs covered $90 per pill for steroids, which did nothing for me, and now, despite the fact my ever improved MS got me disability and retirement, with a lot of stress, and something has really worked, I can't get covered!"

Hence the chagrin.

Al Fine recalled for *The Choice*,[1] the publication of the Committee for Freedom of Choice in Medicine Inc., how he had been misdiagnosed with various ailments before the confirmation that what he really had was MS, one of an ever-growing list of disorders the American medical establishment considers to be "incurable."

He had lived earlier in Hawaii, where he received his initial treatments for the crippling disease — one in which the body's own self-defense system is attacking the myelin sheath around nerve tissue and which gradually leads to paralysis, incapacity, and often blindness and death.

When he saw he was getting nowhere with synthetic hormones, he listened to his wife Marie, who was no friend of American orthodox medicine and indeed had been victimized by it:

Both her breasts had been removed and restorative surgery botched at a major Honolulu hospital long before the "old-boy network" of physicians and lab techs admitted to a mistake in diagnosis. Here was a woman in the prime of life told she had breast cancer — and who did not. Yet she had suffered the physical and emotional trauma of the covered-up mistake.

Her stockbroker husband could not be sure that what had happened to his wife was not just some kind of unfortunate fluke — after all, wasn't American medicine the finest, most advanced (while certainly the most expensive) in the world?

He made contact with another of the MS patients who had trekked to the American Biologics-Mexico SA Medical Center in the Mexican border city who was by then in his sixth year of therapy and impressive improvement. He was one of several patients who, over time, had recaptured enough of his faculties, at least for a time, to be able to walk. He told Fine he would "have a chance" at the Mexican hospital, which specialized in therapies US medical orthodoxy at its kindest called "unproven" and at its worst described as "quackery."

"When I got there in July 1987, I couldn't walk up those stairs outside, or any stairs," Fine told me, as editor of *The Choice*. "I was about to have to make a single decision: between an electric or a hand-guided wheelchair."

At AB-Mexico, Fine became a patient of Roberto Tapia MD, who in turn worked closely with German-born Wolfram Kuhnau MD, a septuagenarian disciple of the late Paul Niehans MD, Switzerland, 20th-century pioneer of a form of treatment widely known in Europe as "live cell" or "cellular" therapy — the subcutaneous or intramuscular injections of suspensions of living cellular material, usually of endocrine tissues, from animal embryos (or other birth-related structures.)

The Mexican hospital, as part of an international medical research network (Bradford Research Institute), had become the first treatment center in North America to utilize this 50-year-old European modality (using tissue from cow or shark sources) together with nutritional and detoxification therapies.

At the Tijuana hospital, Fine received brain, pituitary and other cellular suspensions as well as drops and infusions of the oxidative agent Dioxychlor, the synthetic immune booster isoprinosine, the Rumanian-pioneered "longevity drug" Gerovital, intravenous and oral Vitamin C, various enzyme combinations, amino acids, Vitamin B complex, other nutrients and a special diet.

"Four months later, I got off the steroids," he recalled. By February 1988 "I had put my cane down and didn't know where it was. It didn't matter — I didn't need it."

Family, friends and associates were startled by Fine's ability to walk, let alone his energetic appearance. But his insurance company, which had paid for the initial round of treatments, would not pay for a second because the FDA did not "recognize" cellular therapy and had long balked at nutritional medicine.

Forced into retirement on disability because of the crippling disease, Fine would have benefited greatly through continuing coverage by his insurer. But 15 months had gone by without any payments at all. Frustratingly, the cost of "alternative" therapy in Mexico was far less — on the order of 10 percent of "orthodox" treatments in the USA — so that the Floridian, like so many others, had to wonder whether American health insurance companies were *really* interested in reducing the cost of medicine.

All these elements converged in Al Fine to lead him to make his story as public as he could.

I was delighted to see Al Fine various times years later during speaking tours in Florida. He was still standing, and still angry. Neither he nor American Biologics considered him "cured" of MS — yet he was one of a growing number of people from several countries who had responded dramatically for an extended period of time to useful, non-toxic therapies to which the American public is routinely denied access.

Victims of the system

The Fines unfortunately epitomize the worst in the American medical disaster: they have been victims of misdiagnosis, medical malfeasance, malpractice, institutional coverup, and of a greed-driven, often venal system in which an interlock of vested economic and political interests has denied Americans and their doctors access to freedom of choice in medicine.

Their cases said it all: if Mrs. Fine had even *had* breast cancer in the first place, she would not have been allowed by the medical orthodoxy to know that there are various "unproven" or "unorthodox" approaches to this most rapidly growing "form" of cancer, primarily among women — techniques and approaches which may be used sometimes even in lieu of surgery, let alone of radiation and/or chemotherapy. She might also have learned that a simple lumpectomy — removal of the actual cancerous tissue — has as good or better a five-year-survival rate ("cure" in oncological jargon) as does removal of the whole breast and surrounding lymph nodes (the vaunted and ever-more-unnecessary "radical mastectomy") let alone followup chemotherapy (treatments with toxic, often cancer-promoting drugs) and radiation (burning of the affected area), which are replete with side effects and disfigurement.

She, and countless women, probably would not have been told most of this. Had they sought out "unorthodox" opinions from "questionable" practitioners, they would likely have found rejection from their orthodox medical practitioners and, should they actually have attempted "unapproved" therapies, non-coverage by medical insurance companies, at least in the United States.

In Al Fine's case, here was the victim of a condition US

medical orthodoxy claims is "terminal" yet originally denied access to information suggesting there may be approaches to managing the autoimmune disorder other than the risky administration of synthetic hormones. Not only that, but Fine's insurance carrier was all too delighted to pay for the expensive, side effects-producing treatments which produced no measurable good effect — and then balked at covering the more natural, non-toxic modalities which actually started returning him to near-normal. As we will see, this was all part of "paradigm capture" — the institutionalized mindset of orthodoxy — backed by greed and ego, which has denied medical choice to millions of Americans.

Through roundabout ways, the Fines had heard about a foreign treatment center whose approaches were based on parameters different from those of American medical orthodoxy. Happily, they were there at least in time for Mr. Fine to be helped, and helped considerably, despite the irritating adjuvant reality of non-coverage of his successful "unorthodoxy."

That Fine had to leave his home country to find therapeutic relief is itself an obscenity — by that time the "Tijuana express" was well-known: tens of thousands of Americans had already made the pilgrimage to the border area of northwest Mexico primarily seeking help through anti-cancer treatments either banned or hard to come by in the United States.(2) The fact that various essentially non-toxic therapies are *not* available to Americans, lacking "significant scientific agreement" (the FDA catch-phrase for "acceptance" of a medical claim by proponents), is the greater obscenity in a nation and a society which pride themselves on alleged freedom of thought and inquiry.

Our publication *The Choice* reported in 1990(3) about the well-known legal case in which a 23-year-old woman who had claimed that a mismanaged stomach stapling operation performed at a major Southern California research hospital had damaged her internal organs and left her with infections, scars and a permanent blood disorder. She was "news" when an Orange County jury decided she should receive more than $1 million in damages.

Attorney Mark Robinson explained that his client had suffered from a condition called morbid obesity, and had originally weighed 300 pounds. She had been subjected to a procedure called a "vertical banded gastroplasty." Yet, he added: "They didn't do any of the steps that were supposed to have been done. She came out with a severe infection. She was in the hospital 100 days the first year. Since that time she has had 22 surgeries. They had to cut out half her stomach, and they cut out her spleen."

In 1992, an Ohio appellate court ruled that an $8 million verdict against a physician and clinic for performing an unnecessary cerebral arteriogram that had left the patient quadriplegic had been "proper."

The 36-year-old patient had argued that her total loss of control in all four members had resulted from malpractice in prescribing an unnecessary, unjustified (and, of course, expensive) technique (the arteriogram). An economist had testified that the value of past and future economic loss of the patient's services amounted to over $1,170,000.[(4)]

In 1991, Ohio State University football coach Woody Hayes made some non-sporting news — which also pointed to an underreported medical problem which is more often whispered about than revealed — when it was found that the famed molder of athletes had undergone two operations within a month's time: one to remove his gallbladder, the second to remove a sponge left inside the body following the first operation.[(5)]

In 1995, *The Choice* reported the tip of an iceberg of medical mayhem:

— At a Tampa FL hospital the wrong leg of a patient was amputated and another patient's ventilator was erroneously disconnected — two of 367 "serious incidents" in medical settings reported statewide in Florida in 1994.

— Two male melanoma patients died at New England Medical Center from a "dosage error" involving the cancer chemotherapeutic agent cisplatin.

—A national furor followed an overdose scandal at the prestigious Dana-Farber Cancer Institute in Boston in which two breast cancer patients were accidentally given four times the prescribed dosage of the toxic chemotherapeutic drug Cytoxan. One of these, *Boston Globe* health columnist Betty Lehman, died of heart failure.

The *New York Times* quoted Dr. Marc Lippman, director of the Georgetown University School of Medicine in Washington, stating that overdoses of cancer drugs are almost always lethal: "There are very few drugs that if you take ten times the recommended dose, much would happen to you for too long. You'd get over it. But with cancer drugs, you'd be dead."

—A Wisconsin clinical laboratory entered an innocent plea in homicide charges growing out of the cancer deaths of two women whose Pap smears had been misread. Families of the two victims had earlier won multi-million-dollar settlements from civil suits against the lab and an associated health-maintenance organization (HMO).

—The South Carolina Supreme Court let stand a jury's $2.25 million award against two physicians for misdiagnosing a deadly streptococcal infection that caused a woman's death.[6]

Televiewers watched for months in 1995/1996 as *Court TV* reported on the lengthy second trial of a New York hospital and its staff on charges of negligence growing out of the in-house death of an 18-year-old girl several years earlier. Her demise was in part attributed to a staff error in which she received the antidepressant Nardil and the painkiller Demerol, a potentially lethal mix. There was a split decision in the case in which the hospital had earlier been fined $13,000.

Even the long-used (since 1945) pulmonary artery (PA) catheterization process, whose annual use and sales add $2 billion yearly to the high cost of medicine, came under fire in 1996.

A review showed that not only did its widespread use mostly

not benefit patients but that "there is evidence that it may increase morbidity and mortality."[91]

Questioning their profession

In 1988, some physicians and physicians-to-be took some long looks at their profession in print, and reported on some of the things they did not like to behold.

Wrote a second-year resident in obstetrics at a major hospital in South Florida:

> *I'm working 110 to 120 hours a week. I start by doing c-sections early in the morning and I'll do six or seven of them during the day and continue to do them all night long . . . We're running at the edge, and I'm afraid some patients have suffered for it.*
>
> *We had one woman who was fully dilated and had been pushing for three hours. The baby's heartbeat had slowed down considerably, which is a clear signal that the baby isn't getting enough oxygen. But we were so busy that no one noticed this. It wasn't that it was completely missed, it's just that it didn't fully register because we were so overwhelmed with the other work we had to do. The baby was born dead, but if the right things had been done, he would have been fine.*
>
> *Since there aren't enough residents, you never feel you can call in sick even when you are sick. We've had two residents faint in the hospital. One collapsed in the emergency room. We put two liters of fluid into him, got him up and put him back to work. Another resident . . . had chest pains and was admitted to the hospital. It appeared at first that he had a heart attack, but it turned out he was suffering from exhaustion and dehydration.*[7]

Another, who wrote that he "dreaded" intensive-care medicine "and almost never send my patients to the ICU," recalled a case in which a terminal-stage leukemia patient, expected to expire at any time, was rushed to the intensive-care unit after suffering an event known as a "pericardial tamponade." He wrote:

> *The resident rushed her to the ICU and began giving her drugs and hooking her to intravenous lines. They couldn't revive her, so they cut open her chest and began doing open-chest cardiac massage . . .*
>
> *I yelled "Stop this! What are you people doing here? This girl has leukemia. She is never going to recover."*
>
> *The anesthesiologist yelled back at me, "We can't stop now. We've gone this far. We've got to keep going . . ."*
>
> *I don't think medicine is very good at teaching physicians when to stop.*[8]

A neonatologist lamented that "I feel my ability to use my judgment has been taken away from me, in part by the government and the law, but mostly by the machines — by the shiny promise of what they can do to keep life going." He added: "You have to know when to stop; when to draw the line between sustaining life and prolonging death."[9]

'Healthcare' delivery?

Were the above cases statistical aberrations, their cases might be overlooked. Unhappily, they are reflections of common disasters which undergird what the nation has been calling its "healthcare delivery system" — a mammoth, obscenely expensive, jerry-built edifice of public and private administrative red tape, closing community hospitals, rapidly mushrooming "managed care" plans, gleaming high-tech medical centers, highly specialized medical practices, frequently overpaid practitioners, overworked interns, frequently ignored nurses, research institutions living on public and private doles, a frequently corrupt federal oversight apparatus (FDA), a monolithic medical labor union/trade organization (AMA) which attempts to keep medical practitioners in line, a mixed public-private insurance system swollen by greed and corruption — and, underlying it all, a gigantic gravy train of pills-for-profit in the form of an international pharmaceutical trust and an allied medical devices/instruments industry with vested interests in the continuing ill health of the nation.

With the American judicial system continually running interference for and arbitrating the friction between all parts of the apparatus — which is indeed a "sick business," a "warehousing of the dying" enterprise, a system which does not prolong life so much as it prolongs death with the latest in high-technology devices and gimmicks — the legal aspects of the monster alone add billions to the total "healthcare delivery" bill, one reaching about a *trillion* dollars a year and constituting between 13 and 15 percent of gross domestic product (GDP) in the mid-1990s.

Iatrogenic disease in America

While proponents, defenders and apologists of the American medical apparatus point to "the finest medical system in the world" (and which, particularly in emergency and trauma care, routinely performs life-saving miracles in the midst of human disasters), a huge shadow on the land has been cast through the rise of what, since the 1960s, has been called *iatrogenic* (literally, doctor-caused) *disease.* Reduced to its simplest concept, American iatrogenicity rhetorically asks: has high-technology medicine been a net plus or a deficit — does it now cause as much or more disease as it cures?

The problem was so great by 1981 that even a major "learned journal" of the American medical orthodoxy, the *New England Journal of Medicine*, was moved to observe that

> *Iatrogenic illness has been a well-recognized phenomenon for over a quarter of a century. In 1955, Barr made note of the price we pay for modern medical care. There is a pressing need for a better understanding of the diseases that would not have occurred "if sound therapeutic procedure had not been employed. . . ."*[10]

The *NEJM*, in two controversy-stirring reports in the same

issue, found that "orthodox therapeutic procedures" used on 815 consecutive patients at a university hospital resulted in 290 patients (36 percent) developing one or more "iatrogenic illnesses," with a total of 497 such occurrences, 125 total patients suffering more than one complication, 76 (or 9 percent) suffering major complications — and in 15 patients iatrogenic complications were directly related to their deaths.

In a second report, the *NEJM* found in a survey of all surgical patients who passed through one hospital in one year that there were 36 patients with adverse reactions due to "physician error" — 31 of these dying and five others leaving the hospital with serious physical impairments.

Two years before, Dr. David A. Davis had told an anesthesia research conference that about 550 deaths from anesthesia were occurring annually in the United States and that the record had not improved in the previous 25 years.(11)

As early as 1966, Dr. L.G. Seidl *et al.* had reported that "seventeen percent of Johns Hopkins Hospital admissions suffered one or more drug reactions,"(12) and in 1971 Dr. Oscar Thorup noted that "twenty percent of hospital admissions [at the Mayo Clinic] have at least one medical or hospital induced complication before discharge."(13)

By 1984, Dr. Lowell Levin, professor of public health at Yale University, could aver that "it sounds like a joke, but a hospital is no place for a sick person to be in."(14)

This should not have surprised: in a blistering report by the US Congress' putatively independent Office of Technology Assessment (OTA), it was found in 1978 that "only 10 to 20 percent of present-day scientific medical procedures have been shown to be of benefit by controlled trials."(15)

The other way to read this striking assessment is that between 80 to 90 percent of all approved medical procedures in the country have *not* been shown beneficial through controlled trials. And this information was released in the midst of the national debate over the controversial compound laetrile against cancer —

one of "orthodoxy's" primary arguments being that the long-used medication had never been "proven" by just such trials!

On March 3, 1993, ABC television "Nightline" anchor Ted Koppel seemed to do a double take as his guest declared that 60,000 Americans die annually of "unnecessary procedures" at American hospitals and clinics and that they are among the 15 million Americans who annually undergo unnecessary surgeries. The speaker was gynecologist Herb Keyser MD, described as "a critic of his own profession."

Recruits for the medical-freedoms fight

Of course, iatrogenicity has sometimes had a beneficial boomerang effect by transforming enraged victims into warriors for health freedom:

The health-freedoms movement in general (and the writer personally) lost a good friend in 1996 when Marie Steinmeyer, 71, combative president of the International Assn. of Cancer Victims and Friends (IACVF), succumbed to congestive heart failure.

For the better part of two decades, Marie had been a considerable thorn in the side of the American medical establishment, a gadfly for change and an activist on several fronts, and no stranger to state-and federal-level legislative hearings.

She was an example of iatrogenic mayhem in capital letters: both of her breasts had been removed in the late 1970s under the suspicion that she might have breast cancer (she did not), and she had received enormously debilitating radiation which almost killed her. A few years later, overdosing by antibiotics for treatment of a presumed ulcer *caused* her to have lupus erythematosus.

Once regarded at a Georgia hospital as "a walking miracle" as she overcame her iatrogenically induced illnesses after conducting her own research into "alternatives," Marie Steinmeyer had become a major voice for medical change in America.

While she was a powerful proponent of change, there remained the question of just how many thousands, or tens of thousands, of medically victimized Americans were out there without voice or vote, mutilated or poisoned by a failing medical model and its coverup apparatus.

Impetus for reform

1993 was the year when the American healthcare crisis could no longer be ignored and a new president launched sweeping, ill-considered — and immediately assailed — proposals for a stem-to-stern revamping of a trillion-dollar juggernaut ranging out of control. The "healthcare delivery system," baptized by reformers and health-freedoms advocates as the "sick business," by then was being exposed not only as an expensive monstrosity whose costs had escalated out of all reason but, and far worse, a system which did not deliver the goods:

For, while high-tech diagnostics and treatment devices and awesomely expensive drugs continued to capture much attention, it became apparent that the vaunted "war on cancer" had been lost, with upwards of 1,500 Americans dying per day from this greatest curse of civilization (figures would continue to rise dramatically each year thereafter); that "heart disease" fatality statistics, while plateauing out, still accounted for more medical deaths in the USA than any other cause; and that rapidly escalating diseases which had either not been known of a century before or had been only modest threats, including an alphabet soup of "incurable" diseases of all kinds (CFS, CP, MS, MD), plus Parkinson's, Alzheimer's, and osteoporosis, were advancing in both incidence and mortality; and that the various arthritises had created their own treatment industries, with some 40 million Americans affected by arthritis in some form and the figure expected to be 60 million by 2020. More terrifying, the worldwide pandemic of AIDS had reached a dozen years of institutional existence by 1993 — with neither a single "cure" delivered by standard or orthodox medicine, nor vaccine immediately likely.

And it was in 1993/1994 when political warfare broke out again — as it had twenty years earlier — over the right of the government to set standards for and to control the labeling claims of dietary supplements, to which increasing millions of Americans had turned for health reasons and which constituted a rapidly growing $4 billion per year challenge (to become some $7 billion-plus by 1996) to the far more lucrative but threatened synthetic drug industry, which was increasingly seen as in *de facto* control of organized medicine and of post-graduate medical education. Compromise legislation passed in 1994 essentially put a Bandaid on the problem — but was a step forward.

Death by orthodoxy

1993 was the year when it became notorious that officially approved remedies and devices with the FDA or AMA stamp of approval were causing at least 100,000 deaths per year — as opposed to (depending on who was counting) none or a handful of fatalities from natural products.

1993 was the year when UNICEF reported[16] that the United States was "back up" to 20th place in infant mortality (it had been in recent years as low as 24th) — a shocking statistic which meant that at least 19 other advanced countries were ahead of the United States, self-proclaimed exponent of the world's finest medical system, in the survival of the very young.

1993 was the year when the Physician Insurers Assn. of America (PIAA) reported[17] that medical liability insurers had paid out $340 million over a seven-year period for settlements averaging $104,000 each for "medication errors," mostly bearing on the misuse of glucocorticoids, antibiotics and narcotics. Such "medication errors" were the primary allegations of negligence in more than 7,000 claims in the PIAA data bank and drawn from a study of 100,000 malpractice suits — each of which had of course enriched attorneys. (***See NOTE #1, Page 81.***)

1993 was the year when RAND Corporation researchers announced[18] that 41 percent of hysterectomies — still among the most popular of surgical procedures in America's surgically oriented, knife-wielding medicine — in seven huge HMOs (health-maintenance organizations) had either been "clearly unnecessary," "unnecessary" or "questionable." By then, some 500,000 such surgical excisions of women were still being performed each year at a cost of about $2 billion — yet down from 1991, when a Health and Human Services (HHS) survey set the figure at 700,000 per year, including 2,000 deaths and 250,000 "major complications" among female victims.

(An HHS/*Seattle Times* overview of the problem in 1991 showed[19] that, of course, hysterectomies sometimes really are necessary for the reasons for which they are recommended — incipient cancer, pre-menstrual stress, irregular periods, mild endometriosis, cysts — but that they may be followed by "post-hysterectomy syndrome" which includes overall bad health, a lifetime daily regimen of synthetic hormones and constant antibiotics, leading to yeast overgrowth and the need for drugs to help control such overgrowth. A gynecologist was quoted as calling the procedure a "pelvic housecleaning" which physicians see as "neat and tidy" without taking into account a woman's suffering and loss of self-image — or, said some, being aware of what men might do if "genital housecleanings" were performed upon them in their 20s and 30s in an effort to head off all possible medical problems in that area.)

A year later, research on women patients at Balboa Naval Hospital, San Diego, led to the recommendation that doctors cease performing hysterectomies for asymptomatic benign uterine tumors and the conclusion that some 30,000 of the 175,000 hysterectomies performed annually on non-cancerous benign fibroid tumors were not necessary.

Revolt from within

Ivan Illich's epochal *Medical Nemesis* (1976) had helped bring the concept of iatrogenic medicine to the domestic vocabulary in the 1970s. His multi-phase essay on medical mismanagement — following Ruth Mulvey Harmer's blistering critique of the AMA in 1974 (*American Medical Avarice*) — would swiftly be joined by internal exposés of the medical profession, most particularly Dr. Edgar Berman's *The Solid Gold Stethoscope* and Marcia Millman's *The Unkindest Cut*. By the end of the decade, another exposé from within, Dr. Robert Mendelsohn's *Confessions of a Medical Heretic*, would set the standard for self-criticism by the medical profession.

In terms of growing costs, as early as Illich's research,

> *Since 1950 the cost of keeping a patient for one day in a community hospital in the United States has risen by 500 percent. The bill for patient care in the major university hospitals has risen even faster, tripling in eight years. Administrative costs have exploded, multiplying since 1964 by a factor of seven; laboratory costs have risen by a factor of five . . . The construction of hospitals now costs in excess of $85,000 per bed, of which two-thirds buys mechanical equipment that is made obsolete within less than ten years. These rates are almost twice those of the cost increases and of the obsolescence prevalent in modern weapons systems.*[20]

With the bright star of allopathic medicine beginning to fade noticeably even by the 1970s, medical reporters noted the strange connection between less medicine and lower death rates not only in the United States but wherever standard or orthodox (that is, allopathic) medicine prevailed:

In his own searing account of his own profession, Thomas Preston MD noted in 1981 that

> *In 1973, doctors in Israel went on strike for a month, during which time they attended only emergency cases. The death rate for the country dropped 50 percent — the largest decrease in mortality since the previous doctors' strike twenty years before! In Bogotá, Colombia, doctors were out for 52 days with a concomitant 35-percent decline in the mortality rate. During a strike in Los Angeles, there was an 18-percent decrease in the death rate, with the death rate returning to the usual level when the strike was over.*[21]

Flaying his profession for both over-diagnosing and over-treating, Preston noted that "most patients visiting physicians get some type of treatment. Of these, fully 80 percent do not need the treatment they get, 10 percent get ineffective treatment (because nothing effective is available) and the other 10 percent may get benefit from treatment subject to complications."

As early as 1981, a congressional subcommittee estimated that in the USA there were 2.4 million unneeded operations costing $4 billion and claiming 11,900 lives. At the same time, the independent Health Research Group estimated a minimum of 3.2 million unnecessary operations per year at a cost of $4.8 billion and a loss of 16,000 lives, and estimated also that half the operations covered by Blue Cross might have been unnecessary.[22]

A 1977 report had shown[23] that more than half the widely-used new surgical operations introduced during 1964-72 were not improvements over existing forms of therapy, but were actually harmful.

Despite the image of dramatic new surgical techniques being implemented only after careful scientific investigation patients are often literally used as surgical guinea pigs.

In 1995, Dr. Richard Greene, Agency for Health Care Policy and Research, told *USA Today* that "anything that hasn't been shown with hard data to be an effective treatment is experimental. That would go for virtually 85 percent to 95 percent of all surgical procedures."[24]

Even so, the surgeon remains the apex of the "healthcare-delivery team," a figure often treated with almost religious devotion by patient and medical staff alike.

X-rating X-rays

Concern over the utility and safety of relatively new surgical techniques has not obscured equal concerns with more established medical practices, very much including the inherent dangers of the X-ray machine.

X-ray therapy has become modern medicine's classic

double-edged sword: correctly used, the rays can be of great diagnostic benefit and have limited value therapeutically, particularly in reducing intractable pain. Yet, as in the notorious case of cancer, X-rays can as easily be described as "causes" (that is, inducers or organizers of the malignant process) as "cures" (destruction of tumor masses).

In their major study of the X-ray problem, John W. Gofman and Egan O'Connor observed that "ionizing radiation, even at extremely low dose rates, breaks human chromosomes and inflicts enduring chromosomal injuries."[25]

Since by that time (1985) more than 300 *million* medical and dental X-rays were being taken every year, the degree of possible damage — which often takes decades to show up, as in thyroid cancer — is significant.

Gofman and O'Connor estimated that 78,000 people were getting cancer annually from medical and dental X-rays (a generational statistical derivative: 2,340,000 cancers induced by radiation), and that even if X-rays are designed to "look" only at one organ they enhance the likelihood of cancer in many other organs. Gofman in 1995 argued that X-rays are *the* major cause of breast cancer.[26] (We discuss the mammography and low-level radiation emission scandals in *XI.*)

In 1978, the Senate Subcommittee on Health estimated[27] that more than 30 percent of 240 million X-ray procedures costing $6 billion the preceding year had been unnecessary. The unanswered question was: what damage had they done?

All of which speaks to the constant, nagging problem not only of the unnecessary nature of many medical diagnostics — but also their danger.

Invading the patient

"Invasive" diagnostic procedures are those in which needles, tubes, catheters and the like are inserted into various parts of the body — and of course far more of this is done in the controlling confines of the hospital than in the doctor's office. There seems to be, as some have noted, a virtual frenzy to over-test patients in hospital settings as well as to over-treat them — imperatives which may only in part be answered by the argument that physicians and hospitals must engage in such activities while practicing "defensive medicine" as a protection against malpractice suits.

Yet according to one frequently-quoted study,[28] 14 percent of patients who had undergone an "invasive" diagnostic procedure had suffered at least one complication because of the procedure, and of these three-quarters had required a specific treatment to counteract the complication or extended hospitalization or both.

The "thin-needle biopsy" — in which tiny pieces of tissue are taken from the body for diagnostic analysis (the only "orthodox" way to confirm cancer) — is another practice zealously pursued by the medical profession. Yet one study showed[29] a 32 percent complication rate from such biopsies, with a third of these being classed as "major." And, by the 1990s, there was little doubt that the act of biopsying a tumor often ran a certain risk of *spreading* it.

Impaired physicians and nurses

To which must be added the often hidden problem of incompetent, alcoholic or drug-dependent physicians.

In 1993, *Women's Day* reported[30] that between 5 and 10 percent of American doctors are poorly trained, incompetent, or physically or mentally impaired — and that while their negligence kills or injures between 150,000 and 300,000 patients a year, many of them continue to practice.

Earlier, *Medicine on Trial* (1988) brought the problem of alcoholic or drug-dependent medics into the open.

Various studies in the recent decade made it clear that:

— Of doctors in practice as of 1985, somewhere between 22,600 and 36,600 were recovering alcoholics or soon-to-be alcoholics.[31]

— *The Impaired Physician* pointed out in 1983 that "alcoholism is a primary disease to which physicians, as a group, seem highly susceptible, and often goes hand in hand with drug abuse."[32]

— A 1985 report indicated that "between 10 percent and 13 percent of the nation's physicians will have a substance abuse problem sometime during their lives."[33]

— A 1986 Harvard University study found[34] that 59 percent of physicians and 78 percent of medical students reported use of psychoactive drugs at some point in their lives; 10 percent of physicians admitted current regular drug use occurring once a month or more often; 3 percent of physicians and 5 percent of medical students reported they were drug addicts at some time.

To say nothing of substance-abused nurses. Data released in 1986 by the American Nurses Association's Committee on Impaired Nursing Practice found[35] that of 1.9 million registered nurses at the time about six percent had alcohol or other drug dependencies, that approximately 100,000 "chemically impaired" nurses were currently in the work force and that between 1980 and 1986 1,300 nurses nationally had been put on probation for drug-related problems with 1,038 undergoing license revocations.

That there are far more drug addicts among physicians than the population at large has long been known, if only because physicians have legal access to substances statutorily denied the non-medical population. As early as 1975, a report showed[36] that about one out of every six known drug addicts in the United States, England, the Netherlands, France and West Germany was a doctor.

Omniscience/omnipotence on demand

But another part of the problem may be the screening process by which students are chosen for medical schools — those AMA-approved institutions designed to turn out, with cookie-cutter precision, millions of AMA-molded, AMA-lining, AMA-practicing allopaths.

In his own swipe at his own profession, Thomas Preston MD, among many other critiques, deftly demolished the stereotype of the omniscient, quasi-divine physician, an image cultivated by medicine for centuries. He observed that

> *medical schools get bright students, but not the very brightest (who go into physics or biochemistry). The brightest medical students end up in nonclinical medicine, e.g., research. Some physicians are exceedingly common and dull; within the profession they are easy to spot. But to the laity they all look the same. The patient sees the professional, not the person.*[37]

Michael B. Rothenberg MD and Jo Rothenberg, describing the "omnipotence/omniscience syndrome," observed of the psychological makeup of many medical school students:

> *Medical school admissions committees select groups of students who seem to share certain compulsive, competitive, and egocentric traits. When those students enter into curricula that not only reinforce those traits, but also add to them the expectations of omniscience and omnipotence, then it appears that the people who are responsible for those curricula are, to a large extent, influencing the professional values and capabilities of many of our doctors.*[38]

Needless surgeries, dangerous drugs

A Committee for Freedom of Choice in Medicine Inc. gathering of iatrogenic data in 1986,[39] gleaned from many sources, pointed to 500,000 needless tonsillectomies in children as among the 2.4 million unnecessary surgeries per year, cited a nurses' publication (*RN*) poll claiming that three out of every 10 surgeries were unnecessary, noted an Ohio State University study that 10,000 patients were dying annually from fatal reactions to legal drugs, particularly antibiotics, and general data showing that 60,000 hospitalized Americans were dying annually from drug reactions while at least six million had some kind of drug reactions while hospitalized.

We noted then that iatrogenic disease was at the time

estimated to be the 10th cause of disease in the United States and was adding $3 billion annually to the healthcare bill, that a Centers for Disease Control (CDC) 10-year study had shown that 5.7 of every 100 hospital admissions in the mid-1970s resulted in some kind of new infection, that hospital-acquired infections were striking at least 2 million Americans per year while killing 15,000 of them, that some 30 percent of US hospital patients were estimated to be malnourished and that such institutional malnutrition might be accounting for 50,000 preventable hospital deaths per year.

That the overuse of drugs — that is, the massive incursion into, and by some accounts the controlling factor in, American medicine — had become epidemic was obvious by the 1960s. In 1976, Spencer Klaw reported[40] that "legal" drug reactions were responsible for five percent of all hospital admissions in the United States (1.5 million patients per year — far less than what would be the case 20 years later), and Thomas Preston would later summarize that "there is not a drug on the market with no adverse side effects, unless it is mountain water."[41]

Leading the pack in drug overuse is the family of "wonder drugs" called antibiotics — whose victories over certain infectious diseases of an earlier era are indeed impressive and of historical significance. Yet the idea that if a little dose of antibiotics may actually be good then massive overdosing and over-using such compounds on a grand scale is all that much better has led the medical profession into a considerable problem with iatrogenicity:

It is now fairly evident that no small part of the "substrate" of immune impairment on which such modern calamities as chronic fatigue syndrome (CFS), fibromyalgia, multiple allergenic/sensitivity reactions ("universal reactor syndrome"), various autoimmune conditions and even AIDS may rest is due to lifelong overuse of antibiotics — beginning with their over-administration against childhood disease, advancing through teen years with use against acne, and followed through adult years for use in virtually every medical complaint.

This is because antibiotics (whose very name suggests "against life") may indeed smash many pathogenic bacteria, but, as in the upper intestine, they may also reduce or eliminate benign and useful bacteria which can lead to unleashing *Candida albicans* yeast. The release of pathogenic yeast while impairing benign bacteria may over time lead to immune system dysregulation as the body fights off the internal imbalance between good and bad bacteria while attempting to mount a defense against the poisons (mycotoxins) produced by rapidly advancing systemic yeast infection.[42]

These years-later developments were of course neither known about nor contemplated when antibiotics were rushed onto the market and suddenly made available for prevention and treatment.

Ken Harvey MD has called the physician tendency to over-prescribe broad-spectrum antibiotics "the refuge of the diagnostically destitute," adding that in certain medical minds "in theory it doesn't matter what you treat, if you have a broad agent it will kill all germs." But "the danger of using broad spectrum antibiotics to treat any infection is that you are selecting out resistance on a broad front. If they're selective against 20 micro-organisms, then all those 20 are being put under selection pressures to become resistant."[43]

Hence the multiple plagues, particularly being noticed in the 1990s, of antibiotic-resistant strains of everything from gonorrhea to tuberculosis.

As some dissidents have noted, antibiotics pumped into a patient to prevent the occurrence of an infection that *might* happen, rather than to fight one that is already present, is a major problem, so much so that one study showed that "70.9 percent of prophylactic antibiotic administration to surgical patients was irrational on the basis of proved efficacy," and overall "only 7.6 percent of prophylactic therapy was rational."[44]

In 1995, a "mathematical model" showed that drug-related morbidity and mortality was costing the US more than $75 billion

— and most of this from drug-related hospitalizations.[45]

Some 60 percent of patients prescribed drugs have drug-related medical problems and 28 percent of all hospital admissions are from drug-related illnesses — thus causing 9 million hospitalizations per year, another 1995 study showed.[46]

A multiple-study assessment of what allopathic medicine euphemistically calls "adverse drug events" — ADES — in 1997 found that ADES may account for up to 140,000 deaths annually in the US. And "fatal ADEs" are expected in 0.31 percent of hospitalized patients.[92]

Drugs used in "heart disease" and hypertension have their own inherent dangers as do those used against cancer — the primary irony being that they may cause or enhance the conditions for which they are prescribed (*See X and XI*).

'Emerging' and 're-emerging' diseases — a global threat

By mid-decade it was becoming clear that the problem of antibiotic-resistant bacterial diseases was becoming so severe that much of the world was facing a global health threat of the "re-emerging" pathogens which allopathic medicine had allegedly vanquished or at least could control.

This was paralleled by the explosive development of something somehow even worse — "emerging" new viral diseases, captained by the quick-killing hemorrhagic viruses, particularly Ebola, and for which there was virtually no effective treatment.

The problem of "emerging new viruses" was part and parcel of the AIDS furor (*see XIII*) in which the "company" concept was that somehow an older animal virus had somehow gotten into humans (the "AIDS virus") to produce the most attention-getting pandemic of this century.

Yet, alongside Ebola, Marburg and other hideous viral infections, the "HIV" viruses said to cause the AIDS syndrome seemed pitifully weak — taking years to kill (if they ever killed at all) rather than the hours to days of the "emerging new viruses."

New terror: the antibiotic-resistant germs

Concern over antibiotic-resistant germs came home in triplicate in 1994, as it became obvious that the single biggest contribution by allopathy to modern medicine — the antibiotic wonder drugs — was wearing thin: *Newsweek* reported[47] that in 1992 some 13,000 American hospital patients had died of infections "that resisted every drug doctors tried" — due to mutated bacteria which had developed immunity to antibiotics.

The magazine quoted Dr. Sherwin Nuland (who terrifyingly recounted the development of drug-resistant germs in *How We Die*): ". . . medicine's purported triumph over infectious disease has become an illusion."

In 1997, a Centers for Disease Control and Prevention (CDC) Emory University Rollins School of Public Health study of eight hospitals in seven states surveyed in 1994-1995 showed that excessive use of antibiotics in intensive care units (ICU) had made bacteria more drug-resistant in the ICU than anywhere else.

Levels of antibiotic-resistant bacteria in ICUs reached between 7.7 percent and a stunning 79.9 percent, the study pinpointed.[93]

By 1994, the problem of drug-resistant venereal disease, tuberculosis and childhood ear infections and meningitis was becoming spectacularly noticeable, but so were outbreaks of infectious conditions caused by eating raw or undercooked processed meats which had been treated with so many antibiotics — farm animals reportedly receiving 30 times more antibiotics (penicillins and tetracyclines primarily) than humans do -- that resistance had occurred. By then, at least 500 Americans were thought to be dying annually from resistant microbes in meat and poultry, while some 6.5 million were made ill.[48]

Dr. Stuart Levy (in *The Antibiotic Paradox*) was quoted as saying that "antibiotic usage has stimulated evolutionary changes unparalleled in recent biologic history." Adding to the scandal, the American FDA had deemed as "safe" the levels of antibiotics which a Rutgers University study found increased the rate at which resistant bacteria emerged by from 600 to 2,700 percent!

A sinister parallel development: some 40 percent of *Staphylococcus aureus*, responsible for some pneumonias and for blood poisoning from surgical wounds, was said to be resistant to every antibiotic except one (vancomycin), while resistance to the latter was developing. (In 1997, Japanese research reported the first case of vancomycin-resistant *S.aureus.*)

To say nothing of a surge in "Group A" streptococcal infections in general, including so-called "flesh-eating" necrotizing fasciitis, an allegedly rare disorder suddenly becoming more commonplace by the mid-1990s.

Scientists now understand how bacteria, as if possessed of their own kind of innate intelligence, can develop resistance to antibiotics through the creation of "resistance genes" and the spreading of antibiotic-immune cells through their own filament-based outreach to other cells, a process eventually allowing such resistant bacteria to transfer resistance both to their own progeny and to other bacteria.

The prospects are for a race against time in which high technology will be utilized to outsmart the "smart germs" which, as it works out, were never really eliminated by the wonder drugs but quietly bided their time until wholesale resistance could be developed. The result is the grimmest scientific challenge yet to the allopathic paradigm. ***(See NOTE #2, Page 81)***

(Oddly, *Newsweek* devoted a single sentence to what might be the key to victory: "A healthy immune system easily repels most bacterial invaders regardless of their susceptibility to drugs."[(49)] This is a clear demonstration of media participation in paradigm capture through no obvious intention.)

Group-thought swiftly developed: while antibiotic-resistant bacteria evolved primarily due to specific human problems (overdose, overuse), the "emerging new viruses" were the result of man's destruction of the natural habitat, the ease of international transportation, and political/economical events.

As we shall see (*XIV*) there may be some even more sinister explanations for "emerging new viruses" which at least must be considered.

International attention has swiftly turned to the combined problems of antibiotic-resistant bacteria and "emerging new viruses."[50,51]

The Rockefeller University's Dr. Joshua Lederberg summarized:

> *"We face an ever-evolving adversary: microbes a billionfold more numerous than ourselves, vested with high intrinsic mutability and replication times measured in minutes, not years. Within every infected person, we see a Darwinian struggle mobilizing the genetic diversity of our immune cells to respond to unpredictable invaders . . . But many microbes have learned their own tricks of jamming or coming in under the radar scan, masking their antigens, or simply multiplying faster than our immune system can respond . . . Pitted against microbial genes, we have mainly our wits."*[52]

"Wits," of course, should — indeed, *must* — mean the development of a new medical model, which the problem of the "emerging" and " re-emerging" diseases is also helping to bring about.

Fatal errors, expensive bed sores

In other iatrogenic matters, in 1989 the RAND Corporation claimed[53] that results of a 12-hospital study by researchers had shown that nine common medical errors, ranging from prescribing the wrong drugs to misdiagnosis of stroke, appeared to have caused as many as 27 percent of all deaths from heart attack, stroke and pneumonia among hospital patients.

1990 was a year of further medical disaster revelations:

The International Association for Enterostomal Therapy (IAET) reported[54] that year on the developing scandal of bed sores in hospitals and nursing homes: almost 60,000 Americans per year were said to be dying annually from this widespread problem of nursing neglect. The same data showed that almost 40 percent of nursing home residents were at risk for developing a bed sore, or an estimated 600,000 of the nation's elderly, and that management of this single element alone was adding $10 billion to the health bill since each one cost $5,000 to an amazing $86,000 (average: $45,000) to treat.

The bed sore matter was only among the more prominent of the revelations slowly evolving toward the end of this century in the "warehousing" of the cast-off elderly: local news reports were rife with tales of physical mistreatment, over-medication, and the outright drugging of "senior citizens" in "nursing homes" often staffed by inadequately trained or unlicensed personnel.

Victimizing the elderly

In fact, the abuse of the elderly — and of the very young — had reached scandalous dimensions by the middle of the decade.

In 1994, data from the National Medical Expenditure Survey found that a quarter of all Americans 65 years or older were being given drugs that they should never take, compounds whose effects ranged from inducing amnesia and confusion to causing heart problems and respiratory failure.

The survey found that many of 20 drugs routinely prescribed for the elderly were unnecessary either because there were safer alternatives or they simply were not needed. Key offenses in the study led by Harvard Medical School's Dr. Steffi Woolhandler and colleagues: 1.8 million seniors had been prescribed the blood thinner dipyridamole, which is useless other than for those who have had artificial heart valves inserted — but only 36,000 Americans had had such a procedure and only half of these were over 65. And more than 1.3 million older Americans had been prescribed the addictive narcotic propoxyphene, said to be no better than aspirin in relieving pain.[55]

The over-prescribing of drugs for the elderly was also brought home by the consumer group Public Citizen's *Worst*

Pills/Best Pills II survey: Americans over 60 constituted a sixth of the population but consumed 40 percent of prescription drugs.[56]

At the other end of the scale, childhood behavioral disorders increasingly are dealt with by prescription mood-altering drugs, which by the 1990s had led to scandals in local school districts and raised the specter of drug-dependent children (the "Ritalin generation.") Ritalin — methylphenidate — was being used legally by 2 million American school children, who often called it "Vitamin R," by 1996. The "cheap high" of Ritalin abuse has led to serious side effects and death.[57]

Bombshell from the GAO

In June 1990, in a report which caused immediate negative responses from the overseeing FDA, which seemed to sense guilt by inference, the Congress' General Accounting Office (GAO) claimed[58] that more than half the new drugs approved for marketing in the United States had severe or fatal side effects which had not been found during the testing phase of the compounds, and not been evident until many years after. The GAO had reviewed all 198 drugs approved between 1976 and 1985 and marketed for substantial periods of time: 102 had been found to have side effects serious enough to warrant withdrawal from the market or to have incurred major label changes.

It should be strongly emphasized that the fact *so few* new medical entities had been approved for the American marketplace was because of the world's most expensive, time-consuming, red tape-generating, animal-testing, licensing system for new drugs — one touted as the safest, best and most responsible in the world.

Preventable disease

By the last decade of this century, the numerous research and treatment mishaps among the major killers (cancer, "heart disease", AIDS) had become public knowledge, and we will deal with each of these calamities separately. Each of these overlapping areas of the "healthcare delivery system" had generated gigantic industries in testing, treatment and management, all of which had added up to a majority of the expenses counted in the trillion-dollar national health tab.

It also was becoming clear that so much of disease is *preventable* — that dietary and lifestyle changes alone could vastly reduce risks for cancer and heart disease, and virtually all of AIDS, and that failure to act on the onrush of new information on dietary links to the major chronic illnesses — information somehow unwanted by or irritating to a death-oriented medical establishment and its pharmaceutical support apparatus which drew profit galore from the expectation of death and suffering rather than the promotion of health — was perhaps the biggest single reason for the astronomically high cost of medicine in America.

Indeed, in 1991 a private group called Wellness Watch reported[(59)] that social costs imposed by preventable disease totalled about $680 billion annually (the lion's share of healthcare spending). Wellness Watch referred to studies by the RAND Corporation, Harvard and InterStudy which showed that a fourth to a half of all hospital stays, medical/surgery procedures and prescriptions are unnecessary, and that in-hospital medical care was resulting in injury or death to 3.7 percent of all patients, or about 1.1 million injuries and over 150,000 deaths per year.

Dangerous hospitals

In December 1992, the official Centers for Disease Control and Prevention (CDC) upped the statistics on "nosocomial infections" (medical industry jargon for infections caused by modern medicine and occurring during hospital and clinic stays), claiming that such events involved more than 2 million patients and had cost that year about $4.5 billion.[(60)]

Usually, nosocomial infection means that a patient picked up a fresh infection of some kind simply from *being in* a germ-laden hospital or clinic. This growing element may be the single most pervasive problem within "iatrogenic" medicine and shows no signs of letting up:

As early as 1985 it was reliably estimated[61] that there were at least 100,000 nosocomial-related deaths per year, from the two million or so patients — between 5 to 10 percent of the total patient population — who acquired such an infection. Some 100,000 patients were thought to be acquiring nosocomial bacteremia — bacteria in the blood — at treatment facilities.

A study by V.L. Yu *et al.* indicated that infection acquired by treatment was "the principal cause of morbidity and the second leading cause of death in the population undergoing hemodialysis" (as in kidney treatments), "with infection of the vascular-access site with staphylococcal bacteremia the most common serious complication."[62]

L.S. Elting *et al.* reported[63] in 1986 that "polymicrobial septicemia," or multiple-microbe infection, was the most frequent cause of death in cancer patients — that is, above and beyond the cancer process itself, acquisition of new infections through the act of being treated was claiming the highest number of cancer patients. Other research showed[64] that pneumonia was the most common hospital-acquired infection and might be responsible for as many as 15 percent of all hospital-related fatalities.

Modern medical technology brings with it a huge element in nosocomial infection — catheters, inserted into various parts of the body for the constant intravenous treatment or feeding of the patient and often kept in the body for long periods of time, are themselves important pathways for invasion by new bacteria.

Virulent hepatitis infection from widespread use of dialysis units,[65] outbreaks of such dangerous pathogens as *Pseudomonas aeruginosa* caused by contaminated equipment in delivery rooms,[66] death from rabies occurring after the patient received a corneal implant from a man with undiagnosed rabies,[67] even failure to follow simple rules of hygiene, such as persistent and aggressive washing of hands,[68] and the development of antibiotic-resistant bacteria from mass "prophylaxis" programs in hospitals aimed at cutting down on hospital-ravaging bacteria have added to the scandal of nosocomial infection.

Iatrogenic disease data published in 1988 by the People's Medical Society indicated that about 40 percent of patients suffered side effects from their medications and that such reactions could leave one "blind or dead, afflicted with kidney, liver or brain damage, necrosis, ulceration of the bowel, intestinal hemorrhage, skin scars, extreme sensitivity to sunlight, or other disabilities that may last for months or years."[69]

This, because, as Louise Lander wrote,

> *Introducing the chemistry of medication into an individual's internal ecology is intrinsically risky. Drugs (even aspirin) are inherently toxic and, at dosage levels that vary widely among individuals, will produce a toxic reaction ... And practically any drug will in some people produce a hypersensitivity, or allergic reaction, a danger that is unpredictable unless the reaction has occurred before. Either type of reaction may be as trivial as a transient skin rash, or as final as death.*[70]

• Charles P. Inlander *et al.*, drawing in 1988 from a "selection pool . . . so vast and deep," reported[71] common drug reactions from the medical literature. Some highlights:

• Attacks on the gastrointestinal tract (mouth, esophagus, stomach, small and large intestines, pancreas) — common at some level from virtually *all* oral drugs.[72]

• Drug-induced myopathies (muscle disorders), including the multiple sclerosis-like disorder myasthenia gravis and related conditions.[73]

• Cataracts in children receiving high-dose oral prednisone for chronic asthma.[74]

• Multiple diseases of the liver (cell necrosis, hepatitis, impairment of bile secretion), accounting for some 8 percent of all drug reactions.[75]

• Systemic lupus erythematosus (SLE), an often hideously disfiguring condition of which an impressive 10 percent of cases are caused by medications given to treat other diseases, and described as "an elaborate example of pharmacological provocation of an illness."[76] (*See earlier Steinmeyer case.*)

• Drug reactions diametrically opposed to the stated intent of the drug's action — such as analgesics for muscle contraction headaches which may actually feed the pain, tranquilizers to control schizophrenia which may cause serious mental and emotional problems unrelated to the original disorder, and even common drugs used to treat irregular heartbeat (arrhythmia) which actually *cause* it.[77]

Vaccines: the dark side

Vaccinating children and adults against all manner of microbial diseases has been a major element in state-mandated medicine (US Public Health Service, CDC, etc.) and such immunizations — in which (often) live, "attenuated" disease-producing microbes are injected into the system — have had a demonstrable effect in helping reduce many of the infectious diseases of old.

Such mass immunization programs are part of the AIC social propaganda which attributes great successes to allopathic medicine. Without question, immunizations helped bring the worldwide problem of smallpox to an end and reduced the killer childhood diseases of old, particularly polio.

But end-of-century research and evidence continues to point to dark sides and possible scandals in such programs, not the least of which includes cases of polio (direct or delayed) *induced* by the polio vaccines.

In 1985, the book *DPT: A Shot in the Dark*[78] documented egregious flaws in the whole-cell pertussis (whooping cough) and related vaccines at a time when media attention focused on injuries, deaths (and lawsuits) in highly-politicized immunization campaigns.

In 1992, the CDC's immunization division reported[79] that the pertussis (whooping cough) vaccine had killed 250 children in the 20 months prior to July 31, 1992, while also causing 7,200 reactions. This reality — deaths due to mandatory vaccine programs — was offset by the fact that in pre-vaccine times pertussis used to kill as many as 7,000 Americans per year. Even so, as of late 1992, some 3,200 pertussis vaccination claims had been filed against the US government, according to the US Public Health Service.

Forty states had mandated the vaccine but because actual cases of the disease had dropped over time, there was now the intriguing irony, said Dr. Joanne Hatem, director of the National Vaccine Information Center, that "for an individual child, the risk is greater from the vaccine than the disease."

In 1994, following a 1993 pertussis outbreak in Cincinnati primarily among children previously immunized, it was demonstrated that the vaccine had failed to give full protection.[80]

As we note elsewhere (*XIII,XIV*), researchers looking into either the "accidental" or biological warfare components of vaccine/man-made virus research have called attention to the very strong likelihood that experimental animal-derived viruses capable of causing diseases in humans were introduced into human vaccines.

Lest this be dismissed as political paranoia, it was a well-credentialed establishment scientist who more than any other tried gamely to bring national attention to the problem of "viral contaminants" in polio vaccines.

Dr. W. John Martin, University of Southern California professor of pathology and former director of the FDA's Bureau of Biologics viral oncology branch, warned in 1995 of "the potential introduction of pathogenic viral variants into humans through the use of African green monkey-derived cell lines." He had identified a "stealth virus" in chronic fatigue syndrome (CFS) and noted that CFS, attention deficit disorder, autism and other behavioral problems might have a link to "stealth virus vaccine contaminants."[81]

Summarized vaccine contaminant researcher Leonard

Horowitz DMD MPH:

> *In other words, anyone, and particularly those who received polio vaccines prior to 1964, is at risk of carrying SV40 [simian virus-40] and spreading it to others at home or in the community. The virus is apparently circulating now throughout the human race, and may give rise to more virulent viruses over time. . .*[82]

Whether through error (iatrogenicity) or intent (biological warfare development), such warnings must be taken seriously and call into question state-mandated vaccination programs.

And doubters of the immunizations-eradicate-disease line have began to be heard, particularly the late Dr. Robert Mendelsohn, who argued strongly that medical history reflected that as incidence of a specific disease was beginning to die out on its own, promoters of vaccines often moved in to take the credit for the falloff, thus inflating success for one of the bulwarks of standard Western medicine.

For all the above reasons, it became clear why Dr. Mendelsohn could write:

> *. . . I no longer believe in Modern Medicine.*
>
> *I believe that despite all the super technology and elite bedside manner that's supposed to make you feel about as well cared for as an astronaut on the way to the moon, the greatest danger to your health is the doctor who practices Modern Medicine. . . .*
>
> *I believe that more than ninety percent of Modern Medicine could disappear from the face of the earth — doctors, hospitals, drugs, and equipment — and the effect on our health would be immediate and beneficial.*[83]

Misdiagnosis mayhem

There is also the naggingly persistent problem of misdiagnosis (to say nothing of over-diagnosis), which has contributed in no small way to the epidemic of American iatrogenic disease:

A 32-hospital study in 1985 found[84] a 20 percent error rate in a comparison of 1,800 "clinical" (that is, visual observation) diagnoses made on living patients contrasted with "anatomical" diagnoses made on autopsy. It was estimated that half the errors had led to the patients' deaths. Pulmonary embolisms, peritonitis and pulmonary abscesses were the most commonly overlooked medical problems.

In 1983, a shocking Brigham and Women's Hospital/ Harvard Medical School study in Boston discovered[85] that doctors missed certain diagnoses in dying patients about one-fourth of the time and that one in 10 patients would have lived had diagnoses been made correctly.

Other hospitals came up with 20- and 10-percent diagnostic errors, many leading to death.[86,87]

Part of the problem may be that — as a medical examiners group reported in 1994[88] — only half of the nation's 25,000 emergency medical jobs are staffed by physicians certified to provide emergency medical care.

Revolution in the air

All of which makes it understandable why a majority of Americans — including many physicians and professional healthcare givers — believe that some kind of urgent reform is necessary.

It is understandable why a 1991 American Medical Association (AMA) survey learned[89] that 69 percent of citizens polled believed that "people are beginning to lose faith in their doctors" and that 63 percent believed that "doctors are too interested in making money."

Yet an earlier AMA poll, in 1989, had found[90] doctors not all that happy, either: as many as a quarter of practicing physicians "probably would not go"to medical school if they could start out all over again.

While what we are calling in this study the Allopathic Industrial Complex (AIC) — whose components we also call "The Club" — is beginning to fall apart at the seams, even though state-of-the-art high technology in research springing from that selfsame AIC may yet at least partially save the day, the ever resilient human species, subspecies *americanus*, is beginning to take things into its own hands:

The fight over laetrile against cancer, as we will show, set off a series of irreversible currents in modern American medicine which have led to gradual abandonment of the carefully nurtured myths of the physician as god-like and "medical science" (an oxymoron) as infallible and ever advancing.

Depending on who is counting and from what perspective, either a large plurality or a low majority of Americans either believe in, or have used or do use, some form of non-mainstream or "unorthodox" or "questionable" or "dubious" (these being phrases from the AIC to describe all dissidence from the standard or allopathic line) form of therapy, which proponents are more comfortable calling "alternative","complementary" or "integrative."

Stops on the Tijuana Express

More embarrassing for the AIC, its "quackbuster" propagandists, the AMA, and government medicine, ever greater numbers of Americans are simply abandoning the United States and heading for any place where they might be able to "cure" their incurable diseases — usually, and most dramatically, Mexico. What's more, standard physicians often not only support their decisions but in some cases have actually brought such options to their patients' attention.

By the time this was written, there were an estimated 30 operations (hospitals, clinics, converted motel rooms, houses) in the area of Tijuana, Mexico, offering some sort of "alternative" or "unapproved" therapy to a clientele usually composed in the great majority of Americans fleeing their country, usually for cancer therapy, but increasingly for treatments for virtually all the ever-lengthening list of so-called "incurable" diseases.

It is true that more than half of such places probably did fit the general definition of "quack" operations — the brush with which organized medical "quackbusters" through the deft manipulation of the compliant, and at times just plain lazy, American media attempted to paint *all* south-of-the-border operations. That is because there were and are any number of confidence agents, hustlers and opportunists who ravenously feed along the edges of the cesspool of American medical failure.

As a trained journalist, this writer — who admits moving from alleged objectivity to ardent radical defense of the need for unabashed major medical reform — was always amazed by the capacity of the American media to so often miss the true story about what was going on south of the border:

The *real* story is not how many frauds, quacks and unlicensed practitioners set up shop over the border — it is why so many Americans would abandon American medicine to seek them out. The emphasis on dirty syringes on the floor (as viewable in various "ambush journalism" television shows pandering to organized medicine) and magic-bullet cures for cancer and AIDS that turned out to be useless or fraudulent has always been, in real terms, less vital than the central issue: *why can't America cure these things?*

But while Americans have sought answers elsewhere, growing numbers of US physicians and medical practitioners — often at great risk to themselves, their profession, their economic standing and their physical safety and freedom — have dared to think new thoughts and to challenge the system.

References

1. *The Choice*, XV: 1.2, 1988/1989.
2. Ross, John. "Fleeing to Mexico." *San Francisco Bay Guardian.* April 7, 1993.
3. *The Choice*, XVI: 4, 1990.
4. "Procedure results in quadriplegia." *American Medical News.* July 26, 1993.
5. Mitchell, Gene, "Warning: hospitals may be hazardous to your health." *Alive Magazine.* Fall 1984.
6. *The Choice*, XXI:2, 1995.
7. Pekkanen, John, "The unbelievable confessions of 7 angry doctors." *Redbook*, October 1988.
8. *Ibid.*
9. *Ibid.*
10. *New Eng. J. Med.*, March 12, 1981

11. Mitchell, *op. cit.*
12. Seidl, LG, *et al.*, "Studies on the epidemiology of adverse drug reactions: III. Research in patients on a general medical service." *Bulletin of Johns Hopkins Hospital,* No. 119, 1966.
13. Thorup, Oscar, *Mayo Clinic Proceedings,* 1971.
14. " Talking points." Committee for Freedom of Choice in Medicine, Inc., Chula Vista CA, 1986.
15. *Assessing the Efficacy and Safety of Medical Technologies.* US Congress: Office of Technology Assessment (OTA), Publication P3206-929, 1978.
16. *The Choice*, XIX:1, 1993.
17. McCormick, Brian, "Insurers study drug errors leading to suits." *American Medical News,* July 12, 1993
18. *J. Am. Med. Assn.*, May 12, 1993
19. *The Choice*, XVII: 1, 1991.
20. Illich, Ivan, *Medical Nemesis.* New York: Pantheon Books, 1976.
21. Preston, Thomas, *The Clay Pedestal.* Seattle: Madrona, 1981.
22. *Ibid.*
23. Gilbert, JB, et al., "Progress in surgery and anesthesia: benefits and risks of innovative therapy," in Bunker, JB, ed., *Costs, Risks and Benefits of Surgery.* New York: Oxford University Press, 1977.
24. Friend, Tim "That operation you're getting may be experimental." *USA Today.* Sept. 13, 1995.
25. Gofman, JW, and O'Connor, E, *X-rays: Health Effects of Common Exams.* San Francisco: Sierra Club Books, 1985.
26. Gofman, John, *Preventing Breast Cancer: The Story of a Major, Proven Preventable Cause of This Disease.* Cited in *The Choice*, XXL:2, 1995.
27. Preston, *op cit.*
28. Schroeder, SA, *et al.*, "Frequency and morbidity of invasive procedures." *Arch. Int. Med. 138*, 1978.
29. "MDs flout warning on thin-needle biopsy." *American Medical News*, Jan. 8, 1979.
30. *Women's Day*, Oct. 12, 1993, cited among "ten most underreported news stories of 1993" by San Francisco *Bay Gardian*, March 30, 1994.
31. Watkins, T, "Physicians: a higher risk group." *Medical Tribune*, June 19, 1985.
32. Scheiber, SC, and Doyle, BB, *The Impaired Physician.* New York: Plenum Press, 1983.
33. *Phoenix Gazette*, March 30, 1983.
34. Inlander, *op. cit.*
35. Wolfe, L. "Nurses and drug abuse: new ways to help." *New York Times*, July 26, 1986.
36. Freese, AS, *Managing Your Doctor.* New York: Stein and Day, 1975.
37. Preston, *op. cit.*
38. Rothenberg, MB, and Rothenberg, J. "The omnipotence/omniscience syndrome." *Resident and Staff Physician*, June, 1985.
39. "Talking points," *loc. cit.*
40. Klaw, Spencer, *The Great American Medicine Show.* New York: Penguin Books, 1976.
41. Preston, *op. cit.*
42. Culbert, ML, *CFS: Conquering the Crippler.* San Diego CA: C and C Comunications, 1993.
43. Inlander, *op. cit.*
44. Wang, J, "Antibiotic prophylaxis in surgery — too much or not enough?" *Modern Medicine,* Sept. 1, 1985.
45. Johnson, JA., and Bootman, JL., "Drug-related morbidity and mortality. A cost-of-illness model."*Arch. Int. Med.* ISS, 1995.
46. *Arch. Int. Med.*, October, 1995.
47. Begley, Sharon, "The end of antbiotics." *Newsweek*, March 28, 1994.
48. *Ibid.*
49. Cowley, Geoffrey, "Too much of a good thing." *Newsweek*, March 28, 1994.
50. *Infectious Disease — A Global Health Threat.* Washington DC: National Science and Technology Council, September 1995.
51. Garrett, Laurie, *The Coming Plague.* New York: Penguin, 1994.
52. Lederberg, Joshua, "Infectious disease — a threat to global health and security." *J. Am. Med. Assn.*, Aug. 7, 1996.
53. *The Choice*, XV: 1,2, 1988/1989.
54. *The Choice*, XVI: 2,3, 1990.
55. *J. Am. Med. Assn.*, July 27, 1994.
56. Friend, Tim, "Education on prescribing is 'terrible.'" *USA Today*, July 27, 1994.
57. Stepp, LS, "A wonder drug's worst side effect." *The Washinton Post,* Feb. 5, 1996.
58. *The Choice,* XVI: 2,3, 1990.
59. *The Choice*, XVII: 2, 1991.
60. *The Choice*, XVIII: 3, 1992.
61. Nahata, MC, *Drug Intelligence and Clinical Pharmacy*, October 1985.
62. Yu, VL, et al., "Staphylococcus aureus nasal carriage and infection in patients on hemodialysis: efficacy of antibiotic prophylaxis." *New Eng. J. Med.*, July 10, 1986.
63. Elting, LS, *et al.*, "Polymicrobial septicemia in the cancer patient." *Medicine*, July 1986.
64. Stratton, CW, "Pulmonary infections in critical care medicine — the Wright State University School of Medicine symposium: Bacterial pneumonias — an overview with emphasis on pathogenesis, diagnosis and treatment." *Heart and Lung*, May 1986.
65. Bryan, JA, in Bennett, JV, and Brachman, PS, eds., *Hospital Infections.* Boston: Little, Brown and Co., 1979.
66. Fierer, J. *et al.*, "*Pseudomonas aeruginosa* epidemic traced to delivery-room resuscitators." *New Eng. J. Med.*, May 4, 1967.
67. Anderson, LJ, et al., "Nosocomial rabies: investigation of contacts of human rabies cases associated with a corneal transplant." *Am. J. Pub. Health,* April 1984.
68. Inlander, *op. cit.*
69. *Ibid.*

70. Lander, Louise, *Defective Medicine.* New York: Farrar, Straus, Giroux, 1978.
71. Inlander, *op. cit.*
72. Zentler-Munro, PL. and Northfield, TC, "Drug-induced diseases: drug-induced gastrointestinal disease." *Brit. Med. J.*, May 12, 1979.
73. Lane, RJM, and Mastaglia, FL, "Drug-induced myopathies in man." *Lancet*, Sept. 9, 1978.
74. "High cataract rate tied to daily prednisone dose." *Pediatric News*, November 1979.
75. Keeling, PWN, and Thompson, RPH, " Drug-induced diseases: drug-induced liver disease." *Brit. Med. J.*, April 1979.
76. Kale, SA, "Drug-induced systemic lupus erythematosus." *Postgraduate Medicine*, Feb. 15, 1985.
77. Inlander, *op. cit.*
78. Coulter, Harris, and Fisher, BL., *DPT: A shot in the Dark.* New York: Harcourt/Brace/Jovanovich, 1985.
79. *The Choice*, XVIII: 3, 1992.
80. Christie, CDC, *et al.*, *New Eng. J. Med.*,July 7, 1994.
81. Martin, JW. *et al.*, "African green monkey origin of the atypical cytopathic 'stealth virus' isolated from a patient with chronic fatigue syndrome." *Clin. and Diag. Vir.* 4, 1995.
82. Horowitz, Leonard, *Emerging Viruses: AIDS and Ebola.* Rockport MA: Tetrahedron, 1996.
83. Mendelsohn, RS, *Confessions of a Medical Heretic.* New York: Warner Books, 1979.
84. McDonald, Betsy, "New autopsy study: not even practice makes diagnosis perfect." Washington University in St. Louis Feature Service, September 1985.
85. "Diagnostic errors cited in study." *San Jose (CA) News*, April 1983.
86. "Pathologists build case for more autopsies." *Medical World News*, Oct. 14, 1985.
87. Friederici, HHR,and Sebastian, M, "Autopsies in a modern teaching hospital." *Arch.Path. Lab. Med.*, June 1984.
88. Raeburn, Paul, The Associated Press, Sept. 15, 1994.
89. Gordon, JS, "Healing with feeling." *Washington Post*, Aug. 29, 1993.
90. *Ibid.*
91. Dalen, JF, and Bone, RC, "Is it time to pull the pulmonary artery catheter?" *J. Am. Med. Assn.*, Sept. 18, 1996.
92. Bates, DW, *et al.*; Classen, DC, *et al.*; and editorial, *J. Am. Med. Assn.*, Jan. 22/29, 1997.
93. *Clin. Infec. Dis.*, February 1997.

NOTE #1

According to the AMA-organized National Patient Safety Foundation in 1997, as many as three million medical errors occur in hospitals each year and cost up to $200 billion.

— USA Today, *Oct. 10, 1997*

NOTE #2

The World Health Organization (WHO) reported in 1997 that a study of 50,000 tuberculosis patients in 35 nations had a form of multiple drug-resistant TB. "Untreatable" cases were accounting for 2 to 14 percent of the world total.

— The Associated Press, *Oct. 23, 1997*

III
MILKING AND BILKING THE SYSTEM:
Greed and gouging nourish the medical money machine

"There is probably no area in which deception is more widespread in medicine than the accumulation and dissemination of clinical knowledge . . . Most of the 'knowledge' on which therapy has been based has been incorrect, but, at every stage in the history of medicine, the knowledge of contemporary doctors was considered authoritative. Discarded practices might be disdained as superstition or inaccuracy, but current practices have always been believed to be true and accurate."

—**Thomas Preston MD (*The Clay Pedestal*)**

"The surest way to power in a medical center is to ally oneself with technology . . . In addition, technology reimburses its followers well. The anesthesiologist makes more than the pediatrician, and the internist who performs more procedures to make a diagnosis makes more money than the internist who does only a few. A third lesson, not explicitly stated but obviously followed in practice, was that virtually everyone should be treated . . . medical students are being swamped by science and technology at the expense of healing skills."

— **David Hellerstein**

"There is a need in fulfilling the requirements of medicine to use professionals other than physicians. The concept that the doctor, the physician, is the only professional who can exist in the execution of the function and requirement of medicine is idiocy."

— **Harold M. Schoolman MD**

"Physicians think they are doing something for you by labeling what you have as a disease."

— **Immanuel Kant**

"Doctors are men who prescribe medicines of which they know little, to cure diseases of which they know less, in human beings of whom they know nothing."

— **Voltaire**

The trillion-dollar bill arrives

It became official on December 28, 1993:

On that date the Commerce Department announced[1] that total healthcare spending in 1994 would, for the first time, rise to $1 trillion dollars and would account for a full 15 percent of the nation's total gross domestic product (GDP). The long-feared trillion-dollar figure was suddenly upon the "healthcare delivery industry" sooner than had been warned about only a few years prior.

The official projection was a rise of $118 billion in one year's time to a shocking $1,060,500,000,000 — the highest figure the US government used other than in dealing with astronomical events and the national debt.

The figure meant that, in 1994 as every year preceding for decades, Americans were paying more for healthcare in one form or another than any people on earth.

A reassessment of Commerce's figures by the Health and Humans Services Dept. (HHS) in 1996 claimed the real figures were not quite so bad — $949 billion and 13.7% of GDP.[2] (To which, by 1995, the shocking estimate of the costs of "iatrogenic disease" — $182 billion — would have to be considered. *See II*)

With various estimates of healthcare cost increases of anywhere from 9 percent to 14 percent by 1998, the question remained: just how much *can* we afford?

And this question accompanies an equally important one about value received: in 1993 the World Health Organization (WHO) ranked the US at a mere *18th* place among developed countries for its level of "good health."[2a]

By 1992, the US was already spending an estimated $3,094 per person and the average working-age family was spending, directly or indirectly, $8,821 for what was constantly touted as the finest medical system on the planet.

A benefit-consulting company reported in 1996 that the cost of healthcare benefits had risen to an average of $3,821 per worker in 1995 despite increased efforts to control medical costs.[3]

The trillion-dollar figure arrived just as business, particularly small business, was pondering the ever higher costs of medical insurance for employees — a problem growing so swiftly that it imperiled corporate growth in America and made tens of thousands of small entrepreneurs think twice about opening new enterprises.

In 1994, an updated 1987 National Medical Expenditure Survey calculated in 1993 dollars estimated that hospital stays were the largest component of medical charges ($329 billion per year) and doctor visits were $90 billion annually.[4]

All of which was feeding the revolution in "managed care" — the burgeoning increase in HMOs (health maintenance organizations) and PPOs (preferred-provider organizations) which are dominating medical private payment schemes as the millennium ends.

As bad as the total cost of healthcare had become, it was also obvious that it had a great deal of "fat" which could be removed:

— In February 1993 a survey by the National Medical Liability Reform Coalition claimed that "defensive medicine" — a phrase meaning the ordering of marginal or unnecessary tests and procedures solely to protect against malpractice suits — had cost the system about $9.9 billion in 1991. It added that "tort reform," or overhauling this aspect of the medico/legal system, could save between $7.5 billion and $76.2 billion over five years. The huge span of possible savings was due to the fact that the total dollar impact on "healthcare delivery" involving endless litigation between parts of the system was hard to pin down.[5]

— In 1993 the American Medical Assn. (AMA) estimated that "avoidable" components such as smoking, substance abuse and violence were adding $42.9 billion to the healthcare bill while adding up to $180 billion annually in such "indirect expenses" as lost productivity. The healthcare bite from smoking alone was estimated at $22 billion annually.[6]

—Earlier, the Health Insurance Association of America estimated that sorting, shuffling and processing billions of pieces of paperwork generated by four billion medical insurance claims per year was adding $40 billion annually to the healthcare bill. The Associated Press added that "some say it's more like $90 billion, or about double our annual trade with Japan."[7]

Even in 1992, when "healthcare delivery" reached the $820 billion figure and government statisticians were scrambling to predict just when the magic trillion-dollar figure would arrive, what some call "the sick business" was eating up 14 percent of GDP and, in terms of "real spending" and "adjustments for inflation" as viewed by economists, healthcare delivery was far ahead of the other big components of GDP — both defense and education were around 5 percent.

In 1970, as *The Washington Post* reported,[7] the "big three" budget-busters were still defense, education and healthcare, but all shared about 6 percent of what was then called GNP — with $236 billion going to defense, $218 billion to education and $215 billion to healthcare.

By any definition, by the late 1970s and throughout the 1980s total spending on all aspects of healthcare, ranging from the doctor visit to the latest high-tech diagnostic to the specialized therapy to the intensive-care unit to the hospice, from the cost of a filling to the gigantic strides in private health insurance costs and the uncontrollable, metastatic growth of government programs, made healthcare an out-of-control administrative free radical unable to be reined in because, ultimately, so many vested interests were in play.

By the 1990s, with the nation in the midst of debate over the need for sweeping healthcare cost reform — with no clear idea yet of how to achieve it — the "healthcare delivery industry" could be defined in huge subdivisional chunks — at least $200 billion to cancer and somewhat more to the total of conditions and pathologies grandly lumped together as "heart and circulatory diseases," for example. And these were part of the $659 billion per year spent by 100 million Americans on "chronic conditions."[8a]

There were subdivisions of these, of course — diabetes by

the mid-1990s was up to $105 billion in overall costs. As of 1995, some 16 million were said to have either of the two forms of the blood-sugar disease.[9] Arthritis in its various forms (32.6 million patients), and such conditions of the elderly as osteoporosis and Alzheimer's, afflicting some 15 percent of Americans by 1995, were in the multi-billion-dollar ranges. (Indeed, with Alzheimer's at $82.7 billion in *direct* costs, this malady had become the nation's third most expensive disease by 1994.[10])

Clinical depression, said to be "the most undertreated disease in the USA," was estimated in 1996 to be costing the country $53 billion a year.[11] Ulcer treatments constituted a multi-billion-dollar industry — much of it, it was later learned [*see VIII*], unnecessary.

Projections for AIDS — which necessarily overlapped with those for cancer — and of the rapidly advancing immune disorder CFS (chronic fatigue syndrome) were already multi-billion-dollar sectors of the total healthcare tab.

A 1996 Harvard University found[11a] that a staggering 31 percent of Americans were either uninsured or had difficulty in paying for medical bills — an incredible figure that could mean that more than 80 million citizens were without adequate coverage.

The medical free market isn't

All along, the American public has been fed the myth that the United States has a "private" system of medicine based on free-market principles — one of the major deceptions of the Twentieth Century.

The smokescreen obscuring just what the American medical system is has kept the philosophical arguments about it reduced to a kind of Left vs. Right rigged wrestling match — the Left insisting that the problems of giant medicine are monopoly practices and capitalism itself, things which can only be solved by socialism or the euphemisms therefor more sonorous to American "liberals"; the Right insisting that the real problem is giant government and the regulations, red tape and collectivistic competition-blocking which spring therefrom, key targets of "conservatives."

Yet what has arisen is not really either, and even columnist Robert Samuelson, writing in the *Washington Post,* was conceptually, if not semantically, on the mark, as he opined:

> *We have arrived at socialized medicine in America. I do not report this as either a good or bad event but simply as something that has happened with hardly anyone realizing it . . .*
>
> *Socialized medicine does not mean that government will run every hospital or employ every doctor. Even in countries with national health insurance, the medical complex often remains in private hands. It does mean that most of the critical decisions about health care will ultimately be settled politically.*[(12)]

Jarret B. Wollstein wrote in 1992 that

> *America does not have a free market in health care, and in fact has not had one for 50 years. What we have had is a half-century of mounting encroachment upon medical freedom, leading to more and more health care problems.*[(13)]

And Terree P. Wasley (in *What Has Government Done to Our Health Care?*) was equally perceptive:

> *. . . (a) look at the history of health insurance in the United States reveals not the competitive marketplace that most believe exists but an industry filled with anti-competitive efforts of medical societies and hospitals to suppress alternatives, guarantee their own income, and use government intervention to further their own objectives.*[(14)]

If by 1990 the two major government insurance programs for the elderly and/or the destitute (Medicare and Medicaid) accounted for 28 percent of the nation's total healthcare expenditures, and if, as intermittently has been the case for years, government plans of one kind or another have covered over half of hospital bills, then it is easy to reach the conclusion that even before the Clinton Administration's first-term sweeping and ill-conceived "health-care reform" plan that a kind of "socialized medicine" had, in however awkward a guise, appeared on the scene.

By 1994, it could be reported of medical research alone that

> *The federal government is the mainstay of the nation's giant biomedical research establishment and pumped more than $12 billion into health-related R & D in 1993. About $3 billion of this money is spent in government labs. But the vast majority of federal monies is doled out to universities and private, nonprofit laboratories.*[(15)]

Linda Marsa, who analyzed the above for *Omni* magazine, also quoted Sheldon Krimsky, chairman of the department of urban and environmental policy at Tufts University:

> *"The iron triangle of government, industry and academia constitutes a mutually reinforcing system of self-interest that brings to a close an important period of independence for basic research."*[(16)]

Included here, she noted, is the small amount of drugs produced annually which actually are intended to serve as therapeutic advances, as opposed to a majority of "me-too" or "workalike" or "lookalike" drugs which flood the market. Some 70 percent of the drugs expected to have "a substantial therapeutic gain" are produced with government involvement, Marsa noted.

Socialized medicine?

American fascist medicine

Yet there is a better term to define government intrusion into or regulation of private monopolies (in this case, among the drug industry, the hospital corporations, medical device manufacturers, private insurance giants, and the like). It is what this writer has long defined as *fascist medicine*, the most notorious version of which was announced as the rejected "national healthcare reform" plan launched by the White House in 1993.

Fascism is the better term to define government-regulated or government-controlled, or government-utilized monopolies in the "private sector" in which free markets are *not* free, prices are rigged and, ultimately, as in communism, goods and services can and will be politically rationed. True, fascist medicine lacks the other necessary component — a single dictator. But that personality might also arise.

It was funereally amusing in the 1990s — as it had been decades before — to hear the American Medical Association (AMA) bemoan the coming of socialized medicine, when the AMA has been the primary fomenter of the allopathic medical monopoly and the chief quencher of all competition to allopathy in the medical marketplace (*VII*). It has been equally amusing in the most negative of ways to listen to the pharmaceutical giants, astride the most inflation-proof of industries (*VIII*), defend the medical "free market," as if one existed.

These interests define the elements of what we call the Allopathic Industrial Complex (AIC) or "The Club" — the licensure-sanctioning-education-doctor-training-propaganda arm of the allopathic medical industry itself, as enshrined in the American Medical Association (AMA); the medical research/ treatment components within the federal governmental superstructure, as particularly exemplified by the National Institutes of Health (NIH) and all its subsidiaries, the Veterans Administration, and various overlapping agencies and departments; the powerful, if now somewhat waning, major health insurance companies, whose machinations and policies did so much for so long to obscure the true cost of medicine's uncontrolled inflationary rise; an interlock of research hospitals and research facilities in the public and private domains often sharing public and private monies but nonetheless subject to the parameters and concepts of the AIC and often addicted to the governmental (and private) grants mechanism which by its nature demands instant results and nourishes a "publish or perish" attitude which has often corrupted scientific/medical research and has led to hasty observations, revelations and pronouncements which later turned out to be wrong or fraudulent; a thriving medical devices and diagnostics industry virtually as inflation-proof as the drug business; the pharmaceutical — drug — business itself, perhaps the single largest and certainly most influential factor within the AIC, since it represents a global behemoth of several dozen major pharmaceutical manufacturing conglomerates which, as we shall see, are the more visible remnants or extensions of the greatest international consortium of overlapped industrial entities in human history; the recent dizzying increase in "managed care" doctor-patient-hospital arrangements (HMOs, PPOs) covering up to half the American population, and the would-be monitor or policeman of the whole apparatus, the federal Food and Drug Administration (FDA), a corrupted and compromised agency whose mere existence and (often) outright criminality reflect the truth in the axiom "that government governs best which governs least."

While the media are not themselves *direct* members of The Club, they are so influenced by it (and some of their boards of directors intertwined with it) and have been since the AMA discovered the mother lode of advertising riches at the turn of the century, that they have been "captured by the paradigm" (*IV*) and are the transmission belt through which the message of The Club is constantly beamed: the Marcus Welby Syndrome, or symbol of the avuncular, home-visiting, wise and moral medical mentor, versions of whom have appeared in many a television series, movie and other entertainment endeavor (productions almost always "advised" by the AMA).

The Club: not fudging on divinity

The sum total of The Club's propagandizing throughout the boom era of the Twentieth Century has been to re-clothe doctors with the presumptive magical or divine garb with which they were arrayed in ancient times (*IV*), not because the doctor is necessarily the primary culprit here (actually, he or she is *not* the chief negative factor) but because a total belief system needs a touch of the divine and a greater-than-human symbol around which to rally power and authority. The authorized, sanctioned physician as drug-peddler is as necessary to the international drug trust as television is to the automotive industry.

Generations of Americans have been spoonfed the various medical myths which establish the philosophical underpinnings of the AIC — somehow, the acts of birth and death are supposed to be AMA-approved, AMA-supervised allopathic activities to be carried out in AMA-approved, AMA-supervised allopathic healing (or dying) temples; all major decisions as to the health of the people are to be in the hands of skilled allopathic professionals trained in "medical science" and dispensing treatments, diagnostics and curative measures developed by "vigorous scientific discipline"; the laity is itself too ignorant or busy to be able to make major decisions on general health and healthcare — hence the need for the routine checkup, at the very least; while wholesale failure and disaster are sometimes perceptible through the enormous media and propaganda haze hurled aloft to obscure the truth, American medicine is the best on earth, American science which underpins it is the most competent, and if the answer to a total disaster (AIDS, for example) is not presently found it soon will be.

These are central truths necessary to, and nurturing of, the paradigm of the Allopathic Industrial Complex. Unlike the Middle Ages, when dissenters were burned at the stake, or in openly authoritarian societies of current or recent memory, where they are executed, dissidents of the American AIC are neither burned at the stake nor executed — they simply are ruined professionally and economically. Their works and theories are not likely to be published in the "accepted" (that is, AMA-lining) journals; their techniques and nostrums, even if allowed through some escape clause of local or federal law, will probably not be "covered" by medical insurance, public or private; medical dissenters face, socially at the very least, vilification, peer rejection, humiliation, and, administratively, possible loss of "hospital privileges," and, legally, possible civil and criminal penalties.

Of course, elements of this situation are beginning to change. We will explain which elements and why — and also why the AIC itself is beginning to crumble, much of the crumbling being helped along by some astonishingly courageous physicians and other AIC members blessed with morality and openness of mind in addition to their unquestioned valor.

Step one: birth as an AMA procedure

If there is a beginning point where the AIC paradigm meets its ultimate customer, the human client, it is at the act of birth itself.

Astoundingly, the myth has been spread far and wide that birth is indeed a medical operation and should be in the hands of "qualified experts" — not the farm mothers, lay midwives, *curanderas* and others who for virtually all of human history have "assisted" at a "delivery," often with far greater skill than medically trained personnel of the Twentieth Century.

American reliance on medicine begins with that very first element: the human as a product seemingly conceived almost as much by organized medicine as by the Divine or Mother Nature.

By the late 1980s, "c-sections" — cesarean operations — were accounting for as many as 25 percent of all the births in the United States though known to be four times as risky as non-surgical deliveries.(17) Stephen A. Myers MD, of Chicago's Mt. Sinai Hospital, was quoted by Inlander *et al.*, with what may be the *real* reason: "The bottom line, I think, is that a cesarean is often much easier for an obstetrician. They don't have to stay up all night waiting."(18)

(In 1994, the Public Citizen Health Research Group found that while the "c-section" rate was dropping — to about 22.6 percent of all births in 1992 — the technique still constituted the most common major surgery performed in the USA, some 420,000 instances of which were unnecessary. The unnecessary "c-sections" added $1.3 billion to the total healthcare tab.[19])

From that point on, the human consumer of medical services is grist for the allopathic mill — which, in childhood, may include the needless tonsillectomy and, perhaps later, the needless cataract surgery (of the latter, a 1985 study showed[20] that at least 23 percent of such operations might not be necessary, and many of which were often due to fraud, abuse, kickbacks and "other enticements.") Young women may be conned into a needless hysterectomy, which is itself an entire industry — one involving 560,000 women a year (1997 estimate) and adding $3 billlion annually to the health tab.[20a] Antibiotics, antihistamines, sedatives, the venerable aspirin tablet, will have entered the family medical cabinet in great numbers since early in life — and, yes, they may have saved lives and often will have relieved many a symptom.

But from childhood on, the patient/client is "prepped" for membership in the consumer division of the AIC, like it or not — from state-mandated immunizations, which themselves may be unproven and dangerous, to the use of recently FDA-approved toxic drugs which years later turn out to have been extremely dangerous. Every ailment, minor and major, will be dealt with in some way by the AIC, and at the end of it all the biggest economic "take" will usually be in the final year of life — the 12 months which turn out to be the most profitable for the AIC and the single biggest economic drag on the "healthcare delivery industry cost crisis."

In sickness and in wealth

In 1993, the AMA's own *Journal of the American Medical Assn. (JAMA)* reported[21] that life-prolonging treatments for, as an example, critically ill cancer patients cost a literal fortune and buy little extra survival time, and are by no means always desired either by the patient or his family. In a survey of 150 terminally ill patients, intensive-care hospital bills for such patients exclusive of post-surgical recovery ranged from $82,845 to $189,339 per year of life gained — but most patients who made it home lived less than three additional months and only 20 made it more than a year.

Six-figure and even seven-figure costs for intensive or long-term, protracted care for terminal disease are far more common than rare, as hundreds of thousands of families can attest.

Yet the high cost of keeping a patient alive (depending on the precise definition of "alive," which is often wanting) for days, weeks, months, while hooked up to any number of modern medical marvels, is excused as an adjunct to great breakthroughs in high technology — be it of diagnostics or treatments.

Indeed, it is the high-technology argument (if we're not doing well against cancer, AIDS, a host of heart diseases and stroke, MS, lupus, rheumatoid arthritis, Alzheimer's, Lou Gehrig's disease, Parkinson's, now — just wait, because the troops are on the way) which has still kept a great deal of popular sentiment on the side of organized medicine despite the increasingly prohibitive cost thereof.

Hence "high technology" has become one of the selling points of modern medical orthodoxy — it shows the creative human mind at its most physically and mechanically ingenious. And because there *has* been the payoff of the occasional rescue-from-death's-door, the seeming return to life from certain death due to a pump, infusion, shock or other technique, the downside of it all — the gruellingly expensive and even cruel prolongation of death, which economically means the last few months of a terminal patient's treatments usually cost more than all the foregoing years of therapy combined — may be overlooked.

High tech: high costs, high hopes — and questions

The wielding of high-technology mechanical marvels at the very least creates the illusion that the white-smocked technician knows what he is doing and that the unknowing patient is now securely in the hands of "the best medicine that money can buy."

In 1988, *Fortune* looked at some of America's major high-tech medical gadgetry and research technology leading off with the carotid endarterectomy, which reporter Edmund Faltermayer correctly described as "a kind of Roto-Rooter job on clogged neck arteries" and done on about 80,000 Americans annually as of that year.

He added:

> *Typically costing $9,000, counting the bill for a hospital stay, the operation is designed to prevent strokes. Another triumph of modern medicine? Or an overly risky, overdone alternative to cheaper drug therapy? Incredibly, no one knows for sure and no one is tracking the patients on a systematic basis to find out.*[22]

When the probing RAND Corporation looked into the "appropriateness" of the carotid endarterectomy, it found that only just over a third of such procedures had been truly "appropriate" and that 32 percent were "borderline."

That was only the tip of "appropriateness" studies that year. Several research groups found[23] the vaunted coronary bypass (averaging $37,000 per operation) to be "unjustified" 14 percent of the time and "debatable" 30 percent of the time; that Pacemaker implants at $9,000 per insertion were "unjustified" at least 20 percent of the time and "debatable" 36 percent of the time; that coronary angiography (X-rays of heart arteries injected with dye and averaging $3,400 per treatment) was 17 and 9 percent respectively; and that even the time-honored upper gastrointestinal tract endoscopy (upper GI scan — visual examination with a fiber-optic device, averaging $750 per scan) was 17 and 11 percent respectively.

Fortune quoted InterStudy's Dr. Paul M. Ellwood Jr. of Minneapolis: "Half of what the medical profession does is of unverified effectiveness."[24]

While we deal in greater detail elsewhere with the useless or misleading diagnostics rampant among the top killer diseases (cholesterol counts, mammograms and tumor "markers," for example) — the constellation of disorders called "heart disease" plus all expressions of cancer — there continue to be enough questionable uses of surgical procedures (recall hysterectomies) to keep filling court calendars.

In 1991, for example, a Dartmouth survey of trans-urethral resections of the prostate (TURPs — a form of surgery to remove the tissue of swollen prostates, a problem affecting the vast majority of middle-aged to elderly males in North America, northern and western Europe and other alleged enclaves of civilization) found[25] that 400,000 such operations were being performed annually at a cost of $3 billion, and trailed only cataracts in payouts by Medicare.

But this first sweeping survey of decades of TURPs showed that 20 percent of patients with moderate symptoms before surgery remained unimproved following it, that one out of five needed a second TURP within 10 years of the first, that 25 percent of patients had short-term complications of varying severity, that 4 percent underwent persistent incontinence, that 5 percent became impotent, and that TURP patients were more likely to die from heart attacks within five years of the surgery than were patients who had undergone complete removal of the prostate (prostatectomies), a procedure said to be riskier than the TURP.

Going wrongly by the numbers

To the side effects of high-tech medicine have been added, year by devastating year, the accumulation of laboratory errors in potentially life-saving tests, misread X-rays, misunderstood and complicated laboratory analyses, and outright sloppy lab work which, as a particularly notorious example, the American College of Obstetricians and Gynecologists reported in 1988, failed to catch between 15 and 40 percent of cervical cancers or precancerous conditions.[26]

This should not totally surprise:

In 1985, Jocelyn Hicks PhD, chairman of the laboratory medicine department of Children's Hospital National Medical Center, Washington, found in a survey of doctors' office laboratories in the capital area that 38 percent of the individuals performing the tests had had no formal lab training and that "most tests were being done by receptionists, nurses and physicians with zero lab training."[27]

A year earlier, a California survey of thousands of in-office labs had found[28] that 44 percent of employees in such "unregulated" labs had no formal training to perform lab analyses, that fewer than 30 percent of such in-office labs had adequate quality-control procedures and that 80 percent of the results reported by the "unregulated" labs were "significantly less accurate" than those from regulated laboratories.

None of which, of course, lessens the frequent problems of erroneous, misleading, confusing or conflictive results from *regulated* laboratories — computer printouts on which key life-and-death medical issues may depend and during the wait for which a patient with a fatal disease may be literally gnawing his fingernails off as he awaits "results."

Milking the sacred cows

In a January 1992 survey[29] by the San Jose (CA) *Mercury News,* based both on RAND research and preliminary statistics from the then two-year-old Congressionally-mandated Agency for Health Care Policy and Research, a combination Administration/congressional effort at looking at the costs and outcomes of American medicine, it was found that reducing millions of dollars in unnecessary tests could shave $50 billion a year off the nation's healthcare bill.

The combined research zeroed in on some of the most sacred of medical high technology's sacred cows:

• Magnetic resonance imaging (MRI) — Costing about $560 per scan, this technique was found not to be particularly useful for common examinations of the spleen, pancreas and liver cancer, but widely used for those purposes anyway. (By later in the decade MRIs could cost at least three times more.)

• Computerized axial tomography (CAT) scan: Normally fetching at least $360 per scan, as opposed to $36 for X-rays, CATs were determined to be no better than standard chest X-rays for detecting certain tumors, "but most radiologists use them because they've gotten used to doing so."[30]

• Fetal heartbeat monitor: While normally costing $175, "the device is no more effective than a nurse with a stethoscope and a wristwatch."[31]

By 1992, a major study[32] upped the bad news on coronary angiograms — by then performed about a million times a year at an increased average cost of $5,000 each — to a statistic instantly attacked (but not disproved) by the National Heart, Lung and Blood Institute: virtually half of all such procedures were found to be unnecessary and/or easily postponable until later. (*See X*)

The need for a gimmick

While many procedures — diagnostic and therapeutic — are indeed life-saving, life-extending advances, there is, at the very least, a subconscious drive on the part of medicine to utilize more and more of them.

In a sweeping critique of his own profession, iconoclast Thomas Preston MD noted in 1981:

> *There is not a physician in private practice who does not recognize the need to have a "gimmick" by which he can increase his income almost at will. Endoscopy, bronchoscopy, electro-cardiograms, all laboratory tests, needle biopsies, dialysis, X-rays, catheterizations, scans and even skin tests provide means to amplify income . . .*
>
> *Although physicians may not make conscious decisions based on income, in practice the financial incentives are always in the direction of performing the procedure. These influences may be subtle . . . but they are real and important.*
>
> *Medical tests are expensive and profitable. It is common practice for pathologists to enter into contracts with hospitals under which they receive a percentage of the fees from all laboratory tests. Some*

pathologists make well over $250,000 a year from this source alone . . .[33]

Critical observers of American medicine have long noted that the US medical fee structure, intimately enmeshed with insurance practices, has helped make various procedures far more rewarding to doctors than those which *do not* involve the use of a tube, knife or needle.

As Thomas B. Almy observed in 1981,[34] even under Medicare general practitioners could see threefold increases in income by ordering up various laboratory procedures to be done in the office, and surgeons could receive three to seven times more money per hour spent in the operating room than for each hour of in-office or bedside consultation.

Hence the growth in the medical monolith of the equipment/device business — one which, as *Business Week* assessed in 1992,[35] was a $23 billion-per-year industry growing by 25 percent a year, virtually as inflation-proof as the pharmaceutical industry.

The latter (which we examine more closely in *VIII*), is, of course, a key, chronic, huge component in the "healthcare delivery industry cost crisis," since the cost of medications alone could (and often does) bankrupt patients, and became a significant factor in the mid-1990s moves for "cost containment."

As late as 1993, Philip R. Lee MD, Assistant Secretary for Health (Department of Health and Human Services), told the Senate Select Committee on Aging that "some new drugs have recently reached the market at a cost of $50,000 to $300,000 per patient per year."[36]

'We don't know what we're doing'

The government's Agency for Health Care Policy and Research had begun in 1990 with a $500 million federal grant earmarked to help doctors find out what really "works" or does not "work" in medicine and the launching of a five-year survey to assess medical practices since, at the time (1989 figures), it was estimated that 20 percent of the healthcare bill ($125 billion, a figure then considered big enough to wipe out the federal deficit) was being wasted on unnecessary, inappropriate or dangerous treatments because of a lack of knowledge and consensus as to what is truly efficacious.

Dr. David Eddy, director of Duke University's Center for Health Care Policy and Research, had made the astoundingly honest asseveration that "we don't know what we're doing in medicine."[(37)]

The new survey was set up on the heels of some sobering assessments of the status of American medicine, including these:

• "Perhaps one-quarter to one-third of medical services may be of little or no benefit to patients" — National Institute of Medicine.

• "The link between the process of care and patient outcomes has been established for relatively few procedures." — Office of Technology Assessment (OTA), the US Congress.

• "Uncertainty about the most effective diagnostic and therapeutic approaches is pervasive." — Dr. Dennis S. O'Leary, president, Joint Commission on Accreditation of Health Care Organizations.

• "The embarrassment of our ignorance about the efficacy of health care practices is both hard for us to admit and hard for our clients to accept. It is difficult to face the disillusionment of the patients and the anger of the payers who ask, 'But how could this be? I thought you knew what you were doing.'" — Dr. Donald Berwick, Harvard Community Health Plan.

A considerable amount of evidence that US medicine has been engaging in guesswork stemmed from two decades of research by Dr. John Wennberg, professor of community and family medicine at Dartmouth Medical School.

He and his colleagues for years tracked what the press called "inexplicable treatment patterns between different cities, hospitals and even different doctors without any appreciable differences in outcome for the patient."[(38)]

For example, he found that in one Maine city 70 percent of

women had undergone hysterectomies by age 75 — but in a city only 20 miles away only 25 percent had had them.

Other variations included these:

• In Rutland VT, seven times as many children had their tonsils removed as in Hanover NH, some 50 miles away.

• In one city in Iowa 60 percent of men had had prostate surgery, as compared to 15 percent in another Iowa city.

• In two teaching hospitals associated with the Harvard Medical School and separated by a few city blocks, percentages of births by cesarean section were 19 in one, 30 in another.

• "No difference in mortality" was found between Boston, with 55 percent more hospital beds and an outlay of 70 percent more dollars on healthcare per capita, and nearby New Haven CT.

Assessed Wennberg: "For most common illness and medical conditions, the necessary assessments to establish correct therapy have not been done."[(39)]

The diagnostic-referral scheme

That high technology diagnostics and testing, let alone treatments, might not be all they are cracked up to be is one thing — that they are money machines for doctors or doctor groups is quite another, and constitute yet another considerable chunk of the trillion-dollar "healthcare delivery" bill.

In a study eagerly awaited by health officials across the country, a Florida state agency in 1991 reported[(40)] that doctors' ownership of laboratories, physical therapy clinics and high-tech diagnostic centers had tended to increase the use and cost of such services without improving access to care for poor or rural people.

The Florida Health Care Cost Containment Board survey found that more than 45 percent of doctors practicing in Florida (some 8,500 of a total of 18,250) had invested in joint diagnostic/testing ventures to which they referred patients — with "imaging centers" utilizing MRI, CAT-scans and X-rays leading the field.

Wrote columnists Jack Anderson and Dale Van Atta: the

report exposed "the sleazy profits doctors collect by investing in medical labs where they send their patients for over-priced and needless procedures . . . It shows that residents of the Sunshine State are being bilked through doctors' self-referrals. The only other explanation for the data is that people in Florida have more complicated ailments than the rest of us."

They added:

> *The most attractive investment tool of the 1990s for Florida doctors is the magnetic resonance imaging (MRI) machine. They are as numerous as street-corner vendors in Florida. (Jean) Mitchell and (Elton) Scott found that nearly all the centers in Florida with MRI machines are owned by doctors who refer their patients there. Nearly all exams conducted at those facilities are done on people with insurance.*
>
> *We have to believe either that people with insurance need more complex diagnostic procedures or that poor patients are not being run through the same hoops because they can't pay for it.*
>
> *The number of billings made to patients covered by insurance contradicts the claims of groups such as the American Medical Association and the Florida Medical Association that doctor-owned labs and clinics promote better care for the poor. The three labs in Florida not owned by doctors do far less business than the doctor-owned MRI labs.*[41]

A year later, it was California's turn to fall under the vested-interests glare:

Nearly nine of 10 "free-standing" (that is, not connected with hospitals or mobile vans) high-tech radiological centers in California were found in 1992[42] to be owned by physicians who referred patients to them, according to the same Florida State University economists who had exposed the Florida scandal.

Such ownership was not routinely disclosed to patients and contributed to health costs and unnecessary uses of services, particularly MRIs and CAT-scans, said the researchers.

By then, Jean Mitchell's research on MRI use nationwide had found that a number of physicians were making as much as $200,000 a year simply through referrals to self-owned facilities. And a Center for Health Policy Studies survey found that questionable MRIs performed at joint ventures nationwide added $728 million in additional costs for one year alone.

These were two of the more notorious studies of "self-referral" which came to light in the 1990s. But self-referral — between doctors and doctor groups — for treatment purposes is as pervasive as the problem of self-referral to diagnostic centers.

Reader's Digest reported in 1993 that

> *One man needed treatment for a rare condition that produced toxic levels of iron in his body. His doctor referred him to a joint-venture company. After 18 months, the man's bill reached $86,970 — the limit of his insurance coverage. If he'd gone to a different provider for the identical treatment, the cost would have totalled $27,534, more than two-thirds less.*[43]

Reporter John Pekkanen, a persistent chronicler of physician mischief, also reported how a California physician had been told "right to my face" that should the doctor open up a home-care operation "that for an investment of $5,000 I could count on an annual return of $100,000 — if I referred 20 patients a year to the business."[44]

Pekkanen also reported that a 1991 study in New York City had found that self-referred facilities marked up "home-infusion" drugs and other supplies for domestic home-care use as much as eight times higher than retail pharmacies did.

Insurance: a good idea gone wrong

The misuse and abuse of self-referral joint ventures specializing in high-priced needless tests points directly to one of the more festering sores in the medical miasma:

The third-party insurance scheme (and often scam), whose

presence in the healthcare delivery crisis has been a prime contributor to the astronomical costs of American medicine.

While originally conceived, like so many things, as both a good idea and a convenience (see *VI*), the technique whereby hundreds, then thousands, then millions of people organized as groups, companies, unions, professions or simply as individuals would pool their premiums into group payment plans in advance of actual need over time ran from providing a distinct and genuine service to being a scheme which helped hide the out-of-control costs of medical practice.

By the 1990s, the insurance claims/reporting/billing process was a red tape-generating patchwork nightmare of ever-changing forms, approaches, ideas, state, federal and local guidelines, and, ever so frequently, ever-changing whims of claims processors.

"Acceptance for coverage" of a device, technique, drug, compound, modality or novel medical approach — usually anything not specifically banned by the FDA or by a state law — simply meant the high road to its use. Companies, and groups of companies, could establish "acceptable guidelines" for the costs of everything from a syringe to 10 days of intensive care for brain cancer. As long as physicians, hospitals, administrators and professional billers knew which "codes" to use and what the accepted guidelines were, enormous hospital bills could be designed, passed, certified — and paid off by the "third-party" payers.

This is a proximate reason for the disclosures in the 1980s and 1990s of fifty-dollar aspirins, outrageously expensive doctor visits (these could be put on the bill even if the visiting MD simply walked into the room and said "hello" and, frequently, whether he was even there), and the advent of the thousand-dollar-per day hospital bed (as in California, Florida and New York) irrespective of any treatment connected with the occupant of the bed. The presence of various "caregivers," ranging from night nurse to vocational nurse to anesthesiologist to attending physician, would of course raise the cost of what went on in the bed by an equal or greater amount.

The technique whereby collective or group plans shielded the true costs of medicine prospered in the post-World War II era and through the 1950s and 1960s but began to fall under increasing review in the 1970s. The defense of the system also ran this way: expensive overuse of medicine here is compensated by the lack of it (thanks to healthy people) there; the occasional fraudulent billing here resulting in a huge outlay is compensated for by the underpayment there — somehow it all works out. This line of reasoning was equally rampant in both private *and* public plans.

The US Congress' watchdog General Accounting Office (GAO) reported in May 1992[(45)] — and the FBI confirmed in 1995[(46)] — that health fraud — primarily in the form of insurance billing scams and medical kickback schemes — was such a massive subindustry in "healthcare delivery" that it would reach $100 billion by 1995. This led to efforts at legislation and more belt-tightening within the insurance industry itself and of course helped set the tone for the Clinton Administration's major, if awkward, jab at healthcare reform in 1993/94.

Data reported to the late Rep. Ted Weiss' House Governmental Operations Subcommittee was fashioned around a California scandal (aside from the doctor-owned joint-venture imagery business) in which mobile laboratories providing heart and blood pressure measurements attracted insured patients, waived co-payments and offered doctors kickbacks for referrals. Many of the unnecessary tests were billed, often with phony diagnoses, to insurance companies. This single scheme resulted in $1 billion in fraudulent billings, involved about 20 doctors and led to 12 indictments, the GAO reported.

Investigators said the labs, over a 10-year span, operated under 600 different names and tax identification numbers. After being probed by (and indicted following) a Health and Human Services (HHS) inspector general's investigation, the group had stopped treating Medicare patients and concentrated exclusively on the privately insured.

The GAO said the health insurance system is vulnerable to fraud for a variety of reasons, including as the more prominent:

• Thousands of insurers process some 4 billion claims a year. Hundreds of thousands of medical providers use a wide variety of payment methods and administrative rules.

• The vast numbers of insurers make billing patterns hard to identify. Thus a doctor who bills for more than 24 hours' worth of visits on a single day might not be discovered when claims are split among so many insurers.

• Cooperation among insurers to detect improper billing is made difficult by privacy concerns and incompatible data systems.

• Health providers increasingly own medical facilities and thus supply both the demand for and supply of services, creating potential conflicts of interest.

High on the hog

For many of these reasons, the private healthcare insurance industry was variously reported in the 1990s either to be on the ropes — particularly true for many small companies among the nation's estimated 1,500 insurers and as "managed-care" coverage plans spread exponentially — or to be living high on the hog while the industry itself was poised to go down the tubes.

In January 1993, the American Medical Association weekly *American Medical News* reported that the goal of health insurers had become, "unlike that of other health care interest groups, simply to survive. At stake are their estimated 460,000 jobs, $280 billion in annual premiums and a vital foot-in-the-door product for selling lucrative policies like life insurance."[(47)]

But before too many tears could be shed, July 1993 testimony before the US Senate's Permanent Subcommittee on Investigations called attention to shenanigans within New York Empire Blue Cross and Blue Shield, the combination major private health insurance provider in that state.[(48)]

As the Manhattan district attorney launched an investigation into claims of falsified records and perjury, even as the "Blues" racked up $255 million in losses in 1990, the Senate probers were told that the Blues' ousted chairman made $600,000 a year, rode in a chauffeur-driven Lincoln Town Car, that the insurance combine provided helicopter trips and accounts at Cartier and Tiffany's for various directors and employees, that it had a fleet of 123 cars, some $130,000 in art objects and what *Time* called "$62,832 in tacky silk plants, the $48,000 in computer and security systems in [the chairman's] home . . . and a $20,000 Chippendale desk, which was placed in storage and never used."[(49)]

Reported the magazine: these items were being paid for by "the nation's largest nonprofit health insurer at a time when it was trying to stave off insolvency by drastically raising the premiums of the elderly, the poor and the chronically sick."

It added that "some $70 billion flows annually through the US system of 70 not-for-profit Blue Cross and Blue Shield companies, which control more than 30 percent of the private health-insurance market." In other bad news for the "Blues":

• In 1989 New Hampshire regulators intervened when the state's BC/BS exhausted its cash reserves.

• In 1990 West Virginia Blue Cross ran out of money, leaving 51,000 individuals with unpaid claims. Investigators found that "among other unethical business practices, executives had funneled Blue Cross money to businesses in which they had a financial interest."

• Maryland's Blue Cross plan suffered a drop in net worth from $122 million in 1985 to $25 million by the end of 1992. "The recently departed boss . . . was given $775,000, twice the average for the Blues. In return the plan's policyholders received abysmal service marred by delays and lost claims."

• Between 1985 and 1992 Blue Cross of Washington DC had losses of $182 million while its director "spawned 40 subsidiaries, from a global travel and lost-luggage service to a Blue Cross of Jamaica . . . He enjoyed frequent Concorde flights to Europe and $900-a-night suites in Barbados."[(50)]

In 1994, a television exposé made things even tougher on

"the Blues," noting indictments of various officials in New York and Maryland, toting up the costs of executives' travel by limousine and Concorde jets, and maintenance of executive-suite "skyboxes" at baseball stadiums and "executive conferences" at opulent spas.

It referred to a General Accounting Office (GAO) survey which found 11 percent of the "Blues'" health insurance plans to be "weak" — and reported how the system allegedly policed itself with one of its own divisions, whose top executive made more than $700,000 a year. It also quoted a senator calling the giant health insurors "too big to discipline" yet designed in such a way as to take advantage of tax breaks.[(51)]

Such hijinks make it all the more infuriating to Americans who find it difficult to have "alternative" therapies — usually far less expensive than "standard" or "orthodox" approaches — covered by their private medical plans, written by companies which insist they are interested in keeping down the high costs of medicine and working in the best interests of their patients.

With his two decades of observation and experience with American patients who fled to Mexico to seek "alternative" therapies they hoped could at least extend their lives if not cure them, this author is fully aware of the absolute venality of so many private insurance companies and of their suspicious ties to the allopathic paradigm and the drug business:

By the mid-1990s south-of-the-border clinics — often charging as little as 10 percent on the dollar (or less) even for much advanced conditions as "terminal" cancer — had literally saved American private insurance companies, when they agreed to pay for treatments not approved by the American FDA, *millions* of dollars. Yet many patients, even those obviously benefiting by "alternative" therapy while spending far less on it, found it difficult if not impossible to secure reimbursement for such treatments.

The scenario was indeed riveting: a private plan would swiftly cover an outlay of hundreds of thousands of dollars for cancer therapy based on radiation, the cobalt machine, surgery and toxic drugs, all of which stood a fair chance injuring the patient, but balked at covering the expense of intravenous nutrition, oral supplements and detoxification.

When it became so obvious that nutritionally-based therapies were both effective *and*, in the main, far less expensive than standard or orthodox modalities, the question put by so many enraged premium payers to their high profit-oriented insurance carriers — "why won't you cover this while you'll pay for that?" — usually went suspiciously, and damningly, unanswered.

All of which further made it difficult for long-time observers of the health insurance industry to squeeze out any tears for such companies as they too complained about the high cost of medicine and the nation began a headlong plunge into new "managed care" structures, which covered three-quarters of American workers by 1997,[51a] a major motive for which was the medical industry's defensive response to the failed Clinton Administration's "healthcare reform" try.

To their credit, by late in the decade, some health-maintenance (HMO) and preferred-provider (PPO) organizations were beginning to ponder — and some to implement — coverage of "alternative" therapies, for the most basic of reasons: they simply cost less, often far less, than standard or orthodox therapies. This economically-inspired attention to the bottom line has been among the most salutary elements of the sweeping revolution going on in medical insurance/payments (see *Introduction*) even though it has fueled debates over standard of care vs. financial considerations and has embroiled the AIC in intense soul-searching.

Enter the 'Great Society'

Yet it would be the most arrant of oversights to pin fraud, abuse and mismanagement solely on the private health insurance industry — when it has been the government, or public, sector, which has been by far the bigger component in the cost portion of the healthcare delivery crisis.

The Medicare and Medicaid government insurance programs (*see also VI*) were launched in the Sixties as part of President Lyndon Johnson's "Great Society" with — as usual — the best of motives: guaranteed healthcare for the aged, infirm and economically destitute, a veritable socialist's dream come true.

Unfortunately, the premises on which all such schemes begin — cost controls and orderly demand — began to collapse shortly after the plans started.

With projections of both costs and demand vastly underrated by the government, the cost of the two medical-charity schemes ballooned from $5 billion in 1967 to over $160 billion in 1990.[(52)]

As of 1997, the projected cost of Medicare was $207.7 billion and that of Medicaid $105.8 billion, an aggregate almost doubling the 1990 figures.[(52a)]

As Steven Hayward and Erik Peterson reported in 1993, the original projections of the level of demand for supposedly "free" (that is, taxpayer-paid) Medicare services had originally been for 10-percent increases in hospital admission rates among the elderly "but in fact hospital-admission rates among the Medicare-eligible rose immediately by 25 percent, the rate for surgical procedures by 40 percent, and the number of hospital days by 50 percent."[(53)]

Originally, the House Ways and Means Committee had estimated that the Medicare program would cost about $12 billion by 1990 (or about 10 percent of its true 1990 cost of $107 billion).

Like most government projections, virtually everything originally stated about Medicare has turned out to be wrong:

It did not cost $155 for a day's stay in the hospital in 1985, as originally projected by the planners — but in fact it was over $600 per day. The hospital-insurance part of the program by 1990 was not the $9 billion originally projected — but indeed $63 billion.

As for Medicaid, the Heritage Foundation predicted[(54)] that "if current trends continue, state Medicaid expenses will have increased more than 480 percent by the year 2000" — and in most states, as of 1997, Medicaid was the single biggest expense after education, even when the federal government on the average was paying for 60 percent of Medicaid bills.

In his broadside attack on government in medicine, former AMA President Edward R. Annis MD described the development of the Medicare gravy train:

> *(Once goverment was able to get) all the millionaires, the middle class and paupers over sixty-five riding in the cart together, it began writing rules and regulations governing all doctors and hospitals that treated Medicare patients, meaning virtually all doctors and hospitals. The cost of this administrative burden today — paid for by the people still pulling the cart (the working people) — is greater than all the doctors' fees combined. To cure the rising costs, government added "cost controls," which in turn caused prices to rise even faster.*[55]

In the early 1990s, as the private medical sector felt the heat from protests and efforts at reform, private medical spending, while still high, was actually on the decline.

But, reported the federal government in 1993,[56] Medicaid spending had zoomed by 30.6 percent in 1991 and Medicare by 12.6 percent. Medicare's financial situation was described as so parlous that the Medicare Hospital Insurance Trust Fund was expected to "run dry" sometime between 1998 and the end of the century.

Marcel J. Sislowitz MD, a Manhattan surgeon, put it all together in 1988:

> *When Medicare was first introduced, there was a hue and cry from the medical profession about "socialized medicine." However, when it was quickly discovered that the system paid rather well (much better, in fact, than many patients ever could), especially for surgical procedures, most of the objections abated rather quickly.*
>
> *Certain practitioners, mostly surgeons, who astutely vetted the system early on, turned it into a virtual money machine. They quickly came to appreciate that when a*

third party (the government) pays the bill, the first two parties need not be concerned about costs.[57]

One way of working the system, noted Hayward and Peterson in 1993:

> . . . *If the average gall-bladder surgery costs $10,000 and requires four days of hospitalization, that is what the government will pay the hospital for a Medicare patient, regardless of how long that particular patient may need to stay.*[58]

This is a government version of abuse in private insurance practice: the computerized guideline says that a bunion may be treated for this amount of money for this amount of time, so that is what the claim will state.

Bilking Medicare and Medicaid: big business

That providers who "work the government system" are carbon copies of those who "work the private system"was brought home in 1996 when a Georgia-based "home health care" company agreed to pay $225 million in fines and reimbursements for Medicare fraud while its two major executives began serving prison terms.

Fraud included "inflated and fraudulent bills" and such items as personal expenses for senior managers and lobbying expenses.[59]

The same year, Laboratory Corp. of America agreed to pay $182 million to settle federal charges that it submitted false claims to federal and state health programs for medically unnecessary tests.[59a]

In 1997, the US government's "Operation Labscam" caught SmithKline Beecham Clinical Laboratories in alleged billing frauds involving Medicare and other agencies. The company agreed to pay $325 million to resolve the charges.[59b]

Indeed, the General Accounting Office (GAO) told a Senate subcommittee in 1996 that Medicare fraud was reaching $17 billion a year or 10 percent of the Medicare budget.[60] And Sen.

William Cohen of Maine reported that combined Medicare-Medicaid fraud had reached $44 billion a year.[61]

In 1994, a group called the Medicare Beneficiaries Defense Fund in New York reported[62] that "a small but growing number of doctors" were asking their Medicare patients to sign papers requiring them to pay large sums of money they did not owe—and that such activities meant that "tens of thousands" of Medicare recipients were paying millions of dollars they need not have been paying. The Fund revealed how certain physicians were either pressuring Medicare patients to negotiate private contracts that required individuals to pay for unnecessary services not covered by Medicare or, as waivers, to exempt certain doctors from federally imposed legal billing limits.

But Medicaid has been equally targeted.

In 1995, a national settlement agreement of $161 million was reached for what was called "the nation's largest-ever Medicaid fraud investigation." It involved a home healthcare products company which was doing business in all 50 states and pleaded guilty to charges of defrauding federal healthcare programs by overbilling for certain treatments and supplies and making improper payments to induce providers to refer patients.[63]

To say nothing of bungling-through-bureaucracy, leading to overcharging, and a further negative impact on "healthcare delivery":

— In 1991, the Health Care Financing Administration (HCFA), itself a tax-sapping bureaucracy established in no small degree to monitor the other health-related bureaucracies, acknowledged[64] that the nation's elderly were being overcharged at least $1.7 billion a year in Medicare-related payments. HCFA chief Gail Wilensky pointed out that the agency could not afford to inform all possible Medicare recipients who might be paying extra costs and who were not aware of 1988 exemptions and "caps." This struck some observers as interesting since at tax time the IRS seemed to have no particular problem in informing the entire citizenry that it was time to pay up.

A Senate panel in spring 1994 heard of a litany of complaints against the two major government-subsidized healthcare systems at a level sufficient enough to give even the most starry-eyed advocates of socialized medicine pause:

— Suppliers were charging some elderly Medicare recipients in nursing-care homes as much as $10,000 a month for bandages for bedsores and other wounds, with two particularly notorious cases resulting in $43,000 and $44,000 in charges over a few months' time.

— Health and Human Services (HHS) Inspector June Gibbs Brown showed the legislators a "deluxe" wound-care kit being peddled to Medicare recipients for $45 each when it was a plastic container with sterile gloves, a small roll of tape, gauze, scissors, a pad and a sterile sheet that "you could get for two dollars in a drugstore."

— Maryland Assistant Attorney General Carolyn J. McElroy showed how a supposedly non-profit day-care program and summer camp for disturbed youths churned out fraudulent Medicaid billings for $1,000 a day, including $40-per-day "psychotherapy" visits for youths attending Girl Scout meetings, sewing circles and a St. Patrick's Day party.

— In another Medicaid abuse, a Maryland taxi company was actually billing the government for taking drug addicts to a clinic to secure methadone and providing kickbacks to customers. One woman used the cab service to get to "an open-air drug market to buy her illegal drugs."[(65)]

Also, in 1994 — the information was not forthcoming until 1996 when a Freedom of Information Act request gleaned the data — it was found that a random audit of 21 hospitals had found $50 million in expenditures "improperly charged" to Medicare. They ranged from trips to Europe for a hospital employee to inspect sculpture ($2,433), $5,302 in plane and train flights for executives' wives, memberships in exclusive clubs (including $53,977 in parking fees and $500 in "consulting services for a cooking contest"), $4,653 for meals at swanky restaurants by one hospital's executives, part of a $70,000 yearly housing allowance and $10,082 in insurance premiums for a fine arts collection and his predecessor's car for a university president, to $10,215 in clocks, watches and bowls provided as gifts to a medical college's "employees and friends" and expenses of a "dinner with open bar for 175 doctors" from a medical center.

A General Accounting Office (GAO) official noted that although the audit covered cases in 1994 "I'm sure it's still going on."[66]

In 1996, it was learned that the US Justice Department had entered into "gentlemen's agreements" — essentially meaning keeping the public oblivious — with many of some 4,600 hospitals found during a two-year investigation to have double-billed or over-charged Medicare and for which $120 million in penalties was expected to be collected.

Knight-Ridder News Service quoted the president of the People's Medical Society concerning the apparent effort by the federal side to conduct "quiet" investigations of the Medicare ripoff:

> *"This is typical of how the federal government and Congress . . . have fallen over backwards to protect the identity of doctors and hospitals and the bad things they do with the public money, including fraud and malpractice."*[67]

Piercing the veil

The "third-party insurance" scheme is thus wasteful and inflationary whether it be public or private, for the true costs of medicine have been, until recently, artfully hidden through collective policies paid either by the private sector (as monthly or periodic payments) or the public one (through increased taxes.) The nature of the beast — gouging based on collectivist premiums and payments — is to *encourage* medical overuse, as occurs in virtually any country with "socialized medicine," and to charge the maximum amount for the maximum number of goods and services.

Hence, whether public or private, the system is open to waste, abuse and fraud — as is *any* massively collectivistic endeavor whose *true* costs are obscured by the veil of widely-dispersed funding.

But by the 1980s the real costs of medicine could no longer be hidden — particularly in the "private sector." Individual health-insurance policy holders found their premiums rising dizzyingly every year and sometimes every month. If they were neither old enough nor poor enough to qualify for either federal or state "assistance" they were left with a Hobson's choice: face virtual bankruptcy by pre-paying for services which might never be necessary (the essence of the insurance industry itself) or do without. Many opted to do the latter, gambling that they and their families would "make it" long enough at least for the parents to reach their "senior years," where some kind of mandated coverage would result, without a major medical calamity occurring during the interval.

Hence the various estimates in the 1990s leading to an assumption that between 37 and 41 million Americans (and, by 1997, possibly double this — see earlier) had no health insurance, public or private, at all — a figure used to "excuse" the idea of a national health insurance plan. Yet, as at least one analyst put it,[(68)] perhaps as many as 90 percent of the uninsureds were not currently "in need of a doctor's care" (usually, the young and moderately well-employed), and/or many simply did not want to pay for insurance anyway.

And medical costs also spurred the rapid growth in "managed care" doctor-hospital arrangements. This in turn set off new elements in the national medical debate — whether business practices should take precedence over the "best" medicine, whether cost controls and the muzzling of doctors always benefited the patient, whether the true future of American medicine would evolve into a series of interlocking HMOs and PPOs loosely guided by the government.

It also created a new business elite — wealthy (and sometimes multi-millionaire) executive officers of the leading HMOs with salaries which made the takehome pay of top surgeons look pale by comparison.[68a,68b] Part of this is because "administrative costs" for "for-profit" hospitals (diverting money from patient care to "overhead") has galloped far ahead of such costs for "non-profits" since 1990.[68c]

A VA chamber of horrors

While Medicare and Medicaid reflect socialist components of the existing medical melange called the nation's "healthcare delivery system," it should be recalled that the longest-running, and by some definitions, worst, of these socialist components is the network of "free" (taxpayer-paid) hospitals for military veterans run by the Department of Veterans Affairs (DVA) and military services.

It is sometimes easy to forget that the DVA or VA system of 172 hospitals, 233 out-patient clinics and 122 nursing homes has been a far older government scheme than Medicaid and Medicare, which after all are insurance systems usually conducted in private hospitals, clinics and at home.

Proponents of nationalized (socialized) medicine need only read the ever-lengthening list of complaints of deteriorating facilities, long waiting lines, antiquated equipment, and frequently incompetent personnel which frequently have infested the DVA system and have been subjected to considerable journalistic and even entertainment-industry oversight to question this approach.

As of the mid-1990s, the entire DVA system had an annual budget exceeding $30 billion.

As an information officer for a south-of-the-border private hospital, it frequently fell to me to explain to veterans languishing in VA and military hospitals *why* they could not be accepted at our foreign facility, since it required at least partial payment on admission and was not "covered" by any governmental health insurance.

It was heart-breaking to hear the laments of these ill, wounded or disabled veterans making do in a VA or military hospital, often needing the very things (EDTA chelation therapy, megadose nutritional treatments, dietary control, etc.) that American orthodoxy and, very especially, federally run medicine, denied them. It was even more disturbing to me to have to explain just how and why these individuals, many of whom had risked their lives for their country, could not be treated in a foreign hospital unless they had funds for travel and up-front payments, and how, in their hour of need, their country had let them down.

On Jan. 15, 1992, CBS News captured part of the scenario. As *The New American* reported it:

> *Walter Reed Army/Navy Medical Hospital was refusing to provide some amputees returning from the Gulf War with artificial limbs, while others were being given shoddy prosthetics fabricated with antiquated technology. Further, the hospital was refusing to accept donations of modern limbs for the veterans. When asked why, a Medical Services colonel arrogantly asserted:*
>
> *"We disapprove [of] it because we are primary health care providers and we believe that we provide the best total care to the patient. And the patients belong to us."*[69]

No tyrant could have said it better.

A deluge of paper

It is difficult to calculate just how great the intrusion of the government, through Medicare, Medicaid and state programs, has added to the enormity of the paperwork avalanche which now buries hospital administration, but it is considerable.

Added to the mountain of red tape generated by private insurance and local administration, and involving additional compliance with other agencies and departments, the combined federal-state-local mountain of forms, printouts, etc., meant, as the *New England Journal of Medicine* reported in 1993,[70] that hospital administrative costs were eating up 25 cents of every dollar spent at hospitals.

Even though the number of US hospital patients has decreased as smaller hospitals and clinics have gone out of business, the administrative overhead has zoomed — as the *NEJM* reported, in 1968 US hospitals employed 435,000 managers and clerks and had 1.3 million patients, while in 1990 there was a virtual reversal: there were 1.2 million managers and clerks for 853,000 patients.

Before Medicare, doctors spent an estimated fifth of their time caring for the indigent and destitute, but by 1990s they spent a fifth of their time on mandatory/regulatory paperwork (forms, waivers, reports) averaging 10 pages per patient or, according to an AMA study in 1989, doctors' staffs were spending 46.7 hours per month processing Medicare claims.[(71)]

The International Society for Individual Liberty, noting that the United States has "one of the most regulated medical markets in the world," reported[(72)] that "over 800 federal and state laws (some hundreds of pages long) govern all health care providers and institutions" and that by some estimates two hours are spent filling out government paperwork for every hour spent on providing health services.

The paperwork avalanche, complexed by the high technology of computerization, is a prime target not only for planned abuse but for simple error:

One exposé of the healthcare cost mess in 1994 showed how the "error rate" of hospital billing was typically 5 to 7 percent per bill and that in some assessments *no* hospital bills were found free of error. The estimated cost to "healthcare delivery" through erroneous bills: $28 *billion* a year.[(73)]

The pay's good, too

While the AMA and physicians themselves may rightfully blame a huge amount of the obscene cost of American medicine on the government, and while the government may blame it on drug companies and medical device manufacturers (and the latter return the blame to the government), and while it is also true that many elements of the "healthcare delivery team" are either underpaid or simply adequately paid, the reality is that doctors as a group enjoy more wealth and financial security than many other professionals — save, for example, executives of major drug companies.

Science reported as early as 1978[74] that while in 1939 physicians' earnings were less than twice as high as those of many technological and professional people, by 1975 their earnings had quadrupled and their incomes had continued to (and essentially still do) outpace inflation.

While we note elsewhere (*VII*) the basic salary ranges of physicians, the seven-figure surgeon (orthopedic, neurological, oncological) — apex of the "healthcare delivery team" — is not a rarity. There is now a plethora of medical specialists, each particularly trained in a subdivision of medicine, to whom we are asked to turn over our bodies. Each one will do, or intends to do, that for which he or she has been specifically trained — an impulse Victor Fuchs correctly described as "the technological imperative."[75]

The trip to the doctor's office for a vague complaint means not leaving there, at the very least, without a prescription (usually written in a third-grade scrawl and/or in medical Latin) to be taken to the pharmacist (support system for the AIC — the channel between the prescribing physician and the prescription), and often needing to be refilled depending on the condition being treated and/or the nature of the drug. The initial visit may often mean something far grimmer: the ordering up of a test, or series of tests, relative benefit unknown, which firmly locks in the consumer to the "medical loop" — tests, more tests, more drugs, clinic and/or hospital stays, possibly very expensive, visually impressive and conceivably highly dangerous medical devices, surgeries and other procedures.

In the great majority of cases, all or most of the foregoing activities will be largely paid by somebody else — actually, thousands to millions of somebodies-else — through collective payment schemes so that, as seen, the actual financial impact of it all, however much it may ultimately affect the financial (let alone physiological) health of the consumer, is not immediately felt.

Lawyers circling overhead

There also is merit in the doctors' argument that overuse of diagnostics and therapeutics is their only defense against the malpractice case vultures of the American legal apparatus. While this defense is a long way from adequately explaining the high cost of medicine, it at least accounts for a part of it.

As former US Surgeon-General C. Everett Koop MD told a television program:

> *I didn't mention what money would be saved with malpractice reform because the numbers are incalculable. But you would get rid of the practice of defensive medicine, where I think about one-fifth of everything that is done in America today on patients is done to prevent a doctor's being guilty of a lawsuit someplace down the road.*[(76)]

But even if there is over-priced medicine, and occasional diagnostics and procedures of doubtful merit, even if there are scams and schemes in public and private health insurance, occasionally incompetent physicians and nurses, too many bureaucrats and certainly too many lawyers ready to pounce at the mere suggestion of a lawsuit, at least American medical *research* remains an area of pristine purity and innocence — or at least runs one of the arguments in defense of The Club.

Yet this is hardly the case, either.

Research: frills and frauds

A report by the House Governmental Operations Committee in 1990 referred[(77)] to at least 13 researchers who were evaluating a heart-disease drug with federal research funds from the National Institutes of Health (NIH) who at the time either owned stock or held stock options in the company that had developed the drug.

This in turn was only one of 10 cases which led the

committee to charge that Americans may be misled and even endangered by scientific misconduct and conflicts of interest in federally funded medical research.

The House panel's findings — based on a three-year investigation — claimed that universities conduct inadequate investigations of such possible misconduct and that in several cases they had retaliated against "whistleblowers" — conscientious researchers who report wrongdoing. The legislators also claimed that NIH officials usually accepted the findings of universities and in some cases ignored financial conflicts of interest among scientists who received federal grants.

And none other than Dr. Bernadine Healy, who headed the NIH during the Bush administration, was quoted in *Science* in August 1993 assailing her former domain, which oversees 4,500 in-house researchers in 25 different institutes, as a progress-quenching and bloated bureaucracy run by "dictators."[(78)] The magazine drew on interviews with more than 100 scientists to describe a situation of institutional authoritarianism in many of the component institutes.

In 1993, Rep. Ron Wyden (D-Ore.) brought to light an overlapping problem: the granting to major private concerns of foreign commercial rights to research breakthroughs funded by US taxpayers, usually through the NIH.

This is the tip of a taxpayer-ripoff/drug industry research collaborative scheme in which pharmaceutical companies may achieve monopoly status on compounds developed at taxpayer expense through the governmental-academia interlock. The fruits of such research involve pricey drugs which the American taxpayer is gouged into paying for twice — first, through taxes which subsidize their development; second, through the retail costs of their consumption in America's massively overpriced drug market.

A parallel development may be that such research allows drugs and technology to be shipped abroad while the same are not allowed at home through some red tape foulup involving the FDA bureaucracy.

The sources of infestation in the taxpayer-subsidized, government-protected drug company monopoly scheme are two pieces of legislation:

In 1980, the Bayh-Dole Act (enhanced by further legislation later) gave universities patent rights on federally funded research conducted on their campuses. In 1986, government researchers were allowed a similar privilege through the development of CRADAS (Cooperative Research and Development Agreements).

The US Congress, usually ready to knuckle under to the drug interests, provided corporations with tax credits for investing in university research as well as an additional 50 percent credit for developing "orphan drugs" (those which had lost prior patents over time) against diseases affecting small numbers of patients. According to the Office of Technology Assessment (OTA), such sweetheart deals allowed a $1.4 billion tax credit windfall for the pharmaceutical giants in 1993.[79]

A case study of the situation was the development and marketing of taxol, an anti-cancer agent derived from the bark of the rare Pacific yew tree and of mixed (if controversial) utility in several "forms" of cancer:

The federal National Cancer Institute (NCI), which had already spent $32 million (taxpayer funds) to develop what some called the most important new anti-cancer drug in 15 years, solicited proposals for a CRADA. Rushing in was drug giant Bristol-Myers Squibb (BMS), which, in the words of a magazine report:

> *was awarded exclusive rights to harvest Pacific yews on federal forest land, then the only source of taxol, and monopoly control over the data from federally funded research . . . BMS pays no royalties on taxol sales and a pittance for the yew tree bark. In exchange, the company agreed to a fair-pricing clause. Yet once taxol won FDA approval, BMS set the drug's wholesale price at $1,000 per treatment — roughly eight times what it cost NCI*

researchers to synthesize taxol . . .[80]

Such a maneuver is what led to Congressional oversight and Rep. Ron Wyden's remark that "American consumers who have funded drug development through the gifts of corporate-tax credits and federal lab research should not be bludgeoned by price gouging."[81]

At one of Wyden's hearings, it became common knowledge that San Diego's Scripps Research Institute, the United States' largest private biomedical laboratory, had signed a 10-year, $300 million agreement with Swiss pharmaceutical giant Sandoz whereby the international drug company would receive the right to commercialize breakthroughs made by Scripps — at the time a recipient of $100 million per year in NIH (that is, taxpayer) funds.

This was, wrote reporter Linda Marsa, the equivalent of American taxpayers providing Sandoz with a leveraged buyout of $1 billion in research on which it would have exclusive rights.[82]

So all is far from pristine within the federal research establishment — and elements of it may be just plain foul, particularly as they relate to cancer and AIDS (*XI,XIII*).

The great charity ripoff

If the scent of scandal and corruption wafts ever upward from the research establishment, Americans can usually take heart that in the area of sheer philanthropy a kind of national innocence abounds which, among other things, provides many millions of dollars for research through voluntary donations.

Yet time and the centralized, corrupting influences of the certainty of hard cash turned over for altruistic purposes have greatly besmirched the efforts of organized fund-raisers to feed on the good instincts of the American people, arguably the most generous on earth:

By 1994, two economics professors had found that more than 2,000 ostensibly non-profit organizations in the USA focus on health issues — and that their revenues from public donations exceed $10 billion *annually*, a strikingly modest amount of which actually goes to meaningful research.

In a swipe at American charities' "Big Three" — the bloated American Cancer Society (ACS), American Heart Assn. (AHA) and the American Lung Assn. (ALA) — James T. Bennett and Thomas J. DiLorenzo found that the same had

> *become large, bureaucratic and have strayed from their traditional charitable mission of finding causes of and cures for diseases and helping the needy.*
>
> *Instead, fund-raising is the major concern, and the primary beneficiaries are their executives and staffs and members of the medical establishment.*[83]

Noting that "six-figure salaries and generous benefits are not uncommon for top executives" of the major charities, Bennett/DiLorenzo reported that, for fiscal year 1991, 38.9 cents of every dollar spent by the ACS went to executive and staff compensation, that for the AHA it was 34.3 cents of every dollar spent, and that for the ALA it was 42.5 cents.[84]

By the end of fiscal 1993, they added, the ACS had a net worth of $520.3 million and owned more than $61 million in real estate and equipment (*see also XI.*)[85]

Those who donate to the major charities — whose top executives are easily in the six-figure brackets — should be aware of the Bennett/DiLorenzo findings as to how much of the take goes to direct help and/or research:

AHA "spends nothing to aid people suffering from heart disease," ALA "spends less than 1 percent of its revenues on direct assistance to lung disease patients" and for every dollar the ACS spends on cancer research US taxpayers add another $15, they wrote.[86]

Huge amounts of the donated dollars go to what the major charities call "public education," a sweeping generic term which can mask many a barrel of pork.

References

1 The New York Times News Service, Dec 12, 1993

2. *American Medical News*, June 10, 1996.
2a. "America's vast sick-care economy." *Alt. Med. Dig.*, 17, 1997.
3. *San Diego Union*, Feb. 26, 1996.
4. Morgan, David, *Reuters*, Aug. 19, 1994.
5. *Ibid.*
6. Cited in *The Choice*, XIX: 1, 1993.
7. *Ibid.*
8. *The Choice*, XVIII: 2, 1992.
8a. Hoffman, Catherine, *J. Am. Med. Assn.*, Nov. 13, 1996.
9. *The Choice*, XXII: 1, 1996.
10. *Am. J. Pub. Health*, Aug. 18, 1994.
11. Bowman, Lee, Scripps Howard News Service, Jan. 26, 1996.
11a. Winslow, Ron, "Study of access to medical care finds outlook remains grim for uninsured." *The Wall Street Journal*, Oct. 23, 1996.
12. Cited in Hoar, WP, "The Clinton cure-all." *The New American*, Nov. 1, 1993.
13. *The Freeman*, October 1992.
14. Cited in Lee, RW, "Creating the 'crisis.'" *The New American*, Nov. 1, 1993.
15. Marsa, Linda, "Unhealthy alliances." *Omni*, February 1994.
16. *Ibid.*
17. Inlander, CB, *et al.*, *Medicine on Trial*. New York: Pantheon Books, 1988.
18. Eckholm, E, "Curbs sought in caesarean deliveries." *New York Times*, Aug. 11, 1986.
19. The Associated Press, May 19, 1994.
20. "House report says 23 percent of lens implants not necessary." *Hospitals*, Sept. 1, 1985.
20a. Angier, Natalie, *The New York Times*, Feb. 17, 1997.
21. *The Choice*, XIX: 1, 1993.
22. Faltermeyer, Edmund, "Medical care's next revolution." *Fortune*, Oct. 10, 1988.
23. *Ibid.*
24. *Ibid.*
25. *The Choice*, XVIII: 1, 1992.
26. Weiss, MJ, "Fatal mistakes." *Ladies' Home Journal*. June 1988.
27. *Ibid.*
28. *Medical World News*, April 9, 1984.
29. *The Choice*, XVIII: 1, 1992.
30. *Ibid.*
31. *Ibid.*
32. *J. Am. Med. Assn.*, Nov. 11, 1992.
33. Preston, Thomas, *The Clay Pedestal*. Seattle: Madrona Publishers, 1981.
34. Almy, TB, "The role of the primary physician in the health-care 'industry.'" *New Eng. J. Med.* 304, 1981.
35. *Business Week*, January 1992.
36. Culhane, Charles, "Drug industry hits Clinton price plan." *American Medical News*, Jan. 3, 1994.
37. *The Choice*, XVI: 4, 1990/1991.
38. *Ibid.*
39. *Ibid.*
40. *The Choice*, XVII: 3,4, 1991.
41. *Ibid.*
42. McClatchy News Service, June 1992.
43. Pekkanen, John, "Can you trust your doctor?" *Reader's Digest*, September 1993.
44. *Ibid.*
45. *The Choice*, XVIII: 2, 1992.
46. *The Choice*, XXII: 1, 1996.
47. Quoted in *The Choice*, XIX: 1, 1993.
48. *The Choice*, XIX: 2, 1993.
49. Behar, Richard, "Singing the Blue Cross blues." *Time*, July 12, 1993.
50. *Ibid.*
51. "Sixty Minutes" (CBS), May 15, 1994.
51a. Scripps Howard News Service, Jan. 20, 1997.
52. Lee, RW, "Creating the 'crisis.'" *The New American*, Nov. 1, 1993.
52a. Rich, Spencer, "More for Medicare and Medicaid." *The Washington Post*, Feb. 7, 1997.
53. *Reason*, January 1993.
54. Lee, op. cit.
55. Annis, ER, *Code Blue: Health Care in Crisis*. Washington DC: Regnery Gateway, 1992.
56. *The Choice*, XIX: 2, 1993.
57. New York Times News Service, January 1988.
58. New York Times News Service, cited in *The New American*, Nov. 1, 1993.
59. "Firm settles in fraud charges." *American Medical News*, Nov. 25, 1996.
59a. Johnson, Julie, *American Medical News*, Dec. 9, 1996.
59b. "LabScam scores latest victory." *American Medical News*, March 10, 1997.
60. Green, Stephen, Copley News Service, Feb. 15, 1996.
61. *The Choice*, XXII: 1, 1996.
62. McLeod, Don, "Some doctors bilk Medicare patients." AARP Bulletin, January 1994.

63. *The Choice*, XXII: 1, 1996.
64. *The Choice*, XVII: 3,4 1991.
65. The Associated Press, cited in *The Choice*, XX: 1, 1994.
66. Rubin, Daniel, Knight-Ridder News Service, Aug. 25, 1996.
67. Knight-Ridder News Service, Nov. 24, 1996.
68. Annis, *op. cit.*
68a. Mitka, Mike, "HMO executives claim fat paychecks." *American Medical News*, Feb. 5, 1996.
68b. "A billion-dollar bonus for the CEO of US Healthcare." *Healing Miracles* (Whitaker Wellness Institute), Summer 1997.
68c. Woolhandler, Steffie, and Himmelstein, David, *New Eng. J. Med.* 336, 1997.
69. Lee, *op. cit.*
70. Wool handler, Steffie, and Himmelstein, David, *New Eng. J. Med.*, Aug. 5, 1993.
71. Lee, *op. cit.*
72. Grigg, WN, "Freeing the consumer." *The New American*, Nov. 1, 1993.
73. Marsa, *op. cit.*
74. "Doctors' fees — free from the law of supply and demand." *Science* 200, 1978.
75. Fuchs, VR, *Who Shall Live?* New York: Basic Books, 1974.
76. *The Choice*, XVIII: 1, 1992.
77. *The Choice*, XVI: 4, 1990/1991.
78. *The Choice*, XIX: 1, 1993.
79. Marsa, *op. cit.*
80. "Taxol: the anatomy of a deal." *Omni*, February 1994.
81. *Ibid.*
82. Marsa, *op. cit.*
83. Bennett, JT, and DiLorenzo, TJ, *Unhealthy Charities: Hazardous to Your Health and Wealth.* New York: Basic Books, 1994.
84. "Uncharitable charities." *USA Today*, July 19, 1994.
85. *Ibid.*
86. *Ibid.*

IV
ERROR BY CONSENSUS:
The rise of 'scientific medicine'

"We have built a model of health and illness, birth and death, around an outmoded conceptual model of how the universe behaves, one which was fundamentally flawed from the beginning. While the physicists have been painfully eliminating the flaws from their own models, we have in medicine ignored those revisions totally. We find ourselves, thus, with a set of guiding beliefs that are as antiquated as are body humors, leeching, and bleeding."

— **Larry Dossey MD in *Space, Time & Medicine***

"The efficient physician is the man who successfully amuses his patients while nature effects a cure."

— **Voltaire**

"I firmly believe that if the whole materia medica . . . could be sunk to the bottom of the sea, it would be all the better for mankind — and all the worse for the fishes."

— **Oliver Wendell Holmes**

"The physician's duty is to heal the sick, not to enrich the apothecary."

— **Paracelsus**

"I pleased nobody except the people I cured."

— **Paracelsus**

"It is a common fate of all knowledge to begin as heresy and end as orthodoxy."

— **Thomas Huxley**

Religion, magic and medicine

Medicine has always been inseparable from, and integral to, religion — just as religion has always been inseparable from magic.

Perhaps this is why, even today during the pachydermal death throes of the allopathic system, that "standard" or "orthodox" or "regular" Western medicine (that is, allopathy) still behaves as if it *were* a religion.

Slavish devotion to a set of "scientific" principles now being abandoned in some realms of genuine science constitutes a creed; unswerving allegiance to various areas of linear logic which emanate from the creed serves as a statement of belief; and there is a hierarchy of medical pontiffs, archbishops, bishops, priests and parallel religious orders through which the tenets thrive and are enforced.

Dissenters are not burned at the stake — they are simply ruined professionally.

(One of the victims of the "regulars" — the late Robert Mendelsohn MD — was himself originally a "regular" of the American Medical Assn. variety. It was he who, in *Confessions of a Medical Heretic*[1], did more than any other to redefine modern American medicine as little more than a religion, complete with temples, priests, rituals and sacraments, and whose books and thousands of columns and articles deeply wounded "standard" medicine in the USA. Shortly before his untimely death in 1989, a "quackbuster" group was avidly attempting to force newspapers to drop his column from their pages.

(He followed the earlier tradition of another "regular" dissenter, Edgar Berman MD, who, in *The Solid Gold Stethoscope*[2], similarly took his chosen profession to task.)

If today's "scientific medicine" (an oxymoron, in that traditionally medicine has always been, and so should still be, an art rather than a science) is observable as the last redoubt of rationalism, then it is still a reflection of a creed or belief system, not a fact — the belief being that of *faith in reason*. And all that flows from the premise is thus a shoring up of an attitude, a belief system, a *paradigm*, in which health is held to be the absence of disease, disease is held to be primarily the result of exogenous pathogenic factors, curing is said to be the ridding of these factors, and the human animal on which medicine is practiced is considered to be an intricate machine, a combination of tissues, organs and cells.

As we shall see, this paradigm neatly fits the needs of twentieth-century medical economics, captained by the global pharmaceutical megaindustry and complete with licensure, social sanction, specialized training, a network of research facilities, hospitals, grants-funding processes, medical supplies and devices, insurance schemes, media manipulation, and enormous political clout.

Behind and above, under and through it all, exists the physician-healer, doctor — usually referred to in English without the definite article, rendering "doctor" an intimate member of the family, along with "mother," "father," "sister," "brother," none of which needs carry the definite article, either. (And also above all other professions — whoever says "plumber will see you in a few minutes"?) He is the quasi-divine intermediary between life and death, the terrestrial and the Divine. It is not the fault of doctors if they also are taught to think this way in approved, licensed schools of (allopathic) medicine. Doctor *is* healer in the human mind, regardless of the name of the healing process.

Yet so much of what the modern, organized religion of Western medicine likes to dismiss as heretical and quack has equal roots in the shared human tradition — indeed, modern medicine would not have developed without a prior reliance on medicinal plants (herbs) as the first true medicines on this planet, *together with* the ineffable X factor of spirit or religion. The "laying on of hands," or faith healing of a kind, however derided by the ecclesiastical allopathic orthodoxy as "unscientific," is the first observable manifestation of human medicine — faith healers plying their trade are depicted in the wall paintings of caves in the

Pyrenees which date before 13,000 BC.[3] In fact, both written and oral traditions from many ancient peoples make it evident that human touch was one of the earliest forms of medicine, and that the application of human touch, later organized as acupressure and massage, was usually part of religious, spiritual or philosophical concepts.

Our earliest knowledge of the medicine of ancient Egypt dates from papyri from about 2000 BC in which it was stressed that the duty of the pharaohs was to maintain the health of their subjects — that is, the divinely ordained ruler was physician as well as leader of the state, including King Athotis of the First Dynasty, who was said to practice healing and wrote concerning the human anatomy.

The healing methods of ancient Egypt consisted of rituals, special ceremonies and various religious rites aimed at exacerbating the power of the gods while routing from the patient the negative spiritual forces thought to cause disease. The intermediary was the physician/priest, whose ministrations included prayers and spells as well as physical remedies, which might be in the form of aloe, mint, myrrh, castor oil, opium, cedar, copper, lead and even salt, to which great powers were attributed.

Yet the remedies, we are told, would seemingly not "work" without the incorporation of the X factor — in this case, the incantations or magical words thought to be central to healing. In this ancient time, healing through mind, spirit *and* body — the holistic concept — was dominant.[4]

The first attempt of society to *protect* itself against physicians was enshrined in the Code of Hammurabi (circa 1950 BC), the first historical collection of decrees and regulations, setting forth the duties and rights of all citizens and some of whose concepts date back to ancient Sumer. Included were regulations governing the activities of the physician-priests, including such draconian ones as chopping off the physician's hand should his surgery on a patient's eye occasion the loss of the eye.

At a time when Western medicine is being forced to take a

serious look at live-cell or cellular therapy, long derided by the orthodoxy as quackery and said, as usual, not to be "scientific" (yet now being co-opted by American medicine — *see XVII*), it is often forgotten that one of the oldest medical documents extant, the Eber Papyrus (circa 1550 BC), refers to preparations made from animal organs, and that extracts of organs for medical therapy abound in the *Materia Medica* of Pliny the Elder and Aristotle.[5]

It is convenient to forget that perhaps the oldest surviving organized medical system, the Ayurvedic in India, placed great importance on diet, that Chinese acupuncture, dating back to millennia before Christ, was, as was Ayurvedic medicine, a reflection of a belief system or religion (cosmic dualism or Taoism), and that the various healing systems developed in ancient India and China were *holistic* in nature — that is, they understood healing as applicable to the trinity of mind/spirit/body and treated *people* rather than diseases.

It was Jan Smuts who, in 1926 in *Holism and Evolution*, a philosophical landmark, actually coined the term "holism." This concept — of a "wholeness" in nature — includes the notion that mankind is more than the sum of its parts.

Under current American-led Western medical thinking, man is not really even the sum of his parts — he is simply a mass of parts, ranging from the invisibly presumptive and submicroscopic to the grossly observable (glands, organs, systems). There is now a plethora of medical specialists ranging from the hematologist to the brain surgeon who have access to parts and pieces of a given patient, hence reflecting a multifactoriality of disciplines based on parts and pieces. This has given rise to the humorous observation by allopathic medical heretics themselves that proctologists are to be pitied since their entire field of practice is limited to "one square inch of puckered tissue" beyond which gastroenterologists have more or less established a "thou shalt not pass" line.[6]

American-led Western traditional medicine — and, indeed, most of its opponents in the medical ideas marketplace — traces itself back to Hippocrates of Greece (circa 400 BC), even though stylized treatments of human beings in what one would now think of as medical ways antedate Hippocrates by millennia.

There are, for example, traditions of organized herbal medicine in various ancient cultures, with empirically guided herbal practitioners gathering data on, and using, medicinal plants (herbs) in a methodical way. The *Nei Ching* (dated beyond two millennia BC) and the *Shen Nung Pen Tsao Ching* of China, of uncertain ancient origin, reflect an enormous amount of knowledge by Chinese herbal healers extending back better than 4,000 years. Indeed, the first Chinese emperor (Huang Ti, the Yellow Emperor, circa 2674 BC) was said to be the pioneer of Chinese medicine. A portrait of the god of husbandry, Shen Nung, circa 3494 BC, describes a deity who allegedly sampled all kinds of herbs to determine their healing powers (before himself being poisoned to death.)[(7)]

Traditions of herbal healing appear in most of the ancient civilizations of the Orient and the Middle East, some to this day (as in Persian herbal medicine, very much alive) and in the recently revitalized ancient tradition of Ayurvedic healing from India, a system which appeared more than three thousand years ago and which, among other things, included ancient forms of inhalation anesthesia, vaccinations and dietetics.

The ancient Egyptians, and other peoples of the Old World, codified herbal healing and structured the foundation of herb-based pharmacology. In the New World, the great pre-Columbian cultures (Inca, Maya, Aztec, and related) have left evidence of knowledge of medicinal plants, human anatomy and a wide variety of medical practices. As "white witch doctor" of the Jivaro Wilburn Ferguson, an American, found in South America, native tribes there had an oral-traditional herbal pharmacopeia and considerable knowledge of herbal medicines passed down for generations.[(8)] North American Indian tribes had — and often still have — "medicine men" who were traditional healers who possessed much medical knowledge.

From earliest times, medicine was an integral part of

religion, with the physician-priest, the medicine man, the shaman, the intermediary between tribe, clan or nation and the divine, established as a unique individual, perhaps a mix of the Divine and the secular. This anthropologically oft-observed phenomenon, apparently universal in human nature, may account for the status in which physicians are still held today in various human societies: those to whom we hand over our bodies for healing, curing or treating must be, or must seem to be, somehow elevated over the laity, a sociological paradigm not only not lost on, but nurtured by, organized Western allopathic medicine to its great advantage in the century now ending.

Hippocrates breaks ranks

In the West, though, it was a human thinker, Hippocrates, clearly not a divine being, to whom both modern Western orthodoxy and unorthodoxy turn as "the father of medicine," and whose philosophical impact on the healing arts continues to the present time — despite some wholesale misstatements and misperceptions by which the sage of Cos must also be measured.

Hippocrates may be described as the West's first holistic medical thinker as well as its first allopath and integrative practitioner.

Up to his time, Greek medical belief was invested in Asclepius (continued in the Roman tradition as Aesculapius), offspring of Apollo. It was he who, as mankind's divine intermediary or shaman, had virtually abolished sickness and death before Pluto decided, and Zeus agreed, that the supply of available new human souls to the netherworld had been endangered by too much healing. Asclepius was killed by a thunderbolt, but temples to his craft and memory dotted the Greek peninsula and islands, where the first hospitals or *asklepiea* were built.

Greek healing often was conducted "directly" through the laying on of hands or through the medium of the physician/priest applying a sacred item, relic or animal. It was also conducted "indirectly" through directions provided in dreams and visions, in which higher powers prescribed certain roots, herbs, fasts, baths, ointments, touch techniques and even gymnastics. Tales of impressive cures from the healing deity Asclepius spread far and wide and constituted much of Greek medical thought by the time of Hippocrates.[9]

The ancient symbol of the snake, in more than one culture a manifestation of cosmic power, became the symbol of Asclepius — and one or two snakes wrapped around a winged staff became the symbol of both Mercury, messenger of the gods, and the medical profession itself in the form of the caduceus, an internationally recognized ancestral motif. (Purists would argue that the "staff of Asclepius" is *not* the same as the caduceus, or symbol of the messenger.)

Dramatically removing medicine from the Divine — or at least from a higher-power X factor — Hippocrates taught that disease is a natural process and can be managed naturally. He established the "four humours" and the "four qualities" as the causes and definitions of illness.

Hippocratic medicine — ancient eclecticism — believed, first and foremost, that there was a healing power in nature, and that conditions for healing lay in proper diet, adequate exercise, sufficient rest, fresh air and personalized nursing. Only when this holistic approach failed did Hippocrates suggest the conservative use of "drugs" — that would be some 300 healing plants — and such procedures as enemas, purges, diuretics and bleeding. This general approach, with ever-greater attention to medications, would chart the course of Western medicine for centuries to come.

Hippocrates also attempted to codify ethics and inject morality into the practice of the *art* of medicine, and the first injunction of the Hippocratic Oath — to which physicians, for generations, swore allegiance — was *primum non nocere*: "first, do no harm." In the latter part of the current century, Western medical schools began moving away from the Hippocratic Oath, and at times either attempted to modify or supplant it, inasmuch as so much of what goes by the name of "scientific medicine" is indeed harmful, as in the cutting, burning and poisoning of Western civilization's most awesome killer (and one of allopathy's most notable failures), cancer.

As profiteering, often on an obscene scale, infected the medical/pharmaceutical combine, physicians were also all too frequently induced to move away from the more charitable, population-serving, healing-first musings of Hippocrates. And why not? If he could be wrong about "the humours," perhaps his cogitations on medical ethics also were wrong. Or so some have argued. Yet even at this late date, medical practitioners of most varieties in the Western world delight in seeing themselves as the heirs and champions of Hippocrates.

Dawn in China

In the East, the earliest medical texts of China (in distinction to the legendary beginnings of herbal medicine there millennia before Christ) date from about 540 BC with the *Tso-chuan*, followed by the organization of ritual and administration and the enshrining of the medical physician as separate from priests and magicians. The salient personality of this period, Pien Ts'io (c430-350 BC), may actually be a personification of several people. To him has been attributed knowledge of the pulse rate for diagnosis/prognosis.

In the third and second centuries BC, Chinese medicine borrowed from India and Persia, with Tso Yen (c 305-240 BC) introducing into the Far East the notion of five elements instead of four. After this time, the Chinese medical system incorporated the idea of elements and vital forces just as its ancient Indian, Greek and (later) Arab counterparts did.

The chemical element in what we might call ancient allopathy seems to date from Babylonian times, with the introduction of mercury as a kind of elixir (which would reach outrageous proportions in Western medicine centuries later).

The ancient intercourse between Mesopotamia, Greece, and the Far East helped China's methodical medical system evolve into a mix of knowledge about herbs, mineral remedies, poisons, dietetics, respiratory techniques, physical culture, the study of sex and the quest for immortality. Medicine in China flourished in the first few centuries of the Christian era within a burst of scientific and intellectual inquiry, as would occur later in Europe. The *Annals of the Han Dynasty* included major treatises on medicine, prescriptions in general, immortality methods, sex and general hygiene, yet only Huang Ti's *Classic of Internal Medicine* has survived.[10]

A battle of ideas

In the West, Aristotle (384-322 BC), the philosopher also known as the first biologist, a botanist and the founder of comparative anatomy, changed the direction of post-Hippocratic medicine. Aristotle's notion that there are four fundamental qualities that are linked with four elements said to constitute living matter (earth, air, fire, water) would color medical thought at least until the 17th century.

Galen (131-200 AD), whipsawed between the Hippocratic method and Aristotelian philosophy, while "drowning the substance of the Hippocratic corpus in Aristotelian form"[11] and heretical for his time, made great contributions to Western medical practice even though he may be said to have brought the Greek spirit of inquiry in medicine to an end. Not until the 16th century were the theories of Aristotle and Galen rigorously questioned by Vesalius (1514-64), whose reliance on detailed observations of anatomy and on dissection placed Western medicine back on what its modern-day defenders would consider the "right" scientific track. He also was a heretic in his time.

The success of Christianity in the Western world temporarily moved Greco-Roman medicine away from its rationalistic basis and re-incorporated the Divine into the concept of disease. Evil spirits were thought to lurk behind much of disease as late as New Testament times in contrast to the natural-law view of the Greco-

Romans. With the theological/philosophical triumph of the new religion much of the ancient notion of spiritual retribution through disease reappeared.

It may be said that the mingling of religion with the Hippocrates-founded rationalist view constituted a medical marriage made in hell, with the offspring observable today in the allopathic paradigm: just as in times of old evil spirits needed to be tortured out of the body by fire, surgery, and purges, today the offending entities, better classed as tumors, viruses and other "microbes," and their physiological sequelae, need to be cut, burned and poisoned, the human patient literally tortured back to good health by a priestly physician and his craft.

While the Dark Ages settled over Europe, interest in herb and folk medicine was kept alive both by "wise women" (viewed by Christians as witches) and by Christian monks in continual communication with each other, but it fell to the Arabs to advance and refine what we think of today as pharmacy and medicine, with the names Mesue, Rhazes and Avicenna added to medicine's serpentine history. By 800 AD pharmacy was an independent profession among the Muslims with the first "drugstores" opened in the Abbasid capital of Baghdad.[12]

While the medieval pharmacopeias of Europe and the vast Arab culture borrowed from each other as well as from the work of the ancient Greco-Romans and Mesopotamians, the promotion of toxic minerals as drugs, while a feature of ancient medicine, reached new dimensions due to two events — one philosophical, the other pathological.

Alchemy and syphilis: rallying points

First, through alchemy, scientists and philosophers sought to transmute baser metals into gold — an accompanying system of religion and occultism (transmuting man into God) which persisted for centuries and which often focused on the strange liquid metal mercury. Alchemy (magic) was to some extent the father of chemistry and the uncle of pharmacy.

Second, the return to Europe in the 16th century of sailors from the West Indies brought back to the continent (for it probably had existed in less virulent forms in prehistoric times) the hideous disease syphilis, a scourge second in devastation only to the Black Death (bubonic plague), which had swept across the continent in the 14th century, leaving a vastly reduced human population and evidence of a pestilence which seemed to elude every attempt at cure.

Syphilis, which usually took much more time to maim and kill than had the plague, presented European doctors with decades of physiological challenges. (It should be noted that a brutal cultural "tradeoff" had occurred during the European penetration into the Americas: the Europeans brought smallpox, which, in terms of total scope and devastation, came nearer decimating the entire indigenous population of the New World than did syphilis in Europe.)

While mercury, along with other metals, had been medically used before the onslaught of syphilis, it was the discovery that forms of this metal (now known to be antibacterial) might relieve some of the gross symptoms of the Great Pox which caused its catapulting into fame as a "cure."

In the form of quicksilver, mercury could be taken in fairly large doses and was relatively non-toxic — though continual use of it could and did lead to toxicity. The relentless use of quicksilver by any and all peddlers of cures for syphilis is loosely linked to the words *quacksalver* (peddler of mercury) and eventually "quack" — a pretentious pretender to medical knowledge.

While it has been said that "the use of mercury in the treatment of syphilis may have been the most colossal hoax ever perpetrated"[(13)] in the history of medicine, such use — passionately defended by some, heatedly opposed by others — dominated much of Western medicine for centuries.

With alchemy establishing a philosophical base for scientific investigation into the nature of metals and minerals, and with the scourge of syphilis (the cancer and AIDS of the Renaissance) presenting a major medical challenge, the tone for much of Western medical allopathy was set.

The advent of Paracelsus

The manufacture of medicines and the attempt to isolate single remedies from mineral, plant and animal sources, carried to a high art by the Arabs, helped prepare the medical revolution largely headed by the Swiss-German doctor and mystic Philippus Theophrastus Bombastus von Hohenheim (1493-1541), far better known by the less wieldy title Paracelsus ("greater than Celsus"). He would apply alchemy and chemistry to medicine and his far-reaching concepts both colored medicine for centuries to come and also ironically formed a great part of the philosophical foundation of homeopathy, which would arise as the major challenge to allopathy in the 19th century.

Paracelsus was both the distant father of chemotherapy and a reformer of surgery. He faced head-on many of the fanciful beliefs of sixteenth-century medicine, including the religious notion that witchcraft was often the origin of disease. A free thinker and mystic who managed to ruffle virtually everyone's feathers, he was persecuted by the organized medical regulars — and religious fanatics — of his time and driven from his native Switzerland to Germany, France and Italy.

It was Paracelsus who set the foundation for scientific drug development, ideas which would lead to breakthrough drug discoveries in the nineteenth century. Allopaths, homeopaths and philosophers of various kinds have found in this strange radical a spiritual fellow traveller.

Hence, by the Renaissance, there was a cobbled-together medicine in the West, blending knowledge of medicinal plants (herbs), minerals, and some knowledge of anatomy, together with a hermaphroditic concept of both natural and Divine law. The concepts of "science" and "scientific medicine" had not yet developed to full bloom.

Descartes and Newton: birth of a paradigm

What now stands as the modern medical paradigm in the West is a belief system firmly rooted in the 17th century and deriving its philosophical nutrition from the thinking of Rene Descartes and Sir Isaac Newton, both of whom were "enlightenment" thinker/researchers ready to shuck the religionism of past centuries and to anoint human rationalism as a new creed itself: faith in reason.

The underlying concept, thanks to Descartes, is that of the orderly, mechanistic universe, a clockwork existence divided into never-the-twain-shall-meet compartments of mind and matter, with the material universe constituted as a kind of perpetual-motion machine operated by natural laws, with all things within that universe, including living organisms and man himself, serving as cogs and levers.

Sir Isaac applied this "Cartesian" thinking to an expanded mechanical framework of existence and set the stage for what the West would incorporate as a considerable amount of "the scientific method" — observation, experimentation, reproducibility of outcomes, predictions of the former, and the orderly categorizing of them all. The machine-like human in the machine-like universe became the guiding concept of "the scientific method" and of what would later be classed as "scientific medicine" — at root a nonsense phrase.

Yet, as the Twentieth Century blazed exponential patterns of scientific thought and discovery, with zig-zagging changes in concepts, the Cartesian-Newtonian postulates have mostly survived as interesting relics, for as much raw "science" is now based on the *unseen* (as in quantum mechanics, by which physics has undergone perhaps the deepest philosophical revolution) and the *assumed* as by the known and measurable. Just as physics more and more describes a reality assumed from invisible elements, there is a rush of paradigm shifts from the dualistic universe (Descartes/Newton) to the interconnected, multiphasic universe, the holistic or even — some say — pantheistic Total One.

While Western orthodox medicine has, in the main, stayed locked in the Cartesian/Newtonian mold, real science has slowly (and sometimes rapidly) escaped from it.[14] Yet the verbalizing of the thought-construct, the semantical manipulation of the Old Order tries to persist. It is this adherence to outmoded concepts, however enshrined in orthodoxy and sometimes mandated by the state, that requires a name of its own.

Velikovsky: science vs. scientism

Scientism is the least objectionable term for the adherence to preconceived notions masquerading as pure knowledge ("science") and it became best known in the 1950s in the 20th-century pilloring by the organized scientific hierarchy of Immanuel Velikovsky, whose *Worlds in Collision*[15] and subsequent works challenged many of the standard or orthodox concepts (in their day) of planetary evolution, geology, astronomy, physics and other disciplines. Despite Dr. Velikovsky's eventual vindication on many (but by no means all) points, organized scientific thought at the time, as expressed in "learned journals," other favored publications, and the research community itself, was slow to accept what seemed like a major change (paradigm shift) in some of its belief systems, and loath to forgive.

Velikovsky was reviled and at times humiliated not so much because anything he wrote posed a serious economic challenge to the hierarchy, but because that hierarchy's egos were bruised.[16]

Medical scientism's reaction to its challengers is even worse, for they pose not only serious philosophical/ego problems for the supposed gatekeepers of truth but, worse, a solid economic threat:

What if promotive health overtook "preventive" medicine, or any other medicine, as society's major health goal? What if such promotive health vastly reduced or nearly eliminated the need for a global pharmaceutical cartel? What if adherence to holistic principles in living, eating and thinking kept people out of the medical loop while maintaining them in an essentially healthy state less and less requiring the service of allopaths? What if . . .?

Hence, in the ongoing conflict of medical scientism vs. legitimate science, opponents of the allopathic paradigm must not only be branded as quacks, charlatans, self-deluded, criminals, etc., but denied access to social sanction, "standard literature," licensure, and any sort of arrangement which allows them to mount a serious competitive threat to the "regular" profession. They must be isolated, neutralized and, if all else fails, eliminated.

This has been the outcome of Western organized medicine's incarnation of "the scientific method," the culmination of many events, twists and turns since the rise of the Cartesian/Newtonian postulates, and the rise of error by consensus in the abandonment of the concept of holism.

'Scientific medicine' as a rationalist cult

There were, of course, starts and stops along the way:

The "rationalists," who later would become medicine's "regulars" and, in the USA, the "orthodox" or "standard" practitioners (allopaths), would draw much of their thinking from Galen, and, later, Hermann Boerhaave (1668-1738). But some medical thinkers traced their intellectual lineage back to the mystic/philosopher/healer Paracelsus, who incorporated dieting and mind-over-matter for healing, and, as such, was practicing holistic medicine.

In post-Renaissance/Reformation times, what would ultimately become allopathic medicine owed much to the Galen-based tradition (and "the scientific method" dangling from Cartesian-Newtonian postulates) and to William Cullen and John Brown, 18th century Scots physicians. On the Western side of the Atlantic, the famed American physician Benjamin Rush, a signatory of the Declaration of Independence, despite his "regularist" upbringing warned that the fledgling Republic in the

West would be ill-served by a single school of medical thought which would become, in effect, state-mandated.

As the Renaissance/Reformation era "rediscovered" humanism and freed itself from orthodox religion in the West, the result was a flowering of science (pure knowledge, or the assumption of it) and "the scientific method." The struggling doctrines of Western medicine, be they Hippocratic-, Galen-, or Paracelsus-colored, were deeply influenced by the explosion of "scientific" thought. The practitioners of their day were as eager to prove the sanctioned authority of their craft through science as their forerunners had insisted on demonstrating the sanctioned authority of theirs through religion. There simply was a new religion, rationalism, with its own articles of faith. Cartesian/Newtonian postulates set the intellectual tone, and established the premises, and all that flowed therefrom would serve, over centuries, to bolster the premises.

"Scientific medicine," to be moved a quantum leap ahead by the French medical school in the 19th century, would focus on body parts and pieces, and on the observation and classification of symptoms. It would come to confuse symptoms with disease and devolve into a system of managing symptoms rather than elucidating the causes of disease states, particularly in those conditions for which no simple "microbe" could be found.

Like the other "sciences," "scientific medicine" would slowly remove the healer from the healing under the Renaissance-to-Twentieth Century thought-construct or paradigm that true knowledge occurs only following careful observation, then quantifying and reproducing results. This "scientific" approach would rid medicine once and for all of spiritualism, religion, guesswork or even intuition — all ultimately to be denounced as "unscientific." The art of medicine would be replaced by the "science" of medicine.

Werner Heisenberg has related how Albert Einstein dissented from Heisenberg's (and indeed "science's") view that scientists observe, measure, and then form conclusions dispassionately from the collected data. Einstein argued that the reverse is true: the scientist begins with a belief system or model, a preconceived view, and this preconceived view is apt to determine to a great extent that which is observed.[17]

In the West, doctoring by physicians for a very long time remained a privilege of the upper classes, and, as in British medical practice, was compartmentalized along a guild system. There were surgeons, apothecaries and physicians, but not, in the main, "general practitioners." In fledgling America, the farm mother was the "primary care physician," and untutored "quacks" were available for the dispensing of any number of nostrums. There were also such lay physicians as herbalists, midwives and "natural bonesetters", some of whose healing feats were legendary.

As we shall see, the advent of homeopathy in Germany in the late 18th and early 19th centuries was a major challenge to the "scientific" authority of the rationalist "regulars." It led to disputes over territory, sanction and authorization which eventually gave way to the allopathic monopoly in America which, in turn, has dominated medicine in the Western world.

Western medicine's addiction to "the scientific method" would ultimately carry it into the ultimate contradictions which became clear in the last half of the present century.

As "science" roared ahead full steam in Europe, "scientific medicine" became greatly influenced by the new religion, perhaps nowhere more impressively than in France, whose riveting, 19th-century debates on host-vs-microbe would dominate the thinking of Western medicine that has been followed ever since.

In the conceptual arena, if man was a machine within a much greater machine (the cosmos), then each and every component part of the human machine must also be seen as machines. Anatomy was thus eventually joined by biology and microbiology — tissues, organs, cells and kinds of cells must be taken into account in human medicine. But things could not stop there — parts of cells ultimately came to be of great importance.

The French debate ("is the terrain of the host more important than the microbe?") was settled, we know, in favor of the allopaths. From the latter 19th century onward, in alignment with the primacy of the ideas of Koch and Pasteur, "microbes" would take on a meaning all their own, and medicine swerved violently into an all-out search for "germs" and the understanding of their roles in causing all diseases.

It should be noted that even within the rationalist/allopathic thought-construct or paradigm the healer of pre-microbial medicine was indeed practicing an art and not a science: healers instinctively knew that their interactions with patients, their taking of extensive medical histories, their interest in whether the patient's grandmother had dropsy or not, had a bearing on fashioning a treatment design (protocol) for the individual patient. That is, until the advent of the French medical debates, it was *presumed* that the *terrain* of "the host," the human body or human *persona*, was "more important" than an understanding of "the disease," now thought so often to be caused by a microbe of some kind.

As late as the second decade of the twentieth century, majority medical opinion in America held that scurvy was some kind of microbially caused disorder, and only later would it be conclusively proven that scurvy arises as a Vitamin C deficiency state. But the thinking was linear and reasonable — thus "scientific." If the causative microorganisms of such scourges as syphilis and many other bacterial diseases had been found, then it followed that virtually *all* human disorders involved microbes of one kind or another. By that time, the allopathic fraternity was organized, had recaptured and licensed medical schools, and was beginning to be locked into the vested economic interests which would then guide it throughout the 20th century. Dissidents to the allopathic line on disease conditions in 1915 were — as in the 1990s — derided as "quacks."

Challenges to the allopathic paradigm

The reality has thus been that Western organized medicine

(allopathy) now has at its disposal an awesome amount of knowledge about diseases and their presumed germ-microbial-parasitical-bacterial-viral-genetic causes, and far less knowledge about, and interest in, the patient ("host"). Allopathy can now describe with great detail just how the tuberculosis bacterium "works" — yet it cannot state or explain how many TB-infected persons will have symptoms of, let alone succumb from, this malady if left untreated by allopathic nostrums. It can eradicate yellow fever among a given population, but is unable to state why the causative agent did or did not infect all persons who were exposed to it let alone explain why among those infected some developed symptoms, some did not, and some died while others did not. The reason is simple: organized Western medicine knows "all about" yellow fever, but very little about the host in whom it may or may not flourish.

Faced, now, by multifactorial disorders with multifactorial "causes," the allopathic paradigm has reached its limit: linear thought and the hunt for viruses and even genes can neither explain nor predict the total syndrome that is AIDS, nor that of most of cancer, nor that of virtually all the "autoimmune" disorders and so many "inborn errors of genetics" — diseases, conditions and metabolic challenges either not known about a century ago or in existence in such tiny numbers as to have been overlooked.

Modern allopathy is thus perplexed by philosophical conundrums which suggest that linear thought may be in error: does correlation really mean causation? Does effect prove cause — and vice-versa? Is it not as appropriate to conclude that cancers cause viruses as it is to state (as virologists do) that viruses cause cancer? Does a multiplicity of "new" or possibly reactivated "old" viruses in chronic fatigue syndrome (CFS) argue that this multifactorial calamity is actually the *result* of these submicroscopic structures, or are these submicroscopic structures in abundance *because* of CFS, whose actual cause or causes may lie elsewhere? Is the presence or absence of a gene or a defect therein within a malignant process a *cause* of the process, a *result* of the process, on simply a "marker" for it? /

The allopathic model, to be sure, neatly explained the direct cause of, though by no means the final outcomes of, a host of pathogen-caused diseases, and allowed this school of thought, perhaps justifiably, to seize the high ground. Whole epidemics of infectious disease have been wiped out thanks largely to allopathic thinking (even though infectious disease has yielded to other medical approaches as well). And the great expansion in anatomical knowledge in the 18th and 19th century equipped the "regulars" (usually meaning allopaths) with ponderous structural information about the human body which ultimately brought surgery from the ranks of a minor trade plied at a compensation rate similar to, or less than, that of barbers, to the Olympian apex of the "healthcare delivery team."

Before the advent of the Koch-Pasteur germ theory of disease and its notable triumphs against infectious disease, the "regular" school got along mainly through its precision work with knife and lancet. The historical record of medicine is replete with horror stories of surgeries performed before the era of anesthetics and of the administration of invasive, frightening procedures in "regular" medicine in the form of the bleeding of patients with leeches, their purgings and blisterings with all manner of agents, and a vast array of pokings, probings and poisonings which went on in the name of medicine — reasons why so few people wished to be treated by physicians let alone go to hospitals.

The death of Charles II: 'rationalist' medicine at work

The well documented death of Charles II of England is one of the best descriptions of "regular" medicine at its scientific worst and is a casebook example of iatrogenic mayhem writ large. It is as appropriate to say that Charles II — and George Washington — were probably killed by their doctors as it is to say that many doctors have also saved many lives.

A description of the treatment and death of Charles II

coming from the pens of his doctors and other witnesses is the best reported royal demise.[18] The composite description is a horror show of "rational" medicine at its most gruesome:

Charles II, who actually may have been suffering from a form of Bright's disease, was misdiagnosed since Day One (Feb. 2, 1685) after loss of speech and ensuing convulsions. He was at first bled (16 oz. of blood taken from the right arm), then "cupped" for 8 oz. more, then made to vomit by the administration of "orange infusions of the metals, made in white wine," white vitriol and peony water; given an enema made of "powder of sacred bitters," syrup of buckthorn, rock salt and the "orange infusion;" and "blistered" with various agents all over his head; forced to take various preparations "to give strength to his loaded brain," "excite sneezing," "keep his bowels active at night" — and "spirit of sal ammoniac was applied now and again to His Most Serene Majesty's nostrils" while "cephalic plasters combined with spurge and burgundy pitch" were applied to the soles of his feet.

Charles II miraculously made it through Feb. 3, though much the worse for wear due to the overabundance of "rational" medicine at his disposal, including more bleeding, this time from the jugular vein, and, to counteract a sore throat, a combination of herbs and syrups. Still surviving by Feb. 4, but slipping rapidly, the monarch received a "mild laxative" and a draught of "spirit of human skull, 40 drops."

On Feb. 5, as I described it in an earlier book:

> *. . . to counteract a fever, the body of physicians provided Peruvian bark, antidotal milk water, and syrup of cloves. They continued using extract of human skull in a "pearl julep." Yet on Feb. 6, "as the illness was now becoming more grave and His Most Serene Majesty's strength (Woe's me!) gradually failing, the physicians were compelled to have recourse to the more active cardiac tonics, and to prescribe . . . Raleigh's stronger antidote, an essence of dissolved pearl, and*

goa stone."

A host of remedies followed during the day, including more sal ammoniac and bezoar stones from animal intestines. All these measures failed to alleviate the royal personage and at length he expired . . . the misuse of the blistering agents — including Spanish fly, or cantharides — proved fatal, robbing the kidneys of their last vestige of functional activity.[19]

A description of the death of George Washington, in the form of a criticism of "standard" medicine, was made in 1832 by Dr. Wooster Beach:

Think of a man, within the brief space of little more than 12 hours, deprived of 80 or 90 oz. of blood; afterward swallowing two moderate American doses of calomel . . . then 5 grains of calomel and 5 or 6 grains of emetic tartar; vapours of water and vinegar frequently inhaled; blisters applied to his extremities; a cataplasm of bran and vinegar applied to his throat, upon which a blister had already been fixed . . . is it surprising that when thus treated, the afflicted general, after various ineffectual struggles for utterance, at length articulated a desire that he might be allowed to die without interruption![20]

So by the 18th, and well into the 19th centuries, the two major techniques or devices of "rationalist" medicine, consistently defended in textbooks and speeches, were the lancet (for bleeding) and the administration of mercury, usually in the form of calomel. But along with them came the blistering agents, vomiting-inducers, laxatives, enemas, poultices of all kinds and, as a tactic of last resort, surgical incision by men practicing a trade on an economic par with barbers, who were held to be less dangerous.

The enormous damage done to the American public in the 18th, 19th and early 20th century by mercury (in the form of calomel tablets), aside from the administration of other toxic minerals and metals in the name of medicine, must be laid squarely at the feet of the "regular" practitioners. The attempt to eradicate the multiple sequelae of syphilis over the centuries through the allopathic misperception that it was a skin disease and that treating pustules and poisoning the body with toxic metals would somehow cure the disorder is another low-water mark in the history of the "regular" profession.

A matter of semantics

It is only because the "regulars," who particularly laid claim to rationalism and medical licensure, were challenged by "irregular" practitioners that the term "allopath" evolved — and it was first used derisively by the rapidly advancing primary opponents of the "regulars," the homeopaths, to separate the latter from the former. Yet, as the conceptual and other struggles between homeopaths and the "regulars" advanced through the 19th century, many of the latter came to accept the term themselves, so that in several languages the derivative of "allopath" is an acceptable definition of a follower of a school of medical thought which believes in curing diseases by finding their opposites, the linguistic essence of *allo-pathy*. (In Spanish, for example, the term *alópata* is commonly and frequently used by the "regulars" as a non-derisive, acceptable term which usually means that the practitioner carries an MD degree.)

In fact, in most Western countries the idea that there are various schools of medicine of which allopathy is only one, albeit the primary one, is not alien. It is in the United States where the Allopathic Industrial Complex (AIC), over time, has been so adroit that it has arrogated to itself the terms "doctor," "physician" and "medicine" so that when an American thinks of a "doctor" he really means a dispenser of synthetic drugs or a surgeon — in other words, an allopath, more comfortably called a "physician" by the AIC. The American public is not allowed to know that chiropractors, naturopaths, herbalists, homeopaths and others have an equal linguistic right to be described as "doctors" who practice "medicine," nor is the average American even slightly familiar with the terms "allopaths" or "allopathy."

Allopathy: state-sanctioned medicine

At the philosophical level, American allopathy has the sanction of organized science — it is the medical division of 17th century rationalism, the continuer of a tradition of dualism and the concept of man as machine. It is what is meant when American apologists speak of "scientific medicine" — an indirect way to say that that which is *not* allopathic is, by definition, not "scientific." Actually, of course, while allopathy has described itself as "scientific," it is actually *scientistic*, or rigidly hidebound.

At the social level, American allopathy has sanction, authorization and licensure: an MD degree (for "doctor of medicine") means instruction in allopathic models and concepts, and only MDs, or practitioners of instructional currents which have in effect sold out to allopathy (such as osteopathy, originally an independent line of medical thought in the USA), have full access to the medical-industrial complex: they may draw blood, have "hospital privileges," are referral physicians for the gargantuan third-party insurance payer schemes (or, often, scams), are tied in with medical products, devices and diagnostic and monitoring equipment, and their post-graduate education is due almost exclusively to the economic motor which drives modern medicine — the pharmaceutical cartel — for which MD physicians serve as legalized purveyors of drugs. In America, only licensed allopaths have full statutory access to our bodies.

At the religious level, American allopathy continues the rituals and sacraments of the physician/priest — it is pathogens, rather than devils and spirits, which are expelled or exorcised through the rituals and sacraments of allopathy, and carriers of advanced disease conditions are to be punished or indeed tortured back to good health through ritual mutilation and cutting (surgery), burning (now meaning radiation), and poisoning (chemotherapy, synthetic hormones, etc.). The physician/ priest, backed by the pharmaceutical cartel, now has at his disposal a vast armamentarium of mood-altering chemical compounds to placate, soothe, ameliorate, mitigate, dull or stimulate the "host." In the simple palliation of symptoms which might otherwise go away or take much longer to manage, the administration of such compounds through the physician-to-pharmacist-with-arcane-language mechanism may indeed bring about short-term wonders, and often they really *do* help.

At the economic level, since allopaths are the prime cogs in the pharmaceutical machine, the MD degree carries a guarantee of economic stability and upward mobility despite inroads made upon the profession by malpractice insurance, the litigious society which America has become, and an overgrowth of attorneys (with more than 65% of the world's entire supply of lawyers coming from the USA alone) who professionally mediate the endless frictions between patients, physicians, insurance companies and medical institutions, and whose fees have added no small part to the swollen cost of "healthcare delivery" at the current time.

At the political level, organized allopathic medicine, through the misnomered American Medical Association, has maintained a firm lock on the way allopaths are trained and the way they think, even though the holistic/metabolic/health-freedoms revolution has considerably pierced its armor. The Allopathic Industrial Complex, through political-action committees (PACs) state by state, has largely been able to sabotage health-freedoms legislation, or any perceived threat to its primacy in social sanction and authority.

Professional lobbyists bankrolled by medical organizations at the state and federal levels often represent the primary lobbying forces in major states (as in California, which, while essentially an agricultural state with major aerospace and real estate industries, during the 1980s and 1990s counted organized medicine as its *major* lobbying force during most years.[(21)]) The political hijinks learned years ago by "democratic" machine politicians are utilized by PACs, not only of medicine but all other industrial or economic concerns financially important enough to need legislative protection from "the people." Ballot-box prostitutes have honed to a refined science the guiding, thwarting and alteration of legislation.

The media as co-conspirator

At the public-perception level, organized American allopathic medicine essentially captured the organized media decades ago. Part of the capture, of course, relates to economic vested interests — the boards of directors of media empires (be they of print or electronic persuasion) may be directly or indirectly tied into the same interlock of vested interests which ultimately educates the American public about "medicine" through advertising.

Journalists, largely products of rationalist/humanist education, have "bought" the 17th-century model in medicine as surely as the allopaths have, and are not to be blamed for unconsciously participating in the semantical process whereby the allopathic-pharmaceutical message is beamed to the public.

The media have been ongoing collaborators, if often subconsciously, of spreading the Allopathic Industrial Complex "line" by helping that complex appropriate the terms "doctor," "physician," "medicine" and even "curing."

Journalists from the "straight" media who visibly stray at ever greater distances from the Party Line in medicine (Morris Bealle in *Super Drug Story*, as an example;[22] this writer as a lesser one) can expect rough sailing and, often, peer rejection.

"Doctor" is perceived as the kindly Marcus Welby of television fame; hospital dramas and stories make up a fair portion of passive TV media entertainment; the medical profession, however beleaguered it may be, is still, in the public eye, a popular hero, if an ever more tainted one.

An editor is not to be blamed for accepting as gospel truth a press release from the AMA or the Food and Drug Administration (FDA) while setting aside or holding back a press release from an "unorthodox" group — he simply has been trained that way. That is, he has been "captured by the paradigm."

Paradigm capture and cognitive dissonance

Indeed, *paradigm capture* is an increasingly observed and studied phenomenon in modern psychology, and it, with a parallel factor, *cognitive dissonance* (as socially applied) can help make understandable just how an educated person with a seemingly intelligent and self-described objective mind cannot recognize or understand what he or she is seeing.

Cognitive dissonance — the holding of opposing thoughts at the same time — can also be described negatively as the *inability* or *disinterest* in processing new, unexpected or *unwanted* information.

Negative cognitive dissonance on a grand scale, for example, in many quarters greeted Columbus' epochal achievement in 1492 — sailing West to ostensibly arrive in the East and discovering "the Indies" because the world was round, not flat, when the pillars of orthodoxy (the Church and incipient science) essentially disagreed with the very concepts. For many Europeans at the time, since what Columbus claimed to have done could not be done, so, *ipso facto,* it *was* not done.

Understanding of this phenomenon is essential — it explains how intelligent, avowedly intellectually honest people can absolutely disagree about the rightness or wrongness of observed truth. In the vast majority of conflicts over truth, we are not dealing with conscious dishonesty, simply the consistent human problem of cognitive dissonance, one made all the more difficult to dislodge when there are great vested interests (greed and ego, primarily) in the maintenance of an incorrect paradigm.

In modern "scientific" medicine, for example, if orthodoxy (gatekeeper of presumed truth) has ruled that something cannot be (for example, laetrile reducing a tumor) and yet the objective evidence is that a tumor has indeed been reduced with this agent, then negative cognitive dissonance (inability or disinterest in processing new, unexpected or unwanted information) sets in: the patient must (a) have been misdiagnosed in the first place, (b) be somehow responding to prior standard or orthodox therapy (if this were ever administered in the first place), or if neither (a) nor (b) is tenable, then (c) be undergoing a "spontaneous remission" — that is, "cure" for reasons not presently understood but which must have to do with something, indeed *anything other than,* the "quack" "cure," since the latter cannot "work."

In collective/social terms, the allopathic thought system or construct is nothing more than that — a paradigm, a belief system, rigidly adhered to and believed in with the same fervor with which Christians embrace the Virgin Birth and redemption through Christ's crucifixion. When the paradigm comes acropper based on observed, objective, seemingly measurable phenomena, then the mind of the observer (usually a physician) must enter a phase of cognitive dissonance: it must block out the unwanted new truth or scramble psychologically to explain it away. In rare moments, intellectual honesty — acceptance — may set in.

Only an ongoing onslaught of unexpected (and, at first, unwanted) new information can eventually accomplish the desired processing of new truth in the human mentality.

The current holistic/metabolic/integrative revolution in modern medicine constitutes an onslaught of seemingly new and unwanted information difficult to process by the guardians of so-called scientific medicine (the Allopathic Industrial Complex) — it is at first usually not processed at all (cognitive dissonance) but is increasingly forcing its way into collective reality (paradigm shift).

As the paradigm shifts, media and public acceptance will follow.

References

1. Mendelsohn, RS, *Confessions of a Medical Heretic.* New York: Warner Books, 1979.
2. Berman, Edgar, *The Solid Gold Stethoscope.* New York: MacMillan, 1976.
3. "Faith and the Human Touch," in *Powers of Healing.* New York: Life-Time Books, 1989.
4. Jayne, WA, quoted in "Belief and the healing arts of ancient civilizations." *World Research News,* 2nd/3rd Quarter, 1993.
5. Kuhnau, WW, and Culbert, ML. *Live Cell Therapy: My Life with a Medical Breakthrough.* Tijuana BC, Mexico: Artes

Graficas de BC, 1983.
6. Berman, *op. cit.*
7. Hong-Yen Hsu and Preacher, WG, *Chinese Herb Medicine and Therapy*. Nashville TN: Aurora Publishers, 1976.
8. Ferguson, Wilburn, *Tsanza*, unpublished material made available to the author, and correspondence, 1976 - 1981.
9. Jayne, *op. cit.*
10. Huard, Pierre, and Wong, Ming, *Chinese Medicine*. New York/Toronto: McGraw-Hill, 1972.
11. Preston, Thomas, *The Clay Pedestal*. Seattle WA: Madrona, 1981.
12. Griggs, Barbara, *Green Pharmacy*. New York: Viking Press, 1981.
13. Goldwater, LD, quoted in Griggs, *op.cit.*
14. Dossey, Larry, *Space, Time & Medicine*. Boston/London: Shambhala, 1982.
15. Velikovsky, Immanuel, *Worlds in Collision*, New York: MacMillan, 1950.
16. de Grazia, Alfred, ed. *The Velikovsky Affair* (*The Warfare of Science and Scientism*). Hyde Park NY: University Books, 1966.
17. Dossey, *op. cit.*
18. Crawfurd, Raymond, *The Last Days of Charles* II. Oxford: Clarendon Press, 1909.
19. Culbert, ML, *Vitamin B17: Forbidden Weapon Against Cancer*. New Rochelle NY: Arlington House, 1974.
20. Beach, Wooster, *Reformed Medical Journal* (USA) I: 1, 1832.
21. *The Choice*. XV:3, Summer 1989.
22. Bealle, MA, *Super Drug Story*. Washington: Columbia Publishing, 1962.

V
THE PERPETUATION OF ERROR:
Victory of the Allopathic Paradigm

"The history of medical schools in the nineteenth century is a tale of schisms, conspiracies, and coups, often destroying the institutions in the process."

— Paul Starr, *The Social Transformation of American Medicine*

"The doctor comes with free good will
But ne'er forgets his calomel."

— *Detroit Review of Medicine and Pharmacy,* 1884

"The test to which all methods of treatment are finally brought is whether they are lucrative to doctors or not."

— George Bernard Shaw, *The Doctor's Dilemma*

"Physicians should . . . minister to the sick with due impressions of the importance of their office; reflecting that the ease, the health, and the lives of those committed to their charge, depend on their skill, attention and fidelity. They should study, also, in their deportment, to unite tenderness with firmness, and condescension with authority, as to inspire the minds of their patients with gratitude, respect and confidence."

— American Medical Association Code of Medical Ethics, 1847

"It is not your duty to cheat either yourself or other physicians out of a legitimate practice by supplying this person and that one with a word-of-mouth pharmacopoeia for general use . . . Use whatever strategy is necessary to prevent such persons from taking unfair advantage of your prescriptions."

— D.W. Cathell MD, *The Physician Himself*(1881)

Allopathy: the fight for authority and exclusion

Just as one cannot separate medicine from religion and magic at the philosophical level, neither can it be separated from politics at the social one:

The history of American medicine, culminating in the rise of the Allopathic Industrial Complex (AIC) and the war which has now broken out to dislodge it, is one of greed, arrogance, vested interests, colliding theories, political movements — and, of course, some genuinely good intentions.

As allopathic, symptom-based medicine arose as a natural element within the Cartesian-Newtonian thought process which underscored much of Renaissance "enlightenment," and took upon itself the definition of "scientific" practice, it needed to enshrine its authority in the law, exclude pretenders, establish legitimacy through licensure and, in America, manipulate semantics for the laity so that certain words took on specific meanings in order to bring about desired ends:

Only *licensed* degree holders from *recognized* schools should be able to practice *scientific medicine*. Any dissent from this train of concepts was *unscientific* at best, *quackery* at worst — even though the word "quack" did not always have the same venomous flavor with which it is used today.

The establishment of the Allopathic Industrial Complex in the United States was not completed until the twentieth century, when the allopathic paradigm made comfortable common cause with gigantic wealth, corporate interests and that peculiarly American phenomenon, organized philanthropy as a convenient tax-dodge, power-acquisitor and underwriter of theories (*VI*).

The roots of the complex, however, arose from the philosophical plane (the emergence of the "enlightenment" and rationalism in Renaissance times and thereafter, the Cartesian/Newtonian postulates, the Hippocrates-Galen-Vesalius evolution of ideas relating to medicine, anatomy and disease), the sociopolitical plane (the struggle for legitimacy, authority and sovereignty) and the economic one. The sociopolitical and economic roots are visible in the 18th century; the war for authority and the elimination of serious competition date from the 19th.

British beginnings

American medicine initially drew its inspiration from British medicine — though it was never able to import that system in its entirety.

The British approach had been largely determined in the 16th century when the reign of Henry VIII sought to bring order out of the chaos of medical practice in and around rapidly growing London at a time when "the great imitator," syphilis, was a major problem demanding full medical attention.

Indeed, 16th century medicine in England was a mirror of conceptual and semantical battles yet to come — for there now existed a vast body of medical lore and a rapidly developing apothecary (pharmaceutical) industry, primarily thanks to the Arabs of the Middle Ages. It was probably — then as now — snobbery (ego) which led persons well-trained in the "scientific" medicine of their day, equipped with knowledge of biology and anatomy and already dabbling in pharmacy, to look with disdain on midwives, folk medicine and treatment by "simples," including the practices of the quicksilver-dispensing back-alley practitioners who proliferated in the war against syphilis ("quacks").

The "practitioners of physic" — the original allopaths — took for themselves the grandiose title of *physicians* to distance themselves from the quacks, the amateurs, the dispensers of folk remedies, and even the surgeons, who, while supposedly limited to cutting, increasingly encroached upon the internal-medicine turf of the physicians. Below both were the "barber-surgeons" who practiced primitive dentistry, simple surgery, cupping and bleeding. These were distinct from the literal swarm of semi-skilled amateurs described as "a multitude of persons, of whom the greater part had no insight into physic, nor in any other kind of learning; some could not even read the letter on the book, so far forth, that common artificers, smiths, weavers and women, boldly and accustomably took upon them great cures, to the high displeasure of God, great infamy of the faculty, and the grievous hurt, damage and destruction of many of the king's liege people."[1]

Here allopaths were, typically, in seeming alignment with God, and there was a 16th-century call to "regulate the practice" and banish from it the quacks, pretenders and other agents of healing.

Hence, in 1512 Parliament passed the first of various acts, which continued through the 1540s, to enshrine "physicians," regulate the practice of medicine in London and environs and establish limitations and demarcations between various kinds of practitioners. (One act chastised surgeons who, "minding only their own lucre, and nothing the profit or ease of the disease or Patient, have sued, troubled, and vexed divers honest persons . . . the most part of the persons of the said Craft of surgery have small cunning, yet they will oftentimes impair and hurt their patients."[2])

However, the irony is that these 16th century acts which so instituted *physicians* as predominant in medicine also *protected* freedom of choice in medicine and specifically legalized herbalists (that is, "every person being the king's subject, having knowledge and experience of the nature of Herbs, Roots, and Waters, or of the operation of the same . . .") This particular act, derided by allopaths as "the quacks' charter," is the legal foundation by which herbalism (and, by implication, naturopathy) may be practiced in the United Kingdom today — and is, tangentially, a presumptive defense of such approaches in the United States.

American physicians were never able to transfer the British caste system of medicine to the Western shore of the Atlantic, but even so, the "regular" profession (dispensers of emetics, cathartics, purgatives, bleeding and leeching agents, together with surgeons and anatomists) considered themselves in the forefront of "science" and regarded others as "quacks" and/or "empirics." While the elite British physician was "above" charging for his services (and was sufficiently well off enough to have little interest in migrating to the Colonies), practitioners in British North

America included apothecaries, who followed a trade and were the primeval incarnation of today's pharmacists, and the surgeons, who — like barbers — practiced a craft.

Medicine in the Colonies

From earliest colonial days, though, would-be practitioners of "scientific medicine" were faced by a vast and varied medical folklore from Native Americans and the skilled if uneducated and unlicensed ministrations of midwives, abortionists, bonesetters, nostrum peddlers and the doctor of first resort, the farm mother.

The first American medical society was set up in New York in 1749. The first attempt by doctors to establish bodies with licensing power was that in 1763 by physicians in Norwich, Connecticut, who asked the local legislature to "distinguish between the honest and ingenious physician and the quack or empirical pretender"(3) — an effort that failed, as did John Morgan's initial effort at chartering a medical society with licensing authority in Pennsylvania.

The triumph of the American Revolution led to a flurry of interest in the new States to allow medical societies and licensing. Typical was the Massachusetts Medical Society, incorporated in 1781, established so that "a just discrimination . . . be made between such as are duly educated, and properly qualified for the duties of their profession, and those who may ignorantly and wickedly administer medicine. . ." (4)

Hence medical societies and licensure proliferated in the days of the earlier Republic, but with authority and legality remaining often in a very grey area. The westward movement of Americans and the republicanist trappings of the new "democracy" (a term not found in the Republic's founding documents and, it may be argued, never the real objective of the revolutionists of 1776) did not look kindly on caste systems, professional elitism or any of the other residue of monarchical Europe. The term "doctor" might well cover the apothecary, the general physician, the dispenser of toxic minerals and the to-be-avoided-except-when-all-else-fails surgeon.

The early medical schools were those of four universities (Harvard, Dartmouth, New York College of Physicians and Surgeons, and the University of Pennsylvania) which taught the rationalist/"solidist" doctrines of Galen and Boerhaave and one of whose major guiding lights in the early days of the Republic was Dr. Benjamin Rush, a signer of the Declaration of Independence who left his stamp on medical thought and training in the United States for generations.

American medicine in the 19th century

In the 19th century, American medicine was colored as much by politics ("democracy," particularly during the Jacksonian era, vs. oligarchical elitism, and the early efforts for deregulation, delicensure and medical freedom of choice against presumptive monopoly) as it was by "science" (the breakthroughs in medicine largely occurring in France later in the century) and, to a lesser but genuine extent, by religion (peculiarly born-in-America religious groups favored certain "sectarian," non-allopathic forms of medicine.)

At the level of economics, medicine was not a particularly attractive profession, with annual salaries of allopathic doctors holding steady at around $1000 a year in the middle decades of the 19th century as opposed to several hundred dollars earlier (and this was before rampant inflation). It was natural for educated physicians to resent the seeming profiteering of the sellers of herbal and other elixirs and preparations for the cure of everything from sleeplessness to cancerous tumors and also to be aware that common people regarded hospitals and mercury-dispensing, knife-wielding physicians as dangerous last-ditch resorts for treatment.

As America moved westward and "democracy" swept through the young Republic, the "regular" medical profession was faced with these contenders:

• "Herb doctors," also called "Indian doctors" or "botanics," ranging from uneducated users of the pharmacopeia of American

Indian tribes to allopathic doctors who added herbal remedies to their practices and often preferred them.

• The Thomsonian phenomenon of radical Samuel Thomson (1769-1843), who established a movement often described as a cult, rejecting school medicine and utilizing a treatment system built around the *lobelia* root (Indian tobacco) and steam baths.

• The independent patent medicine hawkers, who might appear anywhere selling a range of lotions, tonics and elixirs of plant, animal or mineral origin.

• The followers of health reformer Sylvester Graham (of "Graham cracker" fame), who advocated a vegetarian diet, sound hygiene, abstention from coffee and alcohol, and whose organization attracted women in considerable numbers at a time when other medical schools of thought were essentially sex-discriminatory.

• The natural bonesetters, who specialized in dislocations and fractures and who, usually without formal training, brought what Paul Starr described as "a kind of mechanical craftsmanship applied to medicine." (5)

• The doctrines of Christian Science as articulated by Mary Baker Eddy.

• And, finally, the homeopathic movement, which was introduced into the USA in 1825 but had been founded in the 18th century by Samuel Hahnemann, a brilliant German physician.

Thomsonians formed the major opposition to the "regulars" in the earlier 19th century — the homeopaths mounted the major challenge later and were involved with the allopaths in a major ideological and territoriality struggle whose conflicts colored much of 19th century medical history.

An "Eclectic" school of medical thought, uniting Thomsonians and some of the "Indian doctors," also flourished for a time, but never mounted the same degree of challenge to the "regulars" that came from homeopathy.

Some of these trends would coalesce later in the naturopathic movement, but naturopathy as a unified discipline was not a major factor in "alternative" medicine until the 20th century.

The conflicting schools of medical thought were often interwoven with philosophical and religious ideas: the Swedenborgians inclined toward homeopathy, Mormons favored Thomsonianism, the Millerites (and subsequent Seventh-Day Adventists) favored the mineral-water treatments called hydrotherapy and later essentially advocated vegetarianism as a way of life (if not as a school of medicine), and Christian Scientists engaged in a form of mind-over-matter medical practice, setting the stage for legal and conceptual conflicts which continue to the present day.

In rapidly growing, westward-moving America, there could be no single monopoly of medical thought, and medical options were as many and varied as were religious and political beliefs. It may be said of the middle decades of the 19th century that there was far more medical freedom of choice for Americans than has ever existed before or since, with the political state essentially adopting a hands-off posture. There also were death, disease and a lower median lifespan than in medical-monopoly times to come, but medicine was yet to turn truly political, and few Americans at the time believed that the Constitution contained any guarantee that either good health or good medicine should be a "right."

The challenge of homeopathy

Homeopathy was quite a different animal from the competing native American medical systems and ideas that sprang up in the wake of "democracy":

Here was a unified medical concept developed by well credentialed physicians (the intellectual and primary pioneer being Samuel Hahnemann, 1755-1843) whose growth in America was primarily accomplished by winning converts from among the "regulars." The theory and practice of homeopathy laid every bit as much claim to "science" as did the "regular" rationalist practitioners, for whom the homeopaths essentially reserved the word "allopaths" (treaters by contraries).

With Hippocrates, Hahnemann believed in and described a "vital force" in nature (*vis medicatrix naturae*), whose disturbance underlay disease and dysfunction.

Like the allopaths, the homeopaths were greatly concerned with the categorizing, cataloguing and understanding of symptoms of disease. But, diametrically opposed to the regular profession, homeopaths followed as a first law the Paracelsian dictum of *similia similibus curantur* — roughly, "like cures like," the "law of similars," a view also attributed to Hippocrates.

Where the allopathic "law of contraries" suggests that the answer to disease is to find an antidote or a *contrary* to suppress a symptom, Hahnemann and his followers (Constantine Hering being the great American articulator of Hahnemann) administered to the ill minuscule dilutions of a substance which, if given to healthy people, would produce symptoms similar to those of the patient. (As an example, ingestion of Belladonna might provoke scarlet fever-like symptoms in a healthy person; a Belladonna dilution hence homeopathically may cure scarlet fever in children.)

Under organized homeopathy, thousands of dilutions of natural substances have been "proven" against thousands of symptoms, and the correct dose or potency elaborated. The classical homeopath is as interested in the mental and emotional state of the patient as he is in the physical symptoms of the illness. Whole groups of symptoms fit mass profiles of pathology and psychology (the homeopathic *miasms* and *psoras*). The development of a homeopathic *materia medica*, whose pharmacopeia is a legal document in the United States, is the result of hundreds of thousands of "provings" of thousands of dilutions on millions of patients since the 18th century.

Homeopathy, first in Europe and later in America, where it spread like wildfire, brought a benign, non-toxic treatment for a vast array of diseases. Therapy consisted of the careful interviewing of the patient, the taking and recording of his symptoms, the consultation of existing information on the ever-growing list of homeopathic dilutions available, and then dispensing, usually orally and in liquid drops, the correct doses of the correct remedies, all without nauseating, blistering, bleeding, or physically disturbing the host. It had everything to which organized allopathy would become ever more resistant: gentleness, non-invasiveness, and economy. Proper homeopathy if properly applied meant that a single round of treatment with infinitesimally minute dilutions of substances should be all that was necessary for cure — not a device to keep the patient ever returning for a constant supply of drugs. The dilutions were themselves so tiny that there could hardly be a justifiable markup in their production and they often could just be given away.

While allopaths might note a similarity to the accepted theory of immunization of Edward Jenner (a gross demonstration of a homeopathic-like process in which a diseased person's immune system is stimulated to protect itself against a disease by the actual administration of the same disease), it would not let the German "new school" infest America without a major fight. In a matter of years, homeopathy became the primary competitor to allopathy in the medical marketplace, the rising star of the "empirics," a foreign implant flourishing in the democratic soil of the new Republic.

As the non-allopathic schools of medicine grew, the control over licensing by "regulars" diminished; and as they diminished some of the "irregular" schools established their own licensing mechanisms.

Georgia's medical licensing law, originally passed in 1825 to empower allopaths, was changed in 1839 to read that it did not operate against Thomsonians, herbalists "or any other practitioner."[(6)] In 1847 Georgia set up a Botanic Medical Board of Physicians and stipulated that only botanical doctors with degrees from botanical colleges could collect their fees in court actions.

Harris Coulter, the gifted chronicler of American homeopathy, informs us that in two decades (the 1820s and 1830s) Delaware, Vermont, Maine, Indiana, Maryland, and South

Carolina repealed their allopathic licensing laws in whole or in part, and that when the then-aborning American Medical Association (AMA) surveyed what for it was the sorry state of affairs in 1849

> . . . *it found, furthermore, that Rhode Island, Pennsylvania, Virginia, North Carolina, Texas, Tennessee, Kentucky, and Missouri had never regulated medical practice, while in Wisconsin, Iowa and Arkansas existing legislation appeared to have fallen into abeyance. The only states in 1849 with any claim to regulate practice were Louisiana, Michigan, New Jersey, and the District of Columbia.*[7]

While Thomsonianism diminished as a major competitor after the 1850s, Eclectic medical institutes or societies existed in Ohio, Connecticut, California, New York, Georgia, Illinois and Massachusetts, an Eclectic Dispensatory had been published (1854) and physicians calling themselves Eclectics would exist well into the 20th century.

But neither Thomsonians nor Eclectics nor herbalists nor nostrum peddlers developed the combined sociopolitical-economic threat that the homeopaths did.

After the first American homeopathic institute was founded (1844) and the (Homeopathic) Hahnemann Medical College was established in Philadelphia in 1848, the "new school" proliferated across the land from its more geographically limited beginnings in the 1820s. Homeopathic doctors frequently joined, or came from the ranks of, existing allopathic medical societies. International in scope, armed with its own journals and education, homeopathy became so commonplace that laymen often could not distinguish between the two major schools — the kindly physician visiting the farm by horse-drawn carriage and carrying a black bag might just as easily be a homeopath as an allopath, and laymen were rarely interested in the schooling of practitioners unless their curiosity were piqued by observing their differing procedures.

A homeopathic journal in 1865 outlined why one physician

turned from the "regular" to the "sectarian" practice: "After having blistered, bled, and drugged my patients for twenty-seven years, I determined to find some more humane mode." (8)

This led the physician to a consideration of homeopathy against cholera, and he found it a highly successful approach to the malady when it hit Dayton, Ohio, in 1849.

By the Civil War, homeopathy had taken on a political hue — the majority of homeopathic practitioners were either Republicans or Abolitionists. The social elites of New York and Boston preferred homeopaths, and homeopaths were earning more for their services than allopaths.

Dr. Tulio Suzzara Verdi (1829-1902), a refugee from revolutionary Italy, became perhaps the most colorful homeopath in American history, and, as the personal physician of Abraham Lincoln's secretary of state, William Seward, would greatly influence the federal government and District of Columbia. He attended various high officials of the Lincoln administration, fought politically with influential allopaths, and found his golden moment in work with the Homeopathic Yellow Fever Commission. This was a board set up to assess medical records in the battle against the New Orleans yellow fever epidemic in 1878 which spread up the Mississippi Valley, causing more than 74,000 cases and 16,000 deaths.

The surgeon general had appointed a commission to assess the causes and prevention of yellow fever, but Dr. Verdi had been unable to have a homeopath placed on it. Hence, with help from a benefactress, Mrs. Elizabeth Thompson, and the American Institute of Homeopathy, he was able to set up the Homeopathic Yellow Fever Commission.

The statistics gathered by the homeopaths were convincing: death rates from homeopathically treated yellow fever victims were between 5.6% and 7.7% as opposed to 16% and higher overall for those in the hands of allopaths. The homeopathic yellow fever victory profoundly influenced congress and also swayed the American people. It also stiffened the spine of the allopathic majority to continue its crusade to "do something" about the "new school," which seemed unstoppable.[9]

Allopathy fights back

During the battles for power and authority in 19th-century American medicine, the non-allopathic "sectarians" never achieved victory by numbers — "regulars" were in the majority in every decade. It was estimated that by 1871 some 13% of all medical practitioners were in the "sectarian" camp, that of 75 medical schools 15 were operated by non-allopaths, and that by the 1880s allopaths operated 76 medical schools, homeopaths 14 and Eclectics 8.[10]

Some of the reason for minority status of course had to do with the "irregulars" themselves — they were often as doctrinaire as the allopaths, as unwilling to compromise, as certain of their "science" as the "old" school. Homeopaths would eventually split into major opposing groups over the issue of which levels of which dilutions were best to prescribe.

But in the meantime, the growing number of non-allopathic physicians — and that considerable segment of open-minded doctors who might indeed be academically trained as allopaths but who also engaged in homeopathy or other "natural cures" which would later be regarded as naturopathy — continually posed a challenge to the orthodoxy at every turn.

The issues bore on economics (homeopaths, particularly, made more money as a group than allopaths), social impact (homeopaths were among the first to offer free medical services) and, strangely enough, openness.

In keeping with European guild thinking, the regular doctors often moved in an atmosphere of secrecy, as if to protect the inner workings of their craft — as had, in earlier ages, the stone masons from whose international, secrecy-shrouded organizations the Masonic movement in part evolved through a presumed group need to protect the secrets of building and architecture. In keeping with the general anthropology of it all — doctors as quasi-divine

— the physicians, particularly the allopaths, seemed intent on insulating themselves from the public through the use of Latin terms and avoidance of answering patient questions, an arrogant and haughty attitude which persists to this day.

In 1881, D.W. Cathell, in a multi-editioned tome (*The Physician Himself*), set the standards for image-building and keeping the (allopathic) doctor at a distance from the patient. Conviviality between doctor and patient, he argued, "has a levelling effect, and divests the physician of his proper prestige."[11]

Be quick in diagnosis, swift to treat under the image of intellectual certainty, wrote Cathell, whose manual depicted doctors as seeming to face a skeptical, even hostile clientele. He also suggested various ways for physicians to mask the contents of their prescriptions: "By employing the terms *ac. phenicum* for carbolic acid, *secale cornotum* for ergot, *kalium* for potassium, *natrum* for sodium . . . etc., you will debar the average patient from reading your prescriptions."

He also firmly argued against helping people treat themselves:

> *Especially avoid giving self-sufficient people therapeutic reports that they can themselves resort to . . . It is not your duty to cheat either yourself or other physicians out of a legitimate practice by supplying this person and that one with a word-of-mouth pharmacopeia for general use. If compelled to give a person his self-conceit and make him feel that he knows enough to practice self-medication and dispense with your services, use whatever strategy is necessary to prevent such persons from taking unfair advantage of your prescriptions.*[12]

While homeopaths often engaged in the same kind of Latin-based professional gobbledegook, the homeopath nonetheless provided the wherewithal for people to treat themselves at home with kits of homeopathic remedies. Housewives in particular became distributors and users of homeopathic remedies, and the latter cost so little to prepare that they were often given away.

The remedies, dilutions of natural sources triturated or shaken (succussed) down to a dose so minuscule that, in some cases, only the "vital force" was thought to remain, were at the very least harmless. The tendency of the homeopathic practitioner to be extremely patient with the client, jot down all signs and symptoms — to spend sympathetic time with the patient — was another strong appeal of "the new school." Homeopaths seemed to care, and their practices did not, nor could they, terrify the patient.

Great were the pangs of self-righteous outrage uttered by the allopaths that "unscientific" individuals, "quacks," be they homeopaths or not, not only actually made money off medicine, but frequently (and in terms of homeopaths, usually) received more pay than did the calomel dispensers.

Intoned the *New York Journal of Medicine* in 1846, as the idea of an AMA was just getting underway: "quackery . . . occasions a large pecuniary loss to us . . . degenerate members of our own body condescend, from the desire of pecuniary gain, to embrace the trade of the charlatan."[(13)]

And, observed another: "The United States . . . must be regarded as the very elysium of quackery . . they assume an equality . . . and by fraud and deception, too frequently triumph and grow rich, where wiser and better men scarcely escape starvation."[(14)]

The Massachusetts Medical Society in 1848 seemed to let it all hang out. It noted that

> *In times long since past there was supposed to be something recondite, mysterious, far above the apprehension of the vulgar, in the knowledge of medicine. The oracular air, and the dictatorial authority which they assumed, were submitted to as rightfully belonging to those who possessed secrets of nature and art of an almost supernatural character . . . The confidence of mankind . . . in the regular profession has changed its character, and has probably much diminished.*[(15)]

Lamented the Michigan Medical Society:

Our noble art . . has indeed fallen so low that there are few to do it reverence . . . quackery and empiricism in divers forms, like the locusts and lice of Egypt, swarm over our state and are eating out the very vitals and sucking the life blood of the community.[16]

And, said the New Hampshire Medical Society: "We are really in less repute with the people than the unblushing, boasting, presumptuous quack."[17]

The regular profession, thus, faced with an increasing decline in public trust, facing economic and ego challenges by the "irregulars," most predominantly the homeopaths, and also aware of the disorganized and sorry state of medical schools and medical curricula, decided that it was time to do something drastic.

Advent of the AMA

Just years before the AMA was formed, though, a survey in 1843-1844 by the Monroe County Medical Society in New York had found that, although "quackery and patent nostrums everywhere abound," it was also "equally evident that public opinion will not tolerate penal enactments prohibiting Empiricism."[18] That is, as late as the mid-1840s the allopathic network accepted the reality of freedom of choice in medicine despite its strong opposition thereto.

That was all to change.

The movement to form a national American allopathic medical association in the 1840s has been defended by apologists as answering more the need for upgrading medical education and practice — admittedly in an organizational shambles as of that decade — than as an attack on homeopathy *per se*.

Yet the central figure in calling for, organizing and serving as spiritual mentor of the AMA in its first half century was Dr. Nathan Smith Davis of New York, a bitter foe of homeopathy and, as Harris Coulter has recalled in detail, "the single man most responsible for the extreme anti-homeopathic orientation of

American medicine."[19]

There were several starts and stops along the way to securing interest from the disparate state allopathic medical societies in forming a national body. The *New York Journal of Medicine* set the issue squarely in 1845:

> *The profession in almost every state in the union is now left, so far as legal enactments are concerned, to take care of itself. . . For if we cannot make rules or laws which will banish stupidity and empiricism, we can, at least, fix our* own *standard of qualification, and thereby say who* we *will recognize as* our *associates.*[20]

Davis noted the same year that

> *all a young man has to do in order to become a physician is admittance into the office of some physician, where he can have access to a series of ordinary medical text-books, and see a patient perhaps once a month . . . and in the course of three years thus spent, one or two courses of lecture in the medical college, where the whole science of medicine, including anatomy, physiology, chemistry, materia medica, pathology, practice of medicine, medical jurisprudence, surgery, and midwifery are all crowded upon his mind in the short space of sixteen weeks — and his education, both primary and medical, is deemed complete.*[21]

The first National Medical Convention convened in May 1846 in New York, primarily to set up committees and agendas to report in 1847 on broader plans for the new national organization. In that year the doctors noted that, in addition to low scholarship standards, general disorganization and the threat of "empiricism," there was also the matter of overcrowding of the profession, with some 80,000 physicians of one kind or another, divided almost evenly between "regulars" and "irregulars," thought to be practicing at that time.

The net result of the jostling and propaganda was the evolution, in 1847, of the American Medical Association (AMA).

Had it been honest at its inception — which it was not — it would have been more properly called the American Allopathic Medical Association. Its appropriation of the word "medicine" would be a guidepost to its continuing zeal for semantical manipulation, co-optation, centralization and destruction of opposition all under the guise of streamlining, organizing, purifying and bringing its own set of standards to "scientific medicine."

The formal title "American Medical Association" was officially adopted May 5, 1847, and the organization was incorporated in Illinois — where it has remained ever since. Dr. Nathaniel Chapman was elected its first president. The AMA's stated objectives were "to upgrade medical education, establish standards for medical practice, advance medical knowledge, promote the usefulness, honor and interests of the medical profession, *educate public opinion*, and encourage concerted action by physicians." The AMA, said Chapman, "presents a spectacle of moral grandeur delightful to contemplate."

Yet 100 years later President Harry S. Truman would refer to the organization as "just another mean trust."[22]

The Michigan Medical Society mouthed in 1850 the new group-think of the AMA and of its continual awareness of its major foe:

> *We are the guardians of the public health . . . We have to defend our interest, the public health, against a worse enemy, even, and one more subtle than disease: an enemy in league with it, spreading desolation and death wherever it goes . . . An enemy who has many strongholds upon the affections of the people; and one who in many places more than rivals us in their esteem. . .*[23]

While American homeopathy's best days still lay ahead, and it remained a strong force in the 19th century, the AMA's thrust for consolidation of the whole medical profession meant that, gradually, much of homeopathy and Eclecticism succumbed to co-optation. This was partly because these two schools shared with the allopaths a desire for protection against untrained practitioners, since allopaths, homeopaths and Eclectics all had their own schools and organizations.

As late as 1892, after all, the homeopaths had established their own treatment network, controlling some 110 hospitals, 145 dispensaries, 62 orphan asylums and homes for the aged, more than 30 nursing homes and sanatoria and 16 insane asylums.[24] They had their own major institute, major medical school, pharmacopeia and medical journals. Eclectics claimed some 10,000 practitioners. They no more relished being undercut by other "irregulars" than did allopaths enjoy seeing their own market share whittled down by "sectarians."

It was not until later in the 20th century that the rise of the Allopathic Industrial Complex (AIC) would all but do away with the "new school," but the seeds of its destruction lay slowly germinating during the time of homeopathy's American heyday, the last half of the 19th century. They included:

— The aforementioned desire of the homeopaths themselves to be protected against medical infidels, even if it might mean occasional accommodations with the allopaths in terms of medical education, medical regulations and medical licensing procedures.

— The fact that the homeopathic movement underwent a severe doctrinal schism at home and internationally — between the proponents of "high" and "low" dilutions of homeopathic remedies. The schism set up mutually insulting and back-biting ideological camps.

The coming of 'scientific medicine'

But far more important were two major trends in medicine in America particularly after 1850:

— The onrush of scientific achievements in medicine within the general parameters of allopathy, paralleled by an explosion of renewed interest in science itself, a kind of "second Renaissance" sweeping North America. The new breakthroughs seemed far more to favor the allopaths, whose linear approaches had suffered severely at the hands of the "irregulars." And

— The early development of the pharmaceutical industry, which would make common cause with the allopaths, sensing (correctly) that homeopathy represented a natural enemy in the medical marketplace. The early wedding of allopathic and pharmaceutical interests would provide organized allopathy (particularly the AMA) with a massive new source of revenue, directly or indirectly, through advertisements in medical publications and the ultimately comfortable relationship between drug companies (be they "ethical" or "patent") and their natural distributors — the allopaths.

The achievements of "scientific medicine" — to which allopaths laid claim — first came in bacteriology in the 1860s-1870s in the work of Louis Pasteur and Robert Koch, who won the raging ideological debates in French medical academe over host-vs-microbe ideology and set allopathy off on a decisive new tack which would come to dominate allopathic thinking well into the 20th century. The idea that *microbes* caused disease, rather than disease being a disturbance of vital forces or something else within the host, deflected attention from concern in general about the patient to a mad rush for knowledge about those microorganisms, those microbes, those *germs*, which must surely be the "cause" of all disease *within* the host. That is, the central error of allopathy — abandonment of the holistic concept — became institutionally perpetuated.

It is known that Pasteur, on his deathbed, essentially recanted. Of his long-time ideological foe, colleague and contemporary, Claude Bernard, who defended host-as-paramount, Pasteur was said to have confessed: "*Bernard avait raison. La germe n'est rien — c' est le terrain qui est tout*" — "Bernard was right. The germ is nothing, the terrain (soil) is everything."[25]

While this reassessment may have been overstated, the great impetus to the study of disease by the discovery that so many (but by no means all) diseases had some exogenous cause that could be detected and then attacked has represented modern medicine's most important fork in the road.

From that point on, full knowledge of the patient (his own health, that of his family and forebears, his diet, habits and attitudes) would take a seat behind knowledge of the "etiological cause" (be it microbe, bacterium, germ, parasite — and later, of course, virus or gene) of the disease.

The "causes" of many of the feared killer diseases of the era (diphtheria, typhus, typhoid fever, tetanus, yellow fever, cholera, plague — and perhaps the most sinister and multifaceted of all, syphilis, "the great masquerader" or "imitator") were not long in being delineated. As Jenner had set the stage for immunization techniques and ideas a century before with the smallpox vaccine, the development of diphtheria antitoxin in the 19th century constituted a major achievement for allopathic thinking. Victories over tetanus, typhoid, cholera and plague were to follow, even though these often could be affected or even eliminated by proper homeopathic treatments.

The rise of antiseptic surgery in the latter 19th century also provided more vindication for allopathy: the use of knife and scalpel, so often associated with suffering and failure, took on some new respect, and mortality from operations significantly declined.

New advances in diagnostic techniques from mid-century onward brought a new range of equipment within the physician's grasp — the stethoscope, ophthalmoscope, and laryngoscope, for example.

Yet it should not be forgotten that most of these breakthroughs were achieved by people who were often assailed mightily by the medical orthodoxy for their efforts — Joseph Lister, father of modern antiseptic surgery, was roundly denounced by his medical peers; Ignasz Semmelweiss, who insisted physicians wash their hands between deliveries of babies, was driven to an insane asylum. In their time, Jenner, and later Pasteur, were, to some, nothing more than "quacks." The road to new concepts is forever strewn with the ideological bones of those who dared to think new thoughts.

Rise of the drug empire

But what would ultimately do in the non-allopaths eventually was the drive for profits and pure greed, as exemplified by the pharmaceutical industry, which began in the United States during the Civil War in Washington's efforts to keep the Union forces supplied with calomel and other toxic "curatives."

Just as the European apothecaries had resented Hahnemann in the century prior, the rising drug business in America instinctively sensed, particularly in homeopathy, its natural enemy: it was a method of tiny dilutions of natural substances in which less was held to be better and more effective and the cost of production was virtually initiated at a point of diminishing returns.

A philosophy that enunciated corrections of "the vital force" by tiny amounts of natural things, possibly never needing to be administered more than once, was a clear and present danger to an industry which needed to produce gross numbers of gross products in which more was said to be better and more effective. And, any system of medicine that said in effect that correct eating, drinking and *thinking* habits, with adequate rest and exercise, were the ways to health or that stressed fasting or detoxifying the body through natural means, or which would oppose the violation of the human temple by noxious substances of all kinds, even in the interest of rooting out a microbe, was a natural antagonist to the thinking and interests of the drug dispensers.

In the Civil War and immediate post-Civil War era, a number of companies competed among themselves for the production of drugs used by allopaths. These included Sharpe and Dohme, E.R. Squibb and Frederick Stearns, as the pioneers, to be joined by Warner, Parke-Davis, Lilly, the two Merrells, Merck, and Abbott Laboratories, among others.

The growth of the "ethical" drug companies (those which provided drugs with known formulas and known ingredients essentially to medical professionals) was matched by an explosion of "patent medicines" — sometimes called *nostrums* — which were remedies whose ingredients were usually kept secret but whose names were copyrighted or otherwise trademark-protected. The patent medicines were pitched directly to the consumer, and claimed to cure everything from baldness to cancer.

The advent of patent medicines would soon provide the excuse for an attack by the "investigative journalists" of their day, the *muckrakers*, to expose the shabby situation of the uncontrolled pharmaceutical industry and, in the popular mind, set the stage for the "need" for government control thereof, eventually leading to the development of the government pillar of the Allopathic Industrial Complex — its enforcer, arbiter, policeman and extortion agent, the Food and Drug Administration (FDA).

The drug companies began publishing their own periodicals but swiftly found it even easier to peddle their wares by setting up ostensibly independent medical journals which became little more than print propaganda for pharmaceuticals.

Harris Coulter recounted the early days of drug-oriented medical journalism in America by examining the publishing antics of Parke-Davis:

Following the company's incorporation in 1875, it set up a publishing department "to maintain its legitimate ties with the medical profession." Its initial publication was called *New Preparations*, to be followed in 1877 by the purchase of the *Detroit Medical Journal*, which was converted into the *American Lancet*, whose long-time editor was, among other things, a vice-president of the AMA, a trustee of the AMA's *Journal*, and president of the Michigan Medical Society.

New Preparations became the *Therapeutic Gazette* in 1880, whose editorship went to a man who would become president of the Philadelphia College of Physicians. There then followed *Medical Age* (1883), *Druggists' Bulletin* (1887) and *Medicine* (1895).

Wrote Coulter:

It is difficult to believe that this large array of

periodicals was needed just to present information on Parke-Davis's contributions to medical science. The probability is greater that this journalistic population surplus was designed to provide paying positions for the leaders of the allopathic profession and thus to guarantee a favorable reception for the company's products.[26]

Aside from mouthpiece journals set up directly by the drug companies, the industry pumped in increasing amounts of paid advertising to "legitimate" medical publications, so that by the end of the century there were approximately 250 medical journals, with only one supported solely by the profession alone. All the other major ones, very much including the AMA's own *Journal of the American Medical Assn. (JAMA)*, the *New Medical Record*, and the *American Journal of the Medical Sciences*, were supported in varying amounts by drug industry advertising.[27]

Which is to say, the allopathic medical journals became a useful and willing conduit for the growing pharmaceutical industry. The "legitimate" journals as well as the mouthpiece publications took turns sniping at homeopathy and other competitors of the allopathic paradigm for, at root, the basest of reasons — allopaths were to be, putting it bluntly, drug pushers.

However much the Allopathic Industrial Complex would later rail against this reality, it could not successfully avoid it — as page after page after page of expertly crafted advertising which now dominates the "standard" medical journals in the United States eloquently attests on a weekly basis. It was known in the last century as in the present that he who pays the piper calls the tune — and in terms of medical journals the primary piper-payer beginning in the last half of the 19th century was the drug industry. It still is.

So the revolutionizing currents in American medicine in the last half of the century were due far more to economics (the growth of the drug industry) and renewed interest in science, than to successful politicking by the AMA — the full brunt of which would not be felt until the 20th century. In fact, as of 1900 the

AMA had only 8,000 members, while the total membership of other societies (including local and state) was about 33,000, with 77,000 practitioners belonging to no organizations at all.[28]

New contenders

Before the century was over, new contenders had arisen to allopathy which did not seem ready for co-optation in the best interests of unified medicine: Christian Science remained outside the pale (and, indeed, the opposition to this organization by older Protestant bodies was one of the social forces in favor of standardizing medicine); osteopathy, founded in the 1880s by Andrew Still, a rural Missouri doctor, focused on repairing the body by placing its parts in their presumed proper relationship; chiropractic believed most of disease was the result of energy disturbances caused by vertebral misalignments (subluxations); and, suddenly, there was naturopathy.

Eventually, in the 20th century the American medical monopoly-to-be would essentially co-opt osteopathy (while leaving the degree intact), but it would find as its major contender for power in the late 20th century the rapidly growing chiropractic profession, which it viciously — and unsuccessfully — sought to suppress.

As a separate discipline, naturopathy arrived in America in 1896 in the person of Benedict Lust of Germany, whose tuberculosis had been resolved by a "nature cure" consisting of hydrotherapy, vegetarianism and "air baths." This European system (with Priessantz, Kniepp and others as pioneers) frequently had been combined with homeopathy. Lust wanted to make the treatments known in America

As naturopaths recall it, Lust, as an idealistic youth, "was shocked to find his natural health message opposed by medical authorities. He was soon arrested and fined $800 for practicing medicine without a license for giving a bath and massage to an undercover agent (*shades of the late 20th century!*). When he complained, he was arrested again, 'carried to the Tombs as if I had committed murder,' indicted for criminal libel, and placed under $10,000 bond."[29]

The man who founded the American School of Naturopathy in New York in 1901 would ultimately be arrested another 30 times on similar charges. He eventually earned an MD degree in order to ward off prosecution. Naturopathy was to fade in and out of the American scene as allopathic medicine took on new power, authority and centralization.

A paradigm in motion

For by 1900-1901, the American allopathic paradigm was well in motion:

Increasingly, scientific researchers were joining hands with medicine. Johns Hopkins University opened its medical school in 1893 with a four-year program and the (at the time) radical requirement that no student could enter without prior college degrees. This was a landmark event in the reform of medical education which had begun around 1870.

The 19th century had begun with a small but organized allopathic cabal in conflict with unregulated and often unschooled practitioners and various claimants to the medical arts. The democratic wave which swept over young America had halted all attempts at centralized authority and had ushered in decades of medical freedom of choice. This freedom had seen the rise of competing schools of medicine, some highly organized, and a general, if glorious, chaos in the polymorphous growth of the profession overall. Bolstered by international currents (the French medical revolution), science in general and other forces, medicine (as captained by allopathy) moved toward cohesion, centralization, authority and sovereignty.

These currents would converge in the rise of the Allopathic Industrial Complex (AIC) in the 20th century.

References

1. Griggs, Barbara, *Green Pharmacy*. New York: Viking Press, 1981.

2. *Ibid.*
3. Rothstein, William, *American Physicians of the Nineteenth Century.* Baltimore: Johns Hopkins Press, 1972.
4. Fitz, RH. "The rise and fall of the licensed physician in Massachusetts, 1781-1860." *Transactions* of the Assn. of American Physicians 9, 1894.
5. Starr, Paul, *The Social Transformation of American Medicine.* New York: Basic Books, 1982.
6. Coulter, HL, *Divided Legacy: The Conflict between Homoeopathy and the American Medical Association.* Richmond CA: North Atlantic Books, 1973.
7. Coulter, *op. cit.*
8. *American Homoeopathic Observer*, II, 1865.
9. Coulter, *op. cit.*
10. Starr, *op. cit.*
11. Cathell, DW, *The Physician Himself.* Philadelphia: FA Davis, 1881.
12. *Ibid.*
13. *New York Journal of Medicine*, VI, 1846.
14. Coulter, *op. cit.*
15. Massachusetts Medical Society, *Medical Communications*, VII, 1848.
16. *Proc.* Michigan Medical Society, 1850.
17. *Transactions*, New Hampshire Medical Society, 1865.
18. *Boston Medical and Surgical Journal*, XXVIII, 1843.
19. Coulter, *op. cit.*
20. *New York Journal of Medicine*, V, 1845.
21. *Ibid.*
22. Culbert, ML, *What the Medical Establishment Won't Tell You that Could Save Your Life.* Virginia Beach VA: Donning, 1983.
23. *Proc.* Michigan Medical Society, 1850.
24. Coulter, *op. cit.*
25. Ornstein, Robert, and David Sobel, *The Healing Brain.* New York: Simon and Schuster, 1987.
26. Coulter, *op. cit.*
27. *Ibid.*
28. Starr, *op. cit.*
29. Boyle, Wade, "Our naturopathic heritage." *The Naturopathic Physician*, VI:3, Fall 1991.

VI
THE INSTITUTIONALIZATION OF ERROR:
The coming of the Allopathic Industrial Complex

"Competition is a sin."

— John D. Rockefeller

"Philanthropy is the essential element in the making of Rockefeller power. It gives the Rockefellers a priceless reputation as public benefactors which the public values so highly that power over public affairs is placed in the Rockefellers' hands. Philanthropy generates more power than wealth alone can provide."

— Myer Kutz, *Rockefeller Power*

"All professions are conspiracies against the laity."

— George Bernard Shaw

"Current Medical Science is nothing but a false dogma, imposed almost universally, by no matter what means, legitimate or not, by a smoothly organized coterie that in all industrialized nations form the Medical Power, in alliance with the Chemical Syndicate. Their purpose . . . is not the people's health, which is just being used as a pretext for extorting large sums of money, but the aggrandizement of their own wealth and might."

— Hans Ruesch, *Naked Empress*

"The institution of medicine has a great deal invested in the perpetuation of the myth of objective evaluation. It underpins the cognitive and social authority of its practitioners and legitimates powerful vested interests, not only in medicine, but in society at large."

— Evelleen Richards *(The Politics of Therapeutic Evaluation: the Vitamin C and Cancer Controversy)*

Emergence of the Allopathic Industrial Complex (AIC)

The emergence of the Allopathic Industrial Complex [AIC] in the United States is a direct result of the following events and historical tendencies, whose sum total now impacts on many millions of people:

— The enshrining of allopathy as "scientific medicine," an outgrowth of several historical trends in the Christian Era (*IV*).

— The eventual victory, in the United States, of organized allopathy over its contenders through centralization, co-optation, politics and the wedding of allopathic theory to the pharmaceutical industry, beginning in the 19th century (*V*).

— The advent of anti-competitive monopoly corporate capitalism early in the this century, paralleled by born-in-America socialist/collectivist ideas (the Progressive Era, the New Deal, American "liberal" incarnations of British-born Fabian socialism.)

— The rise of organized philanthropy, often as a cover for profiteering by corporate capitalism, through which massive funds for "research" and "education" became available.

— The battle against patent medicines socially stimulated by "muckraker" journalism which gave rise to the original Pure Food and Drug Act of 1906 — which led to formation of the incipient Food and Drug Administration (FDA).

— The Flexner Report of 1910, primarily a creature of corporate capitalist/organized philanthropic interests which would extend monopoly control through research and education over American medical schools, greatly aiding and abetting the allopathic concept and converting organized medicine, often, into a conduit for pharmaceutical profits.

— The rise in the 1920s-1930s of gargantuan international trusts and monopolies as primarily exemplified by a marriage of convenience between the Rockefeller interests in America and the German-based I.G. Farben cartel, a spiderweb of economic activities continuing to this day and often enmeshed with the privately directed world banking community.

— The growth of the American Medical Assn. as a monopoly

labor union/trade association for allopaths.

— The New Deal revolution of the 1930s which, among many things, led to the redefined federal Food, Drug and Cosmetic Act (1938), which gave government a far greater hand in health and drugs and also helped institutionalize the medical/pharmaceutical monopoly.

— The rise of private third-party insurance plans in the 1930s as efforts for socialized medicine were defeated.

— The American commitment to an explosion of scientific inquiry and the making available of huge amounts of federal research funds for this purpose following World War II.

— The advent of Medicare and Medicaid in the 1960s, parallel to the growth and development of a medical-industrial complex uniquely American in nature and combining aspects of social insurance while shoring up the enormous profits of medicine and the pharmaceutical industry.

We have examined the philosophical beginnings of allopathic "scientific medicine" and the victory-by-vested-interests of the American medical establishment in the 19th century. Separate chapters deal more closely with the sorry state of affairs at the FDA and the development of the AMA.

The shadows of history

As we have seen, one cannot separate the history of medicine from that of politics and economics. This is all the more evident in delineating medicine's major trends in America in the century soon to end — economic interests, politics and the practice of medicine are firmly embraced like lovers loath to part.

In the 20th century revolution of American medicine the names Carnegie and Rockefeller loom large.

By the first decade of the this century, there was a Carnegie Foundation for the Advancement of Teaching and there was a Rockefeller Institute for Medical Research. Both were philanthropical extensions of multimillionaire families which had already made their fortunes.

Ironically, John D. Rockefeller, whose General Education Board (GEB) ultimately poured millions of dollars into allopathic medical schools — which helped cause the poorly funded homeopathic institutions to die slowly by financial attrition — only accepted homeopathic treatments during his own life.

His lineage is of interest:

His father, William Avery ("Big Bill") Rockefeller, had been what the allopaths of today would call a cancer quack, an untutored salesman of quack cancer medicines primarily composed of crude oil and alcohol, at various times in his colorful life accused of horse theft, bigamy and rape — a self-confessed "slicker" who said that part of his education for his offspring was "I cheat my boys every chance I get."[(1)]

By the early 1900s the Rockefeller oil monopoly, an oil trust reorganized as Standard Oil, was gushing far more than barrels of petroleum, and was seeking to expand holdings in other areas. In the century's first decade, Rockefeller money was present to invest in medicine, and Carnegie money was present to help "reform" education.

Since the allegedly sorry state of medical education was a sore point to the AMA, whose first 60 years of existence had in fact accomplished little, the national body turned to Carnegie money for an avowedly "independent" review of medical education in America. Abraham Flexner, equipped with a bachelor's degree from Johns Hopkins, was picked by the Carnegie Foundation for the job. His brother, Simon, was president of the Rockefellers' medical research institute.

Accompanied by the secretary of the AMA's Council on Medical Education, Flexner visited each of the nation's medical schools (whose number had dropped from 162 in 1906 to 131 in 1910). The Flexner Report, in 1910, found, among many things, that America had too many poorly-trained physicians, that it also had some of the best, and that it could do with lesser numbers of better trained doctors. What the report in fact did was to open the door to the institutionalization of the allopathic medical paradigm while admittedly if arguably updating medical education in general. It became the litmus test for medical education in this century — and adherence to its views meant over the coming decades an influx of enormous sums of money from the huge tax-free foundations, which, by 1936, included $91 million from the Rockefeller GEB alone and millions more from other foundations.[2]

It has been observed that the GEB provided funds to "a select group of medical schools" and that, even though the board claimed to be a neutral monitor of science responding to the wishes of medical schools, "its staff actively sought to impose a model of medical education more closely wedded to research than to medical practice. These policies determined not so much which institutions would survive as which would dominate, how they would be run, and what ideals would prevail."[3]

The tax-free foundation scheme

The formerly fledgling Association of American Medical Colleges, the first version of which began in 1876, became a ready conduit for the use of foundation funds since the organization began setting "a wide range of standards for all medical schools. It determined the criteria for selecting medical students, for curriculum development, for programs of continuing medical education after graduation, and for communication within the profession as well as to the general public"[4] — while funded from early on by the Commonwealth Fund, the China Medical Board (Rockefeller Foundation division), the Kellogg Foundation, and the Macy, Markle, Rockefeller and Sloan foundations.[5]

The tax-free foundation scheme was adopted earlier in this century by ultrawealthy families as a means of protecting their own enormous profits even while an idea utterly alien to the American republic — a graduated income tax — would be superimposed on everyone else.

Viewing the second decade of this century, it is not difficult to reach the conclusion that a bloodless *coup d'etat* occurred in which key ideas of the original American republic were scuttled for new ones. The tax-free foundation artifice allowed for the mass concentration of enormous wealth in few hands, with tax-exempt "contributions to charity" (philanthropy) as the excuse. The sinister development of an organized central bank in private hands in the form of the Federal Reserve and the advent of the income tax accompanied these developments.

By the mid-1970s, it was estimated that "the great tax-free foundations" had invested over a billion dollars in the nation's medical schools, with half of the faculty receiving a part of their own income from foundation "research" grants and some 16 percent funded entirely in this manner. Getting in on the action were the Ford Foundation, the Kellogg Foundation, Sloan Foundation, Macy Foundation, and Commonwealth Fund, described as a Rockefeller "interlock."[(6)]

The foundation maneuver developed in the early Carnegie/Rockefeller days frequently called for "matching funds" on the part of recipients (that is, the "charitable" family trusts would donate an amount to a given institution which would raise from its members or the public an equal amount.)

Paralleling these activities was the honing to perfection of organized fund-raising drives, particularly exemplified by the National Foundation for Infantile Paralysis, the March of Dimes, and the American Cancer Society (*XI*). Organized fund-raising plus the existence of foundation money available through the tax-free foundation scheme often led to situations in which it became more profitable to look for the answer, and to keep looking, than to find it. (One wonders if, had it not been for European research, the Salk and Sabin vaccines against polio would have ever been fully legalized in the USA, where a hunt-for-the-cure polio industry raised enormous sums and usually failed to cure much of anything, even while the crusading nurse, Sister Kenney, had proved that polio could be controlled with entirely natural methods — she was, of course, for years shunned as an eccentric.)

While these events are fodder for conspiracy theories (and

each one was, in fact, a conspiracy of sorts) they also were concurrent with developments in American political thought.

Fabianism in America

One of these trends, as explained in considerable detail elsewhere,[7] was the coming to America of "British socialism" — actually, Fabian socialism — at a time when it was not popular to use the term "socialist." The advent of this basic theory of government and economics, a kind of communism without communists and emphasizing the power of the state to change and direct American society, led to new trends in public education, governmental social policy, and paradigm shifts in American politics — most noticeably the move from the concept of the American government system as a "republic" (rule by law) to the notion that what the Founding Fathers had in mind was a "democracy" (rule by mob). While few institutions (other, oddly enough, than the US military) were willing to differentiate between "democracy" and "republicanism" in the second decade of this century, champions of Fabianism were ultimately as successful in convincing Americans that they lived under "democracy" as allopaths were in convincing the public that allopathy is "medicine."

The advent of a "social agenda" for government in order to correct the manifest inequities and wrongs of human society is of largely Fabian socialist inspiration; the economic machinery to accomplish these aims (deficit spending, graduated income taxes, "guided inflation", "pump priming", subsidies etc.) is equally of Fabian socialist thought and would, in the coming decades, be hidden under the vague term "liberal" in the USA, as to distinguish such thinking from what the British more appropriately called "socialist."

The aforementioned *coup d' etat* in the USA in the second decade of this century allowed for a mass increase in collectivistic theories of government and economics alongside the rise of the tax-free foundations (for the protection of great wealth by a handful of American oligarchic-elite families, and hence the use of vast amounts of money, under the guise — and certainly, from time to time, the actual intent — of philanthropy). Virtually every move made by "dynamic government" since the second decade of this century has, of course, been excused by a perceived collective or national need (political equality of the sexes; racial equality; trust-busting; economic opportunity; rescuing the poor, homeless, elderly and crippled; one-man, one-vote; consumer protection; etc., *ad infinitum*). The net result of concentrating political and economic power to achieve political ends meant ineluctably that the economic power already concentrated (as through the tax-free foundations) would work with, if not outright control, the concentrated political power, and that, at least from time to time, this was the planned outcome.

The resulting structure politically has meant the untrammeled growth in the grasp and reach of government at all levels, with a concomitant decline in *actual* (as distinct from *perceived*) individual liberty, and, for all intents and purposes, the destruction of the non-oligarchic, non-democratic republican model of diffused, non-dynamic, locally-centered government bequeathed to Americans by the framers of the republic and authors of the original Constitution. Economically, it has meant, as in any collectivist system ranging from that of Ramses II to those of Josef Stalin and Adolf Hitler, the eventual and potentially totalitarian concentration of political and economic power in virtually the same hands. In the Western "democratic" models, however, this power is said to be held in check by somehow liberally enlightened political systems vaguely based on "humanism" and "rationalism." The final verdict of history on this *melange* has yet to be rendered.

No single conspiracy

It is inappropriate, however, to blame all rivulets leading to monopoly enthronement and control on a single, well-conceived conspiracy, as monolithic political thinkers of Left and Right are wont to do. Rather, they are a culmination of various concentrations of vested interests and egos (the real stuff of conspiracies) and represent several currents in American society.

In terms of medicine and pharmaceuticals these currents included the growth of organized labor, organized corporations and organized professions. They included the heyday of American journalism, too — a go-for-the-throat activity by journalists, who believed that Article I, Section I, of the Constitution calls for "the public's right to know" (it doesn't) and that part of the profession of the printed word lay in exposing the multifarious shenanigans of the rapidly developing giant corporations and trusts — and the burgeoning market in patent medicine nostrums.

That it suited the incubating medical-pharmaceutical monopoly for enterprising journalists to help expose patent medicines and that the response to these endeavors would ultimately expand the grasp of government itself is now obvious, but it is not demonstrated that there was a cohesive thread of conspiracy to link all these events. The early American Progressives — who themselves co-opted a term from the left side of the French political aisle, hence making government action to secure the rights of "the people" somehow a modern, intelligent, "progressive" thing to do — may or may not have known that the fruit of their well-intentioned endeavors would be the very thing they at least ideologically opposed: the totalitarian concentration of political and economic power in the same hands, protected by the policing power of the state.

For it is now apparent that the "trust-busters" who set out to break up Standard Oil and other monopolies had at best pyrrhic victories — they may have forced political changes which altered the *appearance* of monopolies, but by opening the door to government regulation they wound up allowing monopoly-by-government to accomplish the same objectives.

Since the patent medicine makers were targets of the incubating medical monopoly (for they "mimicked, distorted, derided and undercut the authority of the profession"[(8)]) and of the growing "ethical" pharmaceutical industry (for which they were a direct market threat at the level that really counted: access to consumers), the AMA and early drug companies were only too happy to root for "muckraking" against the nostrum peddlers.

Before Flexner unleashed his famous report in 1910, muckraking reporter Samuel Hopkins Adams printed a series of exposé articles gathered together as *The Great American Fraud*, aimed at exposing nostrums and "quack" doctors, all of this music to the ears of the AMA and most of it music to those of the "ethical" drug industry. The AMA distributed some 150,000 copies of this first-decade series. It was followed in rapid order by Upton Sinclair's *The Jungle*, an exposé of adulteration in the meat-packing industry.

Advent of the Pure Food and Drug Act

Such journalistic enterprises and the wide-open spirit of inquiry, quite aside from vested interests both of ideology and economics, led irreversibly to political reform. The upshot, in 1906, was the first Pure Food and Drug Act, which marked the beginning of federal regulation of foods and drugs and created the excuse — again, and as always, well-meaning at the beginning — of a government agency, which would become the FDA. The early law had few teeth and was designed primarily to halt the most notorious fakers — it did indeed make it illegal for a person to stand on the street corner hawking kerosene as a cancer cure.

The origin of the law, however, was not necessarily sheer altruism. Its primary proponent, Harvey Wiley, a government chemist who railed against frauds and poisons in foods, was at least to some extent spurred on by the organized dairy industry which hoped the government would pass laws to block non-dairy substitutes. Feisty to the end, Wiley was powerless to prevent infiltration into the fledgling FDA by food and pharmaceutical interests and quit in disgust as the agency's head in 1912, or six years after its founding.[(9)]

While one could argue, as some did, that the federal level of government should not be involved in pharmaceuticals, most would assign to government *at some level* a possibly rightful place in the *monitoring of safety* and the nature of claims made for products.

The political lessons of history are inexorable on two points: whenever government enters the market to control something, it usually ends up controlled by that which it attempts to control; and, each and every decision a human being makes to transfer responsibility over what he can or should do for himself to government to do for him builds an equal portion of loss of liberty — that is, tyranny. The FDA's Harvey Wiley was an early victim of this all-too-human reality.

The evolving AMA

While it would be years before federal regulation of foods and drugs would acquire little more than symbolic clout, the AMA — as we shall see — embarked on a period of building its own ties with the pharmaceutical industry, establishing its own pharmacy/chemical research, leading the fight against nostrums, establishing an anti-quackery division, courting the media, controlling medical education and, with the help of major corporate bequests, enabling itself to monitor that education through medical schools and medical licensure. The net result was the evolution of the nation's allopathic organization into an immense labor union for doctors.

Interestingly, the AMA, while usually accommodating dissident minority wings of "social progressives" within its ranks, was heatedly opposed to the notion of national health insurance ("socialized medicine" having first arisen in Germany in the 19th century) and it would remain adamantly opposed to all such measures during its existence. Yet its participation as a major element in an industrial complex engaging in monopoly medicine and rigged, monopoly pricing would only produce over time an equal and opposite reaction leading to calls for the very thing it had spent decades opposing. And, it would move from being benignly perceived by a majority of Americans, and at one time representing a (probable) majority of allopathic medical practitioners, to its mid-1990s position: representing perhaps 40% of the profession, its structure and nature increasingly questioned by much of the public and profession — the "mean trust" description of President Truman.[10]

The American Allopathic Industrial Complex, however, could not have developed only because of born-in-America influences and political currents, however necessary to that complex they have been.

The Rockefeller-I.G. Farben connection

The complex as it stands today has been massively aided, abetted and shored up by its participation in an international pharmaceutical/chemical syndicate, or group of trusts, whose interlocking web of profit-taking companies, corporations and monopolies in a vast array of interests staggers the mind.

As now understood by various researchers and writers who have exposed it, what we may term the International Drug Cartel (IDC) is essentially composed of the ongoing participants of, or fallout from, or entities indirectly aligned with, I.G. (*Interessen Gemeinschaft* — "community of interests" in German) Farben ("dyes"), the German-based conglomerate which had spread to 93 countries and was a major political and economic force on all continents (save, possibly, Antarctica) until World War II.[11] Just as the Standard Oil monopoly was only superficially broken up by trust-busters in the second decade, the original I.G. Farben conglomerate may have altered some of its names and memberships, but it is the great mother of chemical/drug-related monopolies still in the world today.

The origin of the I.G. Farben cartel is at root the same as that of the oil monopoly in the West — for the basic ingredient of a majority of chemicals and drugs is coal tar or crude oil ("petrochemicals"). The discovery of oil, followed by the development of the internal combustion machine, represented steps 1 and 2 in the creation of a vast global enterprise, which, by the early 1940s, was both the largest industrial corporation in Europe and the largest chemical company in the world, with tentacles extending throughout the globe.[12]

In the USA, the Farben combine came to own outright or have a substantial interest in some of the best-known names in the American pharmaceutical industry, some of which were already international in scope (American I.G. Chemical, Lederle Laboratories, Sterling Drug, Winthrop Chemical, Hoffman-LaRoche, Bristol Myers, Squibb and Sons Pharmaceutical, for example.)[13]

And its tentacles included overlaps with some of the best-known names in American chemical, petroleum, rubber, cosmetic, automotive, food and other industries, including Abbott Laboratories, Alcoa, the Borden Co., Carnation, Ciba-Geigy, Dow Chemical, Dupont, Eastman Kodak, Firestone Rubber, Ford Motor, General Electric, General Mills, General Motors, General Tire, Goodyear Tire, Gulf Oil, the M.W. Kellogg Company, Monsanto Chemical, Nestle's, Pet Milk, Pittsburgh Glass, Proctor and Gamble, Remington Arms, Richfield Oil, Shell Oil, Sinclair Oil, Standard Oil, Texaco, Union Oil, and US Rubber, plus hundreds of others.[14]

(None of this is a reflection on any of the products made by these companies and corporations, so many of which have positively impacted on, saved the lives of, or materially and physically enhanced the lives of, millions of Americans. They are reprised here as an indication of the global reach of an international combine which often concealed its interests and often had no national loyalties.)

At the close of World War II, General Dwight D. Eisenhower, then commanding the American Zone of Occupation in Germany, reported that I.G. Farben had stock interests in 613 corporations, including 173 in foreign countries, had assets of 6 billion Reichsmarks and "operated with varying degrees of power in more than 2,000 cartels."[15]

How I.G. Farben reached its cartel agreement with the Rockefellers in the 1920s, and, ultimately, with its final major competitor in America, DuPont, in 1929, makes fascinating reading, and the full story is beyond the scope of this volume, requiring another of at least equal size.

High points are these:

In 1927, the Rockefellers' Standard Oil of New Jersey (Esso) signed a widely ranging cartel agreement with I.G. Farben, under whose terms the Germans would not market petroleum products beyond their own borders and Esso agreed to "stay out of the existing market in all other fields."(16) The two giants also established JASCO (the Joint American Study Corporation) to mutually develop and exploit new scientific breakthroughs, including synthetic rubber. Dissolution of Farben meant that Rockefeller interests inherited a huge amount of the worldwide pharmaceutical business.

Reprising the Rockefeller era:

The Rockefellers first established an oil monopoly in 1870, which was reorganized in 1899 as Standard Oil of New Jersey. In 1911, in a round of alleged "trust-busting," Standard Oil was forced to break up into six separate companies, allegedly (but not really) ending its monopoly. From that point on, the Rockefellers began purchasing oil companies or investing in and ultimately controlling others, so that even as late as 1971 SO of New Jersey would admit to outright control of 322 companies. Included were numerous foreign oil investments.(17)

The oil venture, however, was relatively small when compared to the Rockefeller movement into banking and financial institutions. In 1933, federal legislation — again, in response to a public outcry, engineered or not, this time warning about the concentration of economic power in too few hands — was passed whereby commercial banks divested themselves of all investment banking operations. The net result of this legislation was simply to reorganize the banking monopoly and then expand it, with other powerful, ultrawealthy families now joining the endeavor.

The result of penetration into domestic and international financing and its earlier Farben agreement brought the Rockefeller empire into outright control of, or strong influence in, major corporate structures in America ranging from communications (ATT, ITT, Western Union, RCA), steel (Bethlehem, US Steel), transportation (Florida East Coast Railway, NY Central Railroad, Penn Central, Southern Pacific Railroad, Pan American Railways), major minerals and metals (Anaconda, Kennecott Copper, National Lead), electronics and related (Data Control, General Electric, Hewlett-Packard, Westinghouse, IBM), chemicals (Allied Chemical, Commercial Solvent Corp.), publishing (Cowles, Hearst, Time-Life), automotives (General Motors, Ford), rubber (B.F. Goodrich, US Rubber), foods and food processing (Continental Can, General Foods, Minute Maid), to general merchandise (Sears), and many other brands and names familiar to most Americans, quite aside from petroleum (Shell Oil, Getty Oil.)[(18)]

In life and health insurance the Rockefeller orbit has included the Metropolitan, Traveler's, and Hartford companies.[(19)]

In his monumental *World Without Cancer*, G.E. Griffin noted that:

> *The Rockefeller entry into the pharmaceutical field is more concealed, however, than in most other categories of industry . . . One [reason] is the fact that, for many years before World War II, Standard Oil had a continuing cartel agreement not to enter into the broad field of chemicals except as a partner with I.G. Farben which, in turn, agreed not to compete in oil . . . Because of the unpopularity of Farben in this country and the need to camouflage its American holdings, Standard had concealed even its partnership interests in chemical firms behind a maze of false fronts and dummy accounts. The Rockefellers' Chase Manhattan Bank, however, has always been the principal stock registrar for Farben-Rockefeller enterprises such as Sterling*

Drug, Olin Corporation, American Home Products, and General Analine [sic] *and Film. When Farben's vast holdings in the USA were finally sold in 1962, the Rockefeller group was the dominant force in carrying out the transaction.*[20]

(We will not here digress into other aspects of the Rockefeller empire, which include but are not limited to its enormous importance in American — and hence — world politics through the placing of individuals beholden to Rockefeller interests in the ranks of many spheres of government, other than to state that the Rockefeller-influenced Council on Foreign Relations [CFR] has had a predominant, inordinate effect on American foreign and domestic policy. The connections between international high finance, monopoly corporate capitalism, statecraft, politics and the media make for a fascinating study on their own, and these have been examined in detail as they relate to the Rockefeller phenomenon in American history.[21,22])

The original I.G. Farben apparatus continued worldwide despite some dismantling in 1946 (surviving pieces: Bayer, Hoechst, BASF) and surface divestiture in 1962. The growth of pharmaceutical cartels continued apace, with international drug conglomerates operating in Germany, Switzerland, England, France and the USA, their activities frequently enmeshed with international banking and investments in many other enterprises.

Buying out the opposition

It will be seen from some of the names already mentioned that both drugs *and* foods were recipients of economic munificence from the would-be monopolists, and this economic reality underscores a central element in the current American medical miasma:

In corporate investment terms, the number-one cluster of profit-making enterprises is the totality of corporations, companies and economic endeavors which altogether make up the food processing industry in the United States. Positioned right behind the food processing industrial complex are the pharmaceutical companies, whose profits annually outstrip the rate of inflation many times over in good times and bad (*VIII*).

In the post-Flexner period, with foundation money rushing into the medical schools and medical education reformed to fall along allopathic lines — if, primarily, because this would produce generations of peddlers of pharmaceutical products — all contenders to American establishment medicine began to fall by the wayside. They simply could not survive the green avalanche from the vested interests which saw bright futures in drugs and medical procedures.

As late as 1971, Joseph Goulden could write (in *The Money Givers*):

> *If the foundations chose to speak, their voice would resound with the solid clang of the cash register. Their expenditures on health and hospitals totalled more than a half-billion dollars between 1964 and 1968 . . . But the foundations' "innovative money" goes for research, not for the production of doctors who treat human beings. Medical schools, realizing this, paint their faces with the hue desired by their customers.*[23]

The United States, which had 22 homeopathic colleges as of 1900, had only seven by 1918, and even these stopped homeopathic instruction over the ensuing years.[24] Eclectics were essentially a thing of the past, naturopathy remained excluded, and the war with chiropractic was yet to break out.

In the meantime, as a chronicler of the Rockefeller influence over medicine has detailed,[25] this influence led to a considerable degree of control over the outcomes of efforts made by the Rockefeller-linked foundations.

Medicine in 20th-century America

Various other forces congealed in 20th-century America to invigorate the developing Allopathic Industrial Complex. They included more victories by "scientific medicine" over the infectious diseases, the growing roles played in medical schools by scientists and researchers, the development of sulfa drugs and later of antibiotics — "wonder drugs" all — and the gradual increase in the cost of medicine and medical care, giving rise to renewed debates over whether access to medicine and good health should be "rights."

While homeopathic insurance companies had developed in the 19th century, there was little in the way of private medical insurance in the first few decades of the present century. Socialists and Progressives were among the Americans who first clamored for socialized medicine early in this century, as did New Dealers in the third decade. It was not until the 1960s, however, that actual socialized medicine on the American plan commenced with the Medicare and Medicaid "Great Society" programs, and by that time they simply joined an amorphous, exponentially jerry-built multipartite structure referred to as the nation's "healthcare delivery system."

In earlier years, neither organized labor nor business in general, and certainly not the AMA, embraced the idea of national health insurance, the first organized movement for which had come about in the American Association for Labor Legislation (AALL) founded in 1906 by "social progressives" out to reform, rather than abolish, capitalism.

But by the Great Depression, among economic shifts that were noted and measured, the growing cost of medicine, particularly for the middle class, caused a fresh round of interest in guaranteed health programs. By the 1930s, it was clear that medical care had become a bigger element in family budgets than had income losses, and that coverage of medical expenses was more important than income protection primarily due to the perception that medical advances had become so effective in relieving suffering.(26)

The increasing monopolization of medicine (licensing restrictions and other practices) meant higher salaries for doctors, especially after World War I, and increased costs of hospital care. By 1929, according to a large national survey, hospital charges alone (not including doctors' and private nurses' bills) were 13% of the total family medical bill. By 1934 hospital charges plus physicians' bills for in-house hospital services were estimated at 40% of total medical expenditures.[27]

With various organizations and individuals expressing concern over the costs and distribution of medical care (including the greater migration to urban areas of doctors, leaving rural medical facilities inadequate), a private group called the Committee on the Costs of Medical Care (CCMC), consisting of economists, physicians, public-health specialists, and a past president of the AMA — and more than $1 million in funds from foundations — was set up ostensibly to examine the big picture of medical care in the USA. Among its informational assessments was the first reliable estimate of the cost of medical care in America — $3.66 billion in 1929, or about 4% of domestic income.[28]

The CCMC report in 1932 was actually timid, even though the reception accorded it by both Left and Right made it seem like something else. The committee asked for promotion of group medical practices and group payment plans, while rejecting the idea of compulsory health insurance. Even so, the AMA, criticizing the majority report, called the same an "incitement to revolution."[29]

When President Franklin Roosevelt swept to victory during the bowels of the Depression, it was clear even to ardent New Dealers that compulsory health insurance was an idea whose time had not yet come, and the omission of health insurance from the landmark Social Security Act (1935) is eloquent testimony thereof. As late as 1943, in the midst of World War II, Roosevelt was quoted, speaking of health insurance to a Senate committee chairman: "We can't go up against the state medical societies; we just can't do it."[30] This was a reflection of the continuing strength of the AMA at blocking any major changes in the status quo.

Birthing the Blues

In the meantime, private insurance and medical coverage for members of labor unions was on the move. In 1914, Metropolitan Life Insurance Co. set up a disability insurance plan to cover its home office employees. In 1928 it signed a contract with General Motors whereby the auto giant's 180,000 workers would have disability insurance. But it was in 1929 that third-party insurance schemes on a broader scale got underway — Blue Cross in Dallas, Ross-Loos in Los Angeles, and the first "medical cooperative" in Oklahoma. Blue Shield would follow.

These various measures for group coverage (to devolve into arguments over pre-payment, direct payment, payment arrangements between plans and doctors, doctors and hospitals, plans and hospitals) paralleled continuing rejection by Americans in general of outright socialized medicine while also reflecting society's concerns about the growing costs of medicine, whether those of private doctors' bills or the tab for protracted hospital stays.

Whether filtered through existing government programs (as the Veterans Administration after World War II), company health benefits, labor union plans, or the explosive growth in Blue Cross-Blue Shield private policies of the modern era, all such plans and arrangements, be they pre-paid, fee-for-service, or whatnot, managed for a time to keep the true cost of medical care and fees obscured from private contemplation. Paying premiums in advance, participating in a group plan — allowing a *third party* to administer and shuffle the paperwork — meant that the impact of medical care, for a very long time, was lessened. That a hospital in a group plan might charge many dollars or run useless tests, for example, was in essence hidden by the fact a plan member simply paid an amount per year for coverage which might range from lancing a bunion to managing terminal cancer, and individual cost elements of either treatment were not, for a long time, of great interest to the group plan member.

By the eve of World War II, American insurance companies

had 3.7 million subscribers for various plans involving hospital services and 39 Blue Cross plans then in effect had some six million subscribers.[31] The movement for third-party insurance plans exploded during and after the war, while more efforts for compulsory health insurance (which President Truman said should not be construed as "socialistic") were rejected — the increasingly powerful AMA, often in league with pharmaceutical companies, usually leading the opposition.

Allopathy's American apogee

It may be said that during World War II and for a decade or two thereafter that American allopathic medicine was in its greatest period of social acceptance and indomitable power. It was part and parcel of the growing postwar economy and the direct recipient of breakthroughs in science: penicillin, first of the antibiotics, as a monumental weapon against bacterial diseases; the sulfa drugs; DDT; progress in surgical techniques, and increased availability of blood and plasma for transfusions — elements which by themselves greatly cut death rates since patients who might have died on the operating table a decade before were now more likely guaranteed a new lease on life, for which "scientific medicine" could, and did, take the credit; better vaccines; victories over tetanus, typhus, dysentery, yellow fever, pneumonia, meningitis, and the control of malaria and considerable reductions in venereal diseases.

In allopathic medicine's golden era of great social acceptance (1945-1969), the beginning of overpricing for services went from barely visible to notorious: while the consumer price index rose during those years at an annual 2.8% clip, physicians' fees rose faster, at 3.8%; the average net profit from the practice of medicine rose from about $8,000 in 1945 to $32,000 in 1969.[32]

Not surprisingly, the growth of allopathic medicine was matched by a huge expansion in pharmaceuticals — the synthetic drugs for which the allopathic paradigm served as an ideological basis. It seemed that suddenly there was a drug for every ailment, real or imagined, a feel-good pill for every simple malady and, reaching *reductio ad absurdum*, finally a spinoff industry in the development of drugs to counter the side effects of other drugs!

Dr. Walter Modell, Cornell University Medical College, set the issue squarely in 1961:

> *When will they realize that there are too many drugs? No fewer than 150,000 preparations are now in use. About 15,000 new mixtures and dosages hit the market each year, while about 12,000 die off . . . We simply don't have enough diseases to go around. At the moment the most helpful contribution is the new drug to counteract the untoward effects of other new drugs.*[33]

Two decades later there were some 205,000 medical preparations being marketed worldwide, and the explosion in iatrogenic ("doctor-caused") diseases, often due to overdoses of or inadequate uses of drugs, were increasing in the same proportion.[34] While this went on, the "learned" medical journals told, to any minimally perceptive observer, the story: artfully produced sleek, multi-colored and even multitextured pharmaceutical ads dominated the major medical magazines in a blatant display of control by advertising while the various allopathic editors and boards of consultants of such journals claimed "objectivity" in the acceptance of articles in accord with the belief system (paradigm) of the editors and "peer" consultants which was monolithically the same: allopathic.

'Wonder drugs' and 'scientific medicine'

The advent of wonder drugs — plus radar and the mushroom-cloud presence of the atomic bomb — riveted American attention on the link between a commitment to science and national security. As from a broken faucet, money for science came gushing forth from the federal coffers, a torrent of funds which would ultimately be channeled into a growing medical conglomerate of research facilities, research hospitals, federal agencies, medical products suppliers, research scientists, and any number of new industries (among them the mini-business of learning how to write and apply for research grants and then administering them, together with "creative bookkeeping" techniques aimed at fostering the need to keep and expand such grants.)

Symbolically, the tiny National Institutes of Health (NIH) saw its research budget swell from $180,000 in 1945 to $4 million just two years later. It had ballooned to $400 million in 1960. The federal budget for medical medical research jumped from $3 million in 1941 to $76 million in 1951, while total expenditures for such research went from $18 million to $181 million.[35]

Victories over infectious disease, and better survival rates even at hospitals, seemed to many to be the payoff for the national commitment to "scientific medicine." Yet, new shadows were beginning to loom large over the land — if tuberculosis was under control and, eventually, polio was to be subdued, cancer rates continued to increase alarmingly, as did the whole complex of maladies lumped under "heart disease." Growing numbers of chronic, degenerative disease conditions began to be noticeable, but the excuse normally was that people were living longer due to better "medical science" (certainly the longevity rates were better) so that they were succumbing to more conditions of "old age" (irrespective of the growing rates of chronic disease conditions in children.)

The idea that the wonder drugs would save us from *all* medical problems had begun to wear thin even by the Sixties and, by the Seventies, the holistic medical revolution broke out in full force with the controversy over laetrile and with it a growing rejection of the entire allopathic paradigm.

It was moved along by the avalanche of information in the 1980s and 1990s on the sudden emergence of antibiotic-resistant old bacterial infections and the seemingly sudden — some would say too sudden — appearance of "emerging new viruses" causing hideous fatal diseases[36,37] *(see XIV).*

The great federal power grab

The growing cost of medicine, which (together with the cost of pharmaceuticals) outpaced inflation in the postwar years, led inexorably to renewed efforts for compulsory health insurance and/or some other scheme for socialized medicine. The net result of these renewed efforts was the passage in 1964 of the Medicare and Medicaid programs, which represented a massive intrusion of government into medicine.

Medicare, supposedly, would provide medical coverage for the elderly, as Medicaid would for the indigent. The idea was that by paying for these mass programs out of tax monies there would be some measure of medical cost control, if not outright decrease in cost, for large segments of the population. Going on three decades later, the programs — as wasteful, corruption-fraught and bureaucracy-engendering as any other federal government program — have simply been major contributors to the *increase* of the total cost of healthcare in America, the large government components of the multifaceted Rube Goldberg-like apparatus awkwardly called our "healthcare delivery system" and, as we have seen, better referred to as "the sick business" or even "death management."

By 1990, it could be said that the Medicare and Medicaid programs by themselves constituted 28 percent of the total healthcare budget, and that between 1967 (the first full year of spending on the programs) and 1990 costs had soared from $5 billion to over $160 billion — vastly beyond anybody's prediction at the time they were introduced.[(38)]

As debate over health reform entered a new level in mid-decade, government sources noted that Medicare's projected cost in 1991 of $9 billion was off by $92 billion — since the figure was over $100 billion that year, as we have seen.[(39)]

And the Heritage Foundation projected in 1993 that "if current trends continue, state Medicaid expenses will have increased more than 480 percent by the year 2000."[(40)]

Just as insurance and hospital cost projections for the federal programs proved to be far off-base, so too were the *use* features thereof.

In 1993 it was reported that the "original 1965 cost projections [of Medicare] allowed for a 10-percent increase in hospital admission rates among the elderly, but in fact hospital-admission rates among the Medicare-eligible rose immediately by 25 percent, the rates for surgical procedures by 40 percent, and the number of hospital days by 50 percent."[41]

By then, estimated the Congressional Budget Office, while in 1965 there were 15 workers per Medicare beneficiary, there now were four to support each Medicare recipient.[42]

As we shall see, the government was also greatly strengthened in the medical sector through the 1962 amendments to the Food, Drug and Cosmetic Act, which expanded the FDA's role from alleged monitor of "safety" in the use of drug compounds to chief determiner of the "efficacy" thereof. The extension of FDA power into "efficacy" not only greatly slowed drug development in the USA but even more narrowly restricted the practice of medicine. But such new government muscle hardly bothered the international drug trust: in fact, by helping put smaller companies out of business simply through their inability to comply with the costs and time involved in a vast new production of red tape, the FDA helped remove potential competitors to the giant drug firms.

By the end of the Sixties, the era of good feeling with the developing allopathic industry was beginning to diminish. In January 1970 both *Business Week* and *Fortune*, major journalistic monitors of the American business scene, pronounced the American medical system to be "on the brink of chaos" and costing far too much — if only, in that year, $60 billion.

Intoned *Fortune*:

> *Much of US medical care, particularly the everyday business of preventing and treating routine illness, is inferior in quality, wastefully dispensed, and inequitably financed . . . Whether poor or not, most*

Americans are badly served by the obsolete, over-strained medical system that has grown up around them helter-skelter . . . the time has come for radical change.[43]

Enter the Medical-Industrial Complex

Change came, but not *radical* change. One administration after another sought to grapple with the amorphous monster of giant medicine, giant medical costs, accessibility to giant medicine, and failures of giant medicine. While "health maintenance" and "preferred-provider" organizations (HMOs and PPOs) were launched as a partial panacea for the crisis in "cost containment," for-profit hospital chains grew (Hospital Corporation of America and Humana Corporation leading the way) and the trappings of what some came to call the MIC, or medical-industrial complex, became evident.

While the federal bureaucracy and state governments churned out new regulatory agencies aimed at trying to slow down or redistribute more equitably the galloping costs of medicine while noting the great disparities in access to the same between various economic classes, some social critics helped acquaint the population with the concept of "iatrogenic" disease and argued that modern medicine was causing more disease than it was curing. But criticism could not slow the increase in insurance premiums, the increase in doctors' fees, and the attendant profileration of *hyperlexia* — malpractice suits seemed to increase as exponentially as did the rising "mediglomerates" of hospitals, hospital suppliers, insurance companies, group plans, research centers and regulatory agencies.

Describing the advent of the MIC, Dr. Stanley Wohl wrote in 1984:

Over the last thirty years the health care system had indeed become a haphazard unaffordable compendium of ivory-tower university hospitals; decaying Veterans Administration, state and county facilities; mismanaged private and religious order hospitals and nursing homes; and tax-exempt wasteful "non-profit" community hospitals. The entire system was held together by a plethora of unintelligible government regulations, private insurance company dictates, and the practices of a medical profession primarily concerned in many instances merely with preserving its own prerogatives in the field. All attempts at reasonable controls were crushed under the cascade of escalating costs. Insurance companies kept raising their premiums; government programs and community hospitals were going broke; and the average citizen was left holding the bag.[44]

It was into this morass that "the corporation" stepped and has continued to step. The advent of the corporative approach to American medicine, through for-profit hospital operations and a whole interlock of vested interests therewith associated, now means that, to use a more appropriate Italian term from the 1930s, what has evolved (an interlocking medical-pharmaceutical monopoly in essence protected and often nourished by the state) is, as we have seen (*III*), *health fascism.*

The coming of health fascism has meant that the government (meaning taxpayer funds with taxpayers having little to say in their use) has intruded into the medical marketplace parallel to or as a nurturer of corporate capitalism — a state-mandated industry allowing vast profits and underwritten, in part, by taxpayers.

Award-winning journalist Rochelle Jones properly belled the cat in 1990 in *The Supermeds*[45] with her perceptive account of how taxpayers have unwittingly helped finance "franchised healthcare," with the following changes noted in the Eighties:

— Healthcare changed from being a virtual cottage industry dominated by physicians and non-profit hospitals into a nationwide network of for-profit corporations running a variety of medical enterprises, with such "supermed" conglomerates controlling about one out of every five of the nation's 7000 hospitals.

— Doctors have frequently been forced to choose between the business ethic or the medical ethic, with the business ethic gaining.

— More money than ever has been going into advertising and promotion of hospital services, and hospitals now market themselves with techniques picked up from consumer-product corporations.

And worse, she noted:

— Higher death rates have been documented in "supermed" hospitals for many illnesses; and

— In "supermed" old-age homes there is rampant patient neglect, and improper nourishment and unhygienic conditions prevail. Florida, Arkansas, California and Michigan cited "supermeds" for "serious health and safety violations" in the 1980s.

The corporate drive here is clear: in instance after instance, it is more vital to fill the hospital bed than it is to oversee the care of the patient. Within a system in which "alternative" and integrative medicine is either illegal or discouraged, the situation of monopoly-protected, drug-based medicine, unnecessary medical procedures and tests, many underwritten by the taxpayers through the bureaucracy-laden, corruption-riddled Medicare and Medicaid systems, becomes even more desperate.

To the extent that a slim majority of hospital bills by the 1990s were paid by federal and other government programs, American medicine had achieved its own corporative variety of "socialized medicine," but one which was far from "social" in impact, for between 37 and 41 million Americans (as of 1996 — figures which may have been exaggerated) were neither old enough nor poor enough to qualify for federal and related government programs, or were not wealthy enough to pay for the obscene increases in monthly premium payments for overpriced private health insurance, and hence were without medical insurance of any kind — and some just didn't want it.

Again quoting Dr. Wohl, who in 1984 detailed more than 90 major components (insurance companies, medical suppliers, drug companies, research laboratories, etc.) of the MIC as an illustration of how the private part of the hybrid works:

> *When Johnson & Johnson owns a piece of National Medical Enterprises, Bristol-Myers a piece of Hospital Corporation of America, and Upjohn a piece of Beverly [Enterprises], questions of medical ethics arise. Drug companies are supplying pills to hospitals they partially own. These drugs are prescribed by physicians whose salaries these hospitals pay directly or indirectly by contract. Of course the drug houses deny direct ownership of hospital chains, but a close inspection of their investment wing portfolios leaves nothing to the imagination. It is all legal, of course . . .*
>
> *Johnson & Johnson . . . is involved in animal health, diagnostic imaging products, nuclear medicine, ultrasound, digital X-ray, and CT scanning as well as everyday pharmaceuticals. The company finds itself also at the forefront of technology, with new nuclear magnetic resonance scanners.*
>
> *Johnson & Johnson also owns a dialysis business, a critical care company, and an intraocular lens business. It also sells Vascor heart valves. With so much to sell the medical world, is it any wonder that the president of Hospital Corporation of America was elected to the board of Johnson & Johnson?*
>
> *The true giants of the MIC are the insurance companies such as CIGNA and pharmaceutical companies such as Johnson & Johnson . . .*[46]

The HMO/PPO revolution

The drive for "managed care" and "cost containment" in America's strange medical-cost model broke out in the 1980s and started advancing exponentially with the collapse of the Clinton

Administration's scheme for the (virtual) socialization of medicine in the 1990s.

As small business managers faced bankruptcy over the cost of funding medical insurance for employees and as private insurance plan costs continued to skyrocket, the health maintenance organization/preferred provider organization (HMO/PPO; and even "point-of-service" or POS) plans began to proliferate, linking groups of patients, groups of doctors and groups of treatment centers.

Enrollment in HMOs and PPOs ballooned by 13% in 1995 alone to coverage of 149 million Americans,[47] and it was estimated that by the turn of the millennium more than 100 million would be enrolled in HMO plans alone.[48] Estimates in 1997 were that "about half the population" and nearly three-quarters of American workers were covered by such plans.[49,50]

There developed unanswered questions as to greed, profits and medical quality as the managed-care revolution broke out. Fears of "cut-rate" care[51] began to be heard as HMO/PPO executive salaries soared and those of HMO/PPO-connected physicians in some cases actually began to drop. The rapid transition from old-time Marcus Welby-type medicine to what *Newsweek* called a "Wal-Mart model of health care"[52] represented both challenges and opportunity to the burgeoning movement for health freedoms:

On the one hand, drug-based allopathic medicine was maneuvering to keep control of all medical practice; on the other, a few medical groups, and a few medical insurance plans, as we have seen, were beginning to be open to integrating at least some aspects of "alternative" medicine into their group practices.[53]

And, why not? The reality of it all was clear: "alternative medicine" usually costs not only less but often a *lot* less!

The great drug bonanza

While insurance remains of extreme importance to the Allopathic Industrial Complex (AIC) in the United States, it is the mass profiteering by pharmaceutical firms, organized on an international basis, which is still the engine which drives American allopathy.

The capture of medicine by the allopathic paradigm in the latter 19th century and early 20th century opened the door for domination of the profession by the purveyors of cheaply produced and enormously overpriced synthetic drugs, an era beginning in 1899 with the advent of aspirin — by some measures the "best" and certainly the most economic of all "drugs."

Before the aspirin era, as we have seen, mercury and other toxic substances were "drugs of choice," but there also were opium and its derivatives, quinine for malaria and ipecac for dysentery. With homeopathy slowly being ground out of active competition by "medicine," and with the rise of the trusts and corporations early in this century, the way was pristinely open for the synthetic drug industry — and it developed full force and on an international basis.

In 1970 the American Enterprise Institute for Public Policy Research reported that the pharmaceutical industry in the United States had grown by 100% in this century. In 1973 Consumers Union noted that 20,000 tons of aspirin were being consumed every year, or about 225 tablets per person, the same year that *Scientific American* revealed that drugs which affected the central nervous system (CNS) were the fastest-growing element of the drug business.[(54)]

Even so, as Ivan Illich noted in his pivotal 1976 survey of iatrogenicity in America,[(55)] when the FDA began examining the 4,300 prescription drugs that had appeared since World War II, only two out of five were found to be effective, and many were flatly dangerous. (We examine the relationship between the pharmaceutical industry — the modern incarnation, in no small way, of the Rockefeller-Farben worldwide drug interests enmeshed within a web of alliances with other industries — and the FDA in other chapters.)

As we also note elsewhere, in April 1976, the Senate Select

Committee on Small Business was told that the drug industry was paying for "the bulk of educational information provided to the practicing physician."[56]

These were references to the courting of allopathic physicians by the drug companies through "detail men" who provide useful "samples" of an endless array of new synthetic drug products to their medical clients. By that time, it was evident that the "peer-reviewed" or "standard" or "learned" medical journals were dominated by highly professional advertising from the major players in the global drug combine.

In 1982, this writer reported that the US drug industry, despite an ongoing economic recession, was doing just fine, thank you, with projected earnings set at 20% over the $12 billion profits of 1981.[57] By 1992, and despite a second ongoing economic recession, the profits of the "ethical" drug industry (prescription drugs and over-the-counter preparations primarily pitched to doctors) were at least three times greater than 10 years before.

References

1. Josephson, Mathew, *The Robber Barons*. New York: Harcourt Brace, 1934.
2. Fox, Daniel, "Abraham Flexner's Unpublished Report: Foundations and Medical Education, 1909-1928." *Bulletin of the History of Medicine*. 54, Winter 1980.
3. Starr, Paul, *The Social Transformation of American Medicine*. New York: Basic Books, 1982.
4. Griffin, GE, *World Without Cancer*. Westlake Village CA: American Media, 1974.
5. Weaver, Warren, *U.S. Philanthropic Foundations: Their History, Structure, Management, and Record*. New York: Harper & Row, 1967.
6. Griffin, *op. cit.*
7. Martin, RL, *Fabian Freeway*. Belmont MA: Western Islands, 1966.
8. Starr, Paul, *op. cit*
9. Lucas, Scott, *The FDA*. Millbrae CA: Celestial Arts, 1978.
10. Culbert, ML, *What the Medical Establishment Won't Tell You that Could Save Your Life*. Norfolk VA: Donning, 1983.
11. Griffin, *op. cit.*
12. *US vs. Allied Chemical & Dye Corp., et al.*. US District Court of New Jersey, 1942, in Griffin, *op. cit*
13. Griffin, *op. cit.*
14. *Ibid.*
15. *New York Times*, Oct. 21, 1945.
16. DuBois, JE, *The Devil's Chemists*. Boston: Beacon Press, 1952.
17. Hoffman, William, *David: Report on a Rockefeller*. New York: Lyle Stuart, 1971.
18. Allen, Gary, *The Rockefeller File*. Seal Beach CA: '76 Press, 1976.

19. *Ibid.*
20. Griffin, *op. cit.*
21. Allen, *op. cit.*
22. Flynn, JT, *God's Gold: The Story of Rockefeller and His Times.* New York: Harcourt Brace, 1932.
23. Goulden, Joseph, *The Money Givers.* New York: Random House, 1971.
24. Coulter, HL, *Divided Legacy: The Conflict Between Homoeopathy and the American Medical Association.* Richmond CA: North Atlantic Books, 1973.
25. Brown, RE, *Rockefeller Medicine Men: Capitalism and Medical Care in America.* Berkeley CA: University of California Press, 1979.
26. Davis, MM, in preface to Millis, HA, *Sickness and Insurance.* Chicago: University of Chicago Press, 1937.
27. Starr, *op. cit.*
28. *Ibid.*
29. "The Committee on the Costs of Medical Care." *Journal of the American Medical Assn. (JAMA),* Dec. 3, 1932.
30. Blum, John, *From the Morgenthau Diaries: Years of War, 1941-1945.* Boston: Houghton Mifflin, 1967.
31. Somers, HN, and Somers, AR, *Doctors, Patients and Health Insurance.* Washington: The Brookings Institution, 1961.
32. Goldstein, MS, *Incomes of Physicians, Osteopaths and Dentists from Professional Practice.* Washington: Social Security Administration, Office of Research and Statistics, 1972.
33. *Time*, May 26, 1961.
34. Ruesch, Hans, *Naked Empress,* Zurich: Buchverlag CIVIS, 1982.
35. Starr, *op. cit.*
36. Garrett, Laurie, *The Coming Plague.* New York: Penguin, 1994.
37. *Infectious Disease: A Global Health Threat.* Washington DC: National Service and Technology Council, Sept. 1995.
38. Lee, RW, "Creating the Crisis." *The New American,* Nov. 1, 1993.
39. Connell, Christopher, The Associated Press, Oct. 31, 1993.
40. Lee, *loc. cit.*
41. Hayward, Steven, and Peterson, Erik, *Reason,* Jan. 1993.
42. Lee, *loc. cit.*
43. "It's Time to Operate." *Fortune*, January 1970.
44. Wohl, Stanley, *The Medical Industrial Complex.* New York: Harmony Books, 1984.
45. Jones, Rochelle, *The Supermeds.* New York: Macmillan, 1990.
46. Wohl, *op. cit.*
47. *American Medical news*, July 22, 1996.
48. GHAA National Directory on HMOs, Interstudy, 1996.
49. Church, GJ, "Backlash against HMOs." *Time,* April 14, 1997.
50. Scripps Howard News Service, Jan. 20, 1997.
51. Anders, George, *Health Against Wealth.* Boston: Houghton Miffin, 1996.
52. Spragins, Ellyn, "Does your HMO stack up?" *Newsweek*, June 24, 1996.
53. "Roundup of selected insurance providers offering alternative medicine coverage." *Alt. Ther.*, May, 1996.
54. Culbert, *op. cit.*
55. Illich, Ivan, *Medical Nemesis.* New York: Pantheon Books, 1976.
56. Culbert, *op. cit.*
57. *Ibid.*

VII
THE AMA:
Organized allopathy, the drug industry, and the fight against 'quackery'

"I no longer believe in Modern Medicine. I believe that the greatest danger to your health is the doctor who practices Modern Medicine . . . Don't trust your doctor. Assume that if he prescribed a drug, it's dangerous. There is no safe drug."

— **Robert Mendelsohn MD *(Confessions of a Medical Heretic)***

"As it stands, the drug industry seems to be running the medical profession. Doctors are pushed around and bullied and bribed by the drug industry. They have undoubtedly lost control of their own profession and must consequently be held responsible for all the disasters and errors which bad prescribing produces . . . [T]he medical profession . . . now that it is reduced to receiving instructions and accepting commandments from a trade, can hardly be still described as a profession."

— **Vernon Coleman MD (*The Medicine Man*)**

"The medical monopoly or medical trust, euphemistically called the American Medical Association, is not merely the meanest monopoly ever organized, but the most arrogant, dangerous and despotic organization which ever managed a free people in this or any other age. Any and all methods of healing the sick by means of safe, simple and natural remedies are sure to be assailed and denounced by the arrogant leaders of the AMA doctors' trust as 'fakes, frauds and humbugs.'"

— **J.W. Hodge MD (in Ruesch, *Naked Empress*)**

"Establishment medicine, at least superficially and for public consumption, avows and maintains belief in a free market system — so long, it seems, as it remains the only market and is left free to do as it pleases. The choice and comfort of many sick people thus become at best a tertiary concern."

— **People's Medical Society (*Medicine on Trial)***

"The physician is part of a subculture in which maximizing the number of patients he sees is the socially accepted route to a yacht and a country estate, and wielding his prescription pad with a professional flourish is an apparently more efficient means to that end than attempting to talk things out."

— **Louise Lander *(Defective Medicine)***

A revealing victory by chiropractors

On January 13, 1992, *American Medical News*, the weekly publication of the American Medical Association (AMA), with a modicum of comment published the full text of a permanent injunction order against the AMA issued by US Judge Susan Getzendanner in the matter of *Wilk vs. the AMA.*

It was the final brick in the edifice of a solid judicial achievement by the chiropractic profession in the United States:

Four years prior, Judge Getzendanner had declared that the AMA — the trade organization of allopathic physicians which pompously dares to speak for all of "medicine" — had engaged in a nationwide boycott of doctors of chiropractic by arguing that it was "unethical" for AMA physicians (that is, allopaths) to associate professionally with chiropractors.

The 1987 decision — which led to four more years of fruitless appeals by the AMA and parallel or affiliated collaborators — had been the outcome of 11 long years of litigation by "the Chicago four" (chiropractors Chester Wilk, Michael Pedigo, James Bryden, Patricia Arthur) against the AMA and its allies.

In her 101-page 1987 decision, Judge Getzendanner had simply found the nation's organized allopaths guilty of a conspiracy to destroy chiropractic — that the AMA had engaged in "systematic, long-term wrongdoing and the long-term intent to destroy a licensed profession."(1)

Even so, the 1987 decision and the 1992 published order — making it "ethical" for allopaths to associate with chiropractors — had followed the 1978-1980 federal-level findings that the AMA had been guilty of "conspiracy to restrain competition" and that thanks to AMA pressure "new methods of healthcare have been discouraged, restricted and, in some cases, eliminated."

The 1980 US Court of Appeal decision had upheld an extensive ruling in 1978 by the Federal Trade Commission (FTC) following restraint-of-trade complaints and anti-trust charges by chiropractors.

An FTC overview of the evidence presented in the matter of the AMA, the Connecticut State Medical Society and the New Haven Medical Association contained some of the most damning public evidence ever to be brought forward against an organization that likes to speak of itself in reverential terms. Wrote FTC analysts:

- *(There is) a substantial body of formal and informal actions by the AMA that have the effect of enhancing the economic positions of members of the AMA. The end result has been the placement of a formidable impediment to competition in the delivery of health care services by physicians in the United States. The barrier has served to deprive consumers of the free flow of information about the availability of health care and to stifle the rise of most every type of health care delivery that could potentially pose a threat to the income of physicians in private practice. The costs to the public in terms of less expensive or even, perhaps, more improved forms of medical service are great.*
- *. . . AMA ethical structures were motivated by economic objectives rather than by a need to maintain professionalism among physicians.*
- *The record . . . is overwhelming in establishing the anti-competitive effects of AMA's ethical restrictions, their economic motivations and their consequent harm to the public interest.*
- *The record evidence establishes the existence of a conspiracy between the AMA and its constituent and component medical societies . . . To find otherwise than that the AMA and State and local medical societies were engaged in a conspiracy to restrain competition would be to ignore an abundance of evidence to the contrary. The record evidence contains a more than sufficient quantum of*

independently admissible evidence to establish the existence of the conspiracy.

• *New methods of health care have been discouraged, restricted and, in some instances, eliminated.*

• *The record evidence establishes with clear conviction that AMA has prevented the dissemination of truthful, objective information that could provide substantial benefits to the public.*[2]

A history of 'dirty tricks'

Yet, intertwined with and behind the AMA battle with chiropractic lurked even more sinister realities:

Investigative journalists pried from AMA sources the reality that the organization had been engaging in "dirty tricks" against chiropractic since the middle 1960s, that the organization seems to have had both overt and covert units to undercut chiropractic, and that an ongoing effort to block, thwart or undermine *any* form of medicine other than "standard practice" (meaning allopathy) had involved federal and state agencies and officials, law-enforcement officers and insurance companies and the pharmaceutical industry.

Moreover, the circumstantial evidence became overwhelming that after the AMA had undergone severe internal bickering and an attempt to clean up its image, the organized effort to restrain *all* non-allopathic approaches to medicine continued in the form of "quackbuster" organizations said to be "independent" of the AMA.

These same investigative efforts also helped reveal that the synthetic drug/pharmaceutical industry was and is a heavy contributor to such "quackbuster" activities.

Among the key elements in the campaign to ferret out the AMA anti-quackery conspiracy was William Trever's *In the Public Interest*, a little-known if information-crammed exposé in 1972 which undoubtedly helped set the stage for AMA's internal soul-searching a few years later.[3]

Trever's book, allegedly helped along by a knowledgeable AMA "deep throat" member with a houseful of documentation, was the first major compilation of extensive evidence to outline in classic detail, memorandum by memorandum and letter by letter, an extensive effort by the AMA to maintain an American equivalent of thought police within the ranks of medicine and to engage in any and all activities not only primarily aimed at halting chiropractic but indeed targeting non-allopathic medicine in general.

The book outlined, with copious documentation, the existence of an AMA Department of Investigation (a kind of secret spy network, noted the author) and, in 1963, the establishment of the AMA's Committee on Quackery, which, by the AMA's very own wording, "considered its prime mission to be, first, the containment of chiropractic and, ultimately, the elimination of chiropractic."

A committee memorandum to the AMA Board of Trustees on Jan. 4, 1971, let more cats out of the bag. It read: "The Committee has not previously submitted such a report because it believes that to make public some of its activities would have been and continues to be unwise. Thus, this report is intended only for the information of the Board of Trustees."[4]

This, and numerous other documents, prove that the chiropractic profession had become the AMA's central competitive target by 1963-64, and that no punches would be pulled in slandering, vilifying and libeling chiropractors and chiropractic, with the full weight of organized allopathy in politics and the media and every other way to be used to bury a form of medicine the drug-dispensing allopaths regarded as a major competitor.

Quoting Seneca ("if you would wish another to keep your secret, first keep it yourself "), Trever then extensively revealed how the competing profession (chiropractic) was to be attacked "scientifically," politically, judicially and propagandistically. The machinations of the AMA revealed in *In the Public Interest*, seconded by Administrative Law Judge Ernest G. Barnes on Nov. 13, 1978, in a 312-page initial decision in *FTC vs. the AMA et al.*, made the conspiracy/dirty tricks case against the AMA, its allies and subordinates crystal-clear.

As a long-time foe of socialized medicine (but by no means an equally ardent champion of competitive capitalism, since the AMA has always spoken for allopathic monopoly), the organization nonetheless used its clout federally to influence Medicare and Medicaid against chiropractic, efforts which, noted Trever, have "affected every American's freedom of choice by seeing to it that chiropractic health-care services were excluded in these health insurance programs."[5]

In terms of private medical insurance, for years the AMA opposition to a given form of therapy has meant the virtual certainty that insurors would not reimburse for the method however efficacious and less expensive it might be.

This reality was clear as early as 1971, when Senator Edward M. Kennedy, frequently a proponent of socialized medicine and, while no friend of the AMA often blind to the error of entrusting vigilance to the government, accused the AMA of "obstructing almost every major step to improve health care for Americans while degenerating into a 'propaganda organ for purveying medical politics.'"

Said Senator Kennedy on July 14, 1971:

"The organization of our health services is still in a shambles. Why? Because AMA and its friends in the health insurance industry have stood in the way of every major step towards an efficient, effective, affordable health care system for the American people." Remember, this was in *1971*.[6]

Enter P.J. Lisa

Where Trever left off, investigative journalist P.J. Lisa picked up the thread. He first resurrected and updated the AMA conspiracy against "quackery" in general and chiropractic in particular following an in-depth investigation which led to publication of *Are You a Target for Elimination?*[7]

More revealing, his *The Great Medical Monopoly Wars* (1986)[8] documented the transmutation of the AMA's organized anti-quackery efforts into an "independent" coalition of self-described "quackbuster" organizations working in lockstep with state and federal departments, law enforcement, postal authorities, insurance companies and major pharmaceutical houses.

Most importantly, Lisa revealed the emergence in 1964 (or a year after the AMA had set up its Committee on Quackery) of a shadowy, almost James Bond plot-within-a-plot unit called the Coordinating Conference on Health Information (CCHI), which lasted until 1974 — the same year the AMA began to divest itself of the Committee on Quackery and the Department of Investigation following internal squabbles.

The CCHI, noted Lisa, included representation by the AMA, the American Cancer Society, the American Pharmaceutical Assn., the Council of Better Business Bureaus, the Arthritis Foundation, the Food and Drug Administration, the US Postal Service and the Federal Trade Commission.

Revealed Lisa: "According to the now-published 'Operating Procedures' of the CCHI, an effort was made to obscure the involvement of several government agencies which were members of the CCHI."

Since the medical objectives of the CCHI seemed to be identical to those of the surface AMA, and since the medical objectives of the "independent" organizations which succeeded (replaced?) the AMA-connected anti-quackery bodies were the same, it is not difficult to make the circumstantial (at the very least) case for an ongoing organized conspiracy between elements of the pharmaceutical industry,federal, state and local government and the AMA (The Club — the Establishment — the Allopathic Industrial Complex) to suppress non-allopathic medicine.

Lisa also revealed something this author had heard about, since I was a journalist chronicling a good deal of the "alternative" medicine controversy for various books as well as for the

Committee for Freedom of Choice in Cancer Therapy, Inc. (later the Committee for Freedom of Choice in Medicine, Inc.) and its magazine, *The Choice*:

The appearance of a "hit list" of "high-profile" targets, particularly among the more prominent practitioners of what was styled "alternative" medicine.

That there was such a list surfaced during informal periods of investigation and litigation involving various federal and state agencies and targeted doctors: it became dangerous for one practitioner of "alternative" therapy to travel to another state to testify in behalf of a brother practitioner up on charges in that state because authorities from both states were trading information.

Targets on the 'hit list'

Such was the case of physician Michael Gerber MD of California, who testified on behalf of osteopath Robert Vance in Utah when state authorities came after the latter for EDTA chelation therapy and other "questionable" treatments. Dr. Vance was an internationally recognized metabolic therapist at the time and something of a hero in the Netherlands.

Simply because Dr. Gerber, of California, testified *for* Dr. Vance, of Utah, the former found himself in difficult straits back home. Both respected healers ultimately moved to Nevada to be able to practice as homeopaths.

In the 1980s, virtually every high-visibility metabolic therapist came under severe scrutiny and harassment, particularly if he treated cancer. The State of New York spent untold millions in prosecuting nonagenarian physician/researcher Emanuel Revici MD, a gifted Rumanian emigre doctor who had been open about his non-toxic approach to degenerative disease, and Warren Levin MD, an "alternative" practitioner hounded in wave after wave of harassment over many years. Both men had undergone such lengthy persecution essentially for one reason: they were open, and successful, exponents of "non-mainstream" medicine (*I*).

Ahmad Shamim MD was a target of authorities' wrath for a

solid 10 years in his home state of Maryland primarily because he too was a "high-visibility" practitioner of "alternative" medicine with a swollen caseload of essentially happy patients, including some of the longest-surviving cancer patients in his area.

Indeed, it was the persecution of the softspoken Dr. Shamim which led syndicated columnist Jack Anderson and his staff to take an investigative reporter's-eye view of the plight of the nation's "alternative" or "holistic" healers.

With Maryland's ongoing efforts to strip Dr. Shamim of his license well within view, Anderson wrote:

> *"Across the country, at least 1,500 physicians practicing [holistic] medicine are under attack by state disciplinary boards . . . These are not quacks, but medical doctors with all the right diplomas and credentials. But they treat patients with vitamins and enzymes. They shy away from too many X-rays and too many drugs. They believe diet can effectively treat some degenerative diseases.*
>
> *"Their more traditional peers worry that the patients of holistic doctors aren't getting the best care, and some holistic doctors think traditional doctors are conspiring to silence them because holistic medicine threatens the multibillion-dollar surgery and drug business in this country.*
>
> *"The conflict has doctors on both sides afraid to talk for the record. One mainstream doctor from New York told our reporter . . . 'The reason behind the attacks is called group mindset. You learn in medical school to treat each malady separately, like fixing a machine. And you practice that way for years. Then a doctor comes along and says all that money you waste on chemotherapy and surgery is crap, and I'm going to cure you just with diet. The doctor will be labeled a quack whether he is one or not. It's not premeditated conspiracy against alternative therapy.*

It's a subconscious one'".[9]

This was a reasonable attempt to explain both negative cognitive dissonance (inability or lack of desire in processing unexpected or unwanted new information) and paradigm capture (indocrination by and to a core set of beliefs and practices.)

That there was a "hit list" became more evident when reporter Lisa uncovered what he called "new and startling information" in March 1986 while conducting research at the California Department of Health. He wrote:

> *According to documents discovered in Sacramento, an entire underground medical network had been meeting secretly with members of the US Postal Service, the Food and Drug Administration, the Federal Trade Commission, and others, in an effort to launch attacks against chiropractors, nutritionists, vitamin companies, and individuals . . . in addition to chelation therapy, homeopathy, naturopathy, alternative cancer remedies, and so on.*[10]

He listed some of the best-known names among the rapidly burgeoning healthfoods movement and the "alternative" medical cause.

They included Bruce Halstead MD, Colton CA, vice president of our Committee for Freedom of Choice in Medicine, Inc., who was under heavy attack for his high-visibility involvement with or defense or advocacy of EDTA chelation therapy, laetrile, DMSO, and other "must kill" items on The Club's list. Dr. Halstead, a renowned World Health Organization scientist as well as a popular physician, was a globally recognized expert in, among other things, Chinese herbs, marine biology and plant toxicology — and was widely respected in mainland China for doing much to bring herbology from that country to the attention of the West.

He knew, because various agents over the years told him, that the powers that be were out to "get" him on any grounds whatsoever.(*I*) Eventually, Halstead — after his clinic and research center were subjected to an early-morning SWAT-team ra 1983 by two dozen local and state authorities from several jurisdictions — was finally convicted on a charge of providing Japanese herbal tea as a non-specific immune booster in the management of cancer (!) which finally got him several months' jail time in 1997 — an incredible *14 years* following the raid. The herb tea charge was the upshot of well over a decade of continual threats, harassment and vilification aimed his way primarily by California medical authorities, representing a state medical dictatorship approximately the equal of the tyranny practiced in New York.

Never one to be cowed, Dr. Halstead, who saw (among many negatives) the loss of at least $2.5 million in research grants to his well-respected World Life Research Institute as he gravitated in and out of court over an eight-year period, told his supporters in 1991:

> *The American people are being held hostage by a venal medical establishment that denies them access to information on many things that could help save their lives as we increasingly face a plague of radiation, cancer, AIDS and other disasters . . . And then they are denied access to useful treatments . . . The man in the street is asleep as to what's going on, but once he finds out that he has been condemned to death because of a handful of vultures that are making billions of dollars by suppressing the scientific fact that there are better healthways to go, all hell will break loose.*[11]

Laetrile sparks a revolution

The historic background must be added here:

The internal shakeup at the AMA which led to the seeming demise of the Committee on Quackery and the Department of Investigation in the mid-1970s was accompanied by the nationwide furor over laetrile (the precipitating cause of the

Committee for Freedom of Choice in Cancer Therapy and the fight for medical freedom of choice which it engendered) and the parallel rapid development of the healthfoods and dietary supplements industries. As we describe elsewhere, the laetrile controversy provided organized allopathic medicine with a challenge even potentially greater than that of chiropractic.

From an industrial/economic standpoint, the fact that laetrile was in the process of being legalized state by state in open defiance of the FDA, the AMA, state medical boards, the medical media, and such officious if unofficial organizations as the American Cancer Society posed several challenges:

— To the concept of centralized authority for a single school of medicine (allopathy), as enshrined in the AMA.

— To the concept that drugs and surgery are America's best medical options. Few things would terrify drug companies more than the notion that the proper use of natural nutrients and other products could be a healthy and dramatically inexpensive alternative to synthetic drugs, whose marketing produced recession-proof profiteering.

— To the grasp and reach of the federal government, particularly through the FDA, as ultimate arbiter of what compounds should be classed and used as medicines, and to the notion of federal centralism itself. After all, laetrile was eventually "decriminalized" in 24 states representing more than half the nation's population even while the federal government described it as "illegal" and "unproven."

The continuing persistence of chiropractic as a medical specialty being turned to by millions of Americans, together with the explosive growth in the supplements industry, together with a populist upsurge against federal authority — these were congealing events which were certain to excite a coordinated response from vested political, economic and ideological interests.

That response was almost certainly the disappearance from within the AMA structure of its quack-quashing apparatuses and their re-emergence later, under "independent" guise along virtually the same lines, and with essentially the same targets, and using essentially the same *modus operandi* of, the old Committee on Quackery and the Department of Investigation.

We pause here to note that hundreds, if not thousands, of AMA members were never a party to, nor necessarily in favor of, such entities or their tactics. It was because the AMA allowed enough internal debate that it could help to rid itself of its worst excesses. As the years have passed, it has become obvious that many otherwise AMA-lining MDs have attempted to bring new thought, new ideas and a reform mentality to an organization which has often been hidebound in its adherence to primeval medical beliefs.

By the middle 1980s, with the rise of an entire movement for medical freedom of choice and a concomitant exponential increase in sales of dietary supplements, healthfoods and the appearance of many more practitioners of "alternative" medicine and dissidents from within the allopathic camp, and with the enormous profits of the drug cartel undermined by natural therapies, it was clear that something had to be done.

The "public awareness campaigns" ostensibly aimed at "health fraud", "quackery" and the like, and involving the same players, but under a non-AMA and "independent" facade, were mostly to be funded by major pharmaceutical houses while deriving their basic format from the "congresses on quackery" held in the early 1960s by the AMA, when quackery essentially meant chiropractic.

The 'quackbuster' coalition appears

Reporter Lisa's documents review found that individuals later to emerge as major "quackbusters" had met with representatives of government organizations in May 1984 to plan a "national health fraud" campaign along the lines reminiscent of the earlier AMA groups. Eventually, the Pharmaceutical Advertising Council (PAC), one of whose leaders was described by Lisa as the originator of the latest "public awareness campaign," and the

US Food and Drug Administration would become prime movers of what on the surface seemed to be an alliance between public and private sectors to alert the American public to the dangers of "health fraud" — that is, any departure from allopathy, a term to which the American public remained almost entirely oblivious.

The need to coordinate a national campaign against "quackery" and "health fraud" followed on the heels of a failed legislative juggernaut: aging US Representative Claude Pepper, who at one time had fought for freedom of choice in cancer therapy and who was now seen as a veteran defender of "senior citizens," introduced three bills in 1982 which (as Lisa analyzed) seemed almost a carbon copy of a memorandum from the old Coordinating Council on Health Information (CCHI). The bills would have established a "national clearinghouse for consumer health information" from public and private sources, increased penalties against "quacks", and would have developed a "strike force against quackery" to involve the FDA, Justice Department, FTC and the US Postal Service.

These bills were craftily presented to the public as a way to defend gullible "senior citizens" from evil health fraud promoters waiting to divest them of their last dimes.

Again, recalling history:

In the mid-1970s, the synthetic drug trust, startled over the growth of the dietary supplements and healthfoods industries, attempted to equip the FDA with massive new police power to stamp out the presumed economic threats. Health-freedoms proponents stopped this effort and the Proxmire Act was passed (1974) to keep such items out of the purview of the FDA.

But just a few years later, with the new industries continuing to flourish at the same time the hubbub over laetrile had helped lead to a stimulus for medical freedom in general, the economic powers-that-be decided to have another go at it:

What could be more beguiling than legislation to protect the elderly from the promoters of health fraud?

But the health-freedoms movement was "on" to this ploy, as

well. Proponents of the "Pepper bills" were inundated with a barrage of letters, telegrams, and communications from an outraged citizenry. The bills died. The Club had been halted once more.

Hence the importance of secret meetings of The Club in 1984 and 1985 along the lines of "what shall be done?"

By the time of such meetings, 24 states had decriminalized laetrile, some were attempting to do the same for EDTA chelation therapy and the expatriate Burton IAT anti-cancer treatment. Homeopathy — the original demon the original AMA had sought to exorcise in the 19th century — was on the rise again along with naturopathy, which was seeking (and gaining) accreditation in several states, with acupuncture, herbalism and other taboos moving out from the wings.

That is to say, the profits of the international pharmaceutical cartel were being challenged as never before by competitor industries, the allopathic medical concept was being challenged as never before by new ideas, and a 1960s-originated general distrust of central authority itself was in full bloom against the notion that the state (or any monopoly nurtured by the state) should make healthcare and medical decisions *for* the population.

All of these currents were flowing, and the only way to stanch them would be a stem-to-stern, coast-to-coast, highly visible "public awareness campaign" seeming to be unbiased, independent, and fusing together public and private entities. From that time forward, the organizations, whose members proudly styled themselves "quackbusters," denied time and again any link to the past or any control of their organizations by hidden forces. They simply "spontaneously appeared" in the mid-1980s to save the nation from a tidal wave of quackery.

Although such investigations as Lisa's revealed information directly linking major pharmaceutical houses with helping to fund the multi-million-dollar campaign, it was the taxpayers who indirectly paid for it through the presence therein of federal and state agencies.

Food and drug companies could shield themselves from *direct* involvement by simply making donations to other organizations some of whose members later appeared as leading "quackbusters."

For example, top "quackbusters" have often belonged not only to their quack-quashing groups but are members as well of the more vintage (and more respected) American Council for Science and Health (ACSH), another one of those semantically adroit organizations whose title *suggests* a degree of authorization and official sanction representing the whole of the United States.

Yet the ACSH — which has indeed taken some reasonable positions on various issues — has never denied (because it cannot) its considerable donations from the processed-foods, chemical and drug interests.

The (Naderite) Center for Science in the Public Interest (CSPI) was the first to note the links of the drug and food industries, in donation form, to the ACSH, in 1982. Reporter Lisa updated these in 1986, and they were further updated March 6, 1989, by the *Des Moines Register*. Said the latter:

> *. . . Most recognizable among its (ACSH's) major funders are NutraSweet, PepsiCo Foundation, Pfizer Pharmaceuticals, Adolph Coors Foundation, Dow Chemical Canada, Monsanto, General Mills, the National Agricultural Chemical Association, Archer Daniels Midland, Coca-Cola, Exxon, Union Carbide.*[12]

It is not surprising that the ACSH, as well as certain "quackbusters" who identify themselves as ACSH members, would come out foursquare against "food faddists", "environmental terrorists" or anyone remotely suggesting that the nation's plastic food supply is not necessarily safe, that the population has been over-drugged and that there is a vast amount of man-made pollution.

Even so, the ACSH itself did not *directly* engage in the name-calling, vituperation and outright social neurosis of "quackbusters" in the new "public awareness campaign" to destroy what the AMA meant by the word quackery: any departure from the allopathic line in medicine.

The 'health fraud conference' follies

This author sat in at various anti-quack meetings in the 1980s to get a feel for the goings-on:

Magicians were on hand to prove how easily the public can be duped, speakers pointed to the history of medical fakery and charlatanry in days gone by (carefully forgetting the charlatanry aspects of allopathy in the 20th century), alleged experts revealed the terrors of "unproven" remedies (with no reference ever made to the horrors of such "proven"remedies as chemotherapy, radiation, surgery and drug reactions), and there usually were attacks on "quack clinics" along the US-Mexican border. As a journalist, I was intrigued at the absolute failure in such meetings on the part of the organizers to attempt to explain just *why* Americans would seek out "quack clinics," particularly in the Third World, if in fact their own medicine at home were so effective.

I was also present at the two major "national health fraud conferences" staged — and "staged" here should be dressed in its full semantical apparel — in one of anti-quackery's apparent safe havens, Kansas City MO.

The first of these, in 1988, was openly — and indeed outrageously — co-sponsored by the FDA, a reality which brought heavy criticism from those who knew the conferences were actually dog-and-pony shows heavily weighted *against* "alternative" medicine and heavily *for* the pharmaceutical industry and allopathic medicine.

At the 1988 conference, your servant and other health-freedoms apostles were followed from place to place by burly security guards as if we represented some kind of physical threat at a meeting which was allegedly "open" as long as a fee had been paid.

The well-attended 1988 conference was liberally sprinkled with representatives of state law enforcement agencies, federal bureaucrats from the FDA and other agencies, insurance companies and allopathically minded doctors. But it also included what was for the organizers an irritatingly high representation of health-freedoms proponents, none of whom disrupted the various meetings and workshops, which were clearly biased propaganda shows and none of which allowed dissent.

By 1990, with AIDS clearly on the agenda and dispensers of "unapproved" AIDS remedies a new target of the Club, the new "national health fraud conference" was to focus on the new killer syndrome. This time, the FDA — chastened over its prior open co-sponsorship of the 1988 confab — was no longer a co-sponsor, and the turnout was considerably lower than expected. More importantly, AIDS activists had "telephone-zapped" conference organizers to express their concern over the conference's contents and backers. The AIDS activist organization ACT-UP had also done its homework, and provided conference visitors with background information on the sponsoring group and on various of the leading "quackbusters."

The AIDS activists caused enough of a stir, and seized sufficient press attention, for the media focus on the conference to shift to them. The result was a determination not to hold any more health fraud conferences in Kansas City — at least "any time soon."

This was the "high" point of the series of "national health fraud conferences" which grew out of the mid-1980s meetings between stakeholder groups opposed to "alternative" medicine.

In the mid-1990s, essentially the same coalition reappeared under the aegis of the Federation of State Medical Boards of the US.

(In 1997, the Federation, in connivance with the Federal Trade Commission [FTC] and the National Assn. of Attorneys General, approved an 11-item set of "recommendations" aimed — once again — at eliminating "questionable medical practices.")

They turn to book-burning

But in the meantime, "quackbusters" — if defeated conceptually, propagandistically and politically — learned they could do a good deal of damage in the courts through omnibus nuisance lawsuits, such as that aimed — unsuccessfully — at P.J. Lisa's book *The Great Medical Monopoly Wars*.

In 1992, James P. Carter MD, Tulane University, a courageous physician and researcher, published a landmark book, *Racketeering in Medicine*,[13] which has some of the data contained here and is overall a treasure trove of information and fact-finding, much of it having to do with The Club's long-standing attack on EDTA chelation therapy. As this was written, Dr. Carter was under legal attack by "quackbusters" since he had obviously touched some important nerves and had bruised some very pompous egos.

Indeed, book-burning — at least symbolically — seems to be part and parcel of the totalitarian get-the-quacks mentality:

A "quackbuster" group newsletter in spring 1990 warned members that "a distressing amount of quackery seems to have found its way onto the campuses of the nation's schools." It ominously reported "the steady influx into school libraries of books that promote unsound health practices." This of course begged the question of just how many "sound" health practices there are and just who is to determine which ones they are.

Oddly, the same article observed: "We wonder if a basic flaw exists in higher education itself. Several authorities have noted that susceptibility to quackery seems to increase with education." [14]

This dumbfounding remark suggested an answer: perhaps it is *because* people are better educated (as "authorities" did in fact report in the 1980s in terms of what kind of people seek out "alternative" medicine for cancer) that they dissent from tyrannically imposed medicine and seek options.

Only by understanding how organized allopathy and the organized quackbusters were wedded to a single concept (all dissent is quackery) could an article in a 1989 food industry newsletter, *Food Nutrition News,* make any kind of sense:

In it, a "quackbuster" used the words "quack", "quacks", and "quackery" a breathtaking 50 times in 48 paragraphs — possibly aware of Pavlovian brainwashing techniques bearing on ever-repeated words and phrases.[15]

Such has been the establishmentarian attack against unwanted new truth — if it cannot be beaten back through propaganda and politics, then at least symbolic book-burning and ad-hominem legal attacks through America's lawyer-happy court system can slow it down.

AMA's spotty history

If the modern "quackbusters" are little more than the reincarnation of AMA's zealous quack-hunters from an early era, it is necessary to wonder just why allopathy feels so threatened.

Other chapters of this study trace the development of the paradigm or mindset of the allopaths, and how this thought system acquired new force through licensure and political manipulation. It would not have had the fuel to become the *single* school of "approved" medicine, however, without the advent of the giant pharmaceutical combine for which the allopathic concept is a handy apparatus for drug distribution and profit.

Once equipped with authority and funds, allopathic education in this century purged medical schools of the presumptive heresies of non-allopathic medicine.

As we note elsewhere, a primary impetus of the AMA, when established in 1847, was to undercut and ultimately vanquish homeopathy, the major foe of drug-based and mechanical medicine in the 19th century. The decades-long attack on chiropractic a century later was simply a replay of an old melody, although with much greater noise.

The allopathic regulars, whether in Britain or America, liked to denigrate their opponents as "quacks" and "charlatans," so the fact that this line of thought was carried to greater rhetorical perfection in this century should not surprise.

The first 50 years of the AMA were mostly spent in bickering and in-fighting between jealous state medical societies and competing medical schools.

However, as Dr. Bruce Halstead has observed,[16] "a prophet arose in their midst known as 'Doc' George H. Simmons, who was soon to lead the moribund association out of the wilderness into a land flowing with milk and honey . . .

"The politically astute 'Doc' Simmons was an advertising quack, an abortionist, and a diploma-mill licentiate who became the unscrupulous boss and dictator of the official trade organization of organized American medicine — the AMA. He reigned supreme as the editor and general manager of the AMA from 1899 to 1924 . . . It is paradoxical that this advertising quack was later to set the standards of the 'code of ethics' of the AMA, which for decades has prohibited physicians from advertising."

His protege, Morris Fishbein, then became the AMA's editor/leader for ensuing decades. Within his interesting c.v. was helping guide the AMA attack on "unproven cancer therapies," particularly the Hoxsey herbal treatments — and losing to Harry Hoxsey in court.

Of the flamboyant Morris Fishbein, who became editor of the *Journal* of the AMA in 1924, it has been said that he gave organized allopathic medicine its voice and "opened up to it the real sources of power, money, legislative action, and public assent" while arguably managing "to hold back the twentieth century for 50 years for the benefit of organized medicine."[17]

The AMA's heyday was marked by two obsessive concerns: opposing socialized medicine and/or compulsory health insurance in any form, and beating back the forces of "quackery" and "cultism" — that is, anything which did not fit the allopathic mold.

By this time, the early AMA's somewhat leery distrust of the drug industry was mostly, if not entirely, over and both the drug industry and the allopathic monopoly had found ways to use each other (*VIII*). The greater ogres of physicians and their leaders were the non-allopaths and the haunting historical movements for some form of universal healthcare.

By 1931 the AMA could pompously declare:

"All opinions made to the public on the general, social, legislative, and economic relationship of medical practice should be made only through approved channels of the American Medical Association."[18]

The organization fought tooth-and-nail against government medicine, including President Truman's request for national health insurance, which occasioned a huge AMA advertising/ political campaign (55 million pamphlets were distributed which bore the famous painting by Sir Luke Fields of a physician bending over the bed of a sick child — and captioned "keep politics out of this picture"). In so doing, the AMA for a time (1949 and 1950) became the major national lobby in Washington.

Along the way, the AMA came to terms (prodded by a California Supreme Court decision) with osteopathy, which essentially led to that profession's essential absorption into organized allopathy, and even with optometry, whose practitioners had been called "cultists" by the allopaths inasmuch as they were not (as were the competing ophthalmologists) medical doctors (that is, allopaths).

It also remained wary even of nurses, since by the very nature of their profession these heroic individuals might actually encroach on allopathic turf and "practice medicine" when not specifically licensed to do so. And the AMA remained vigorously opposed to nutrition as a form of therapy.

The Simmons and Fishbein eras represent the golden age of the AMA, now an assemblage, practically on the model of the former Soviet Communist Party, of local, state, and regional medical societies, with the equivalents of a Chairman, Supreme Soviet and Politburo at its head. A czar-like chief executive officer, the Board of Trustees, the House of Delegates, dozens of working committees and close working relationships with state and regional affiliates comprise the well-oiled AMA organizational machinery.

When would-be health reformer First Lady Hillary Rodham Clinton was introduced to the AMA in 1993, the spokesman who made the introduction claimed the organization "represents ninety percent of medicine." As only about 40 percent of the nation's allopaths were represented by AMA at the time, this was a drastic misstatement, since as the organized allopathic lobbying force AMA may indeed speak for a large plurality of *allopaths,* whether they are members or not — but never "ninety percent of medicine."

Following several years' decline in members, AMA membership was back to 720,000 at the end of 1995, a 17 percent rise since 1990.

Even so, the organization was engaged in soul-searching about its membership, since despite more members the number of those involved in "primary care" — rather than in "specialties" — continued to fall.[(19)]

A profitable seal of approval

To be an allopathic physician since earlier in this century has always meant the ability to beat the rate of inflation. Certainly the AMA sets the standards and defends the allopathic monopoly.

And being an AMA member, Oliver Garceau wrote, also saves the doctor "the awkward predicament of having to think."[(20)]

Interestingly, the AMA does not like to talk about how much physicians earn — as evidencd both by a 1993 decision not to issue press releases on the latest salary figures and a 1994 decision to "juggle the books" (in the Associated Press' words) as to the last public salary figures announced (1992). Hence, non-AMA and AMA doctor salary assessments may vary.

In what the Public Citizen Health Research Group in Washington called "unabashed deception of the public or anyone else who would want to know what physicians make" and what the AMA secretary-treasurer admitted was "an accounting change . . . to show the whole picture", the national body decided to mingle the salaries of private practitioners, government doctors and young physicians in training. Inclusion of the latter two groups would tend to deflate salaries overall, conceivably deflecting from public view the spectacle of million-dollar-a-year oncological and cardiovascular surgeons, for example.

Salary calculations reported in 1994 and based on 1992 figures showed US doctors in private practice with a mean income of $177,400 a year, ranging in categories from the $111,800 mean for general practitioners to $253,300 for radiologists (and, as earlier estimates showed, about $233,900 for surgeons). "Mean" salaries even as of 1992 of course meant numerous surgeons — apex of the "healthcare delivery team" — had far higher incomes.[21]

By 1997, the AMA's review of salaries showed average surgeon incomes of $316,000, and that of general family practice physicians at $159,000.[22]

In 1996, the Medical Group Management Assn. (MGMA), described as a "group practice trade association," brought in more financial perspectives in reports based on 1995 data:

Family-practice and pediatrics *group* physicians were at the lower end of the median annual salary spectrum ($129,000-plus respectively) while cardiovascular surgeons' mean annual income was $490,000, with orthopedic surgeons second at $302,000. Starting (first-year) salaries were headed by orthopedic surgeons ($227,000).

The assessment of these non-AMA figures was that group-practice specialists "are working harder but have little to show for it"(!) primarily due to the rapidly advancing commitment to "managed care." MGMA data also showed some glaring gaps for physicians *in general*: upward-range salaries for neurosurgeons were at $600,000 as contrasted to lower-percentile salaries of pediatricians, family physicians and internists (all under $100,000).[23]

By 1997, the reported "dip" in general medical salaries over the prior two years seemed to have been overcome. The "median net income" reported by the AMA — the doctors' trade group —

was set at $160,000.[24]

These varying sets of data served to underscore an ever-present reality in American medicine: specialists make a lot more than do generalists — yet it is generalists, more than specialists, who are apt to see the patient as a whole person rather than as an organ or tissue type.

At the same time, US physician fees are the envy of the world:

In 1993, a Knight-Ridder survey comparing US doctor fees with those in Canada and Germany found the Americans not only ahead but *far* ahead of their counterparts in the other two Western countries. Examples:

A 15-minute consultation with an American general practitioner was averaging $41, vs. $20 for the Canadian medic and $5 for the German; an endoscopy fetched $267 for an American doctor, $70 for a Canadian, $64 for a German; a needle biopsy procured $125 for the American, $27 for the Canadian and $17 for the German. All three paid high taxes, but it could be argued that the Americans were more at the mercy of high-priced lawyers and malpractice insurance than their counterparts — though not always by much.[25]

What does being an "MD" mean in America — whether the MD is actually a member of the AMA or not?

It means membership in a major closed society within The Club — where the MD degree can usually only be granted by a medical school accredited by the AMA. The student's education of course is almost entirely allopathic, and internship is only allowed at a hospital meeting AMA criteria as a teaching institution.

Whatever state the allopath works in, his or her medical practice is strictly in accordance with laws promulgated by AMA-lining, AMA-determined, or AMA-friendly state, county or regional medical boards. His membership in AMA-lining, AMA-determined or AMA-friendly state, county or medical societies helps establish "ethical" credentials, and post-graduate education is in the hands of a raft of AMA-approved magazines, monographs, research papers and the like — and visitations galore by drug company sales representatives.

The MD doctor does not stand alone — medical technicians, nurses and others in the "healthcare-delivery team" must have the AMA seal of approval.

As long ago as 1958, Richard Carter in *The Doctor Business* observed:

> *On the national level, the AMA extended its authority far beyond the medical schools. As custodian of medical standards, it began determining the eligibility of hospitals to train new physicians. It gave authoritative advice on the training of nurses and technicians. . .*[26]

The MD degree thus carries a virtual certainty of economic success — despite the high fees charged for malpractice insurance — and existence within a recession-proof industry, a reflection of the even safer economic confines of the even more recession-proof drug industry.

Dissent from within

The AMA has had some of its worst criticisms arise from within its own ranks — by trained allopaths blessed with honesty.

Though such outsiders as Trever and Lisa (with help from insiders) helped detail the organization's obsession with dissent ("quackery"), the AMA has come in for scathing denunciations on even broader fronts.

Even before the premature death of Robert Mendelsohn MD, whose epochal *Confessions of a Medical Heretic*[27] did more than any single book to damage the credibility not only of the AMA but of organized allopathic medicine in general, there had been some important sorties:

Richard Kunnes MD, who after openly declaring that the AMA acronym should actually stand for the "American Murder

Association," set fire to his membership card at an AMA convention, wrote the exposé *Your Money or Your Life* in 1974.[28]

Hans Ruesch, whose *Slaughter of the Innocent* and *Naked Empress* recorded this event, also quoted Niagara Falls NY physician J.W. Hodge MD:

> *"Every practitioner of the healing art who does not ally himself with the medical trust is denounced as a 'dangerous quack' and impostor by the predatory doctors' trust. Every sanitarian who attempts to restore the sick to a state of health by natural means without resort to the knife or poisonous drugs, disease imparting serums, deadly toxins or vaccines, is at once pounced upon by these medical tyrants and fanatics, bitterly denounced, vilified and persecuted to the fullest extent."*[29]

Perhaps the first major whistle-blower of the links between organized allopathy and the drug industry was a journalist — Morris A. Bealle, former city editor of the now defunct *Washington Times and Herald*, who learned — as this writer, also a former newspaper editor, would learn decades later — just how great is the pressure of vested interests to keep certain things from public view.

Bealle's baptism into the way things are began in the 1930s with an editorial fight in favor of those who had been given poor service by the local power company. One thing led to another, and Bealle ran headlong into an assessment of the combination of vested interests we describe elsewhere as the Rockefeller-I.G. Farben combination, the all-encompassing umbrella over, among other things, the international pharmaceutical cartel (*VI*).

He put it all together in 1949 in *The Super Drug Story,* which he found he could not sell to major publishing houses. This eye-opening volume (variously retitled thereafter as *The Drug Story* and *The New Drug Story*) was available only to those who found Bealle's own self-publishing company — and, decades later, through the health-freedoms movement, which did much to resurrect Bealle's work. It had made it through almost three dozen printings by the 1980s.[30]

In his factual exposé of "the House of Rockefeller" in the USA and its pervasive presence in an enormous area of corporations, companies, businesses, and research grants, Bealle (and later Ruesch) noted that the *Journal of the American Medical Assn. (JAMA)* had boasted as early as 1940 that the old United Press news syndicate had been forced to issue a directive requiring all articles on cures and human health to be "cleared" through *JAMA's* New York bureau and science editors. The same editors accepted the powerful Morris Fishbein, the long-time leader of the AMA and editor of the *JAMA*, as an expert on medical matters — even though, as records in the matter of Harry Hoxsey vs. Morris Fishbein would reveal years later — the "expert" had never actually practiced medicine!

Bealle also quoted Charles Lyman Loffler MD as one of those first victimized by the cancer industry wing of the Allopathic Industrial Complex: "Since the regimentation of medicine by quacks and medical gangsters in control of the American Medical Association, this organization has become one of the most vicious rackets in the country."

And this was long before chief heretic Dr. Robert Mendelsohn would say of medicine in general: "I no longer believe in modern medicine. I believe that the greatest danger to your health is the doctor who practices modern medicine."[31]

But while Bealle and others had to get into self-publishing and direct-mail to get their points of view across, Mendelsohn produced mass-market best-sellers which mightily stung the establishment. At the time of his quite unexpected death in 1989 a "quackbuster" group was devoting time and energy in attempting to force the several hundred newspapers which carried his column to drop it — another manifestation of book-burning in the Land of the Free and Home of the Brave.

The AMA and politics

As the voice of organized allopathy, the AMA and its state medical board allies make donations, as hefty as legally possible, to politicians who in turn are beholden to establishment medicine, and who may be counted on either to shore up the existing monopoly or legislatively deflect attempts to curb it. The allopathic industrial contribution to politics often overlaps with those of pharmaceutical, chemical and food interests, but can also be spotted on its own.

The AMA's American Medical Political Action Committee (AMPAC) and similar political action committees (PACs) state by state have raised millions of dollars to support candidates expected to be friendly to organized industrial allopathy. For example, it became a notorious fact that in California (variously described as the seventh or eighth economy in total GDP in the world), in which agriculture is paramount followed by several other major industries, during most recent years the state's *medical* PAC has usually been the chief lobbyist in Sacramento.

Only such a happenstance explains why the State of California administratively could seek to suppress the tide of progressive medicine within the Golden State's own borders while the Legislature frequently looked the other way. He who pays the piper calls the tune:

California Common Cause reported in 1991 that in the prior decade the medical, pharmaceutical and dental interests had contributed more than $23.1 million to candidates for state offices. Of this figure, more than $5 million came from the state's number-one PAC — the California Medical Assn. (CMA)[(32)]

At the federal level, it is of course the same:

In 1990 healthcare industry PACs doled out $8 million to congressional candidates in that single year alone, with the AMA's AMPAC leading the PAC-pack with $2.1 million out of reported total receipts of $4.7 million from 65,000 AMPAC members.[(33)]

(All of which made it strangely humorous to hear

"quackbusters" in recent years rail about the "well-oiled quackery dispensers" and the "big money in quackery," while painting themselves as selfless popular heroes to whom CARE packages should be addressed.)

The AMA and the private health insurance companies also funded the lion's share of propaganda against the admittedly flawed Clinton Administration healthcare reform effort, defeated in 1994.[34]

As the People's Medical Society put it in 1988: "The 'bottom line', according to one AMA document, 'is election of legislators favorable to AMA positions.' This is curious, for should not the bottom line be the best and most complete care options for the patient?"[35]

That the AMA engages in conspiracy became diaphanously clear with the victory by the chiropractors. Yet, AMA watchers could point to a much earlier, ongoing, unsavory conspiracy by the national organization:

The AMA, always heatedly opposed to government medicine, came out against a collective health insurance program, the Group Health Association of Washington DC, and went so far to halt the GHA that the Department of Justice warned the organization to cease and desist in its tactics.

On Dec. 20, 1938, 21 individuals (including Morris Fishbein), the AMA and three affiliate societies were indicted for violating the Sherman Antitrust Act. A guilty verdict on the charge of conspiracy was handed down in 1941. The appeals procedure reached the US Supreme Court in 1943. The lower court decisions were upheld.

Had the AMA connected its distrust of government medicine with a defense of the free market in medicine, it might have gone down as a champion of liberty. Instead, it has defended allopathic medical monopolism at every turn and has thus become a major obstacle to the development of new thought.

Under the guidance of such personalities as Simmons and

Fishbein, it honed to perfection manipulation of words and alteration of language — the very thing American patriots long criticized the Nazis and Communists of doing.

Corrupting the lexicon and peddling drugs

Corrupting the lexicon has become a high political art, and the Allopathic Industrial Complex — conceptually guided by the AMA —has learned the lessons well.

With almost gnat-like persistence, it has referred to its opponents and dissidents as "frauds" and "quacks" while defending its own approaches as "rigorously scientific," "responsible" and "proven."

Worse, in American English it has co-opted the very words "doctor", "physician" and "medicine" to give them a narrow definition. Its journals and publications — laden with pharmaceutical and/or hospital product advertising — speak of the AMA as "medicine's" voice, and present the AMA position on this or that matter as "medicine's" view.

Worse yet, the AMA, as the organized voice of allopathic medicine *even* while representing well under half the nation's allopaths, has been a prime mover in allowing the domination of medicine in the United States by the drug cartel — setting the stage for the modern spectacle of physician as legal drug-pusher.

It was bound to happen, of course, just as soon as the incipient drug business began filling the pages of allopathic medical jounals with huge amounts of advertising, which allowed the journals, and the medical societies behind them, a vast new source of ready revenue.

In April 1976 Chairman Gaylord Nelson of the Senate Select Committee on Small Business reported that "the almost complete takeover by the drug industry of post-graduate medical 'education' is cause for alarm." Nelson's committee had heard from FDA whistle-blower Richard Crout that the drug industry selected and paid for "the bulk of education information provided to the practicing physician."[36]

Added Nelson: "The pharmaceutical industry spends over a billion dollars a year on the promotion and advertising of drugs — or $5,000 per physician per year. That's about twice as much as we spend each year to educate our doctors in our country's 116 medical schools."

"Post-graduate medical education" actually means the courting of physicians by drug company "detail men" as well as the hard-and-soft-sell approaches whereby drug companies sponsor symposia in exotic locales and organize promotions of all kinds which will ultimately associate physician recall and product names.

We explore in *VIII* the outrageous lengths to which the drug industry goes in the wooing of physicians.

It was all summed up for me by an aging defecting allopath some years ago:

> *"We (allopaths) have become whores for the drug boys. We are in the drug-dealing business. Maybe we didn't mean to, but that's where we are. If we keep our noses clean and don't gripe about it, life is wonderful for us. But we can't raise a fuss. If we downplay drugs and upgrade vitamins, we're in big trouble. Everybody knows this."*

Taxpayer-subsidized gouging

The perhaps well-intentioned idea that the rush into medicine of government-mandated health plans would somehow ameliorate the situation (the extreme cost of modern medicine, profiteering by the drug companies) has turned out, as libertarians feared, to be nonsensical and contributory to the problem:

The advent of Medicare and Medicaid — government add-ons to the unwieldy apparatus of American medicine — naturally provided both greedy companies and greedy doctors with vast new possibilities for gouging to be underwritten by taxpayers.

Like any other government-run, government-supervised or government-monitored scheme or agency, these two well-intentioned programs to provide medical relief for the aged or economically desperate would constantly run out of money. Why not? The government-agency scheme has always meant open checkbooks, budgets to be expanded yearly and a continual raid on Congress for more funds. Since the ultimate funder is usually the IRS-raped taxpayer from the American middle class, there is always a bottomless pit of possible revenue as long as there seems to be some rational or humanitarian need for the agency.

While Medicare/Medicaid regulations were also used *against* non-allopathic or integrative practitioners across the country (i.e., the government made it difficult if not impossible for doctors in government programs to prescribe vitamins, herbs or chiropractic *in lieu of* toxic synthetic chemicals, surgical procedures, radiation, and other "standard" techniques), they were bent to allow abuse by mainstream medics at the same time.

In 1989, a subsidiary of giant SmithKline Beecham agreed to pay the federal government $1.5 million to settle an investigation of alleged kickbacks to California physicians — some 100 of whom were allegedly rewarded with thousands of dollars for referring Medicare/Medicaid patients to laboratories in which the doctors were limited partners.

The Office of Inspector General of the Department of Health and Human Services (HHS) had made the probe. The final settlement was said at the time to be the largest under the Medicare anti-kickback law, a 1987 statute designed to help curb such offenses.(37)

As we observe elsewhere (*III*) in the multi-billion-dollar overall problem in fraud and kickback schemes involving physicians and insurance plans, both public and private, the above case was child's play compared to later scandals.

Ethics begins at home

Throughout its serpentine history, the AMA, which has laid so much claim to organizing the (allopathic) profession along the lines of ethics and integrity — while continually beating the drums against all dissent ("quackery", "unscientific medicine", "questionable" or "unproven" treatments) — has had its own continuing internal ethics problems, as we have seen.

The AMA rarely washes its linen in public, though at times it has had to:

In 1993, the organization admitted it had had a "substantial drop" in membership since 1990 and that part of the drop (to 293,988 members representing only about 40% of all physicians; in recent decades the AMA has never had a *majority* of allopaths among its members) was due to the financial problems of former AMA Executive Vice President James H. Sammons.

Sammons resigned in 1990 after 15 years as the AMA's top executive because, as the organization's weekly newspaper put it, he had "approved questionable transactions to two AMA executives." This included the former president of American Medical Services Inc., a holding company for the AMA's "for-profit" subsidiaries.[38]

The organization has also had an ongoing problem with conflicts of interest, even aside from the worst one: its serving as a propaganda channel for the international pharmaceutical cartel.

In its 1993 annual meeting, the AMA "formalized" a policy to reject revenues from tobacco companies "but not necessarily from the companies' non-tobacco subsidiaries" which helped fund AMA "health campaigns."[39]

The 1993 policy statement was a decades-late finale to the open scandal of the 1970s, when the public learned that the AMA held $1.4 million in tobacco company stocks. The situation had indeed become ludicrous: the public had before it the spectacle of AMA doctors grudgingly joining the national anti-cigarette smoking campaign while their trade organization/ labor union was making money off a stock portfolio including R.J. Reynolds and Philip Morris. By 1981, the AMA had divested itself of such stock, a spokesman noting that "the publicity hurt."[40]

In the ethics area, the AMA has spent far more time assailing dissidents as quacks and charlatans than it has in cleaning up its own house — a central reason, perhaps, why state medical boards (directly or indirectly in the thrall of the AMA) spend so much more time harassing "alternative" therapies than chastening allopaths who make mistakes.

In 1984, for example, a report by the Department of HHS' inspector general claimed that somewhere between 20,000 and 45,000 of the nation's nearly 400,000 patient-care doctors "are likely candidates for some level of discipline" — yet only 391 disciplinary actions had been taken by state medical boards.[41]

Said a California justice in a case dissent:

> *Physicians who are members of medical societies flock to the defense of their fellow member charged with malpractice and the plaintiff is relegated, for his expert testimony, to the occasional lone wolf or heroic soul who, for the sake of truth and justice, has the courage to run the risk of ostracism by his fellow practitioners and the cancellation of his public liability insurance policy.*[42]

That is, organized allopathy does not like whistle-blowers. Those who step out of line, let alone those daring to consort with medical dissidents and actually practice non-allopathy, will face shunning and expulsion from the church of organized allopathic medicine. Their conceptual burning at the stake will be economic ruination from loss of license and hospital privileges.

Business as usual

In the meantime, the AMA is itself big business. With its percentage membership of physicians generally having dropped since the early 1970s, though rebounding by 1995, it is obvious that the organization's main source of income could hardly be membership dues alone.

Even by 1974, it was estimated that advertising through its 12 separate journals was earning the national body $10 million a year, or half its total revenues.[43]

By 1993, the AMA could report that in 1992 it had total operating revenues of $197.5 million, up $10 million from 1991 even though "operating expenses" had ballooned to $193.5 million.

The organization's weekly reported that the increase in revenue was largely due to a $7.6 million increase in advertising take, $3.5 million in book and product sales, $1.5 million in subscriptions, and a paltry $1 million each from "royalties" and dues. It also spent $2.3 million promoting its own "health system reform package."

The $9.2 million increase in operating expenses was largely due to $5.1 million in salary increases — including an increase in pay to $442,024 for the AMA's executive vice president.[44]

As the United States entered a period of extreme soul-searching over medical reform in the 1990s, it became customary for conservatives and the Right to defend the AMA as victims of government interference — and for liberals and the Left to champion government management as somehow being the answer to the various problems of runaway inflation in general and the high cost of delivering medical goods and services in particular.

Yet both sides were able to miss the mark:

While government interference in and regulation over medicine had led the United States, even by the end of the 1960s, to a form of crypto-socialized medicine that this writer styles "fascist medicine," and while it is obvious that government, by its very nature, can neither solve the problem(s) nor claim it is *not* the central element in the high cost of medicine, it is also true that the international pharmaceutical cartel has reflected an unfettered drive for profits and that the AMA has nurtured and defended medical monopoly in America.

There is, thus, plenty of guilt to go around on all sides, and no simplistic single-ideology quick-fix solution to a multifaceted problem. Common sense is required for authentic change — and it sometimes appears in unexpected places.

Hitting a nerve

In summer 1978, a Nobel Prize-winning economist struck at the AMA's central nerve:

Why license physicians in the first place?

In a historic address at the Mayo Clinic, Dr. Milton Friedman accused both the AMA and the FDA of hampering the healthy growth of medicine in America. (The FDA, he said, was a "killer" because its restrictions had been keeping life-saving drugs, particularly against heart disease, from Americans.)

The former presidential adviser stunned his audience by arguing that physicians should not be licensed and that it had been by governmental intrusion into medicine that the AMA medical monopoly had grown and prospered in the United States, much to the detriment of health care.

"The control over that [medical] licensure procedure is what has enabled the American Medical Association to exercise its monopoly for these many decades," he said, adding that his opinion was based on "considerable evidence, considerable examination of the effects" of licensing procedures on state medical boards and the monopolistic practices of the AMA.

"You cannot have an open field and an elimination of these monopolistic restrictions unless you eliminate the power of government at that crucial element," he said of licensure. "If we continue with the licensure of medical practice, then either government or organized medicine is going to have monopoly power in the future."[45]

It also must be stressed that not all allopathic doctors not only are not necessarily members of the AMA but are often at odds with its agenda.

One open-minded essentially allopathic organization in the USA is the Association of American Physicians and Surgeons Inc. (AAPS), which as of 1997 claimed about 5,000 members.

The organization has stated:

For more than 50 years, AAPS has operated on the principle that physicians are partners in the care of their patients. If your doctor is a member of AAPS, that means he embraces the Oath of Hippocrates and believes that his duty to the patient comes first. He works for the good of the patient, not that of the government, an insurance company, or a managed health bureaucrat.[46]

AAPS has established a "patients' bill of rights," including such keystone ones as the right to refuse medical treatment and the right to refuse "third-party interference" in medical care, which places the organization at ideological odds with the Allopathic Industrial Complex (AIC).

Allopathic quackbusting goes international

Just as the international drug cartel, chief nourisher of the AIC, is global in scope, and just as AMA-nurtured allopathy is global in scope, so too are the "quackbuster" alliances — governmental/drug company/policing combines.

Their presence is felt wherever non-allopathic therapies loom as important threats to pharmaceuticals — which is now practically everywhere, especially in the Western world, where allopathy became the reigning medical model. As we shall see (*VIII*), the global drug industry seeks to knock out its competition under the color of international law.

Recent decades have marked the rise in Europe of more interest in what Europeans call "biological" medicine, even though such techniques were never as viciously fought as in the United States. Non-allopathic modalities continue to spread across the Western world, with homeopathy in a new phase of research and development and such techniques as radionics and various Eastern healing systems usually legal if officially frowned upon in many Western countries.

In no country, of course, have "unconventionals" been so ruthlessly squelched as in the alleged "home of the free, land of the brave," where the spectacle of doctors hauled off in handcuffs for providing vitamin therapies to patients is simply not believable to a civilized European.

Even in Canada, whose medical establishment has usually been slavishly devoted to the tetrarchs of allopathy south of the border, despite vigorous "quackbuster" activity against Canadian maverick medics daring to step out of line, the degree of tyranny in place against medical free thought pales alongside the Gestapoid activities of the Americans, particularly in New York and California.

In 1993 it was reported that a stunning seven out of 10 general practitioners in Germany practiced some form of "alternative," "unconventional" or "complementary" therapy and that the nation's Federal Science Ministry was providing research grants based on a report the ministry itself had commissioned.

The top five most common "unconventional means" were homeopathy, anthroposophy, physiotherapy, balneotherapy and acupuncture. A group led by Dr. Peter Matthiessen had spent two years researching some 130 "unconventional" therapies and found that "the main principle of unconventional therapies — the stimulation of the natural healing forces of the body — deserves investigation."[(47)]

This was symbolic in that Germany had, since ancient times, been a center of free thought in medicine.

Also in 1993, the *London Daily Telegraph* reported the urging by the "medical establishment" of controlled trials to attempt to determine which "complementary therapies" were safe and effective, that there were by then "well over 100 [such] therapies competing for recognition" and that a "chair of complementary medicine" would be installed at Exeter University.

The *Telegraph* also noted that even in a country where socialized medicine has supposedly modified the cost of medicine public outcry over both "the soaring cost of orthodox medical treatment" and "mounting dissatisfaction" with the results were leading the National Health Service to a consideration of "alternatives."[(48)]

This too was symbolic, for it was the English under Henry VIII who, in what allopaths would later deride as "the quacks' charter," set the legal basis for herbal and natural treatments in the United Kingdom (*V*). It was also symbolic in that homeopathy has long been an accepted form of treatment, and of particular interest to the Royal Family.

The United Kingdom has thus been a leader in at least keeping an open mind to alternatives. In 1982, the British Research Council on Complementary Medicine was established — 10 years before a similar effort would be made in the United States — which was a direct response to the British public's increased use of "unorthodox" therapies.

The Council's first report, covering 1983-1988, was candid in finding the socialized National Health Service (NHS) to be in crisis (the demand for medical services was outstripping the supply of available services) and that reliance on science and high technology rather than the time-honored practicing of the "art" of medicine had led to blind alleys.[49]

The Council's recommendations, and the forces behind them, pointed to the need for a radical new approach to the provision of medical services, called for more self-help care and greater access to validated "complementary" medicines. This important move forward in a country which also serves as a major headquarters of the Allopathic Industrial Complex (AIC), of course, would not go unchallenged.

A major counterattack to medical freedom of choice occurred in England with a "quackbuster" organization which investigative reporter Martin J. Walker found had strong ties to the United States.

In *Dirty Medicine,* Walker exposed the organization HealthWatch, a prime opponent of "alternative" medicine, as tied in with sectors of allopathic medicine, industry and government. The propaganda campaign raised by this coalition against non-allopathic "unconventional" practitioners was a carbon copy, on a lesser scale, of the "quackbuster" blitz in the United States.

Noting the comfortable relationship between socialism and capitalist monopoly, Walker pointed out that the "biggest drug companies will side with and support socialized medicine over private practice simply because government contracts give assured and stable profits without the threat of competition."[50]

In the Netherlands in 1993 there was a replay of the long-raging war going on in the United States over food supplements:

The director of a Dutch group called Foundation for Orthomolecular Education reported that the Dutch secretary of state for public health was about to sign a law classifying all food supplements containing more than 1½ times the RDA (recommended daily allowance — an American conceptual import) of vitamins as registered medicines.

The organization's Dr. R.A. Nieuwenhuis claimed the official "bases this view on reports of official Dutch institutes, like the Food Council, Health Council and the Dutch Consumers Union. Needless to say, all these institutes are very conservative and can be seen as mouthpieces of the pharmacists and pharmaceutical companies."[51]

References

1. *The Choice*, XVIII:3, 1987.
2. *The Choice*, VI:3, 1980.
3. Trever, William, *In the Public Interest*. Los Angeles: Scriptures Unlimited, 1972.
4. *Ibid.*
5. *Ibid.*
6. United Press International, July 14, 1971.
7. Lisa, PJ, *Are You a Target for Elimination?* Huntington Beach CA: International Institute of Natural Health Sciences, Inc., 1985.
8. Lisa, PJ, *The Great Medical Monopoly Wars*. Huntington Beach CA: International Institute of Natural Health Sciences, Inc., 1986.
9. United Features Syndicate, March 17, 1991.
10. Lisa, *The Great . . . op. cit.*
11. *The Choice*, XVII: 3,4 1991.
12. *Des Moines Register*, March 6, 1989.
13. Carter, JO, *Racketeering in Medicine*. Norfolk VA: Hampton Roads, 1992.
14. *The Choice*, XVI: 2,3, 1990.
15. *The Choice*, XV: 4, 1989.
16. Halstead, Bruce, unpublished MS. made available to the author.
17. Harmer, RM, *American Medical Avarice*. New York: Abelard-Schurman, 1975.
18. *Ibid.*
19. Mitka, Mike, "Doctor ranks grow 17% in 5 years." *American Medical News*. Feb. 3, 1997.
20. Garceau, Oliver, *The Political History of the American Medical Association*. Cambridge MA: Harvard University Press, 1941.

21. *The Choice* XIX: 1, 1993; The Associated Press, June 17, 1994.
22. Mitka, Mike, "Physician pay back up, but two-year trend still shows loss." *American Medical News.* Jan. 6, 1997.
23. Mitka, Mike, "Working hard for the money." *American Medical News,* Aug. 19, 1996.
24. Mitka, Mike, "Physician . . ." *op. cit.*
25. Knight-Ridder Tribune News, July 1993.
26. Carter, Richard, *The Doctor Business.* New York: Doubleday, 1958.
27. Mendelsohn, RS, *Confessions of a Medical Heretic.* Chicago: Contemporary Books, 1979.
28. Kunnes, Richard, *Your Money or Your Life.* New York: Dodd, Mead, 1974.
29. Ruesch, Hans, *Naked Empress.* Zurich: CIVIS, 1982.
30. Bealle, MA, *The Super Drug Story.* Washington DC: Columbia Publishing, 1949.
31. Mendelsohn, *op. cit.*
32. *The Choice*, XVII: 3,4 1991.
33. *The Choice*, XVII: 2, 1991.
34. *The Choice.* XX:2,3, 1994.
35. Inlander, CB, *et al., Medicine on Trial.* New York: Pantheon Books, 1988.
36. Culbert, ML, *What the Medical Establishment Won't Tell You that Could Save Your Life.* Norfolk VA: Donning, 1983.
37. *The Choice*, XVI: 1, 1990.
38. *The Choice*, XIX: 1, 1993.
39. The Associated Press, June 18, 1993.
40. Culbert, *op. cit.*
41. Inlander, *op. cit.*
42. Bok, S, *Lying: Moral Choice in Public and Private Life.* New York: Pantheon Books, 1978.
43. Griffin, GE, *World Without Cancer.* Westlake Village CA: American Media, 1974.
44. *American Medical News,* July 5, 1993.
45. Culbert, *op. cit.*
46. Orient, JM, and Kathryn Serkes, *Rx for Patient Power: the Patients' Handbook.* Tucson AZ: Assn. of American Physicians and Surgeons, Inc., 1996.
47. *Lancet,* cited in *The Choice,* XIX: 1, 1993.
48. Cited in *The Choice*, XIX: 2, 1993.
49. Carter, JO, *op. cit.*
50. Walker, MJ, *Dirty Medicine.* London: Slingshot Publications, 1993.
51. Cited in *Townsend Letter for Doctors*, July 1993.

VIII
THE DRUG INDUSTRY: Riding the recession-proof gravy train

"After 1899, the flood of new drugs continued to rise for half a century. Few of these turned out to be safer, more effective, and cheaper than well-known and long-tested therapeutic standbys, whose numbers grew at a much slower rate . . . Many of the new drugs [after World War II] were dangerous, and . . . few were demonstrably better than those they were meant to replace. Fewer than 98 percent of these chemical substances constitute valuable contributions to the pharmacopeia used in primary care . . . Opinions vary about the actual number of useful drugs; some experienced clinicians believe that less than two dozen basic drugs are all that will ever be desirable for 99 percent of the total population. . ."

— Ivan Illich (*Medical Nemesis*)

"The pharmaceutical industry is extremely competitive but the profits that accrue to the successful participants are enormous. [The industry giants'] salesmen try to maintain contact with every physician in the country, and there is hardly a physician alive who hasn't received a gift or free sample from one of them; many a physician's 'black bag' was a pharmaceutical gift."

— Stanley Wohl MD (*The Medical Industrial Complex*)

"Pharmaceutical R & D is a costly and risky business, but in recent years the financial rewards from R & D have more than offset its costs and risks."

— US Congress Office of Technology Assessment Report, 1993

"When will they realize that there are too many drugs? . . . About 15,000 new mixtures and dosages hit the market each year, while about 12,000 die off . . . We simply don't have enough diseases to go around. At the moment the most helpful contribution is the new drug to counteract the untoward effects of other new drugs."

— Dr. Walter Modell, Cornell University Medical College, 1961

The drug industry: impervious to inflation

Beginning in 1993, American magazine readers — as distinct from physicians and others in the medical profession for whom such things had become routine — were treated to a barrage of sleek, professionally produced full-page advertisements from the Pharmaceutical Manufacturers Assn. (PMA) and various drug companies.

A similar television blitz began in 1994.

The message was that nobody — meaning the government — should tamper with Americans' right to the injections, capsules, tablets, caplets, lotions and gels of the pharmaceutical industry which were *in toto* described as life-saving, disease-blocking and virtually as down-home American as the perennial (and increasingly absent) "mom's apple pie."

The advertising campaign was staged as the newly ensconced Clinton Administration began a serious look at the entire healthcare calamity in the United States — which went nowhere — and as the drug industry, never too far from public scrutiny, was coming into sharper and sharper focus as a central player in the runaway costs of American medicine.

The industry had even bypassed physician income (modest by comparison) as a perceived public culprit in the skyrocketing healthcare cost crisis.

Two 1993 reports — as well as a flock of media reports on how Americans were fleeing, primarily to Mexico, to secure both prescription and over-the-counter drugs at prices substantially lower than those charged at home — had set the industry (Number Two in Wall Street profit-taking, right behind the total complex of elements generally considered food production, food processing and food distribution) on its heels:

— The US Congress' putatively independent Office of Technology Assessment (OTA) had reported that drug manufacturers were reaping enormous excess profits on prescription medicines, and that they were spending too much to promote their products while earning an average of $36 million over their costs on every drug they developed.[1]

— The General Accounting Office (GAO) of the Department of Health and Human Services had found that drug prices in other countries were anywhere from 10 percent to 70 percent lower than those charged by American pharmacies.[2]

At about the same time, the US Department of Labor Statistics was reporting that drug prices had tended to rise twice as fast as the benchmark Consumer Price Index (CPI) in the 1980s, and nearly three times as fast in 1991 — or during a time when many other industries were strongly buffeted by recession.

Both public and private organizations had by then pegged the total US revenues from the drug industry at $59 billion in 1992, based on figures from the top 122 pharmaceutical companies, 20 of which manufactured lower-priced "generic" drugs.[3]

The same figures showed that pharmaceutical marketing costs were about $13,000 per physician (as opposed to about $5,000 in 1976), that drug companies were spending about 22 percent of their total sales on advertising ($20 billion a year), and that industry political action committees (PACs) had been scattered across the political spectrum to influence legislation.

The big PAC contributors in 1992 to sway the lawmakers were Pfizer Inc. ($115,650), Abbott Laboratories ($108,475), Glaxo Inc. ($107,100) and Merck and Co. ($75,600).

By any definition, the drug industry — both American and international — is an inflation-proof, recession-oblivious activity.

The PMA's estimate for US companies' worldwide drug sales in 1992 was a stunning $75.2 billion, or 11.7 percent over 1991. Global sales of "ethical" pharmaceuticals (prescription and over-the-counter medications) were in turn said to have been $63 billion in 1991, or 12.1 percent over 1990, with the US market share in 1991 set at $43.5 billion. By 1996, Americans were spending more than $80 billion a year on prescription drugs — about 8.5 cents out of every healthcare dollar.[4]

Even sales of the ostensibly less-profitable "generic" drugs in 1991 were said to have been between $4 billion and $8 billion, depending on how "generic" is defined.

Other ways to define the gravy train have included these:

— The American Medical Association's *American Medical News* found that between 1980 and 1990 prescription drug prices rose 150 percent even though the general inflation rate was 58 percent.[5]

— In 1990, *Time* Magazine reported that the cost of prescription drugs in the United States had soared to $40 billion annually, a jump of 135 percent over the inflation rate of 53 percent in a decade, while noting that the US drug industry actually dominated the $130 billion world pharmaceutical market and constituted the one industry in which American firms were the biggest and growing the fastest.[6]

— In 1991 the Senate Committee on Aging heard testimony that drug manufacturers made an average profit of 15.5 percent in 1990, more than three times the average profit for the top Fortune 500 companies, and that price *increases* for prescription drugs had outpaced inflation in the 1980s by a monumental 300 percent. At the same hearing it was also learned that in 1990 Americans were paying 62 percent more than Canadians for drugs and about 50 percent more than Europeans — and that about 60 percent of American "senior citizens" were without insurance to pay for the pricey compounds.[7]

— In 1992 the consumer group Families USA Foundation (FUSAF) reported that the prices of the top 20 prescription drugs had risen by as much as four times (400 percent) the rate of general inflation in the prior six years, and that between 1977 and 1987 average consumer use of prescription drugs had risen by about 15 percent while spending on them rose by 237 percent.[8]

Even with "cost containment" and "managed care" bywords by mid-decade, drug prices kept on soaring. By 1995, prices of 20 top-selling prescription drugs were up 4.3 percent against an inflation rate of 2.7 percent, FUSAF reported.[9]

The 1992 FUSAF survey had found huge price increases between 1985 and 1991 including, among the top 10, Premarin

(148% price increase), Inderal (128%), Synthroid (110%), Xanax (106%), Feldene (91%), Procardia (90%), Ceclor (82%), Clinoril (72%), Zantac (66%) and Dyazide (65%).

FUSAF pointed out in 1995 that while cumulative inflation between 1989-1994 was 22 percent, makers of 11 top drugs increased their prices at more than double the rate of inflation. The cost of the antihistamine Seldane had gone up 63 percent in the prior five years.[10]

To say that drugs dominate Western medicine is to overstate the obvious.

They are an intimate part and parcel of the entire doctor-patient relationship (such as it is), and their massive over-prescription for the very young and the very old eliminates a great deal of painstaking chitchat and symptom-taking — the mainstay of the medicine of old.

Said Dr. David Himmelstein, who participated in a 1994 study which found that a quarter of American "senior citizens" were being given drugs which were either unnecessary or potentially dangerous (*11*):

> *The quickest and easiest route to get the patient out of the office is to write a prescription. And in the day of the seven-minute office visit, that's what doctors resort to. I'd like to see every elderly American saying, "Do I really need to be on these pills?" and push their doctors hard about it.*[11]

At any given point in the 1990s, then, and as viewed by various sets of data and statistics, the pharmaceutical industry, as grouped in several dozen major houses, most of them international in scope, was turning in enormous profits in the United States which far eclipsed inflation and profit-taking by virtually all other industries.

The worldwide AIDS pandemic now provides the drug industry with its juiciest of possibilities — expensive, toxic antivirals which *may* "slow down" but not "cure" AIDS, and a rapidly developing list of pharmaceuticals to treat, but not "cure,"

AIDS' 30-some opportunistic manifestations (*XIII*).

For the record, neither this author nor most thinking people deny the life-saving effects and frequent miracles attributable to pharmaceuticals — untold lives that would have been cut down by diseases, accidents and inborn conditions in an earlier era have indeed been saved.

The high cost of 'modern medical miracles'

But the "modern medical miracles" in which synthetic drugs have played a role come at an awesome price.

In an illustrative review, the *Orange County Register* in Southern California in 1993 gave a thumbnail sketch of four high-cost, high-tech cases: a diabetic woman with a stomach ailment and high blood pressure was keeping these problems "in check" with drugs costing $150 a month, or more than she was spending for food or her mortgage. A heart transplant patient was taking $50 a day in pills to keep his new heart from being rejected. Emergency-room doctors treating a heart attack patient shut off the attack with a clot-busting drug costing $2,000 for a single treatment. A Gaucher's disease patient was staying alive with drugs costing $270,000 a year.[(12)]

These were costly "wonder drug" uses for maladies above and beyond those involved in the enormous annual costs of cancer and AIDS treatments.

Attempts have been made over the decades to pin down the actual costs of producing the synthetic compounds which now dominate Western medicine. It is understood in market economics that the actual cost of producing an item bears little relationship to the cost of the end product to the consumer, so such figures are often misleading — but by any comparison, the drug business (that is, the "legal" drug business) is a good one to be in:

Estimates of cost-of-production over cost-to-user have varied per item over time from 1500 percent to 7500 percent — with perhaps the lowest markups involving the first major drug marketed worldwide, aspirin (acetylsalicylic acid), and rising to enormous costs for medications which may run from hundreds to even thousands of dollars per injection.

The inflation-proof nature of the bulk of the vast, worldwide market in 400,000 drugs, medications, pills, tablets, capsules, etc. ground out by the endlessly productive drug industry since earlier in this century is readily visible by visiting pharmacies in foreign countries:

Top-of-the-line antibiotics from American and international pharmaceutical firms have long been available in Mexico for prices ranging from 50 percent or more below their cost in the United States. The Third World has been a major "dumping ground" for US and internationally produced pills and potions at prices which — while often unconscionably high for the host countries — are usually far cheaper than when sold in US drugstores. It is also shockingly true that the prescription and side effects information demanded by the US (giving the FDA here its share of credit) for medications is often lacking in foreign countries, and dozens of medications which may be highly addictive, dangerous in specific doses or when mixed with other medicines may be peddled in the same stand or on the same sidewalk cloth with herbs and natural products.

As we have noted (*VI*), voices decades ago warned about the excess production of medications that even then seemed to be a glut on the market. The highly profitable drug industry never sleeps.

Yet, aside from the iatrogenic disasters implicit in many synthetic drugs, either by themselves or because of inadequate dosing or because of incompatibility with other drugs, or simply because the noxious effects of medications may take years to show up, there is a certain incestuousness in the overproduction of drugs:

Health Information Designs Inc. reported in 1989 that, as President M. Lee Morse put it, "we spend $2 billion yearly on pharmaceuticals whose sole purpose is the treatment of adverse effects from other drugs" (!)[13] That is, the health-oriented drug industry itself has produced a spinoff industry of drug-induced disease which has called for a parallel new industry: drugs to treat drugs.

This technological reality should not be separated from the general doping of the Western world by the chemical industry *in toto* — the thousands of chemicals added to the altered food supply for a vast variety of reasons, together with the chemicals also added thereto as herbicides, pesticides and insecticides together with synthetic hormones and antibiotics in meat production and in the cultivation of hybrid plants and vegetables.

'Me-too' drugs: waiting for the breakthroughs

Our focus here, however, is the synthetic chemical industry as it applies to medicine — the exponential increase since the advent of the Allopathic Industrial Complex (AIC) of all manner of medications essentially and originally derived from petrochemicals — an ancillary industry to the petroleum trusts of old.

The earlier alluded-to 1993 OTA report pointed out that drug company profits significantly exceed those earned by industries which bear comparable risks.

But the OTA pointed to a more amazing figure: only 42 percent of the new drugs developed between 1975 and 1989 were classified as "medical improvements" (!)[(14)] This meant that, often, drug companies were simply spinning wheels — grinding out lookalike and similar drugs for the seemingly insatiable market of medical consumers.

Some 53 percent of the 259 drugs approved in the USA in the decade ending in 1991 were classified as "me-too" drugs — that is, in FDA terms, 1-C drugs offering little or no therapeutic gain over existing remedies. Only 6 percent were classified as 1-A, indicating "significant improvements" over drugs already on the market.[(15)]

A key reason to invest in lookalike or "me-too" drugs is, as one researcher put it,[(16)] "driven by the need to generate quarterly earnings for investors" in companies which know the big payoff in research and development is "blockbuster" drugs which will ultimately bring in $500 million a year or more in worldwide sales. Income needs to flow while laboratory scientists work on "the big breakthroughs."

A devious defense

The drug industry defends itself from charges of price-gouging and profiteering in several ways, all of which have enough truth to them to mislead the observer, as long as he doesn't look too closely.

It is quite true, as the drug industry argues, that the high cost of government interference in medicine — an extensive network of federal and state regulation of prescription drugs — has much to do with the hiking of pharmaceutical prices and that the cost of research and development is mind-numbing. It is also true that in terms of the impact of the cost of prescribing drugs as part of the overall healthcare hydra (about 8.3 percent of total US health spending in 1991) the US *percentage* is lower than that of many other developed countries. But these are dodge arguments to obscure the fact that drug production under *any* scheme is excellent business.

In the 1991 hearings of the Senate Committee on Aging, for example, the Pharmaceutical Manufacturers Assn. (PMA) was on hand to testify that the inflation-proof rise in drug prices could be explained by the high cost of research while still being "the best bargain in health care."[(17)]

Which is one of those rhetorical artifices which has some substance: the cost of *some* drugs as contrasted with the cost of *some* medical procedures and the incomes of *most* physicians may not always seem to be out of line at all, depending on what is being treated:

A diabetic may find it economically irritating but not devastating to stay on two insulin shots a day for the rest of his life, whether he or an insurance premium is paying for the treatment. A patient under "experimental" AIDS and/or cancer therapy, particularly one not covered by insurance, may swiftly be reduced to penury.

The PMA is long in assailing the FDA-generated red tape and endless government requirements which go into the presumed general costs and time lapses in bringing a new drug to market — but is equally short on explaining just how this came about and what the accompanying benefits of the system are.

The outlandish cost of drug development

The earlier (1990) PMA estimate of an average $231 million investment to bring a new drug to market over about 12 years may have been, in global terms, well off the mark, the 1993 OTA report on pharmaceutical research and development estimated.

Indeed, by recalculating all aspects of drug development "to the point of market approval," OTA found that "a reasonable upper bound on the fully capitalized cost of R & D per successful NCE [new chemical entity] at the time of market approval is $359 million."[18]

But, added OTA, "the effective cost to a company of bringing a new drug to market is substantially less . . . because they do not account for the taxes the company is relieved of paying when it invests in R & D."

The "true costs," then, in 1990 dollars of bringing a drug to market are somewhere between the earlier estimate of an average $230 million and $359 million — a staggering figure. But OTA added:

> *The cost of bringing a new drug to market is very sensitive to changes in science and technology, shifts in the kinds of drugs under development and changes in the regulatory environment. All of these changes are occurring fast. Consequently, it is impossible to predict the cost of bringing a new drug to market today from estimated costs for drugs whose development began more than a decade ago.*[19]

Even so, OTA assessed: "Pharmaceutical R & D is a costly and risky business, but in recent years the financial rewards from R & D have more than offset its costs and risks."

A Hoover Institution assessment in 1996 set the global drug development cost at a staggering $500 million.

So lamentations about the monstrous cost of drug development (used to mute the alleged net profits on each new item of about $36 million each) are not without a basis in reality.

The inane bureaucracy of the FDA is indeed a costly, progress-inhibiting labyrinth to deal with, as noted in *IX,* but it is a response, however serpentine, to the needs of the gigantic drug combine, particularly of an earlier era, to set up a system which protected its own profits while making it extremely difficult for small companies to compete. It is simple economics: a start-up company with a good idea and a good product, as case after case has shown, simply cannot play in the American drug system unless it can front a minimum $230 million per product and afford to wait up to 12 years for approval. This chilling effect is the proximate cause of the choking of drug-development progress in the USA and the increasing transfer of much American drug production knowhow overseas.

The system which costs so much to license a new painkiller is the same one which stands in the way of nutritional and metabolic therapy, preventive and promotive medicine and the use of nutrients against disease. In a classic "he who rides the tiger" scenario, the tiger of government regulation may indeed consume some of its handlers or anyone silly enough to get off it, but in the main it protects the forest against interlopers — i.e., competitive small companies and promoters of natural therapy products.

The PMA estimated that in 1991 the drug industry spent $10.9 billion in "research and development," a 13.5 percent increase over 1990, and that of each of 30 new drugs approved by the FDA in 1991 an average of 11 years were lost in development and "regulatory review" — a reality to which any small drug producer with the patience and pesos to wait out the FDA drug approval process can attest.[20]

There simply is no doubt that the drug industry *does* spend a lot in the research and development of new products — and huge amounts on conforming to the incessant paperwork caused by the byzantine bureaucratic processes of the FDA and other agencies.

Dodging the question

Yet these costs still cannot explain the huge "take" by the industry, which at every turn likes to avoid discussing how drug prices are arrived at.

The industry was stung during testimony of a Senate Committee on Labor and Human Resources hearing in 1991 when the ever-simmering subject of drug prices and the elderly came up.

Chairman Edward M. Kennedy (D-MA) asked PMA President Gerald J. Mossinghoff to explain just how the retail prices of drugs were crafted.

The media reported Mossinghoff's response:

> *"There's one area that we stay completely away from, and that's the pricing of the drug."*
>
> *Kennedy: "These products are absolutely essential to the health and well-being of patients in this country, and you, as the leader of that organization, are prepared to say here that as a matter of policy you're not going to indicate your sense of indignation or outrage?"*
>
> *Mossinghoff: "I'm saying we are not and we cannot under antitrust laws."*[21]

None of the foregoing should suggest that simply because the drug cartel is effective at getting non-drug competitors out of the way corporate peace abounds within the cartel. In fact, there is slash-and-gash competition among the corporate players, industrial espionage and all the other trappings of limited competition. The competition among synthetic drugs is an allowable activity — it is simply non-patented and unpatentable drugs and natural products which are not even to be allowed to play.

Drug warfare, drug monopoly

Typical of the warfare between high-priced drugs was the late 1980s/early 1990s fight over "clotbuster" medications for heart disease.

At one point, the *dramatis personae* consisted of:

German drug giant Hoechst AG and Astra AB and Kabi Pharmacia of Sweden, producers of Streptokinase, which was administered for about $300 per treatment. In the opposite corner was T-PA (tissue plasminogen activator), which could fetch a whopping $2,200 per shot for British pharmaceutical house Wellcome PLC. After six years of costly research it had halted work on T-PA, largely leaving the field open to the pioneering American biotechnology firm Genentech, partially absorbed by Roche Holding Inc. Then there was Eminase, SmithKline Beecham PLC's "new kid on the block," aimed at cutting into the T-PA market.

By 1990, according to the *Wall Street Journal*, Genentech held about two-thirds of the American clotbuster drug market with its 1989 T-PA sales totalling $196 million. Hoechst's Streptokinase held about a third.

Reported *The Choice*:

> *No sooner had SKB launched Eminase than the company started complaining about, and the FDA began probing, Genentech's marketing of the expensive drug.*
>
> *But right off the bat, results of a trial of 20,000 patients from 13 countries which claimed to show no difference in life prolongation in heart disease victims between recipients of T-PA and Streptokinase were challenged by Genentech and several leading American cardiologists as misleading and flawed.*
>
> *But far from resolving the issue of which drug was better, the Italian study appears to have reheated the*

controversy over how best to treat heart attacks.[22]

In 1993, results of a 2½-year, 40,000-patient, 15-country study showed a slight edge for T-PA.[23]

Unspoken in such conflicts were the realities that the long-damned EDTA chelation therapy is arguably a *preventer* of heart attacks, as are Vitamin E and other nutrients [*X*]. Yet these approaches cannot come close to approaching the profits from heart disease drugs — which is not to say such drugs are not effective and have no legitimate place in therapy.

Most Americans do not think about the cost of a prescription drug until they walk into a drugstore, hand over a prescription to the registered pharmacist, and then get in return a very small bottle and a very big bill. Since the drugstore is the site of the transaction, the druggist gets the blame.

"The fact is that the cost of a prescription drug is determined primarily by the manufacturer," a study by a California newspaper noted in 1993.[24] It quoted University of Minnesota economist/ pharmacist Stephen Schondelmeyer as noting that 69 cents of every sales dollar goes to the manufacturer and that

> *[I]n the world of prescription drugs, the normal rules of the marketplace don't apply. Here, the person who pays for the product — the patient — isn't the one who selects it. And the drug consumer, confronting pain, illness or death, doesn't have the option of doing without.*[25]

Because there actually *is* limited competition among giant drug companies, there is often a facade of down-home free-market capitalism for the worldwide profiteers. Yet there are broad aspects of monopolism and they occur in two areas:

— First, the patent process, which guarantees market exclusivity for 17 years to a drug developer and which can be extended by five years while the compound is under "review" by the tortoise-like FDA, constitutes, said a Smith Barney, Harris Upham & Co. financial analyst, "not only an ironclad barrier to competition" but also provides protection against "anybody scooping your discovery during the long product-development period" — which may be up to 12 years.[26]

— Second, there is a difference between the total industry worldwide (in which no single one of the 20 largest drug giants controls more than 7.6 percent of the market) and "specialized markets" in which a company's "patents and strengths have been developed." In such specialized markets, a single company's presence may be 50 percent or more.[27]

By 1975, journalist Ruth Mulvey Harmer assessed:

> *The drug industry has, by taking advantage of every legal loophole and by perpetrating criminal actions, successfully established all the essential elements of monopolistic control. It has concentrated power in a few hands, enabling the giants to dominate the marketplace and bring possible competitors into line. It has controlled prices through "fixing" agreements and by lobbying through laws that make it illegal for consumers to know how much they are being overcharged. It has corrupted and captured government agencies financed by the public to protect them against exploitation and hazard. It has stimulated a tremendous demand, all out of proportion to need. And it has cloaked all those activities with a thick whitewash of advertising and publicity, persuading victims that the doses administered are for their own good.*[28]

Cashing in on socialized medicine

The drug industry has played two-step with America's fling with socialized medicine — having learned at home when it already had learned abroad: there is so much money to be made in drug production that prices for drugs can be established and monitored by governments at prices far lower than in the United States without the drug company losing any appreciable amount of profit.

In the US, government medicine up to now has been channeled through the Veterans Administration plus the Medicare program for the elderly and Medicaid for the destitute — all three textbook examples of mismanagement, swollen budgets, waste and inefficiency.

On Jan. 1, 1991, congressional action to cut prices for Medicaid recipients went into effect, an action which the industry could not fail to recognize as hostile.

Even so, reported columnists Jack Anderson and Dale Van Atta[29] as well as the *Bulletin* of the senior lobbying group AARP, a decline in Medicaid drug prices as mandated by Congress simply meant a rise elsewhere, the industrial equivalent of sticking the fat lady into a corset.

The US Department of Veterans Affairs, which already had received discounts for drugs at its 172 hospitals, complained that the drop in Medicaid drug costs would be offset by a 21 percent increase in VA hospital prices (or $150 million a year), with spokesmen for the private health-care organization Kaiser-Permanente predicting that "just about everyone will end up paying more."

Anderson/Van Atta wrote that "the drug lobbyists made sure (Arkansas Senator David) Pryor's victory (to reduce drug costs for 27 million Medicaid recipients) was circumvented by hiking drug prices" even to such other governmental customers as the VA apparatus.

"The cost of a key painkiller went up 800 percent for the VA soon after the measure passed," they wrote.

Noting that then Health and Human Services (HHS) Inspector General Richard P. Kusserow had indicated that if the USA adopted Canada's drug-pricing system Medicaid could save $474 million a year (perhaps wishful thinking given government's own track record at holding down costs), they added that "there is an army of profit-first drug manufacturers bent on making sure that never happens. Drug prices skyrocketed 150 percent in the 1980s, three times the rate of inflation. Drug makers were reaping pre-tax profits of about 18 percent." They described the government's Health Care Financing Administration (HCFA) as "cowering before the drug lobby."[30]

Cancer and AIDS: opportunities for The Club

As we argue throughout this account, the drug industry, as a key pillar of The Club (the Allopathic Industrial Complex, the "establishment") was from earliest times the anticipating recipient of largesse from the victory of the allopathic theory of medicine — contraries to treat disease symptoms and pathogens.

It has thus stood to gain from virtually every "new" disease entity to be identified, with the complex of conditions generally considered to be "heart disease" leading the field (with ulcers not far behind). So it is no surprise that the killer complexes of modern times, cancer and AIDS, have provided an almost endless treasure trove for the pharmaceutical giants.

We deal with both of these entities in separate chapters, but suffice it to say the comfortable relationship between the allopathic theory ("microbes cause diseases; hence, ridding the patient of the microbe results in health") and the industry it helped so much to spawn (pharmaceuticals) has continued apace.

If chemotherapy has largely been a blind alley in halting the cancer pandemic in the Western world (though at times of an adjuvant benefit in early cases), then that very same approach against AIDS had, by 1997 — or a full sixteen years after the definition of the syndrome — failed to produce a single cure.

But opportunities abound:

The hasty 1983 announcement that "the cause" of the acquired immune deficiency syndrome had been found and that it was an unusually pesky retrovirus named HTLV-III, later called HIV-1 (*XIII*), led to a Club frenzy of research and development: ways to block, thwart, inhibit or "kill" the "AIDS virus."

In what some have seen as irresponsibly and even suspiciously premature, an "AIDS drug" — a "nucleoside analogue" anti-retroviral agent — was rushed onto the market and whisked through the FDA's approval process. (We note elsewhere how resistant FDA is to whisk anything *other than* a toxic synthetic drug with good Club credentials through that process.)

The hero of the moment was AZT (azidothymidine, zidovudine, Retrovir), lofted to the market by drug giant Burroughs Wellcome.

Interestingly enough, AZT was actually an "orphan" drug — it had been developed as a toxic chemotherapeutic agent years before to be used against cancer. It had mostly failed there, and was awesomely toxic, so it gathered dust until The Club looked around for an agent which might have an effect against "the AIDS virus."

While we discuss the AZT controversy elsewhere [*XIII*], we should pause to see the effect it and another "orphan," pentamidine, taken out of mothballs for use against the form of pneumonia which was rapidly establishing itself as the major killer disease of the AIDS syndrome, had on the drug industry.

By the time AZT was approved in 1987 (after the National Cancer Institute claimed to have found antiretroviral properties in this failed cancer drug), the agent became the most expensive drug ever marketed — a devastating synthetic which originally cost at least $10,000 per year per patient, and whose price was said to have been "compassionately" cut by Burroughs Wellcome after AIDS activists and medical freedom-of-choicers expressed their outrage.

In 1988, the US Congress' Committee on Government Operations reported that both the NCI and the National Institute of Allergy and Infectious Disease (NIAID), both government agencies,

> *not only participated heavily in the development of the drug, but also supplied Burroughs Wellcome with large amounts of thymidine, a scarce and expensive ingredient. However, because the Federal Government has granted the company an exclusive patent on AZT, the Government will not share in profits from its sale, nor is it in a position,*

under current law, to affect the cost of the drug to the public.

Burroughs Wellcome has never agreed to make public its portion of the cost of development and producing AZT, nor adequately justified the extremely high price of the drug. Company representatives testified at a Congressional hearing in March 1987 that research and development costs had been $80 million. The cost of AZT to Federal and State governments under the Medicaid Program was $20 million by 1987 . . .

Burroughs Wellcome lowered the price of AZT 20 percent in December 1987. This was possible, according to company spokespersons, because of the decreased production costs. This would certainly suggest that the profit margin on the drug is quite comfortable. In fact, by April 1988, the value of the parent company's shares had quadrupled from the date the company went public in February 1986.[31]

By 1993, Burroughs Wellcome was earning $400 million annually on AZT, the same year the drug's fortunes began to sag [*XIII*].[32]

While US-produced anti-AIDS drugs coming from smaller companies (Isoprinosine as a major example, Ribavirin as another) were not allowed FDA clearance, AZT charged ahead full throttle.

Pentamidine, an "old drug" approved for use against AIDS-related pneumonia (*Pneumocystis carinii*), had been classed as an "orphan drug" because it had been developed prior to the amended Food, Drug and Cosmetic Act in 1962. It was brought back to production by LyphoMed, a small generic drug company — one of a growing group of enterprises beginning to crowd into the standard drug industry — at the request of the government's Centers for Disease Control (CDC).

The same governmental operations committee reported:

When it was first marketed under the Orphan

Drug Act in October 1984, pentamidine retailed at $24.95 per vial. By August 1987, the cost per vial had reached $95.49 . . . LyphoMed seized an opportunity to develop a marketing and sales staff for the company and resolve its problems at the expense of this one drug. At a cost of at least $100,000 per year to hire, train, and maintain just one physician sales specialist, LyphoMed hired 27.[33]

Rep. Ted Weiss, chairman of the Human Resources and Intergovernmental Relations Subcommittee, summarized:

You saw a good thing which could be used to build your company to a size that you'd never anticipated. And how do you pay for it? You pay for it by soaking the clientele. I think it's really unfortunate that you decided to take this . . . approach . . . to meet CDC's challenge.[34]

(To both Burroughs Wellcome's and LyphoMed's credit it should be noted that the companies occasionally made their drugs available on a charitable basis).

By 1996, the AIDS division of the Allopathic Industrial Complex (AIC) had brought "protease inhibitor" drugs into the AIDS armamentarium (*see XIII*). Yet the optimism-producing "cocktail" combining the older "nucleoside" drugs with the newer "proteases" and another class of drug could easily cost $15,000 per year per patient.

For the vast majority of HIV-infected (and hence potential "AIDS" patients, by the thinking of allopathic medicine) the cost of AZT and pentamidine *alone* — let alone these plus protease inhibitors and any number of drugs to treat "opportunistic infections" — could easily bankrupt most of them within a few months.

The third-party insurance scheme *plus* socialized medicine (through Medicare and Medicaid) have been present to hide the true (and outrageous) costs of these medications and to cause them to be paid either by other policy holders in huge private groups or, more usually, by the taxpayers. The drug companies themselves, of course, are not troubled by *who* pays for the products as long as *somebody* does.

The AMA and the drug industry

AIDS and cancer drugs are simply notorious examples of drug company greed as protected by the pharmaceutical police force (the FDA) and sustained by the underlying mindset (the allopathic paradigm in medicine).

But they are only recent expressions of the same.

In the 1950s, or during the heyday of acceptance by Americans of the American Medical Assn. (AMA), voice and conduit of allopathic medicine, an AMA spokesman described a "prime directive" of the "medical" profession:

> *Both the medical profession and pharmacy must shoulder one major public relations objective: to tell the American people over and over that nearly all of today's drugs, especially the antibiotics, are bargains at any price.*[35]

Yet the AMA — just as the FDA, another major bulwark of The Club — has flirtations with honesty and reason, even involving pharmaceuticals.

In 1972, the AMA's Council on Drugs, wrapping up an in-depth study of the then most commonly prescribed medications, came up with some data which were distasteful both to AMA leadership and the drug industry: some of the most profitable drugs were held to be "irrational" and should not be recommended. Worse, the council's chairman and vice-chairman told a Senate subcommittee, the huge income the AMA took in from drug manufacturers had made the AMA "a captive arm [of] and beholden to the pharmaceutical industry."[36]

It is a graphic example of The Club at work that the AMA's response to these unsettling findings was to . . . abolish the Council on Drugs.

Behind this move lurked the more hidden story of how the AMA and the drug industry were not always in accord. Indeed, the relationship of these two forces of the AIC has been stormy from time to time. They reached their in-tandem balance in the current era out of need: the allopathic system had monopoly control over medical education, training and application while the drug trust needed organized medicine as its major purveyor of products.

In its earlier history, the AMA had relied on the medical profession to monitor drugs and indeed the AMA in 1905 had set up a Council on Pharmacy and Chemistry, allegedly to separate the propaganda wheat from the chaff of the early drug industry. The AMA had begun publishing its *New and Unofficial Remedies* list in 1907 to be supplemented in 1913 by the *Useful Drugs* handbook. By 1929 the AMA Council on Pharmacy and Chemistry had set up a "seal of acceptance" for AMA-approved drugs — an approval which sometimes flew in the face of what drug companies wanted to market.

It was in the 1950s when the drug industry, occasionally smarting under AMA independence through the "seal of acceptance" tactic, found a chance to set things — in its view — right. At the time, the AMA was seeking new revenue sources to fight its old bugaboo, compulsory health insurance programs. The industry moved in immediately to explain how the sale of drug-related advertising in the AMA's *Journal* and other publications could be enhanced: pharmaceutical companies would increase advertising spending if the AMA would submit to certain "policy changes."

Among these was abandonment of the "seal of acceptance" and the *Useful Drugs* handbook. In the latter's place, the drug industry would publish and distribute the *Physician's Desk Reference* — a "Bible" of allopathic drug descriptions which the industry presented as a "medical" guide and index to drugs but which was, and is, little more than an advertising catalogue.

As Ruth Mulvey Harmer detailed in her numbing attack on

the AMA:

> *In [*the PDR*] all the material about every drug listed was prepared, edited, approved and paid for by the manufacturer. As an indication of its objectivity and completeness, in the 1962 edition Parke-Davis deleted from the Chloromycetin entry all references to hazards, and inserted a statement that doctors could get all necessary information from the package insertion and from the salesman.*[37]

These moves led to the final takeover of the allopathic paradigm by the drug industry, despite some modest reforms imposed by Congress. They explain the beautifully produced, full-color, glossy ads now appearing in allopathy's major journals.

By 1971, cooler heads within the AMA and its Council on Drugs had put together the *AMA Drug Evaluations* manual in an effort to replace the drug industry's *PDR*, with $3 million allotted to do so. This more balanced guide to prescribing was widely hailed by physicians but criticized by the Pharmaceutical Manufacturers Assn. (PMA), united lobbying voice of the drug industry. The net effect was that all work was halted on a second edition and the AMA Council on Drugs was abolished.

From then on, the AMA and PMA were usually in lockstep for the greater good of the AIC.

In 1993, a pharmaceutical executive newsletter called *The Pink Sheet* estimated that in 1991 American drug companies spent $10 billion to promote their products, or about $1 billion more than was reportedly being spent on research.[38]

This was only a recent exposé in a series of "bad press" items for the drug industry, which, by the 1990s, was not doing anything essentially distinct from what it had been doing earlier in this century — courting organized (allopathic) medicine like a zealous and jealous lover.

In spring 1992, HHS Inspector General Richard Kusserow reported that a survey had indicated that 8 out of every 10 doctors had said drug company salesmen had offered them gifts to encourage them to prescribe their products.[39]

Two years earlier, Scott-Levin Associates, a tracker of drug company "detail men," said such individuals in 1989 had made 27.4 million products-connected calls or visits, with Bristol-Myers Squibb leading the effort with 2.1 million such contacts. For its famous anti-ulcer drug Zantac alone, Glaxo led in the calls-for-a-single-product category with 928,000. Behind BMS for total visits for products contacts were American Home Products, Merck Sharpe & Dohme and Eli Lilly & Co., tied for second place at 1.6 million calls or visits each.[40] The efforts ostensibly paid off: Zantac was the most profitable drug in America and in the history of the pharmaceutical industry with sales in excess of an estimated $3 billion by 1992.[41]

Scott-Levin found that the number of reps had increased by 40 percent between 1980 and 1990 to some 45,000 "detail men" waiting to descend, vulture-like, on physicians.

Dr. Douglas R. Waud, pharmacology instructor at the University of Massachusetts Medical School, was quoted as saying: "This reliance on detail men is disturbing, particularly since in 1988 less than 5 percent of these people had formal training in pharmacology."[42]

With about 20 cents of every dollar spent on brand-name drugs going to promote and market them, the question arises: "Just what do doctors actually know about the products and how can they distinguish between them — when there are so many 'me-too' drugs on the market?"

Noted the *Orange County (CA) Register*:

> *A doctor treating arthritis may prescribe Voltaren if he trained at Hospital A and Naprosyn if he trained at Hospital B. That's because Hospital A's formulary lists Voltaren as its primary choice for arthritis and Hospital B stocks Naprosyn.*[43]

In 1991, a Public Citizen Health Research Group newsletter reported that in 1988 the drug industry had spent more than $163 million to wine, dine and impress doctors, frequently at such exotic locales as Palm Springs, Monte Carlo and Acapulco, and that the outlay represented a 500 percent increase over 1976.[44]

The breakdown included $85 million for various medical specialty conventions and meetings, $24 million in outright gifts to physicians, and $54 million for "reminder" items, aimed at keeping the name of a company or product ever in the thoughts of workaday doctors.

Despite moves by the AMA and the Accreditation Council for Continuing Medical Education to halt "flagrant promotion practices by some companies in their attempts to increase revenues by influencing doctors' prescribing behaviors," the newsletter noted the following:

> *One pharmaceutical promotion, entitled "The Road to ACOG (American College of Obstetricians and Gynecologists) Sweepstakes," was marketed by Abbott Laboratories through "CAP Pharmaceuticals" to send several obstetricians and gynecologists to their annual meeting.*
>
> *Another incident involved the Collagen Corporation of Palo Alto CA, offering to send 55 dermatologists who were the largest purchasers of injectable collagen on an 8-day cruise to the South Pacific.*
>
> *Most recently, Warner Lambert was cited for a "lasting impressions" sweepstakes in which physicians are sent on a "Texas style" vacation. All of these practices have come under attack by AMA and individual physicians . . .*
>
> *(Reversely), in August 1991, the AMA's American Medical Television announced it would buy lodging (and food and entertainment) for drug and advertising industry executives to come to Chicago to learn about the wonders of advertising their drugs on this AMA cablevision series.*
>
> *For those who suspected that the AMA was in*

bed with the drug industry, here was evidence that they were at least providing beds in return for prescription drug ads that not only doctors but patients will view.[45]

Then there is the considerable element of the life-long drug:

Diabetics, hypertensives, some thyroid patients, many women on "estrogen replacement therapy," cancer and AIDS sufferers and an ever-lengthening group of individuals trapped in the medical (allopathic) loop, are routinely told by their physicians that they need these synthetics to stay alive — and, truth to tell, some of them probably do.

Yet life-long drugs enormously inflate the nation's health-care bill and in those cases where it is not truly demonstrated or proved beyond a shadow of scientific doubt that such medications are needed forever they are major contributors to that bill.

The system is incestuous: it is usually in the best interests of a physician to continue prescribing drugs to a patient — it keeps the patient coming back at at least one charge per visit, and it keeps profits high for the drug involved, one which can only be dispensed by a licensed pharmacist. There is no internal mechanism which induces the practitioner *not* to prescribe drugs, since that is what the system is, after all, all about.

Typical is the case of Warner-Lambert's Tacrine, the first drug "officially approved" for Alzheimer's. By 1994, the cost of the drug was $112 a month. Allegedly, the drug must be continued "indefinitely," lest symptoms reappear, but the costs do not stop there — frequent liver function tests are needed at an additional cost of $148 a month.[46] Since Alzheimer's patients survive an average of nine years, by simple mathematics each Alzheimer's patient is averaging in costs over $28,000 in medicine and tests alone during his remaining years.

Also typical is the case of HRT (hormone replacement therapy) in which women who have undergone hysterectomies and/or "medical management of menopause," as if the latter itself were a disease, face the prospect of life-long dependency on forms of female hormones (typically, estrogen and progestin.)

The debate on the endless use of hormones sharpened in the last half of this decade as dilemmas became obvious:

Long-term use of the hormones in women after menopause seemed to be correlated with lower incidence of heart disease and the hip fractures common in osteoporosis. Yet their use also correlated with possible endometrial and breast cancer later.

The issue is more serious year by year. As of 1997 almost a third of all American women were 45 or older, these figures expected to increase annually as the "baby boom" generation further slipped into middle age. By the middle of the decade estrogen had become the most widely prescribed drug in the US. Some 45 million women were taking the hormone product Premarin as of that year.[75]

But because of unresolved questions about their long-term use, such informed dissidents as Susan Love MD suggest women should not be on hormones "unless there's a very good reason to be on them." And breast cancer activists believe that studies touting HRT benefits simply allow drug companies to dupe women into lifelong use of more compounds the long-term effects of which are still not known.[76]

For cancer and AIDS patients, who in the "terminal" phase are expected to live far less time, the costs of drugs remain astronomical.

Side-stepping science: the Synthroid, Tagamet, Zantac stories

That the drug industry can "get around" unflattering scientific research and block worthwhile information which impacts on the lives and health of millions of people came home in the mid-1990s with the sorry sagas of Synthroid, Tagamet and Zantac, virtually household names to generations:

Synthroid, a medication for thyroid problems said to control 84 percent of the US market while used by 8 million Americans, had long been a major moneymaker for Boots Company, a British drug company later involved in a $1.4 billion buyout by

Germany's huge BASF-AG.[71]

Cimetidine, sold as Tagamet by SmithKline Beecham, and ranitidine, sold as Zantac (Glaxo/Roche), for years were used to treat some 90 percent of all peptic (duodenal and gastric) ulcers (as symptom-maskers, not as cures) and were among the top money-making drugs in the world.

But in 1996, Synthroid's $600 million lock on the thyroid market was on the way to being challenged by research from five independent medical experts who were about to publish an unflattering article in a major medical journal — namely, that Synthroid "worked" no better than three other lower-priced drugs. Publication was delayed 15 months — but took place.

Reportedly, the manufacturers spent $250 million to finance the research and then "did everything possible to discredit the study and block its publication."[72] The latter might have helped consumers save $356 million in drug costs.[73]

In the matter of Tagamet and Zantac, science also was forced to take a back seat for years.

In *1983*, two Australian physicians proposed that their newly discovered bacterium, *Helicobacter pylori*, was the real cause of peptic ulcers — at a time when the Western world was largely convinced that ulcers might be due to a combination of mental stress, "nervous stomach" and spicy foods.

But the antacids cimetidine and ranitidine were well in place and were being constantly sold to millions of ulcer sufferers.

In the decade following the discovery of *H.pylori* it was found that the germ is the main cause of stomach ulcers (overuse of aspirin and the "non-steroidal anti-inflammatory drugs" [NSAIDs] are others) and that a "cocktail" of the antibiotic tetracycline and similars plus metronidazole and bismuth subsalicylate eradicated *H.pylori* up to 98 percent of the time and was curing ulcers with a relapse rate of less than 5 percent.

In 1994 the National Institutes of Health (NIH) advised American physicians to discontinue prescribing Tagamet, Zantac and similar drugs for ulcers and to treat them instead with antibiotics, antibacterials and bismuth compounds. Tagamet lost patent protection that very year.

Noted a *Fortune* writer, Tagamet and Zantac

> *let doctors treat ulcers effectively as chronic problems and enabled drug companies and gastroenterologists to make such good money that they seemed less than thrilled at the prospect of eradicating ulcers. The treatments that grew out of [Barry] Marshall's research often used generic, low-margin antibiotics whose manufacturers rarely spent money to educate doctors on their new use.*[77]

This was a major reason why so little attention was given to the original 1983 research. It fits confortably under the rubric of "medical economics."

Never without an ace up its sleeve, the pharmaceutical industry reacted swiftly: while the public remained essentially uninformed about the truth about ulcers, the drug giants — scrambling to preserve an estimated $8 billion antacid market — struck a deal with the FDA to allow their anti-ulcer drugs to be sold without a prescription.

Noted a Canadian journal:

> *With this master stroke the drug companies freed medical doctors from the the ethical burden of prescribing ineffective, costly drugs while at the same time expanding their market among the broad segment of the population which had never heard of* H.pylori, *much less the NIH advice.*[74]

In the US, the "freeing" of Tagamet and Zantac to be sold over the counter was even hailed as a sign of a more liberalized FDA yielding to popular demand.

The testing trap

Aside from medications, the drug industry also has a stake in the allopathic obsession with endlessly testing human beings for everything — particularly obscure proteins and various "markers" which may drive an otherwise healthy person into a continual state of high anxiety because of an allegedly "suspicious" number.

Needless tests are a large part of the total picture in America's onrushing bankruptcy over "healthcare delivery." But there is also a vast grey area of "possibly useful" tests, the utility of which depends primarily on the whim of the physician and the intensity with which a company pushes a product.

It became obvious in the 1990s, for example, that virtually every male 50 years or older in North America (and probably in Northwest Europe, Australia, New Zealand and other "advanced" countries) might very well come down with prostate cancer if he lived long enough (and even, failing that, it was unlikely he would escape unscathed without at least a touch of benign prostatic hyperplasia [BPH], or non-malignant swelling of the fig-sized gland.)

It also became evident that standard oncological intervention against spreading prostate cancer (frequently involving such total physiological disasters as castration and radiation to be followed by administration of female hormones) was failing to enhance five-year survival ("cure") rates.

Hence, orthodoxy turned to blood markers in an attempt to find some evidence of prostatic cancer before there were symptoms. *Voila* — the prostate-specific antigen (PSA) test — which by 1993 was estimated to be generating, *by itself*, a $28-billion-a-year industry based also on followup biopsies, other tests and treatment.

The message rang loudly, clearly: beginning at age 50 (or maybe 55) all American men should start having PSA tests to spot an early indication of activity which might signal the early presence of prostate cancer. And, without question, there have been cases where a rapidly rising to substantially elevated PSA *has* accompanied or immediately foreshadowed a clinical diagnosis of this swiftly growing cancer in Western males.

Yet, the PSA test helped place standard oncology on the horns of yet another decisional dilemma — since study after study has shown that overall cancer-survival rates and life expectancy (from prostate cancer) have not yet been essentially impacted by therapy, then what is the presumed global good of "finding out" — say, at age 65, or 74, or 80 — that a rising PSA may indicate, at some future date, possible cancer?

In the early 1990s, panic over the spiralling growth of prostate cancer and the sudden availability of the new test caused doctors' offices to be flooded with calls from the middle-aged and elderly: a mature man might feel perfectly fine yet would now have yet a new number to worry about — an increase in the PSA.

While the jury is out on just how many lives will be saved by the mass terrorizing of men over 50 by PSA tests, what is clear is that the national campaign for PSA tests had an interesting origin.

As *The Wall Street Journal* reported in 1993:

> *Some troubling questions have emerged about the role the healthcare industry played in influencing the [American Cancer] society's recommendation [that men over 50 have PSA tests] . . . and about the reliability of the test itself, which costs from $30 to $70.*
>
> *Aside from the charge, possible related expenses include biopsies, ultrasound tests, repeat biopsies, treatment for complications from treatment. Thus, the total cost of mass screening has been estimated at $28 billion a year in the US alone.*(47)

The *WSJ* noted that "the crucial step" prior to the ACS recommendation had come in October 1991 at a urological conference held by the American Cancer Society to discuss the experimental PSA test. Reported the *WSJ*:

> *The healthcare industry picked up the entire $86,649 hotel tab for that four-day symposium at The Cloister, an elegant Sea Island GA resort.*
>
> *Among those paying for the hotel stay were the Hybritech Inc. unit of Indianapolis's Eli Lilly &*

Co. and TAP Pharmaceuticals, a joint venture of Japan's Takeda Pharmaceutical Co. and Abbott Laboratories. Hybritech and Abbott . . . are the only two companies with prostate blood tests approved by the US Food and Drug Administration.

Others helping pay the bill were major players in the business of treating prostate disease: Bruel & Kjaer Instruments, which makes ultrasound equipment; and prostate drug sellers Merck & Co., the Kabi Pharmacia unit of Sweden's Procardia AB, the Schering Laboratories unit of Schering-Plough Corp. and the ICI Pharmaceuticals unit of Imperial Chemical Industries PLC of Britain.[(48)]

Hardly a disinterested group.

Front organizations

And there are times when the drug industry, fully aware of the suspicion it excites in some eyes, can out-do the old Communist Party in setting up fronts which seem to be the very antithesis of anything the founders are really interested in.

In 1993, for example, in the heat of the Clinton Administration's allegedly deep look into the nation's healthcare crisis while also looking at ways to trim the federal budget, the prices of drugs consumed by the federal Medicaid program became a central concern for the industry.

In those heady days of early 1993, what should appear but a group calling itself the Coalition for Equal Access to Medicines — a supposed union of poor people, "minorities" and public-health advocates and styling itself an "ad-hoc volunteer organization."

But, as the *New York Times* reported, the "volunteer" group was in fact "created and financed by another interest group, one with perhaps the biggest stake in the outcome (of budget debates):

the prescription drug industry."

Reported Robert Pear:

> *Public statements of the coalition, like its letters to Congress and the White House, give no clue as to its origins. But its purpose is clear: to defeat a measure the federal government believes would help control Medicaid spending on prescription drugs.*
>
> *The drug executive who inspired the coalition acknowledged in an interview that one reason the group was formed was the industry's belief that consumer advocates and minority members had far more credibility on Capitol Hill than drug companies.*(49)

In the meantime, CARE packages need not be shipped to drug industry executives. Noted the *Orange County Register* in 1993:

> *Richard D. Wood, who retired recently as chief executive officer of Eli Lilly & Co., received \$10.1 million in 1991 — \$2.21 million in salary and bonuses and \$7.89 million in stock — making him the 12th best-paid executive in the United States, according to a* Fortune *survey . . . P. Roy Vegalos, chairman and chief executive of Merck & Co . . . received \$9.7 million.*
>
> *Wood's compensation was 2½ times more than that of Campbell Soup Co. President David Johnson, 50 times more than that of the president of the United States and about 250 times more than the median income of a family of four.*(50)

Also in 1993, a Knight-Ridder survey comparing what Americans estimated drug company, hospital executives and medical specialists earned vs. what they actually earned found the top executive of Bristol-Myers Squibb making \$12.8 million per year, that of Abbott Laboratories $4.2 million, and that of Eli Lilly $2.8 million.[51]

None of this is a crime — it is only suggestive of a high-on-the-hog industry unaffected by the cross-currents of inflation/recession which whiplash all other sectors of the economy. And it also leaves small wonder, as we note in *IX*, that employment in the drug industry is so attractive to FDA bureaucrats upon retirement.

The worldwide drug cartel

In *VI* we examined the vast overlap between the US drug industry in general with the mind-boggling global interlock of enterprises, conglomerates, combines, syndicates and trusts of the I.G. Farben-Rockefeller complex, the essential wellspring of the pharmaceutical industry worldwide and domestically.

One of the first chroniclers of the international drug cartel (IDC) was journalist/reporter Morris A. Bealle who, as we have seen, could not publish his findings through normal channels and had recourse to establishing his own publishing house — which eventually brought his *Super Drug Story* through many editions since its inception in 1949.[52]

While subsequent writers and journalists have exposed both the inordinate influence of the Rockefeller interests in the global and domestic drug marketplace as well as that same power in other areas which directly impact on the lives of every American, Bealle's painstaking review of data found that the combination of international pharmaceutical profit-takers he simply abstracted as "the drug trust" had, by the time of his exposé's first edition, come into virtual "control" of various "health-related" agencies. Whether "control" is the right word or not, "influence in" them can be perceived.

He mentioned the FDA as well within the Drug Trust orbit, but the tentacles of influence did not stop there. The US Public Health Service, the US Veterans Administration, the National Research Council, various medical entities within the Armed

Forces and the National Academy of Sciences — supposedly as open-minded and objective a body as can be imagined — were all under Drug Trust influences, he wrote.

Bolstering this assertion, Bealle reported that at one time the head of the latter agency was Alfred N. Richards, one of the largest stockholders and directors of Merck & Co., even then one of the world's largest drug companies. As another exposé — Hans Ruesch's detailed attack on the vivisection industry and what lies behind it (*Naked Empress*) — observed: "When Bealle first pointed out this fact in his book, Mr. Richards resigned forthwith, and the Rockefellers appointed in his place the president of their own Rockefeller Institute . . ."[57]

While the American expression of the Drug Trust is the focus of this chapter, the international nature of the pharmaceutical octopus cannot be overlooked, for it has played a role, both openly and behind the scenes, not only in endlessly producing toxic synthetic compounds for human consumption but in helping bar the development, use and distribution of natural therapies at every turn.

It was Frederick II of Hohenstaufen, King of Sicily and Germany, who — in the 13th century — first legalized state-approved "doctors" with the excuse that the people should be protected from charlatans, which frequently meant Hippocratic doctors who "threatened to ruin the lucrative medical trade with inexpensive natural treatments that benefited *only* the patient."[54]

As early as 1974, Kurt Bluchel exposed the dark side of the drug trade in Germany, one of its primary foci. He argued in *Weisse Magier* (*White Magicians*) that the drug business was the main reason for the rise in chronic diseases, deformities and cancer then being seen throughout the Western World.[55] As Ruesch related it in *Slaughter of the Innocent*, the original publisher of *Weisse Magier* was "persuaded" to take the book off the market, though it was later re-issued by a different company, and Bluchel followed with another Drug Trust exposé in 1978.[56,57]

While in *IX* we enumerate various drugs and medical

techniques the FDA has approved in the USA, and which had to be altered or withdrawn due to fatalities or severe side effects later, the American experience is only a fairly sizable tip of a much greater iceberg.

Pharmaceutical disasters: a global problem

For example, a "safe" painkiller, Paracetamol, was approved in Great Britain — but 1,500 people had to be hospitalized due to side effects in 1971. A year later, the drug Isopropterol, packaged in Great Britain, was found to be responsible for the mysterious epidemic which may have killed as many as 3,500 asthmatics during the 1960s.

In 1976, British drug giant ICI (Imperial Chemical Industries) announced it was paying compensation to the victims or their kin of the cardiotonic Eraldin, whose preliminary seven years of "very intensive laboratory tests" *on animals* had found it to be safe. But it was countless *human* consumers who suffered severe damage to the eyes and digestive tract, with many dying.[58]

The same year, Salvoxyl-Wander laboratories of Swiss drug giant Sandoz withdrew Flamanil, a claimed fighter of rheumatism which turned out to cause loss of consciousness.

Ruesch also described how the "pep pills" Preludin and Maxiton were withdrawn from the market after causing serious heart and nervous system damage; how the tranquilizers Pronap and Plaxin, which killed many babies in South Africa, were pulled in 1970; how Marzine, used for nausea and travel sickness, was withdrawn in several countries in 1971 because of severe side effects, particularly in children; and how even bismuth, prescribed for both diarrhea *and* constipation, was linked in France in 1974 with a thousand cases of intoxication and at least 28 deaths.[59]

The early 1960s worldwide clamor over the German company Chemie Grunenthal's Thalidomide — which was within a whisker of approval by the American FDA and the scandal over which led to a strengthening of the federal agency through a series of amendments covering both safety *and* efficacy (*IX*) — is among the better known international pharmaceutical calamities.

The drug, offered as a tranquilizer for pregnant women and breast-feeding mothers and which left a trail of deformed babies across Europe, was marketed in October 1961 by Great Britain's Distillers Company under the name Distaval following the usual extensive animal tests. Indeed, said the distributors, "Distaval can be given with complete safety to pregnant women and nursing mothers without adverse effect on mother or child."[60]

In December 1970, at what was at the time the longest criminal trial in German judicial history, Chemie Grunenthal was acquitted on the basis of testimony from "international experts" that animal tests *are never conclusive* for human beings, and that the company had undertaken the required tests in good faith.

In a seeming replay of the Thalidomide story, Americans and Britons learned in 1979 that drugs suspected of causing birth defects had been approved in both countries — under the names Bendectin in the USA and Debendox in Great Britain.[61]

Merrell's drug for morning sickness in pregnant women was the focus of an exposé by the *London Observer* in 1980, which found, among many things, that a "professional relationship" had existed between Merrell and a Leeds University pediatrics professor who had completed a study which cleared the company of any responsibility for increased birth defects among the children of Debendox-using women.[62]

In the USA, the Bendectin label was changed to read that the drug "should be used only when clearly needed" — and stayed on the market.[63]

Perhaps the greatest international drug scandal, though, dealt with Ciba-Geigy's "miracle" drug Oxychinol, a/k/a Clioquinol, an anti-"traveler's sickness" drug launched in the 1970s and sold under several hundred brand names, including 168 in Japan alone.

The launching of this dangerous drug provided evidence of the unintentioned manufacture of a man-made disease — in this case SMON, an acronym for subacute myelooptical neuropathy, which in Japan was found to be the cause of an estimated 30,000 cases of blindness and/or paralysis in that country alone. But cases of death, blindness and paralysis traceable to Oxychinol-containing drugs were also recorded in Holland, Denmark, Germany, France, Great Britain, and Sweden.

In August 1978, a Tokyo court found Ciba-Geigy Japan and two collaborating Japanese drug companies, as well as the Japanese government, guilty of selling drugs containing the deadly ingredient. The defendants were ordered to pay $17 million to 133 plaintiffs on the basis of the first round of cases. There were 5,500 plaintiffs by 1980.(64)

In a searing exposé of Oxychinol, Swedish medical doctor Olle Hansson, Goteborg University, an expert in pediatric neurology who testified at the Japanese trial, disclosed that Ciba-Geigy's own research which dated back to 1939 had shown how toxic Oxychinol was in laboratory animals. A SMON press conference in Geneva in 1980 revealed that the drug giant had disregarded the ill effects of the compound in animals.(65)

With such drug scandals as the above in mind, together with ongoing knowledge of the years-later side effects of all manner of sedatives, tranquilizers, antibiotics, antihistamines and other "miracle drugs" on the market, one can understand why the late American medical heretic Robert Mendelsohn MD could make such a sweeping statement as: "Don't trust your doctor. Assume that if he prescribed a drug, it's dangerous. There is no safe drug."(66)

Those who have traced the development and history of the international pharmaceutical cartel and the related vested interests of which it is a part are to be forgiven for what some see as paranoia:

The belief that *anything* that is useful medically and is *not* a patented, registered synthetic drug of some kind will be blocked, hidden, bought off or taken over — whether it be oxidative therapies against microbes (whose track record goes back to the early part of this century), bioelectrical and magnetic "energy medicine" or the herbs, amino acids, vitamins, minerals and enzyme combinations that integrative/holistic/metabolic doctors choose today over the "miracle drugs" offered by the global drug trust.

An international threat to free choice

Hence the growing concern going into the end of the millennium over activities by transnational pharmaceutical behemoths to attempt to stamp out medical freedom of choice on an international basis.

The effort to make the world safe for synthetic drugs by banishing natural remedies is being carried out under the color of international laws and agreements, the usual allegiance to "science" and the need (euphemistically relayed at this point) to "regulate" substances for "safety."

In the drugs vs. natural remedies arena, the United Nations and international agreements have played schizophrenic roles: on the one hand, the UN and the World Health Organization (WHO), bowing to reality, have had to face up to the fact that a majority of the world's population turns to "lay practitioners," medicine men and the like for medical decisions, that they prefer herbal and natural treatments, that the latter are certainly far cheaper than synthetic products, and that huge sectors of the populace simply cannot afford the synthetics at *any* price.

On the other, global international monopolists have sought to use developing international law and agreements as machinery through which to extend their control over all medicine and even seeds (*see XV*).

In the 1990s, increasing attention was focused on the Codex Alimentarius Commission, part of the UN's Food and Agriculture Organization (FAO) and the WHO, particularly after its nutrition panel voted (in 1995) in favor of the German delegation's proposal for "guidelines for dietary supplements."

The Codex, whose delegations are topheavy with drug-and food-industry representatives, allegedly has no implementing power, but nationalists in many countries fear that UN-backed "recommendations" can have *de facto* force of law through implementation of such binding international pacts as the General Agreement on Tariffs and Trade (GATT) and the North American Free Trade Assn. (NAFTA).

The German recommendation — reflecting the pharmaceutical interests of a nation which is a major source of the global drug empire — was that no dietary supplements could be sold for preventive or therapeutic uses (!), no such supplements could exceed potency or dosages levels as set by the Commission, that Codex regulations would be binding, and that new supplements would automatically be banned unless they passed through the Codex process.[67]

While the vote was only one step in a process said to take many years, and which US governmental officials claimed would not be binding on domestic law, German-born physician/researcher Matthias Rath MD of the USA was apoplectic.

In a bold move, he called on German Chancellor Helmut Kohl and the German Bundestag to cancel all Codex meetings in Germany and to "declare publicly that you will protect the health interests of millions of people worldwide against the plans of the German and international pharmaceutical corporations."

He called the suggested guidelines "a desperate act by the pharmaceutical companies to protect their worldwide drug market against naturally effective and more affordable vitamins."[68]

A Codex vote in 1996 advanced the procedure — hence speeding the day when international pharmaceutical control over natural products might occur — then a 1997 vote set it back a step.

In both the US and Canada in the 1990s governmental authorities, in seeming response to the demands and needs of the drug giants, flexed their muscles against the growing supplements and herbal markets by alleging "safety" problems — as we have seen in the L-tryptophan matter — and also in clamping down on ephedrine-containing products.

For long-time observers of the drug industry and government manipulation of medicine, the concern over "safety" in natural products, however genuine it might be, paled alongside the seeming lack of concern over so many dangerous synthetic drug products marketed for so long both domestically and internationally which had killed or poisoned so many people.

The discernible tactic globally is, first, to regulate or control dietary supplements and herbal preparations as if they were drugs (in the interests, of course, of "safety") and gradually remove them from all access by the general public, or to allow some nutrient monopolies to exist which are in turn linked to pharmaceutical interests.

The blocking moves to all this, of course, are the political enshrinement of freedom-of-choice legislation and the exerting of state and provincial independence from centralized federal authorities. By 1997, eight of the US states had made this decision, as had two Canadian provinces.

The war was on.

A shifting paradigm

In the unfolding war over concepts and therapies, the allopathically aligned "quackbusters" have attempted to score points off the practitioners of "alternative" or "holistic" or "nutritional" therapy by baiting them with the reality that patents on the production of various vitamins are held by a few giant drug companies.

Yet the attack also made the point for the other side: perhaps it was *because* patents were held on certain natural derivatives that progress in their use had not been made before and was in fact controlled — so that any implied threat to the synthetic drug industry could be at the very least "managed" at the source.

When the metabolic therapy revolution broke out in the 1970s, largely stimulated by the laetrile controversy (see *XII*), a chain of unstoppable events was set into play which altered the medical research landscape forever. Research, first largely foreign, and then increasingly American, tended to prove in case after case what the "quacks" had been saying for so long: nutrients *do* play roles, probably *key* roles, in health and disease. The trickle of information on this subject in the early 1970s had become a roar of Mississippi flood proportions by the 1990s.

So, why shouldn't the drug giants cash in on the inevitable turning of the tide toward nutrients, and claim their share of the prize?

The fact that the integrative medical side was beginning to win the debate was flashed first by drug giant Hoffman-LaRoche in 1988.

The international house already had vitamin interests, but it had not bothered to do much with them until the metabolic revolution started turning in undoubted successes in research and application.

In the Nov. 18, 1988, *Journal of the American Medical Association (JAMA)*, there was an advertising supplement which caught many of us in a spasm of eye-rubbing: here was Hoffman-LaRoche explaining the "possible" immunological and other benefits of its favorite ... nutrients. These were B-vitamins in general, Vitamin B6 by itself, Vitamin C, Vitamin A (and its "precursor," beta-carotene), and Vitamin E.

In some of the most tortured semantics we have ever pondered in the area of transconceptualization, the Hoffman-LaRoche copy writer inscribed this unforgettable rationale for the company's actually taking out space in the allopathic medical journal to sell vitamin tablets, long damned as the province of quackery:

> *It seems clear that specific vitamins . . . play important roles in the immune responses of laboratory and farm animals, and limited human data offer the possibility of future insights in both basic and clinical science in immunology and nutrition. For now, at least, the data support a heightened consideration of these interactions in patients who are nutritionally and/or immunologically compromised.*[69]

This was virtually an edict from Olympus, a finely crafted linguistic artifice from a major role player in the international pharmaceutical universe signalling an ever-so-dainty explanation for a major switch in concepts.

The proper translation, in 1988, was simply this: "Since a majority of American adults now pop vitamin pills, why should the big drug companies be left out of the feeding frenzy?"

The rationale stood in stark contrast to the observation in the *Harvard Medical School Health Letter* of approximately a year earlier:

> *The naturopathic claim (that nutritional remedies bolster the immune system) is simply not supportable . . . The use of herbs or nutrition to stimulate or strengthen the immune system is a nonsense claim . . . and to the extent that people wind up believing such claims, we can say that their brains are damaged.*(70)

Clearly a chink had been perceived in the armor of the Allopathic Industrial Complex. It was to widen.

References

1. *Pharmaceutical R & D: Costs, Risks and Rewards.* Office of Technology Assessment (OTA), US Congress, February 1993.
2. *The Choice*, XIX: 1, 1993.
3. *Ibid.*
4. *The Boston Globe*, March 8, 1996.
5. *The Choice*, XVIII:1, 1992.
6. "The price isn't right." *Time*, Jan. 8, 1990.
7. *The Choice*, XVII: 3,4, 1991.
8. *The Choice*, XVIII: 3, 1992.
9. The Associated Press, cited in *The Choice*, XXI:2, 1995.
10. Tanouye, Elyse, "Prescription drug prices rose 4 1percent in third quarter exceeding inflation." *Wall Street Journal*, Dec. 7, 1995.
11. Friend, Tim, "Education on prescribing is 'terrible.'" *USA Today*, July 27, 1994.
12. Drake, DC, and Marian Uhlman, "Making money making medicine." *Orange County* (CA) *Register*, Jan. 31, 1993.
13. *The Choice*, XV: 1,2, 1989.
14. *Pharmaceutical R & D . . ., op. cit.*
15. "Me too approach lessens firms' risks." *Orange County* (CA) *Register*, Jan. 31, 1993.
16. *Ibid.*
17. *The Choice*, XVII: 3,4, 1991.
18. *Pharmaceutical R &D . . . . op. cit.*
19. *Ibid.*
20. *The Choice*, XVIII: 2, 1992.
21. *The Choice*, XVII: 1, 1991.
22. *The Choice*, XVI: 2,3, 1990.
23. *Wall Street Journal*, May 3, 1993.
24. Drake DC, *op. cit.*
25. *Ibid.*
26. Heuer, Christina, in *Orange County* (CA) *Register*, Jan. 31, 1993.

27. Drake, DC, *op. cit.*
28. Harmer, RM, *American Medical Avarice.* New York: Abelard-Schuman, 1975.
29. *The Choice*, XVII: 2, 1991.
30. *Ibid.*
31. Culbert, ML, *AIDS: Hope, Hoax and Hoopla.* Chula Vista CA: The Bradford Foundation, 1990.
32. *American Medical News*, July 12, 1993.
33. Culbert, *op. cit.*
34. *Ibid.*
35. Carter, Richard, *The Doctor Business.* New York: Doubleday & Co., 1958.
36. *National Health Federation Bulletin*, October 1973.
37. Harmer, *op. cit.*
38. *New York Times*, Feb. 21, 1993.
39. *The Choice*, XVIII: 2, 1992.
40. *The Choice*, XVI: 2,3, 1990.
41. Drake, DC, *op. cit.*
42. "Doctors face powerful sales pitches." *Orange County* (CA) *Register*, Jan. 31, 1993.
43. *Ibid.*
44. *Health Letter*, Public Citizen Health Research Group, October, 1991.
45. *Ibid.*
46. "Drug an example of cost dilemma." *American Medical News*, April 25, 1994.
47. *Wall Street Journal*, Feb. 16, 1993.
48. *Ibid.*
49. *New York Times*, July 1993.
50. Drake, DC, *op. cit.*
51. Knight-Ridder Tribune service, April 1993.
52. Bealle, MA, *The Super Drug Story.* Washington DC: Columbia Publishing, 1949.
53. Ruesch, Hans, *Naked Empress.* Zurich: Buchverlag CIVIS, 1982.
54. *Ibid.*
55. Bluchel, Kurt, *Weisse Magier.* Munich: Bertelsmann, 1974.
56. Bluchel, Kurt, *Das Medizin-Syndikat.* Germany: Rowohlt, 1978.
57. Ruesch, *op. cit.*
58. *Ibid.*
59. *Ibid.*
60. *Ibid.*
61. "Common drug causing deformed babies," *National Enquirer*, Oct. 9, 1979.
62. "New thalidomide-style drug fear." London (UK) *Observer*, Jan. 9, 1979.
63. Ruesch, *op. cit.*
64. Izumi, Hiroshi, in *Proceedings*, Geneva Press Conference on SMON, Tokyo, 1980.
65. Hansson, Olle, *Arzneimittel-Multis und der SMON-Skandal.* Basel: Z-Verlag, 1979.
66. Mendelsohn, RS, *Confessions of a Medical Heretic.* Chicago: Contemporary Books, 1979.
67. "Propaganda war over the Codex Alimentarius." *The Choice* XXII: 1, 1996.
68. Life Extension Foundation, November 1996.
69. Hoffman-LaRoche supplement, *Journal of the American Medical Assn. (JAMA)*, Nov. 18, 1988.
70. *Medical Tribune*, cited in *The Choice*, XV: 1,2, 1989.
71. King, RT, "Bitter pill: how a drug firm paid for university study, then undermined it." *Wall Street Journal*, April 25, 1996, cited in *Alt. Med. Digest* 14, 1996.
72. *Ibid.*
73. Coleman, BC, The Associated Press, April 16, 1997.
74. Larsen, HR, "The great ulcer drug rip-off." *Alive* #173 (Canada), March 1997.
75. Krieger, LM, "Hormone therapy found to boost life expectancy." *San Francisco Examiner*, April 8, 1997.
76. Love, Susan, *Dr. Susan Love's Hormone Book.* New York: Random House, 1997.
77. O'Reilly, Brian, "Why doctors aren't curing ulcers." *Fortune*, June 9, 1992.

IX

THE FDA: Storm troopers for the drug trust

(HOW A GOOD IDEA WENT WRONG)

"The American public does not have the knowledge to make wise health care decisions . . .FDA is the arbiter of truth . . . Trust us. We will tell you what's good for you."

— Former FDA Commissioner David Kessler MD (on "Larry King Live," 1993)

"I need the power to order products recalled. I need the power to seize adulterated or misbranded material. I want the power to hire 100 criminal investigators, and I want the power to impose civil money penalties on violators."

— Former FDA Commissioner David Kessler MD (1992)

"The thing that bugs me is that the people think the FDA is protecting them. It isn't. What the FDA is doing and what the public thinks it's doing are as different as night and day."

— Dr. Herbert Ley, former FDA Commissioner (1970)

"The issues that are put to the FDA as to whether foods and drugs are safe and effective have no answer because what is safe for one person is not safe for another; what is effective for one person is not effective for another; and what is a desirable regulatory policy in one person's view is unacceptable to another."

— Peter Barton Hutt, former chief counsel, FDA, 1971-75, quoted in *The FDA* (1978)

"The FDA [is] the police arm of the medical establishment, which consists of physicians trained in allopathic medicine, in which drug therapy, radiation and surgery are the only accepted means of treating patients . . . The greatest resistance to change has been exhibited by the FDA, which is the last and most influential bastion of blind dogmatic bias against dietary supplements in the United States. . ."

— Saul Kent, Life Extension Foundation, before the FDA Dietary Supplement Task Force hearing (1991)

"Giving government the power to control the market for medical goods has been a bargain with the Devil, and so long as the FDA continues to exercise its malignant power, the deadly toll will continue to mount."

— Dr. Robert Higgs, Washington State University

The Fedstapo at work

What much of the American public perceives as the Food and Drug Administration (FDA) was crystallized by media attention in spring 1992 when federal agents, backed by local police, guns drawn, kicked in doors and ripped out telephones as they raided a metabolic therapy clinic in the state of Washington (*1*).

Their targets: "foreign" B vitamins and other nutrients and natural substances.

While this kind of outrage had been going on for years, most of the FDA misbehavior had failed to make the six o'clock news. This time, however, video cameras caught the Feds in the act.

Unfortunately, the image of flak-jacketed federal officers in hot pursuit of intravenous vitamin B complex obscured the fact that there are also honest, dedicated bureaucrats at the FDA and that the agency's painstaking humdrum work in attempting to oversee the purity of foods and cosmetics as well as drugs does not always get the limelight.

For many, the raid in Tahoma WA was indeed the straw that broke the camel's back — it was simply the most obvious and best-reported SWAT-team hit on an "alternative" practitioner by the FDA up to 1992.

It was not only an investigative raid against relatively innocuous substances but indeed a punitive attack — for Dr. Jonathan Wright had sued the federal agency for the return of uncontaminated L-tryptophan it had seized from him during the earlier scare over the link between deaths from a rare disorder and a Japanese version of L-tryptophan produced by new techniques (*see 1*).

But to FDA-watchers, there was nothing new here: when the FDA strikes it does not like to be sued in return. An arrogant federal agency running out of control, the FDA already had a record of punishing citizens for fighting back against it. Even as the Wright raid was going on the FDA was in and out of court over its attempts to put out of business Dr. Stephen Levine's

Nutricology/Allergy Research Group in Northern California — primarily because the plucky Dr. Levine, a producer of quality dietary supplements, had dared to stand up to the Feds and fight back in court after the FDA began harassing him (*1*).

Veteran FDA watchers were not surprised during 1989-1992 as yet another scandal unraveled at the controversy-mired federal agency which, on paper, is supposed to be the nation's guardian of purity and authenticity in foods, drugs and cosmetics:

This time, various FDA officials quit or were reassigned as grand jury indictments kept linking agency officials with a bribery scheme involving the "generic" drug industry.

("Generic" drugs are those compounds known by their common chemical names, in lieu of brand-name pharmaceuticals, and in general are considerably cheaper than the latter. The drug giants have not particularly liked generic drugs. The then-fledgling industry had fallen within the purview of the Food, Drug and Cosmetic Act of 1938, as amended in 1962. The scandal involved allegations that various FDA officials had taken bribes to assure the purveyors of the same of better handling of their products by the federal regulators.)

As that plot unfolded, the agency was hit by more bad news: the Department of Health and Human Services (HHS), itself an enormous bureaucratic satrapy with enough employees and budget to constitute a small sovereign state, claimed FDA's internal controls were inadequate to insure integrity in the drug-approval process, leaving the agency open to "manipulation and preferential treatment."

In the midst of it all, the Bush administration announced the departure of the FDA commissioner-in-turn, Dr. Frank Young, with no reasons given. Ho-hum.

A history of scandal

Earlier, in 1976, the then commissioner-in-turn had announced *his* resignation just as legislative investigators issued a blistering indictment of the agency and 34 of its current and former key employees for "failing to fully protect the public."

Congressional investigators that year had issued a report charging the FDA, pharmaceutical manufacturers, various doctors and research scientists with unnecessarily exposing humans to risks in the testing of new drugs. Various FDA witnesses told the probers that the agency was still failing to protect the public health two years after the Senate had launched an inquiry into charges that the FDA was biased toward the pharmaceutical industry.

And months earlier, the General Accounting Office (GAO) had reported that 150(!) FDA officers had violated federal "conflict of interest" rules by owning stock in drug companies which the agency supposedly was monitoring. (In 1969, a congressional study had revealed that 37 of 49 top FDA officials who left the agency took jobs with food and drug companies.[(1)])

Also in 1976, a House committee rapped the FDA's use of "advisory committees," charging that such committees were sometimes subject to "improper influence" from drug manufacturers.

But it was ho-hum again.

In 1960, the Senate held a highly publicized probe of the drug industry, among whose findings was the fact that many FDA officials had been receiving certain financial "incentives" from the companies they were supposedly regulating.

A particularly notorious example: Dr. Henry Welch, director of the FDA antibiotic division, had received $287,000 in "honoraria" (better known as kickbacks) derived from a percentage of the drug advertising produced for leading medical journals.[(2)]

Again, ho-hum.

Indeed, FDA employment preceding drug industry employment became enough of a revolving door so that various investigators and writers, quite aside from congressional investigative bodies, had a field day exposing the connection.

Ambruster,[(3)] Garrison,[(4)] Griffin,[(5)] and Moss[(6)] have been among the reporters who have brought to light such FDA-industry relationships as these:

—During the chloramphenicol scandal, Dr. Joseph F. Sadusk was director of the FDA's Bureau of Medicine. He could have used his clout to get the dangerous FDA-approved Parke-Davis drug off the market. Instead, he "used his official position to *prevent* the drug from being recalled, and even ruled against a precautionary label."[7] By 1969, when it was ready for recall (and had made a handsome profit for Parke-Davis) and had been replaced by another drug, FDA allowed Parke-Davis to get off the hook by distributing a letter to doctors claiming it was no longer the drug of choice for treating various infections. Sadusk left the FDA and shortly thereafter became . . . vice president of Parke-Davis.

—Sadusk's successor at the FDA, Dr. Joseph M. Pisani, shortly resigned thereafter to work for The Proprietary Association, a trade organization for manufacturers of non-prescription drugs — that is, an industry that the FDA was supposed to be "regulating."

—In turn, Dr. Pisani was replaced by Dr. Robert J. Robinson, who, after a brief stay, left to become a major executive at Hoffman-LaRoche, a major pharmaceutical house.

Omar Garrison, in *The Dictocrats*, added to the list:[8]

—Dr. Howard Cohn, former head of FDA's medical evaluation division, joined Ciba Pharmaceutical.

—Dr. Harold Anderson, chief of the FDA's division of anti-infective drugs, joined Winthrop Laboratories.

—Morris Yankowitz, head of FDA case supervision, joined Smith, Kline and French Laboratories.

—Allen E. Rayfield, former director of the FDA's regulatory compliance division, became a consultant for Richardson-Merrell Inc.

And Ralph Moss recalled[9] that:

—FDA Commissioner Charles C. Edwards later became senior vice president for research at Becton Dickinson, a medical supply company; and

— FDA Commissioner James L. Goddard became chairman of the board of Ormont Drug & Chemical Co.

(Which should not surprise, since former US Surgeon General Leonard Scheele became president of Warner-Lambert's research laboratories.)

In fact, in 1964, and only under congressional pressure, the FDA revealed that in the preceding five years 83 of 813 FDA officials (more than 10 percent) had joined companies they had, as FDA bureaucrats, previously regulated.[(10)]

Ho-hum, ho-hum.

None of this was illegal in any way.

The comfortable relationship between the Food and Drug Administration and the major industries it is supposed to monitor (namely, drugs *and* foods) was by the latter decades of this century so notorious that the agency was undergoing the greatest crisis of confidence since its establishment as a minor government office in the first decade.

As in any other good idea gone wrong, and as in virtually any case in which government efforts are aimed at "solving" a problem, it has been absorbed by the problem: the directorate over foods and drugs has, at least in the drug sector, become every bit what this writer baptized "the Fedstapo" — a policing organization whose "compliance" section is largely designed to protect in the USA the interests of the international pharmaceutical syndicate and its component cartel members while putting out of business all serious competitors to the drug behemoths in the domestic marketplace.

Even while fending off the generic drug scandal, the Fedstapo was engaged in a veritable orgy of healthfoods industry-bashing and dietary supplements persecution and prosecution in the 1990s on a scale that could only be appreciated by a Communist commissar or a Nazi gauleiter.

Whatever else the agency may be doing or may have done in terms of overseeing the safety of foods, drugs and cosmetics, and it has indeed at times operated in the public interest and responsibly in these areas, its domination by the pharmaceutical and food-processing interests and its own incestuous bureaucratic aggrandizement have allowed it to become so befouled with the stench of bribery and payoff that it is a fair assessment that the agency should be dispensed with entirely or restructured along very different lines. Currently, it is often simply a pestilential open sore on the body politic.

We observed (*VI*) that the original Pure Food and Drug Act of 1906, the "enabling legislation" which created the administrative excuse for what would become the FDA, was an outgrowth of some genuine concerns about food impurities and an increased awareness of the possible threats posed by the unrestricted use of patent medicines.

We also noted that the father of the FDA, Harvey Wiley, left the agency six years after its founding, already upset by its behavior.

Dr. Wiley didn't just walk out — he continued to monitor the agency he had done so much to build. As a believer in good nutrition, he was outraged to see the FDA become an instrument of the food monopolies it was supposed to be watching. In 1929 he published *History of a Crime Against the Pure Food Law* which detailed the perversion of the agency.

In a prophetic conclusion, he wrote:

> *The resistance of our people to infectious diseases would be greatly increased by a vastly improved and more wholesome diet. Our example would be followed by the whole civilized world and thus bring to the whole universe the benefits which our own people had received. We would have been spared the ignominy and disgrace of great scientific men bending their efforts to defeat the purpose of one of the greatest laws ever enacted for the protection of the public welfare. Eminent officials of our government would have escaped the indignation of outraged public opinion because they permitted and encouraged these frauds on the public. The cause of a wholesome diet would not have*

been put back for fifty or a hundred years.[11]

He was outlining here only the *foods* division of FDA responsibility. Perversion by the drug industry, already aborning by the time he wrote his exposé, would shortly take on a much greater dimension. Indeed, by the post-World War II era, it became increasingly obvious that the totality of the foods-producing, foods-processing, foods-distribution industry was the single biggest component in profit-taking in America, followed in number two position by the pharmaceutical industry. And the FDA was the supposed monitor of both.

It would not take on its current role (major bulwark of The Club, the policing division of the Allopathic Industrial Complex) until after the synthetic drug industry had massively invaded and captured American medicine and the Rockefeller-I.G. Farben global apparatus was in place (*IV*).

Perversion of a good idea

The original intent of the Food and Drug Act, passed in 1906, was to help consumers by requiring that ingredients be listed on the packaging labels of medicines — and to oversee the purity of foods, since "muckraker" journalism had exposed scandals in the meat-processing industry.

The law remained essentially unchanged and the agency relatively small until 1938, when the injectable form of the drug sulfanilamide reached the American marketplace and its solvent was found to contain a lethal substance. This discovery was the catalyst for the Food, Drug and Cosmetic Act (FDCA), which meant that from then on a drug manufacturer had to submit to the FDA an NDA (new drug application) in which it could be demonstrated that the compound was safe for its intended use.

The most important ancillary effect of the 1938 legislation was the establishment of the prescription-drug apparatus, even when — it has been argued — this consequence was apparently neither foreseen nor was it the central motive in the law.

By interpreting an FDCA provision that drugs be labeled

with adequate instruction for safe use, the FDA ruled that year that certain drugs were difficult to explain on a label in layman's language and that the label should carry the warning "Caution: to be used only by or on the prescription of a physician."

The FDA then ruled that the sale of any such medication without a prescription would be illegal.

While Congress had claimed it was not attempting to interfere with the right to self-medication — which *was* a right until that time, it should ever be recalled — the FDA suddenly equipped itself to provide to allopathic medicine the kind of total control (decisional disenfranchisement of the consumer) the latter had avidly sought since the 19th century.

From 1938 on, the MD physician essentially received the monopoly right to prescribe. These prescription-drug restrictions were formalized into law by Congress with the passage of the Humphrey-Durham amendments of 1954.

As a private research group stated in 1986:

> *A perverse consequence of the prescription-drug system was to deprive patients of potentially valuable information on drug usage and risks. Unlike consumers in many foreign countries, Americans do not receive manufacturer labeling with prescription drugs. Although the FDA required that manufacturers publish technical "package insert" information for physicians, it is typically discarded by the pharmacist before it reaches the patient. The theory is that doctors will provide the appropriate prescription-drug information themselves; in practice, physicians commonly neglect to provide important drug warnings. According to a recent FDA study, 80 percent of the patients surveyed received no drug information whatever from their physicians. There is ample evidence that prescription-drug misuse and misprescription are widespread problems.*[12]

It is also true that many foreign countries, particularly

"developing" ones, may receive no meaningful "package insert" information at all on certain drugs — at least none that reaches the consumer. It is also true that drug manufacturers are required to describe in detail possible side effects and adverse reactions from their products — if the consumer is subscribing to the medical journals in which drug advertising commonly appears and if, with less than 20-20 vision, he has a magnifying glass to read the 6-point type (usually on the overleaf or reverse of the display ad) in which such information is indeed available.

The Kefauver amendments: prescription for chaos

It was not until 1959 that the Senate Antitrust and Monopoly Subcommittee, chaired by Sen. Estes Kefauver, began hearings based on concerns that the 1938 legislation had allowed drugs of uncertain or dubious efficacy and high costs into the US marketplace. While there were other reasons for such concerns, it was the breaking of the Thalidomide scandal, 1961-62, which gave the Kefauver hearings an impetus which ultimately resulted in amendments to the law. These required that new medications to be brought to market should be proven both safe *and* effective.

Ironically, the triggering event — the Thalidomide scandal — dealt with *safety* rather than efficacy. The rush to approve this medication in Europe had left a residue of deformed and crippled babies, and the argument was raised that such compounds could reach the US market in the absence of inadequate testing.

The result was the famous Kefauver amendments — again, a good idea gone wrong — in which enormous new regulations and paperwork were generated for the licensing of new drugs.

The time between drug development and drug marketing, and the cost involved, would soar to produce the "drug lag," whereby the USA fell well behind other industrialized nations in the development of useful new modalities.

Whatever else the FDA has become, few thinking Americans would deny the need for some monitoring by some governmental agency at some level of the *safety* and *purity* of foods and drugs. Yet, the FDA, as the current incarnation of the Food, Drug and Cosmetic Act, carrying the heavy administrative baggage of changes and additions in 1938 and 1962, has become far more than that:

As the arbiter of safety *and* "efficacy," particularly since the 1962 amendments went into effect, the FDA is, on paper, empowered to oversee the elaboration, production and distribution of medications, medical devices and drugs in general. In effect, because the suffocating costs and paperwork generated by the bureaucracy have increased exponentially over the years and can only be implemented by gigantic companies which can afford to get through the licensure/drug approval process, the FDA has thus served as a major stumbling block to innovative small companies while eliminating competition for the international synthetic drug syndicate — that is, the drug cartel, which as of the 1990s consisted of several dozen corporations and conglomerates, often interlocking, which are international in scale.

The pharmaceutical connection

The fact that 150 FDA officials would or could own stock in companies which the FDA was mandated to monitor is old hat in government and was matched, in the Vietnam War and post-war eras, by disclosures that officials from various federal agencies and departments were immersed in bid-rigging and outright profiteering from the enormous American defense industry, the only accumulation of vested interests and corruption which could even come close to equalling the vested interests and corruption in foods and drugs. That federal officials from the defense sector would, on federal retirement, enter the defense industry itself was paralleled by the revolving door of foods/drugs officials entering the private foods/drugs sector, at one level or another. Monopoly breeds opportunity.

During its frankly scandalous history, the FDA's growing power, said to be mandated by its "enabling legislation" (Washingtonese for providing a bureau or department with ill-defined parameters and, often, a blank check from taxpayers to "go solve the problem"), has meant that the drug cartel could grow and prosper in the USA as chief purveyor to and of the Allopathic Industrial Complex (AIC). FDA power has consistently and irreversibly been used *for* the extension of pharmaceutical power and *against* the healthfoods and dietary supplements industries. It has consistently been used to crush minor competitors to the drug giants. Its policing authority has been used on an interstate basis to attempt to thwart resurgent homeopathy, the growing holistic medical revolution, chiropractors involved in Medicare payments, "alternative" physicians and all other enemies of, or challengers, real or imagined, to, the AIC.

Its behavior, in the laetrile and post-laetrile era, has been that of an out-of-control bureaucracy which would trample on any civil right, tell any lie, twist any statute, corrupt any agent and rig any meeting always under the color of the law of its "enabling legislation," despite a string of court setbacks in which judges ruled that, surely, the framers of the original Act and the subsequent amendments never intended the federal government to control the practice of medicine.

FDA as mass-murderer

In a hideous history of lopsided bias for the drug profiteers and of eager and ruthless suppression and repression of natural nutrients, the FDA's red tape-generating machinery has been so often utilized to exclude the medicinal use of natural substances (vitamins, minerals, enzymes, amino acids, naturopathy, herbs, homeopathy, chiropractic, etc.) while allowing the drug giants to license and sell their products to the American public that it can be said that the agency is guilty, at least after the fact, of murder and genocide. For so many of the substances it has allowed on the market, those which have gone through the "safety and efficacy" requirements of the Food, Drug and Cosmetic Act, have killed, maimed, and poisoned the population on a gross scale.

Indeed, in a 1993 House Subcommittee on Health and the

Environment hearing on proposed dietary supplement legislation, the National Nutritional Foods Assn. (NNFA) used data from various official sources to indicate that the death rate from adverse reactions to FDA-approved drugs in the USA averaged 100,000 a year — or between 60,000 and 140,000 — as opposed to no deaths from vitamin products or from "uncontaminated" amino acids.[13]

The NNFA, a healthfoods industry group, gathered its information from the American Association of Poison Control Centers, National Center for Health Statistics, the *Journal of the American Medical Assn.* (*JAMA*), Centers for Disease Control and Prevention, Consumer Product Safety Commission, *FDA Reports*, and the National Highway Traffic Safety Commission to come up with the figure — one some held to be conservative, since some other estimates have placed the FDA-caused death toll substantially higher.

The data appeared as the FDA rekindled its attack on dietary supplements and herbs as potentially dangerous substances, wrapping the attack around the scare over contaminated L-tryptophan.

At the same hearing, a Public Citizen Health Research Group study (*Worst Pills/Best Pills II*) was inserted into the record to indicate that 9.6 million Americans annually suffered adverse drug reactions from substances most of which were FDA-approved, that 659,000 older Americans were hospitalized annually due to such reactions, that 163,000 suffered serious mental impairment from such drugs, and that some products had caused 61,000 cases of drug-induced Parkinsonism and 73,000 cases of drug-induced tardive dyskinesia.[14]

For instance, between 1983 and 1987, or on the eve of reports about deaths from the use of a single variety of the amino acid L-tryptophan, some 1,182 deaths had been reported from the use of certain FDA-approved drugs (and these to 16 Poison Control centers covering only 11 percent of the country) — as opposed to *no* deaths, and no meaningful side effects, from the consumption of vitamin and nutrient pills.[15] These data surfaced as the FDA sought to implement the Nutritional Labeling and Education Act (NLEA) of 1990 by setting up a "task force on dietary supplements" to make it appear that the federal agency was hearing from all sides before arriving at a consensus of what to do about the rapidly growing dietary supplements industry (by 1996 a $9 billion activity — and, with the total of healthfood products involved, as high as $17 billion.)

The FDA, as policeman for the drug interests, was attempting in the early 1990s to replay its behavior of the early 1970s, when it was poised to wipe out American citizens' access to vitamin/mineral tablets, a business already perceived as a threat to the drug cartel. Only a storm of protest led by health-freedoms advocates had headed off the FDA then, and sparked the passage of the Proxmire Law (1974) which protected such preparations from federal control. The existence of such products, which had geometrically expanded in number just as the laetrile furor began to break, was seen as a continuing market threat by the drug merchants, and the AMA/FDA/pharmaceutical combine engaged in heavy propaganda for almost 20 years in attempts to thwart, denigrate or overturn Proxmire.

(There was of course a certain schizophrenia within the drug monopoly, since several of its major participants also owned patents on vitamins, and the booming vitamin supplement business was a growing profit-maker in itself, so that a diversified conglomerate handling drugs, medical devices *and* vitamin/ mineral pills was left with the dilemma of not wanting to shut off the minimal profits of the latter simply because, eventually, they could conceivably cut into the profits of the former as the medical paradigm moved from treating sickness to promoting health.)

Giving the devil his due, it is true that the honest FDA official (not always a contradiction in terms) has had every right to feel frustrated by the agency's seeming charge from Congress — it has been severely criticized at times for being too lax in the safety area just as it has taken its lumps for being over-zealous in "compliance." Some political forces, which believe government interference in, and management of, the private sector is a net social good, have argued for the need to strengthen the agency, however corrupt it may be; libertarian thinkers and small-government advocates have been just as assiduous in arguing that it needs to be reduced, if not eliminated. In the last decade of the century, the agency might get a "C" in protecting the public from certain unsafe elements in foods, drugs and medical devices and an "F" by furthering monoply, quenching freedom of choice, and undercutting innovation in the medical/pharmaceutical market-place.

Before the advent of AIDS, the only syndrome which ever seemed to demand the FDA's total attention and had so severely shaken the nation that, in a few years, it had caused the agency to loosen its awesomely slow drug-approval process several times, the FDA was usually deemed guilty of denying Americans access to useful, proven remedies available in other countries against many of the chronic, degenerative diseases growing exponentially in the American population. At the same time, it was held responsible for having approved thousands of drugs and medical practices that either did not work or whose risks far outweighed their benefits. It was, indeed, damned if it did, damned if it didn't.

By the 1970s, FDA bureaucracy in the pachydermally bulky and ponderously slow drug approval process (the "Investigational New Drug" [IND] and "New Drug Application" [NDA] machinery) led to both public and private studies which suggested that consumers were being hurt by the inordinate delay in approving useful new drugs.

In 1979, Congress held hearings on the by-then-evident drug lag, and in 1980 the General Accounting Office (GAO) issued a scathing report on the drug-approval process.[16] These actions led to a series of reforms aimed at speeding up drug approval, including, in 1982, the Orphan Drug Act, which allowed the FDA to make certain drugs eligible for special approval and tax credits.

The reform efforts did speed up drug approval somewhat and allowed for an increase in new chemical entities to reach the

American public, but the process still remains slow, spotty and strongly weighted in favor of the huge pharmaceutical interests which can afford the time, investment and wait.

In 1986, the private Cato Institute, in a "policy analysis" overview of the FDA, assessed that

> *new drugs still take years to reach the market, during which time they are largely inaccessible, and hundreds of foreign drugs remain legally unavailable. After 48 years of agency regulation, there is no scientific evidence that the FDA approval system is on balance beneficial to public health. The cost of a mere one-year delay in new-drug approval can be estimated at as much as 37,000 - 76,000 lives per decade — several times the worldwide toll of all new drug accidents.*[17]

By the mid-1990s, there were dozens of useful foreign drugs for everything from AIDS, cancer and aging to cataracts and alcoholism to which Americans had no legal access at home, primarily because the promoters of same had no reason to attempt to get through the dauntingly expensive FDA approval processes even should they be perceived as fair.

Indeed, even drug giant Hoffman-LaRoche noted[18] that between 1992 and 1994 some 60 percent of all FDA-approved drugs had first been approved in other countries. Whether they were good or bad, they were left out of the reach of Americans by the FDA's chronic, snail-paced approval process.

And there remained plenty of controversy in the time-lag matter as well:

In 1995 the General Accounting Office (GAO) reported[19] that the time the FDA was taking on new drug approval had dropped from an average 33 months in 1987 to 19 in 1994 (with a drop to as low as 5.8 months in some cases by 1996) but spokesmen for drug businesses big and small argued that even those figures did not take into account the full amount of time it was really taking to bring a new compound from conception to market.[64]

In 1996, an analyst claimed that "under (FDA Commissioner David) Kessler, the average amount of time it takes to develop a new drug has climbed to an all-time high of 15 years" and that FDA claims of a reduction in "review times" were based on only a part of the agency's lengthy assessment process. The FDA called the report "absolutely untrue," and Congress remained confused.[20]

(After suddenly announcing his resignation late in 1996, Kessler took credit for bringing more "breakthrough" drugs to market in less time than his predecessors.)

In the meantime, noted a newspaper editorial, between 1989 and 1994 the FDA's budget authority "increased by 52.6 percent after inflation . . . a real increase of more than 10.5 percent a year" while, during the same timeframe, the agency's roster of full-time employees increased from 7,000 to 9,000.[21]

FDA as obstacle to progress

As I reported extensively in 1983, as of that year the FDA had been blocking chymopapain (admittedly a controversial product) as a non-addictive pain-killer; sodium valproate, which can control epileptic seizures; beclomethasone, for asthma; bethanidine, minoxodil and oral diazoxide for severe hypertension; a host of substances for rheumatoid arthritis; lactulose for liver disease; carbenoxolone for ulcers; verapimil for heart disease; chenodeoxychloric acid for gallstones; and a wide variety of substances for high blood pressure, asthma, arthritis, tuberculosis and other conditions. It consistently opposed the use of EDTA chelation therapy in cardiovascular disease (despite EDTA's legality as a chelator of lead), laetrile for cancer and an ever-growing list of nutrients found useful against an ever-growing list of degenerative diseases, metabolic challenges and inborn errors of genetics.

While it turned out there was some reason to keep some of those things off the market, the "drug lag" in the United States had become so notorious that informed Americans were running off to foreign countries, including Canada and Mexico, to secure medications they could not acquire in the USA. By 1983, the Pharmaceutical Manufacturers Assn. (PMA), voice of the American drug lobby, estimated it was taking drug companies about $55 million and at least five years to get a new drug entity approved through the FDA, with estimates of the paperwork generated in the process climbing to as high as 200,000 pages.

The paperwork engendered by the 1962 amendments — quite literally truckloads — served to cause a drug-development roadblock which, intentionally or unintentionally, meant that only huge enterprises could possibly comply. Only they would have the resources to wait for years, grapple with the red tape, and endlessly test new modalities on live animals before advancing to "clinical" (that is, human) trials. The investment in time and paper-shuffling would, hopefully, result in 17-year patents for companies with huge capital reserves.

Less than a decade later (1990), a Tufts University study found[(22)] that — despite several vaunted changes in the FDA's drug-approval process and various measures aimed at decreasing paperwork — it was now taking *12* years and costing on the average a whopping $231 million to research, test and secure approval for a new drug in the United States. The report by the Center for the Study of Drug Development had the blessing of the PMA and adjusted cost figures for inflation into 1987 dollars. (An Office of Technology Assessment [OTA] study — see *VIII* — set a much higher figure in 1993: $359 million.)

In 1996, as we have seen, a Hoover Institute research fellow calculated the global cost of drug development — from "synthesis of the molecule to marketing approval" — at $500 million, adding that such costs had increased by 40 percent during the Kessler administration.[(65)]

The AIDS crisis led the FDA to approve "compassionate uses" of drugs for ostensibly life-threatening diseases (primarily AIDS and cancer) which essentially helped a handful of toxic AIDS drugs get to market much faster. But other than shaking up the agency over a condition the entire Western medical establishment seemed unable to cure, the new syndrome failed to make much of a dent in FDA bureaucracy overall. As the final decade of the century began the situation remained stagnant: only companies with enormous financial reserves could afford to attempt to license anything, be it a corn plaster or a new anti-cancer therapy, through the awesomely expensive and frightfully complicated and labyrinthine bureaucracy of the FDA.

And, as for the attempt to license nutrients or other natural substances as medical treatments, the message was clear: forget it. There was no financial incentive for a company to attempt to license a natural substance through the FDA.

Noted the Cato Institute in 1986:

> *Because of its monopoly powers over drug testing, the FDA has been able to influence the direction of pharmaceutical research. In general, it has been agency policy to discourage the investigation of drugs that are not devoted to treating disease, such as drugs to extend memory, promote longevity, prevent cancer and degenerative diseases, or improve cosmetic appearance. Research on psychoactive drugs . . . has been virtually forbidden, although there is strong evidence that these drugs may have unique medical or psychological benefits.*[23]

The change in drug licensure/drug development also greatly spurred the vivisection industry — huge profits for the breeding of animals to be used in testing drugs which ultimately would be for human administration only. This entire matter is a scandal so brutal and horrendous that it needs its own treatment elsewhere. The anti-vivisectionist movement, stimulated by such major reportorial coups as *Slaughter of the Innocent* and *Naked Empress* and shocking if highly revealing videos from interested groups, brought this sorry story to the forefront. If Americans learned how few truly useful drugs have ever been developed through the torture of live animals, and how the use of vivisection has itself become a huge industry, they might better understand why various activist groups in the 1980s stormed research labs to "liberate" experimental animals.[24]

Since the 1962 FDA amendments — more red tape and government control based on good intentions — not only did the drug lag between the development of useful medicines in the USA and the rest of the world become apparent, but it was also noted — by then Congressman Steve Symms and others[25] — that had aspirin, penicillin, insulin and digitalis been introduced after 1962, they would still be waiting to clear FDA regulations for "safety" and "efficacy."

The change in the FDA mandates, giving the bureaucrats-for-life seemingly an endless *carte blanche* entry into the field of medicine, was matched by the carefully honed public assumption that a newer, bigger FDA meant better drugs, more protection, more "public service."

Nothing could be further from the truth.

In 1978, an Office of Technology Assessment (OTA) survey estimated that only 10 to 20 percent of medications approved by the federal agency had ever gone through the totality of the ponderous new procedures required by the 1962 amendments. Which really meant that 80 to 90 percent of medications on the American market were actually "unproven," even by the FDA's own definition thereof! Yet when opposing a new item for market (particularly if from a small and struggling company) the agency would always insist that the would-be manufacturer adhere to the most stringent requirements of the Food, Drug and Cosmetic Act.

In 1990, a 10-member blue-ribbon "national committee to review current procedures for approval of new drugs and AIDS," chaired by Louis Lasagna MD, Tufts University, found that "the FDA has the legal authority to approve, and in fact has approved, new drugs on the basis of one scientifically valid study, and on the basis of phase I and phase II clinical studies without the need for a phase III clinical trial."[26]

This was an adroit way to accuse the FDA of selective

approval — pandering — whenever it wanted to, a reality of which champions of laetrile and other "unproven" cancer remedies in the 1960s and 1970s were fully aware: the FDA could seem to rush to the market an expensive, toxic chemotherapeutic agent primarily on the basis of selected foreign research, while closing the doors to a list of less expensive, and certainly less toxic, remedies already in use, if often surreptitiously.

In 1983, I reported that

> *"The direct effects of the Food, Drug and Cosmetic Act have been the elimination of medical competition from the marketplace, the notorious drug lag, and an increase in the operations of the FDA — which now costs taxpayers about $1 billion a year — and a geometric increase in suffering and death. It has been estimated that 24 times the number of Americans who died in Vietnam expired at home because of the amended food and drug law."*[27]

A record of disaster and deceit

While denying Americans access to useful drugs, and indirectly discouraging them from visiting healthfood stores for dietary supplements and muzzling doctors from prescribing such supplements for the prevention or management of a wide array of conditions (aside from the specific vitamin deficiency diseases), it is instructive to examine some of the products which, in times past, the FDA *has* allowed, and what they have done:

— In 1992/93, the FDA took only a tepid position on the growing scandal of side effects from silicone-gel breast implants in women, some of which were said to be linked to cancer and autoimmune disease. The largest product liability settlements in history were announced by implant producers between 1994 and 1996.

— In the early 1990s, plaintiffs were winning lawsuits against the government by claiming that the FDA-approved live oral polio vaccine, not one dose of which was said to have met federal standards, actually *caused* the disease in several patients.

— Aspirin, by many lights the best and certainly the cheapest of the over-the-counter drugs, is associated annually with hundreds of deaths and many thousands of side effects.

— More than 20 years ago, it was detemined that Orabilex caused kidney damage and death, MER/29 provoked cataracts and methaqualone caused severe psychiatric disturbances leading to more than 360 deaths, mainly through murder and suicide. All had been approved by the FDA.

— Drug companies in mid-decade were still paying off awards to victims of the synthetic hormone diethylstilbestrol (DES), developed with much hoopla as a drug to prevent miscarriages. DES has been associated with cancer in girls whose mothers had been prescribed the drug during pregnancy. The full effects of the widespread use of this once-legal drug have yet to be measured.

— Thousands of suits against manufacturers were on the way to resolution by mid-decade in the matter of the Bjork-Shiley convexo-concave heart valve, which the FDA had allowed to be inserted for seven years while deaths and injuries from the device were reported. By 1990, the valve — implanted in some 86,000 people between 1979 and 1986 — was said to have been responsible for 310 deaths and came under fierce attack, along with its manufacturer and the FDA, by a House subcommittee. A "settlement" plan of about $200 million was announced in 1992.

— In 1991, Bristol-Myers Squibb announced withdrawal of Enkaid (encainide hydrochloride) because of higher death risks among irregular-heartbeat patients.

— In 1975, federal probers found that the widely prescribed drugs Aldactone and Flagyl (G.D. Searle & Co. — the tenth largest drug house in the country at the time with sales on these two items alone of $17.3 million) were correlated with cancer in test animals. As Ralph Moss reported: "Further investigation revealed that Searle had known about the tumor-producing potential of these items but had simply given the FDA fraudulent data."[(28)] This was going on while the FDA was in a frenzy of outrage over laetrile and alerting the American population to the evils of this supposedly quack "cancer cure."

(Moss also noted that at least three other companies — Ciba-Geigy, Ayerst Laboratories, Lederle Laboratories — withheld pertinent information or simply fed the agency false data, events which kept begging the question of just who was running the FDA. Even though either strong administrative sanctions or criminal prosecution might have ensued had FDA so wished, FDA Commissioner Alexander M. Schmidt told Senate probers that "the cases somehow went into some bottomless pit that we have not been able to identify."[(29)])

— In 1977, Ciba-Geigy, a member in good standing of the international drug cartel, withdrew Phenformin, a diabetic drug, from the American market since it had been linked to about a thousand deaths annually.

— Phenacetin, taken off the American market more than a decade ago, was a painkiller sold in various compositions under 200 brand names. It turned out to cause kidney blockage and destruction, kidney tumors and destruction of red blood cells.

— Doctors in the USA were prescribing chloramphenicol (Chloromycetin) in the 1950s to almost 4 million people a year for acne, sore throat, the common cold, typhoid and other things despite evidence the drug— one of the top earners at the time for Parke-Davis — could kill patients through inducing aplastic anemia. (*See earlier.*)

— Clofibrate, a "miracle drug" used extensively for 13 years in the USA, was removed in 1981 after a 10-year World Health Organization (WHO) study found that men who regularly took the drug were 25 percent more likely to die of cancer, stroke, respiratory disease and heart attack (ironic in that this was marketed as a heart remedy) than those who took placebo capsules.

— As we point out in another chapter, virtually every toxic chemotherapeutic agent on the American market as a treatment *for* cancer has the capability of either causing cancer in laboratory animals (to the extent such research is germane at all) or, worse, of helping produce "secondary" human cancers later.

— The literature is vast on the subject of immune-depressing and other side effects from the most common antibiotics and synthetic steroids, whatever short-term and indeed at times life-saving effects they may have. The overuse of "legal" antibiotics and steroids is as much a stage-setter for chronic fatigue syndrome (CFS) and AIDS as are "illegal" drugs, I argue elsewhere.[30,31]

— The taker of the cake, however, is Valium, flagship of a class of addictive drugs known as the benzodiazepine family. Profiteering from it, its widespread use in medicine (even today, although it is no longer among the top-ranked drugs, other benzodiazepines having taken its place), the way it was marketed, and its apparent ease of passage through the FDA, usually referred to as "the most reliable" or the most highly developed consumer-protective apparatus in the world, is a story in itself.

During the 1970s and part of the 1980s, Valium was one of the most often prescribed tranquilizers, routinely recommended for both major and minor complaints, and, for years, the top drug of its class in the world in sales. As the late Harold Harper MD and I pointed out in a book,[32] it was oh-so-easy for a physician to dash off a prescription for Valium in just a few seconds after listening to a hypoglycemic reel off a list of vague symptoms, particularly when it was much more time-consuming to subject the patient to a six-hour glucose tolerance test to ferret out the real reason for his complaints.

Yet by 1974 the real markup for Valium was estimated to be from $50 per kilogram when produced in Switzerland to a stunning $75,000 per kilo in the USA, where it was — in the hip parlance of the time — "cut" for sale as tablets. In that year, it was dispensed 22.5 million times at an average of 60 tablets per prescription.

In 1979 the Senate Health Subcommittee was told 68 million prescriptions for Valium, Librium and other related benzodiazepines had been written in the USA in 1978 with a wholesale market value of $360 million, including 44 million for Valium alone. Far worse, the solons learned, addiction to benzodiazepines could cause withdrawal symptoms more prolonged and severe than those from heroin.[33] A spate of various side effects from these drugs continued to be reported, yet each one had made it through the FDA's "responsible" and "scientific" screening machinery and monitoring process. (As did, as we shall see, Halcion and Prozac, controversial sedative/antidepressants.)

As Ivan Illich reported in *Medical Nemesis*,[34] Valium's producer, Hoffman-LaRoche, had spent (before 1976) some $200 million over 10 years and commissioned 200 doctors a year to produce favorable scientific articles about Valium's properties — frequently in the "peer-reviewed" and "learned" journals in which page after page of glossy, full-color ads could be found touting the product(s).

Indeed, by the 1980s, even with the benzodiazepines falling from top spots in world pharmaceutical profits, it could still be said that the markup on Valium alone often was enough to outpace the profits in either gold or cocaine!

Approving the bad, blocking the good

Yet, approving *bad* drugs is one thing; barring potentially *good* ones is another.

The President's Biomedical Research Panel, which convened in 1974 to report on the National Institutes of Health, concluded, "There is a different kind of hazard to public health, posed by the prolonged delays and great costs of developing new and potentially useful drugs which the FDA's own protective system has imposed. In some respects, the agency has become a formidable roadblock."[35]

For example, according to the *Congressional Record* for July 21, 1976, a man from Louisiana

> *devised a product which is useful in filling decayed and abscessed teeth. According to dentists using the product, they would have been unable to save the teeth without the product. Because the cost of*

obtaining an NDA (New Drug Application) approval was too great for this single innovator, he reached an agreement with a nearby dental school to have their researchers conduct the testing. However, FDA refused to grant this innovator an IND (Investigational New Drug application) despite the clinical data he had been able to obtain. Without the IND, the dental school will not touch the product. The upshot of this is that the product will be manufactured and marketed overseas. Americans will have to do without it, perhaps indefinitely.

In the same *Congressional Record,* Idaho's then Rep. Steve Symms, the author of key legislation to reform the FDA, bared the plight of a small drug company in Georgia:

> *They manufacture heparin sodium injection, which is an anticoagulant that has been on the market since the mid-1930s. The major use of the drug now is for open heart surgery and in maintaining life for kidney dialysis patients. All companies manufacturing the product had to submit new drug application data.*
>
> *They* [the companies] *were not able to pool their resources for a combined NDA. This small firm had to cough up $10,000 to, in their words, "tell the FDA officials, most of them completely inept, what the drug did, how it worked, and why it was safe. Now this is something that people in pharmacy, medicine and nursing already know, and we found it difficult to translate the information to the officials of the FDA."*[36]

Not only that, but simply to comply with red tape, FDA regulations have required such items as storing bottlecaps 24 inches from walls, cleaning toilet facilites in a specified manner, filing 18 sets of reports along with quarterly summaries, maintaining written records regarding the cleaning of laboratory beakers, maintaining housing space for test animals whether or not the drug company involved does its own animal toxicity studies or even *keeps* animals, etc., etc.

The result of all this is not only the evils of the drug lag and the removal of competition, but the creation of a super bureaucracy that, like all bureaucracies, not only eventually becomes friendly with the very industry it is supposed to be monitoring, but also has the effect of interfering with the first sacred tenet of medicine, the privacy of the physician-patient relationship itself. It has taken expensive federal court cases by doctors and patients seeking access to freedom of choice in medicine to establish what should be a mother's-milk bit of wisdom: Congress never intended the FDA and the Food, Drug and Cosmetic Act to interfere with the practice of medicine.

Spitball bureaucrats at play

A peek at how the federal agency works was provided in testimony April 9, 1976, before the Panel of New Drug Regulations of the Department of Health, Education and Welfare by whistle-blower Dr. Richard Crout, then director of the FDA's Bureau of Drugs:

> *I want to describe to you the agency as I saw it. No one knew where anything was. There was an enormous documents room — I don't know whether you believe it or not, but this was a place where people said fights went on in a literal sense. There was absenteeism; there was open drunkenness by several employees, which went on for months; there was intimidation internally; and there was a great deal of what I would call feudalism in bureaucracy. I can tell you that, in my first year at the FDA . . . going to certain kinds of meetings was an extraordinarily peculiar kind of exercise. People — I'm talking about Division directors and their staffs — would engage in*

a kind of behavior that invited insubordination; people tittered in the corners, throwing spitballs — now I'm describing physicians; people would slouch down in their chairs and not respond to questions; and moan-and-groan, the sleeping gestures. This was a kind of behavior I have not seen in any other institution from a grown man . . . FDA has a long-term problem with the recruitment of personnel, good, scientific personnel.[37]

And John O. Nestor, a pediatrician with the FDA who spoke out against deficiencies in the agency, told Senate investigators as early as 1963, or just after the Food, Drug and Cosmetic Act was amended, that the FDA "worked too closely with the giant drug companies to be effective."[38]

Inanity, asininity and wordplay

When the FDA is not barring useful drugs, or preventing the use of one "cleared" substance in a situation for which it was not originally licensed, it seems to revel in plain silliness, based primarily on the American obsession with animal tests.

For example, gigantic quantities of saccharine administered to animals in doses equivalent to a human's ingestion of 800 to 1,000 cans of diet soda every day for many years resulted in scattered cases of bladder cancer in the poor animals. This led the FDA to announce a ban on saccharine in 1977 — a move which endangered thousands of diabetics and obese people. The Swiss Medical Association promptly noted that "saccharine has helped countless people to avoid obesity and has aided diabetics marvelously for decades . . . Because it is to be banned on the basis of a scientifically baseless test order and a wrong interpretation of results the FDA has lost credibility on both sides of the ocean."[39]

Of course, the FDA's odd moves against saccharine helped protect the refined sugar (sucrose) industry — the probable cause of its interest in the first place.

The FDA pursued a similar line with its flip-floppery over

cyclamates.

Its troubles with artificial sweeteners did not stop there: by 1990, as the consumer group Citizens for Health noted, federal officials had received 5,500 reports of adverse reactions to Searle's NutraSweet (aspartame), or 80 percent of all consumer complaints involving a food or food additive for that year.[40] The complaints ran from mild effects to seizures. The consumer group wanted to know why the FDA was not checking into aspartame when at the same time it was moving, often viciously, against aloe vera, effervescent Vitamin C, and evening primrose oil — against which no complaints had been filed.

In testimony before a House subcommittee in 1993, it was pointed out that the NutraSweet matter between 1977 and 1983 seemed to be a case of the government approving something at the behest of the drug industry — and that it involved key members of the Gerald Ford presidential team, three ranking FDA officials and two former FDA commissioners.[41]

In 1996, a study statistically linked aspartame and human brain cancer, though the FDA and manufacturer Monsanto were quick to assail the information and reaffirm the product's safety. The revelations were redolent of earlier research in which a breakdown product of aspartame was associated with brain tumors in test animals.[66]

And FDA's activity against evening primrose oil and black currant seed oil in the late 1980s, which caused as much laughter as tears, reflected how the FDA would use its power to keep out sources of natural substances which could be medically used (and which thus threatened the pharmaceutical industry).

In 1988, the Feds started seizing batches of evening primrose oil, arguing that the substance was not on the "generally recognized as safe" (GRAS) list as a dietary supplement. The same year it seized drums of black currant seed oil imported from England. The overzealous FDA policing in the latter matter involved the agency in a running legal battle with Traco Laboratories of Illinois.

What was almost certainly behind the federal agency's concern over both products:

The presence in them of the polyunsaturated fatty acid known as gamma-linolenic acid (GLA), which research suggests may help curb heart disease, stroke, diabetes, atopic eczema, alcoholism and even premenstrual syndrome in persons with low-level concentrations of it.

The galaxy of conditions for which supplemental GLA might be useful thus brings it into direct conflict with such "approved drugs" as aspirin, the non-steroidal antiinflammatory drugs (NSAIDs), and even expensive cholesterol-lowering drugs.

Under the odd semantics with which the FDA has felt itself empowered since 1962 (obscuring meanings of the words "food," "drug," "food additive," "supplement," "claim," etc.) plus the Food Additive Law, the FDA, when it wishes, can assume that a claim (however valid) for a nutrient (or anything else) that can be construed medically will magically transmute the same into a "drug" which, should it not have gone through the FDA bureaucracy for clearance, can then be further construed as "unlicensed" — and hence open to prosecutory action and seizure. (Ostensibly, even water could be so construed if a medical claim is made for it — as in its suggested consumption by a diabetic.)

And, it is perfectly true that naturopaths and nutritional medics have long felt that evening primrose oil and similar substances are useful in the above disorders — which the federal agency has construed as "claims" made for "unlicensed drugs."

In its frankly idiotic, tax-wasting, time-consuming move against Traco, the FDA had wielded the argument that when black currant seed oil was added to a capsule as a supplement the oil mysteriously became a "food additive" that was not "generally recognized as safe" and was hence subject to FDA control — a vaguer approach than attempting to make of the oil itself an "unlicensed drug."

Traco twice won summary judgments against the FDA (as we have seen, the agency never likes to lose in court and, equipped with the endless treasure trove provided by American taxpayers, can hurl waves of litigation against individuals and companies). In his Nov. 28, 1991, ruling, US Judge Harold Baker was specific:

> "*The definition of food additive urged on this court by the FDA would obscure any distinction between 'foods' under section 321 (f) and 'food additives' under section 321 (s) . . . the FDA's reasoning suggests that all foods that are not generally recognized as safe are food additives and Congress could not have intended that result.*"[42]

Yet, as of this writing, semantics remains a powerful weapon in the FDA's hands:

The attempt to manipulate the definitions of "foods", "drugs", and "food additives" has been used consistently by the federal agency to stop, hinder or reduce the full range of healthfood products, natural nutrients and dietary supplements which the FDA (and, thus, the major drug interests) wish to keep out of the medical marketplace. Compromise legislation passed in 1994 at least temporarily ameliorated the situation.

Indeed, it became commonplace among health-freedoms proponents in recent years to wonder, when they saw the FDA suddenly moving vigorously and viciously against a given vitamin, mineral, herb, amino acid, or whatever, just what industry or product the Feds were protecting.

Behind the L-tryptophan grab

The conclusion is inescapable that the uproar over the amino acid L-tryptophan in 1989-90, which led to this natural substance's banning across the United States, served two key purposes:

(1) It gave the FDA a "smoking gun" against "unregulated" nutrients in general and amino acids in particular, an excuse to renew the debate over the need to "regulate" the growing supplements industry, identified as a clear and present threat to the pharmaceutical interests. And

(2) It helped remove a competitor to the huge market in expensive, side effects-causing synthetic drugs, such as

tranquilizers, antidepressants and sedatives, used to treat many of the same conditions for which holistic or integrative medics were using L-tryptophan, at least adjunctively.

The fact that L-tryptophan had been safely consumed by millions of people over many decades was obscured by The Club as it reveled in the 38 deaths from the rare disorder EMS (eiosinophilia-myalgia syndrome) and more than 1,500 cases of the same linked to alleged L-tryptophan use. Worse, the fact that the suspect L-tryptophan was traced to a single Japanese manufacturer and was almost certainly contaminated due to a change in production techniques was glossed over.

And even worse than that was the fact that the FDA, despite its claim of having recalled all the "suspect" L-tryptophan, had inadvertently not recalled all supplies of *parenteral* (that is, intravenous, and/or for use in infant formulas) L-tryptophan products. At least one infant died from parenteral-formula EMS, while virtually all *oral* L-tryptophan, "uncontaminated" or not, remained off the shelves.[43]

In the meantime, the FDA did *not* move against the benzodiazepine Halcion, described in 1991 by *Newsweek* as "Upjohn's second biggest moneymaker (after the closely related tranquilizer Xanax)" with "annual sales of $250 million — $100 million in the United States alone."[44]

The journalistic interest in Halcion, a sedative generically called triazolam, was that Upjohn had "quietly settled out of court" a $21 million civil suit brought by a woman exonerated of killing her mother while on the drug — and that reports of side effects from Halcion had recently led to its banning by England and removal from the market in the Netherlands.

It was also true that the majority of seven million Americans taking the prescription sedative had not reported serious problems.

The Halcion controversy simmered just as the debate over Eli Lilly's controversial Prozac (fluoxetine), an antidepressant, was rising to a fever pitch:

FDA officials had admitted that the use of this perfectly legal drug had led to 14,100 reports of adverse reactions since it had gone on the market in 1987, and that 500 of these had involved suicide attempts. Anti-Prozac forces, notably members or allies of the Church of Scientology, which has long had a running conflict with allopathic psychiatry, unreeled case after case of alleged connections between bizarre behavior, suicide, serial killings and Prozac.[45]

Even so, an FDA advisory panel voted against recommending label changes for antidepressant drugs. It should be understood that this was going on at the same time the federal agency was clamoring for label changes on dietary supplements and foods in general.

In 1991 the Church of Scientology-founded Citizens Commission on Human Rights told FDA Commissioner David Kessler that the FDA oversight committee's favorable findings on Prozac should be nullified because "five of the committee members and four of the consultants of the committee have interests in drug companies which manufacture antidepressant drugs."[46]

It is also true that Prozac — whose world sales reached $2 billion in 1995[47] — has stout defenders among the nation's allopaths and numerous patients of depressive illness who believe the drug has worked wonders for them.

At issue for health-freedoms advocates, however, was the fact that while profits for Prozac, Halcion and Xanax soared, the citizenry was deprived, through a lack of L-tryptophan, of a natural nutrient which many doctors believe can be as useful, without the side effects, as the synthetic antidepressive, sedating and tranquilizing drugs.

FDA's world of 'cleans' and 'dirties'

FDA favoritism for synthetic drugs ("cleans") over natural products ("dirties") continues to be notorious.

A graphic example was the FDA's 1992 approval of Merck's "blockbuster" drug Proscar for the treatment of benign prostatic hypertrophy or hyperplasia (BPH), a prostate gland-swelling condition common in (mostly Western) middle-aged to elderly men.

As Alan R. Gaby MD reported in the *Townsend Letter for Doctors*, the FDA was fully aware that a *natural* non-toxic product (saw palmetto berry extract, a/k/a LSE Seronoa or *Seronoa repens*) was even more effective, and certainly less expensive, in the treatment of such prostatic swelling — but FDA blocked the product as an over-the-counter treatment for BPH.

Concluded Dr. Gaby:

> *The argument put forth by the FDA to reject LSE seronoa cannot be defended by any reasonable scientist. Indeed, the FDA position on this matter would be grounds for flunking [an] eighth-grade science class. As most FDA officials have advanced beyond this level of schooling, one can only conclude that the FDA position on LSE seronoa is a deliberate distortion of the facts.*[(48)]

When the FDA is not banning helpful remedies and preparations, it seems able to literally rush onto the market products from certain companies — in some cases substances for cancer therapy that may actually *cause* the disease.

Also, should a natural substance prove too popular, particularly when another, patented, product is waiting in the wings, the FDA can move with great dexterity. Ponder, for example, the strange case of ACE (adrenal cortical extract), available in this country by the 1970s under various brand names for 60 years.

ACE had been found useful as a general metabolic product in the management of hypoglycemia, adrenal cortical insufficiency, stress, shock, burns, and in building resistance to viral diseases. It had, thus, been used for a variety of things across the board, especially by those practitioners who considered themselves metabolic therapists. But in January 1978 the FDA suddenly classified ACE as "a new drug in violation of the Federal Food,

Drug and Cosmetic Act."

An incensed *small* drug manufacturer told me,[49] "What this all means, of course, is that ACE is a product whose popularity has grown so much that it is now threatening the major drug companies." He warned that the attempt to substitute for ACE — which is nontoxic and relatively inexpensive — synthetic cortisone (cortisone being only one of the fifty or so hormone-like substances found in ACE) was a way to enrich at least three major drug producers, while turning hundreds of thousands of Americans into "cortisone addicts." To take the natural product (originally prepared in China 3,000 years ago) off the market and replace it with one or more synthetic products would, he said, produce "a new generation of captive patients for physicians who don't bother to read the printed inserts."

It was known that cortisone had "hooked" or deranged thousands of users and created a drug dependency worse than that of amphetamines and many other drugs. More than a generation of ACE users, according to metabolic therapists, had never needed to use the steroid drugs usually given to treat the conditions for which ACE had long wielded dramatic and positive effects.

(The production of synthetic steroids is already a multi-million-dollar industry, and although these drugs carry a variety of harmful side effects, dispensing medics may often not read the warnings in the inserts after they have been visited and given a pitch by drug company "detail men.")

After decades of use in this country, ACE suddenly fell under the FDA axe. The "regulatory letter" of Jan. 8, 1978, claimed that the federal agency had "reviewed available data concerning the use of adrenal cortex extract . . . and concluded that the low level of corticosteroid contained in these drugs represents a substantial risk that these serious conditions will be *undertreated*. [*Emphasis mine.*] These drugs therefore pose a significant potential hazard to patients."

This is one of the few instances I am aware of in which the FDA used the argument of "undertreatment" to bolster its claims of hazard in the use of a compound. Distributors were given ten days to discontinue the marketing of ACE and, failing this, "FDA is prepared to initiate legal action to enforce the law."

If the FDA was *just then* determining ACE's safety and efficacy, it could mean only one thing: it was under pressure from big drug firms to remove from the market a product that substantially cut into their profits. The ACE matter showed once again how an important tool in metabolic therapy could be blocked by giant government operating in the interest of giant business.

In terms of laetrile for cancer, with the onset of the victories accorded the apricot seed derivative and the entire area of metabolic therapy in the mid-1970s (*XII*), FDA "compliance" officers went into a frenzy of activity to attempt to smash the entire metabolic program of which laetrile is only a part. Bottles of material, including emulsified Vitamin A, Vitamin B15, and other substances — even, for a time, shipments of apricot kernels! — were tracked down by the FDA across the country and "notices of recommended prosecution" went to firms and individuals involved in the shipment of a whole series of products when it was assumed such items might be used for the metabolic therapy of cancer.

The continued federal harassment of distributors, pharmacists and physicians for their use of or trafficking in substances that are construed as "unproven" had the effect of further criminalizing such individuals. The use of chelating agents such as EDTA and of the absorption agent dimethyl sulfoxide (DMSO) has often landed such people in hot water. Physicians who dared to use medicines licensed for one malady to treat another were — and are — hounded by their state medical boards with the same venom accorded those who dared to involve their patients with laetrile.

The victories of 1978

The year 1978 included two important court battles that served notice that the FDA had overreached itself. Chelation therapy pioneer Ray Evers MD and his patients went to court to secure the use of the chemical EDTA and similar agents in cardiovascular (heart) disease even when they had not been "approved" for such use. Ohio pharmacist Steve Michaelis, enraged over the seizure from his store of laetrile, peach kernels, laetrile publications, and even $740 of his son's money by federal agents, won a return of these items at the federal court level.

In Montgomery, Alabama, US District Judge Robert E. Varner denied the FDA a temporary restraining order against Dr. Evers, a long-time champion of metabolic therapy. Judge Varner held that a physician may use medicines for purposes other than those that are indicated in the medicine's package insert. In a 19-page opinion, he observed, "Congress did not intend the Food and Drug Administration to interfere with medical practice and the [Food, Drug and Cosmetic Act] did not purport to regulate the practice of medicine as between the physician and his patient."[(50)]

Dr. Evers' patients had filed suit for injunctive relief and a declaratory judgment that their constitutional right to privacy and their presumptive constitutional right to receive treatment from a physician of their choice by a system of his choice had been violated by the FDA. The federal government had sought its injunction on the grounds that Dr. Evers promoted and administered calcium disodium versenate in the treatment of hardening of the arteries when the substance "is recommended for heavy metal poisons but not for other things," that patients so treated had been "subjected to an unwarranted risk of grave physical injury or death" as a result of the treatment, and that Evers' use and promotion of the drug, after having utilized interstate commerce in obtaining it, amounted to "mislabeling."

Judge Varner denied all these assertions in what stands as a landmark ruling and pointed out

> "*When physicians go beyond the directions given in the package insert it does not mean they are acting illegally or unethically and Congress did not intend to empower the FDA to interfere with medical practice by limiting the ability of physicians to prescribe according to their best*

judgment."[51]

A day later, Judge Robert M. Duncan, US District Court, Eastern Division, Southern District of Ohio, ruled that the seizure of materials and money from pharmacist Michaelis on July 14, 1977, had been illegal. The seizure had occurred after what Judge Duncan called "an intensive, six-month surveillance of Michaelis and his business operations." The pharmacist was a known distributor of laetrile and a leader in the Committee for Freedom of Choice in Cancer Therapy. At the time of the raid, the FDA sent a dozen agents to his home and store to seize 1,500 vials and 4,000 tablets of laetrile, as well as ten cases of peach kernels and a stack of laetrile-related publications. They also stole $740 of his son's money, an irate Michaelis charged.

Judge Duncan ruled, in an opinion that sent reverberations through the FDA and slowed its 1978 crackdown on laetrile distribution within the United States: "The validity of the July 14 search and seizure of plaintiff's property . . . depends upon the validity of the preceding searches of his packages at various common carriers" in Columbus, Cincinnati, and Hebron, Ohio. "Whether the search is characterized as administrative or criminal, it is encompassed by the Fourth Amendment. The governing principle . . . is that 'except in certain carefully defined classes of cases, a search of private property without proper consent is unreasonable unless it has been authorized by a valid search warrant. . . '" He then went on to say that "the manufacture and distribution of foods and drugs has not yet been specifically held to be among these exceptionally regulated industries to be included; however, this court does not believe that the searches at issue in this case are authorized by statute."[52]

In both the Evers and Michaelis decisions, the FDA received setbacks and warnings that it had gone too far as a federal regulatory agency. These court victories for laetrile and EDTA helped force the FDA back into constitutional constraints.

But it is constantly breaking out of such bonds, primarily because of vague areas in federal vs. state law.

The laetrile and EDTA matters raised a thorny legal issue: just what *is* the jurisdiction of the federal law when it confronts a combination of state laws which say something contradictory?

FDA vs. GH3 and DMSO

The way the FDA operates in this legal limbo has virtually always turned out to be in favor of the synthetic drug industry and against either natural substances or those developed outside the parameters of The Club — witness not only laetrile and EDTA but GH3 (Gerovital) and DMSO as well.

The latter two, just like the former, were held to be threats to mainstream medicine and the nurturing pharmaceutical money pump because of their broad application and, worse, their potentially low cost.

Gerovital, or GH3, the late Rumanian longevitivist Ana Aslan's procaine hydrochloride product, is a clear example of a useful modality falling through the statutory cracks.

As noted earlier (*I*), in the 1990s the FDA moved violently against presumed importers and distributors of "illegal" (that is, foreign-produced) Gerovital, increasingly being used by metabolic/biological physicians as a safe agent not only for life-prolongation but for energy stimulation and a host of other positive benefits.

Homes were raided, some distributors indicted, others jailed — even though GH3 remained legal as an over-the-counter "vitaminic" product in Nevada and was legally available in an estimated 40 other countries.

It had been in regular use in its early form since 1905 and in a buffered form since 1949. Assumed thus to be in the public domain it was not patentable by a single pharmaceutical company and, due to US laws, hence not likely to need approval as a "new drug." Whatever the legalistic niceties, it is an essentially natural compound that thousands, if not millions, of people swear by and that many doctors have recommended. It is not a social threat — but it *is* a presumptive threat to drug companies. Only this reality can explain the vigorous prosecution of Gerovital in the 1990s.

The DMSO saga is a fair epitome of the problems of FDA oversight of drug development and use in a "free country":

In the 1960s, Oregon Health Sciences University surgeon Stanley Jacob MD wrote the first article about dimethyl sulfoxide (DMSO), a colorless liquid originating in lignin, part of the woody tissue of trees and hence a byproduct of the pulp/paper/newsprint industry. Since then, some 10,000 articles in the scientific literature have appeared touting a huge range of biological benefits from this simple, natural, and potentially inexpensive, compound.

Within a few years of the original Jacob article, thousands of Americans were finding relief from arthritis (and many other) pains, sprains, and burns simply with topical DMSO alone.

The FDA strangely halted human trials of the substance in 1965, but pain sufferers continued to have access to it through veterinary (particularly when used as a horse liniment) and underground sources.

Just as several researchers were beginning to note that the compound apparently had a vast field of benefits — ranging from scavenging of free radicals to simply acting as a "carrier" for many other medicines — the FDA finally approved the product (as RIMSO-50) for a single human malady, the painful bladder condition interstitial cystitis, in 1978.

Throughout its history the FDA has often "gone after" DMSO with the same vigor with which it tried to suppress Gerovital, laetrile and EDTA. As one of the most promising developments in modern medicine, it collided with the allopathic paradigm in being a naturally derived substance of multifarious uses (rather than a synthetic toxic drug to be used against a single condition.) Federal and state agencies at times even raided healthfood stores by using the "labeling" argument *ad absurdum* — a copy of a book touting DMSO's benefits within any proximity of a bottle of the multi-use product converted the latter into an "unlicensed new drug" for which a "health claim" had been made.

GH3 and DMSO have intermittently been suppressed, of

course, because they are not single-modality patented synthetic drugs developed within The Club and because they represent potentially inexpensive alternatives to the massively overpriced "regulated" drug industry.

As long as the FDA is empowered to do whatever it pleases, it will be used as a Fedstapo to remove competitors to the synthetic drug industry. Until it is reformed stem-to-stern (if not abolished) it will represent both the policing wing of international vested drug interests and a bumbling, bureaucratic stumbling block to medical innovation in this country, for which millions of Americans will pay a ghastly price.

FDA bias: paying the price

The price is often paid in the side effects from the "legal drugs" which the FDA approves.

The agency, and the pharmaceutical industry, reacted angrily when the General Accounting Office (GAO) reported in 1990 that more than half of the new drugs approved for marketing had severe or fatal side effects which had not been detected during the FDA's allegedly "rigorously scientific" and "thorough" review and testing system — or not reported until years after the medications had been widely used.

The GAO, an investigative arm of the US Congress and thus not directly tainted by The Club, reviewed all 198 drugs which had been approved between 1976 and 1985 and subsequently marketed for a substantial period. FDA would only dismiss the charge of side effects serious enough to warrant either withdrawal from the market or major label changes on 102 of the drugs as "the worst piece of stuff ever to come out of there."[(53)]

Indeed, labeling — which is supposed to clarify the actual nutrient contents of foods and all doses of all ingredients in drugs — became the lever through which the power-mad FDA started to grab for more control than ever going into this century's final decade.

While the tale has many twists and turns, in synthesis the

congressional believers in Big Government in the late 1980s were in tandem with the drug industry in attempting to enhance FDA powers — once again — against the upstart healthfoods/supplements industries. But consumer groups were also targeting the food processing industry, a combination of vested interests even vaster, in their totality, than the drug industry and constituting the other major economic area over which FDA is supposed to exert some surveillance and supervision.

The passage of the Nutritional Labeling and Education Act (NLEA) of 1990 was the usual can't-please-anyone outcome of a vested-interest tug-of-war and, once again, had at least vestiges of a good intention: insisting on honesty in labeling.

The labeling legislation, which equipped the FDA with even more power, was a parallel development to efforts by big-government legislators to provide the agency with even vaster powers for search/seizure/confiscation — weaponry essentially to be aimed at the healthfoods/supplements industries.

It was only an outcry by the organized supplements industry in 1992 which won a brief reprieve for that industry from provisions of the NLEA — one which, the industry feared, would have the effect of putting a significant sector of that industry out of business — and led to compromise legislation approved in 1994.

The FDA's food follies

For the food giants, however, the NLEA was also no friend — and it involved more inanity-based empowerment for an agency which already had far too much clout. It was one thing to be concerned over outrageous health claims made by some food products — quite another to state that using words and phrases like "fresh," "lite" and "no cholesterol" should be reasons for wiping out whole companies through the expenses incurred in making label changes.

Hence, the American public did not know whether to laugh or cry when, in an early sortie against the food industry, the FDA moved against "mislabeled" orange juice (mislabeled primarily because of the word "fresh") in 1991.

These moves came on the heels of a weird incident in 1989 in which the FDA, upon learning that exactly *two* grapes in a shipment from Chile contained a small amount of cyanide, seized two million crates of all kinds of Chilean fruit, one of a series of actions which threw some 20,000 Chileans out of work.

Reasons for this have fueled various conspiracies theories — one, that the FDA, at some level, needed an incident to prove to the American people that it really, truly *was* looking out for their interests; another that the agency, perhaps by error, was itself probably responsible for introducing cyanide (as in laboratory tests) in the grapes, and covered up the mistake.

The agency then charged on with plans to inflict labeling changes on the food industry ranging from the possibly appropriate to the overtly ridiculous. Sweeping food-label changes went into effect in May 1994 with the projected cost of such changes estimated at more than $2 billion.

The American Council on Science and Health (ACSH) which, as we indicate elsewhere, is, while often anti-government, far too chummy with the drug, food and chemical industries, nonetheless was on-target with a 1992 assessment of the NLEA as it applied to foods. Quoth ACSH President Elizabeth Whelan:

> *"What possible enlightenment would the average consumer gain from learning that a serving of macaroni and cheese at lunch contains 13 grams of fat and 30 milligrams of cholesterol that, respectively, account for 20 percent and 25 percent of the amount of those components deemed by the government as OK for us to eat? . . . .*
>
> *"The labeling scheme is 'lite' on science, 'reduced' in common sense and 'high in fat' of the type that will inflate consumer costs."*[54]

All the while, President Bush's appointee to head the FDA, David Kessler MD, was clamoring for more power for the corrupt agency. In a *New York Times Magazine* interview[55] he used the phrases "I need the power" or "I want the power" four times in search of muscle for product recall, seizure of "misbranded or mislabeled" material (the "labeling" device by which the FDA was already intimidating much of small business), and the hiring of "criminal investigators" — which had become a reality by 1993.

It was symbolic of Club interests above bipartisanship that Commissioner Kessler, perhaps the power-hungriest of the power-hungry FDA commissioners, was a holdover in the first Clinton administration.

Just before the second Clinton administration Dr. Kessler resigned under a cloudlet of suspicion involving travel vouchers and expenses,[(67)] though he was hailed as an anti-tobacco champion.

Delaying new devices

The FDA has also wielded a mailed fist against "medical devices" and has been as guilty of blocking progress in this field as it is in attempting to suppress nutritional supplements and herbs.

In 1996, as Electromedical Products Inc. of Texas was attempting to keep its market share of the cranial electrotherapy stimulator (CES) market at a time when the FDA was forcing all CES producers to submit a "premarket approval application" (PMA) or go out of business, its chairman noted:

> *FDA has already chased 24 percent of the USA medical device industry out of the country with its arbitrary and capricious policies over the past three years, leaving the USA five to seven years behind Europe in medical technology.*[(56)]

Dr. Daniel L. Kirsch pointed out that CES — a method of using very small levels of electrical currents applied across the brain stem as a painless, safe, and (according to many) effective method for the control of stress, depression and insomnia — had been clinically used and researched in the USA for 30 years before the FDA decided to crack down.[(57)]

The agency published its "proposed ruling" in the *Federal*

Register in 1993 and the "final ruling" in 1995. This is FDA *pro forma* — " proposed rulings" are published, input is allegedly invited from interested parties, hearings may be held to provide the necessary patina of democratic input, a "final ruling" is circulated and then the agency pounces.

In 1997, and after the Alpha-Stim Company sued the federal agency for "failure to follow its own procedures when dealing with medical devices," the FDA agreed to reconsider.

In recent years the FDA has been particularly sensitive to the increasing presence of electrical, biomagnetic and related treatment or diagnostic devices which, while often researched here or long available in Europe, are regarded as "new" machines which need "premarket approval," meaning that small companies forced into the paperwork simply cannot afford to comply therewith and — like so many others — leave the country.

What is seemingly behind so much of the FDA's (which is to say, the AIC's) sensitivity to such machines is the stunning reality that *natural energy* is a great healer (*see XVII*), cannot be patented, is universally available and is therefore an extreme threat to the synthetic drug industry and the medical model it nourishes.

Blowing it with animals, too

FDA missteps, frequently attributable to plain bumbling, do not stop with surveillance over foods and drugs for humans. They also appear in the area of animals:

Another GAO study, this one in January 1992, claimed that the FDA might be approving drugs for food-producing animals on the basis of "invalid, inaccurate or fraudulent data" supplied by private laboratories. Reviewing FDA activities in this area between October 1985 and September 1990, the GAO reported that the FDA had not conducted inspections to verify data supplied to support more than half the animal drugs it approved, and that the agency's "inadequate procedures" could mean that the FDA "may be unable to fullfill its mission to protect the health and safety of animals and people."[(58)]

To which should be contrasted the fact that a California woman who supplied nutritional supplements to *animals* eventually was jailed in a maximum-security federal prison over a labeling dispute with the FDA (*I*).

Do we need the FDA?

Hence, the growth of FDA power is a sorry history of blocking useful medications while clearing those which often can poison, kill and maim and many of which turn out to be useless.

The drug wing of the agency functions as an appendage of international pharmaceutical profiteers who have a vested interest in the hundreds of thousands of manufactured medicines, drugs, potions and related compounds awash on the world — and American — market.

The argument has been raised again and again that, whatever the shortcomings of the FDA, it or something like it is clearly necessary for consumer protection — that government monitoring (if not control) of the drug industry is an absolute necessity.

In fact, claimed economist Sam Peltzman in a 1974 survey[59] of the agency, the very premises on which the extension of federal regulatory power are based are in error:

Drug development was predominantly safe before 1962 and needed less regulation rather than more, Peltzman argued. Market forces alone generally made it unprofitable (before 1962) to develop and market ineffective or harmful drugs.

The essence of his critique, based on a thorough review of the agency, was that vastly more people suffer or die waiting additional time for new drugs to be approved than are harmed by drugs released too early — a point seized upon by AIDS activists in the 1980s to press for speedier clearance of drugs, however toxic or ineffective they might turn out to be. "Even a moderate increase in the gestation period for beneficial drugs costs far more than the savings from complete suppression of harmful drugs," he wrote.

The Peltzman view was reaffirmed by a Heritage Foundation April 1988 report by attorney Sam Kazman.[60]

The latter argued that the FDA should no longer have the power to block or approve new drugs but rather simply to "certify" drugs for safety and efficacy. "Uncertified" drugs could be marketed under a system which assured an "acceptable degree of professional control" over their availability and full disclosure of risk to patients. Licensed physicians would be allowed to prescribe such "uncertified" drugs as long as their patients had been provided informed consent. Such drugs could only be used in exceptional cases.

Law student Ken Brief — who withdrew from school due to health reasons and whose forced trip to Germany to secure "unconventional" therapy for his non-Hodgkin's lymphoma that he could not have available to him in the United States led to his incisive review of the FDA — noted that, "as I learned more, it became clear that the fundamental criticisms of the FDA could not be addressed by reforms within the agency itself. [They] must come from a redefinition by Congress of the FDA's purpose."[(61)]

A move to de-regulate?

The Congressional elections of 1994 and 1996 brought to the US Congress a new generation of conservative Republicans who captured a legislative majority and set about implementing sweeping reforms which included — at least at the level of high-decibel rhetoric — de-regulation of much of the federal government, including the ponderous FDA. The *Washington Post* noted that the latter "regulates one-quarter of the nation's economic output."[(62)]

In the rapid-fire order new House Speaker Newt Gingrich denounced FDA Commissioner David Kessler as "a thug and a bully" for heading an agency whose red tape had blocked medical progress. And the 1994 Congress made it an anti-big government victory by rejecting the FDA's $890 million plan to relocate from its Rockville MD headquarters to a huge new site.

This, and other FDA-hampering measures, brought with them a suggestion of some honest efforts at reforming the food-

and-drug policeman. Modest reforms were worked out in 1997.

But the new majority, while apparently aware of the pitfalls of giant government, did not seem equally sensitive to those of industrial monopoly, and it was not clear whether simply ganging up on the FDA — however welcome — would have much to do with reinstituting the concept of medical freedom of choice.

In the meantime, "what to do about the FDA" contains notions ranging from simply junking the whole thing and starting from very small scratch, or "privatizing" a good deal of its functions.

Such organizations as the Progress and Freedom Foundation note that the FDA's progress-inhibiting review-and-approval functions could entirely be placed in private hands, and that the idea is far from radical:

Underwriters Laboratories (UL), established in 1874, has for years provided a kind of non-official approval for the safety and efficacy of devices ranging from TV sets and electric razors to hot tubs. The UL "seal of approval" is a coveted cachet from what amounts to a private, independent, third-party entity which sets standards for building materials, fire prevention equipment and a myriad other things — its label goes on a striking nine billion products.[63]

There is relevance in the idea that a federal entity might indeed establish and to a certain extent enforce guidelines, but that the private sector is competent to deliver safety and efficacy in medicines as well as anything else.

References

1. Culbert, ML, *What the Medical Establishment Won't Tell You That Could Save Your Life*. Norfolk VA: Donning, 1983.
2. Griffin, GE, *World Without Cancer*. Westlake Village CA: American Media, 1974.
3. Ambruster, Howard, *Treason's Peace*. New York: Beechurst Press, 1947.
4. Garrison, Omar, *The Dictocrats*. Chicago: Books for Today, 1970.
5. Griffin, *op. cit.*
6. Moss, RW, *The Cancer Industry*. New York: Paragon House, 1991.
7. *Ibid.*
8. Garrison, *op. cit*, quoted in Griffin.

9. Moss, *op. cit.*
10. Griffin, *op. cit.*
11. Quoted in "FDA — friend or foe of our nutrition?" KW Dilling in *Stop the FDA* (Morgenthaler and Fowkes, eds.) Menlo Park CA: Health Freedom Publications, 1992.
12. Gieringer, DH, "Compassion vs. control: FDA investigational drug regulation." *Policy Analysis*. Washington DC: Cato Institute, 1986.
13. *The Choice*, XIX:2, 1993.
14. Testimony of William Doell DO, House Subcommittee on Health and the Environment Regarding Legislative Issues Related to the Regulation of Dietary Supplements, Washington DC, July 29, 1993.
15. Testimony of Saul Kent before FDA Dietary Supplements Task Force, National Institutes of Health, Bethesda MD, Aug. 29, 1991.
16. *Report to the Subcommittee on Science, Research and Technology of the House Committee on Science and Technology*. Washington DC: General Accounting Office, May 28, 1980.
17. Gieringer, *op. cit.*
18. *The Choice*, XXII:1, 1996.
19. *Ibid.*
20. Goldberg, RM, *The Wall Street Journal*, cited in *The Choice*, XXII:2, 1996.
21. *San Diego Union*, cited in *The Choice*, XXII:1, 1996.
22. Center for the Study of Drug Development, Boston MA, 1990.
23. Gieringer, *op. cit.*
24. Ruesch, Hans, *The Naked Empress*. Zurich: CIVIS, 1982.
25. Lucas, Scott, *The FDA*. Millbrae CA: Celestial Arts, 1978.
26. *The Choice*, XVII:1, 1991.
27. Culbert, *op. cit.*
28. Moss, *op. cit.*
29. *New York Times*, July 10, 1976.
30. Culbert, ML, *AIDS: Hope, Hoax, and Hoopla*. Chula Vista CA: The Bradford Foundation, 1990.
31. Culbert, ML, *CFS: Conquering the Crippler*. San Diego CA: C and C Communications, 1993.
32. Harper, HW, and ML Culbert, *How You Can Beat the Killer Diseases*. New Rochelle NY: Arlington House, 1978.
33. Culbert, *What the . . . . , op. cit.*
34. Illich, Ivan, *Medical Nemesis*. New York: Random House, 1976.
35. Culbert, ML, *What the . . . op. cit.*
36. *Ibid.*
37. *Ibid.*
38. *Ibid.*
39. *Ibid.*
40. *The Choice*, XIX:1, 1993.
41. Testimony of William Doell, *loc. cit.*
42. *The Choice*, XVIII:1, 1992.
43. Carter, JP, *Racketeering in Medicine: The Suppression of Alternatives*. Norfolk VA: Hampton Roads Publishing Co., Inc., 1992.
44. "Sweet dreams or nightmare?" *Newsweek*, Aug. 19, 1991.
45. *The Choice*, XVII: 3,4 1991.
46. *Ibid.*
47. Kotter, Julie, "Relighting the inner flame." *Townsend Letter for Doctors and Patients*, Aug./Sept. 1996.
48. *Townsend Letter for Doctors*. Oct. 22, 1992.
49. Culbert, *What the . . . op. cit.*

50. *Ibid.*
51. *Ibid.*
52. *Ibid.*
53. *The Choice*, XVI: 2,3, 1990.
54. *Wall Street Journal*, December 1992, cited in *The New American.*, May 17, 1993.
55. Hoar, WP, "The FDA Follies". *The New American*, May 17, 1993.
56. "Another business being forced out of USA by FDA 'technocide.'" *Townsend Letter for Doctors and Patients*, Aug./Sept. 1996.
57. *Ibid.*
58. *The Choice*, XVIII:1, 1992.
59. Peltzman, Sam, *Regulation of Pharmaceutical Innovation: the 1962 Amendments.* Washington DC: American Enterprise Institute for Policy Research, 1974.
60. Kazman, Sam, *Red Tape for the Dying: the Food & Drug Administration and AIDS.* The Heritage Foundation, April 8, 1988.
61. Brief, Ken, *The Food and Drug Administration and the Consequences of Over-regulation.* Vermont Law School, Dec. 9, 1988.
62. Cited in *The Choice*, XXI:2, 1995.
63. Sevrons, Don, *San Diego Union*, Oct. 1, 1995.
64. Borzo, Greg, "Speedier drug approvals." *Am. Med. News*, Jan. 13, 1997.
65. Miller, Henry, "Oh commissioner, we knew ye well." *San Diego Union*, Nov. 27, 1996.
66. Olney, John, *et al., J. Neuropath. and Exp. Neurol.*, November 1996.
67. Miller, *loc. sit.*

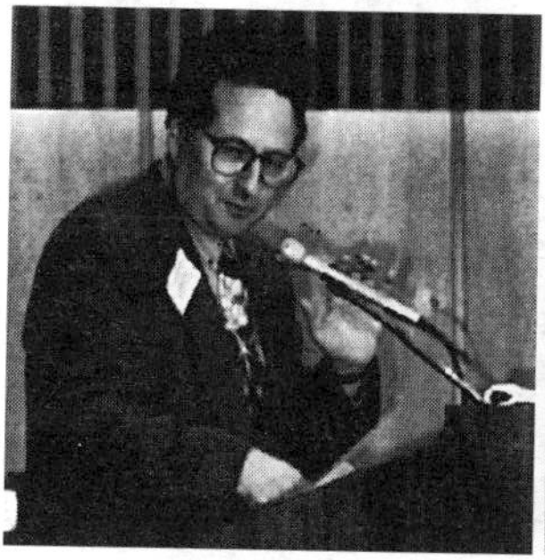

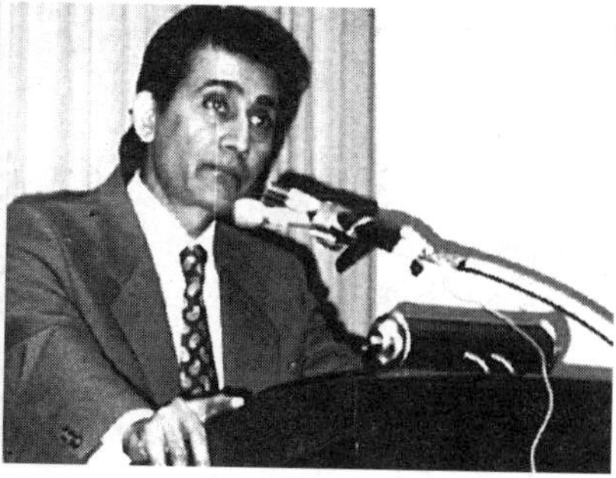

FOR NEW THOUGHT—*Ralph Moss PhD, L, whose exposé books on the cancer industry have helped the fight for change. R, Columbia's Majid Ali MD, arguing strongly for a new medical evaluative model.* — Mike Culbert photos

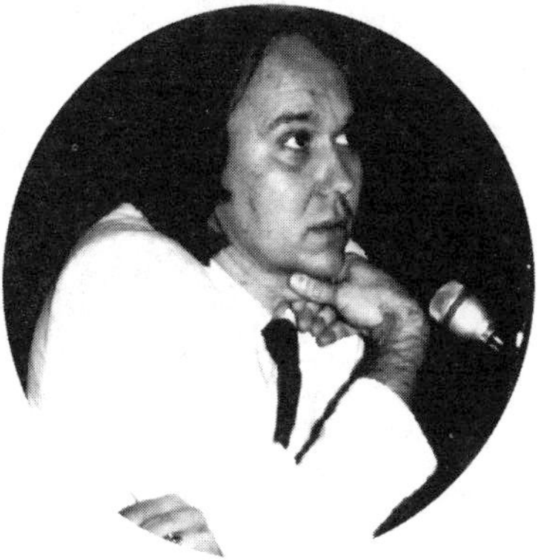

People Against Cancer's Frank Wiewel: spurring evaluation of "unorthodox" cancer treatments

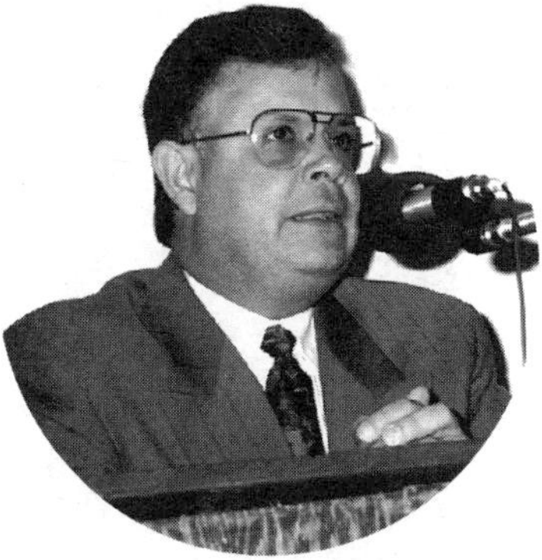

American Biologics-Mexico's Rodrigo Rodriguez MD: applying integrative protocols against disease

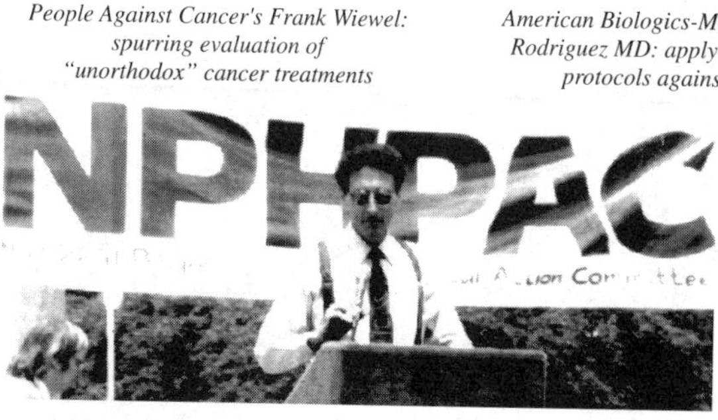

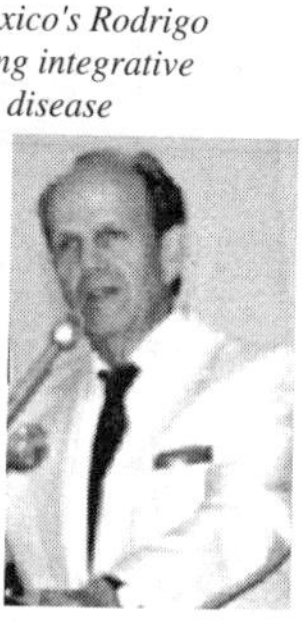

ACTIVISTS—*New York radio commentator Gary Null, L, carries freedom-of-choice message to Washington rally; at R, long-time health-freedoms lobbyist Clintin R. Miller, National Councel for Improved Health (NCIH), makes a point.* —Mike Culbert photos

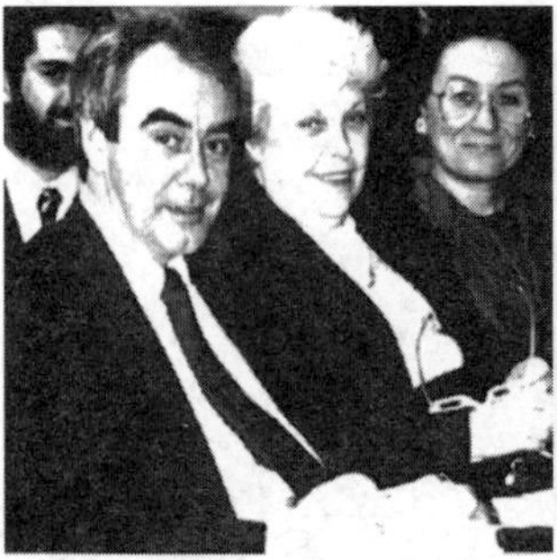

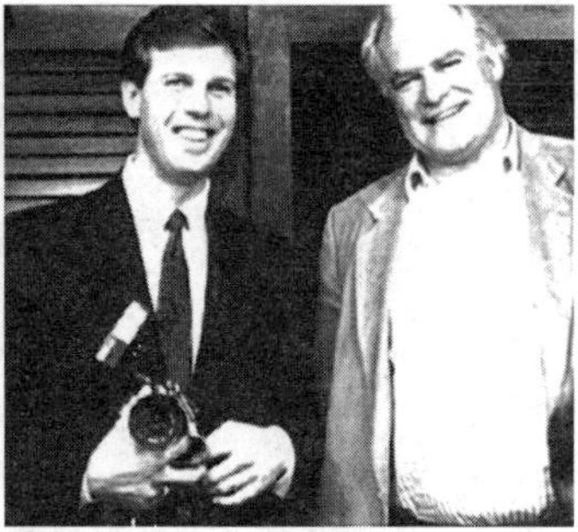

PIONEERS FOR CHANGE—*Left photo, L to R, the late Bob DeBragga, who founded Project Cure; Marie Steinmeyer, president, IACVF; long-time health-rights activist Catherine Frompovich; right photo, L, freedom-of-choice advocate and attorney Mike Evers and R, CANHELP's Patrick McGrady.* —Mike Culbert photos

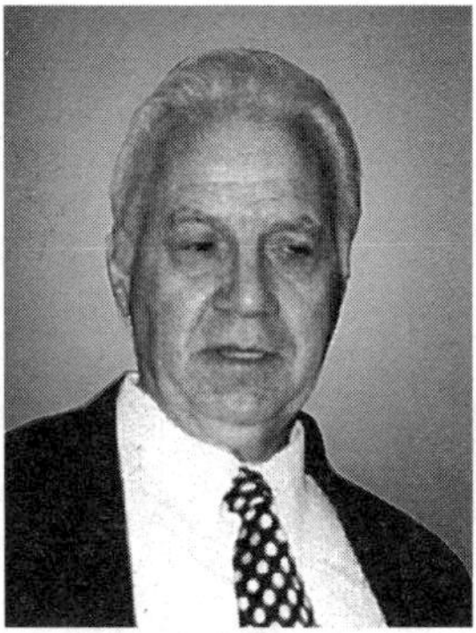

Former US Congressman and Staten Island Borough President Guy Molinari, who brought "alternatives" to congressional attention

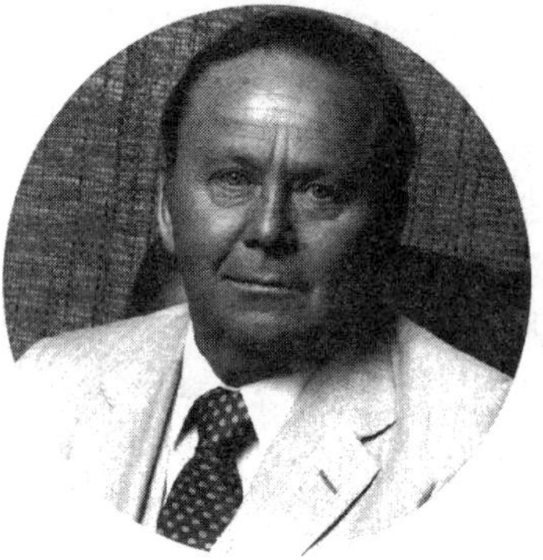

Dr. Robert W. Bradford, pioneer of axidology, advanced medical microscopy, fighter for medical freedom of choice.

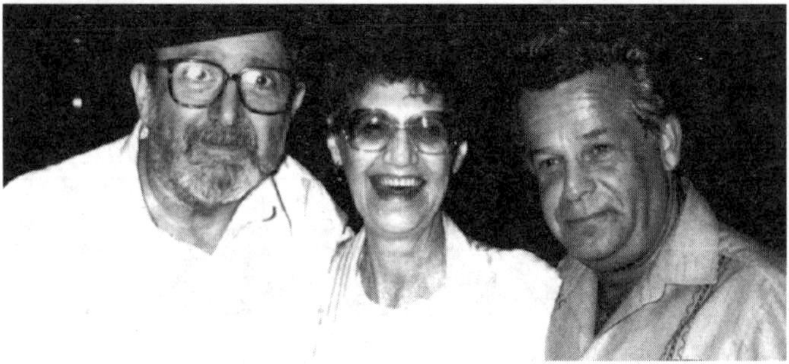

COMPARING NOTES—*At L, Harold and Arline Brecher, key authors of chelation (and other) books; at R, medical writer/activist Michael L. Culbert, as the three met at pre-OAM meetings in Virginia.*

X
HEART HUSTLE:
Schemes, scams and big bucks in the cardiovascular industry

"The moment one has offered an original explanation for a phenomenon which seems satisfactory, at that moment affection for his intellectual child springs into existence and, as the explanation grows into a definite theory, his parental affections cluster about his offspring and it grows more and more dear to him . . . there springs up unwittingly a pressing of the theory to make it fit the facts and a pressing of the facts to make them fit the theory."

— George V. Mann PhD

"The evidence shows that high fat consumption, when accompanied by plenty of the essential nutrients that all cells need, does not *cause atherosclerosis or heart disease."*

— Dr. Roger J. Williams

"The use of the term invasive *is right-on. Somebody is going to be invaded and it isn't going to be the doctor. People who have seen these [*balloon-wielding*] mavericks in action claim the slickest ones can stick a catheter into a groin and wind it around inside the body until it finds a wallet."*

— Charles T. McGee MD

". . . A program that may have begun in sincere but misguided zeal for the public good became intertwined with greed. The world was learning how much money could be made scaring people about cholesterol."

— Thomas J. Moore

Killer number one: 'heart disease'

By any measure, the combination of conditions lumped together as "heart disease" (heart and circulatory disorders, coronary artery disease, arteriosclerosis, peripheral vascular disease, heart attack, stroke, congestive heart failure, etc.) still constitutes the major killer in American medicine, as it does in most of the Western world:

About a million Americans die every year of some form of heart disease, between 400,000 and 500,000 of them from the estimated 700,00 heart attacks each year. In the early 1990s the American Heart Association (AHA) estimated cardiovascular deaths as 43 percent of *all* fatalities, with one American dying of a heart-related condition every 34 seconds.[(1)]

Worldwide, heart disorders caused up to 60 percent of all male deaths and 70 percent of all female deaths in the 60-plus countries reporting in 1995, according to the World Health Organization (WHO).[(2)]

Even so, in terms of the chronic disease plague sweeping the Western world, heart/ circulatory disease for a time had seemingly been the single brightest light — for, at least in terms of fatalities, death rates from heart attack and stroke declined for several years (having fallen steadily in the US they were back up in 1993, again nearing the million mark.[(3)]) This had been seen as a positive trend in disease-survival statistics which would constitute some kind of social triumph were it not eclipsed by the relentless rise in cancer deaths, the spreading AIDS pandemic, the rapidly advancing immunological disorders rampant in the "civilized" world and the fact that heart and circulatory diseases themselves continue to rise in incidence.

It is difficult to estimate the true numbers of individuals who have slowly developing fatty buildups of blood vessels (atherosclerosis) which may not be reflected as true hardening of the arteries (arteriosclerosis) for years or decades, just as it is difficult to assess how many Americans truly have "the silent killer," high blood pressure, whose hypertension also may not be detected for decades, if ever. If both diabetes and its far more prevalent predecessor condition, hypoglycemia, are added to the picture — with diabetes (8 million diagnosed in the USA out of a probable 16 million as of 1995[4]) considered contributory to heart disease — then it is a good estimate that at least a low majority of Americans have a pre-heart disease condition which, if left unchecked should they not expire due to something else, will become "heart disease."

Data from the AHA, Health Care Financing Administration, American Health Information Management Association and the WHO confirmed in 1992 that by 1988 the US cardiovascular disease death rate had continued to show impressive declines — myocardial infarctions (heart attacks) had dropped from 226.4 per 100,000 population in 1950 to 120.1 per 100,000 that year. As of 1992, it was estimated that about 70 million Americans had some form of cardiovascular disease and that the combination of disorders was costing about $109 billion both in health services and lost productivity.[5]

A year later, with fewer actual cases, the nation's heart disease bill was set at about $117 billion. This included $75 billion for hospital and nursing home services, $18 billion for physician and nurse services (as apart from institutional costs), $7 billion in drugs, and an estimated $17 billion in lost productivity.[6] The tab was estimated at $138 billion for 1995.[7] Congestive heart failure, afflicting 3 million Americans, was estimated to cost $60 billion a year to treat.[8] By 1994, the cost of approximately 400,000 coronary bypasses, 300,000 balloon angioplasties, 58,000 repairs to damaged heart valves, and 2,000 transplants of healthy hearts into patients whose own hearts were considered irreparable was an estimated $50 billion per year, or almost 6 percent of the "healthcare delivery" tab.[9]

What all these figures add up to are boosts in overall healthcare cost inflation, mammoth profits for the Allopathic Industrial Complex (AIC), a considerable drag on the economy — and, yes, unquestionably, at least some lives saved.

Mysteries in the victories

Clearly, the medical and governmental orthodoxy has not known what to make of declining deaths from "heart disease" because so many mysteries lurk in the statistics:

An AHA science writers' seminar was told in 1993 that "about half of all deaths from heart disease are sudden and unexpected, regardless of the underlying disease. Thus, 50 percent of all deaths due to atherosclerosis (fatty buildup of the coronary arteries) are sudden, as are 50 percent of deaths due to degeneration of the heart muscle, or to cardiac enlargement in patients with high blood pressure."[10]

This was a roundabout way of saying that despite a multi-billion-dollar annual campaign based on the cholesterol hypothesis of heart disease causation and the multi-billion-dollar industry in heart disease diagnostic devices and techniques, which frequently turned in erroneous or misleading figures, including nationwide efforts to count cholesterol in as many citizens of all ages as could be induced into a mobile lab for such purposes, the actual precipitating reasons for heart fatalities were *unknown* in perhaps as many as 50 percent of cases.

By some other reliable estimates the commonly accepted risk factors for coronary artery disease — excess saturated fats and cholesterol, cigarette smoking, diabetes, high blood pressure, inadequate exercise, obesity, emotional stress, alleged genetic predispositions — are not present in 40 percent of people who die of heart attacks.[11]

In the meantime, the development and application of synthetic compounds (drugs) to be used against heart disease and stroke have continued to constitute a growth industry of extremely profitable dimensions, and the heart-diagnosis, heart-treatment devices and techniques element of "healthcare delivery" are alive and well even if it cannot be demonstrated that, overall, they do very much good.

In the 1990s, while the combination public-private effort to curb the nation's number-one killer seemed to be paying off, it became obvious to observers, statisticians and social critics that the figures were declining primarily because of what people were doing themselves.

They were indeed smoking less (cigarette smoking being broadly accepted as a major risk factor for heart disease), they were exercising more (although, oddly enough, research on physical exertion as a block to heart disease was surprisingly thin in conclusive results), they had drastically altered their eating habits — and they were consuming vitamin pills and other dietary supplements in ever-growing numbers.

What was not clear in the 1990s was just how, let alone if, the change in dietary habits (fewer animal fats and animal proteins, more fruits and vegetables, fewer refined carbohydrate "junk foods") alone accounted for the decline and if so which foods or combinations were doing the trick. Even so, the change in dietary habits promoted by any number of food faddists, nutritionists and a hodgepodge of reasonably scientific studies did indeed correlate with overall declines in heart-disease fatalities.

The heart disease death-rate decline has provided the Allopathic Industrial Complex (AIC) with a propaganda victory that seems justified as long as one does not look too closely.

A major study in 1997 — condemned by elements within the cardiology community — argued that better treatments were more important than dietary and other lifestyle changes in the 25 percent reduction in US heart disease rates between 1980-1990.[141]

The trouble(s) with angiograms

Death from heart attack seems to occur whether or not diagnosis of the disease has been made correctly, if at all.

The gold standard heart-disease diagnostic for years has been the coronary angiogram — or arteriogram — insertion of a catheter up the aorta just above the heart, injection of a dye-like tracing material into the heart arteries, and observation of this material by X-ray.

While many medical critics and even some cardiologists

have long wondered about just how accurate, useful or necessary a procedure the angiogram (first introduced in 1963) is, by 1992 the facts were beginning to come in:

A *Journal of the American Medical Assn. (JAMA)* reported[12] that nearly half of all coronary angiograms were either unnecessary or could have been postponed. But why do so? The 1992 estimates were that one million angiograms were being performed that year at a cost of about $5,000 each — that is, a roughly $5 billion industry in angiograms all by themselves.

Even though cardiologists had embraced the coronary angiogram (angiograph) — allowing them, for the first time, to see minute obstructions in the main arteries of the heart as a kind of road map — serious doubts had been raised within a decade of the launching of the test:

Major studies in 1974,[13] 1976,[14] 1979[15] and 1984[16] found huge swings in interpretations of the test. One analysis (1984) was quite specific:

> *The physiologic effects of the majority of coronary obstructions cannot be determined accurately by conventional angiographic approaches. The results of these studies should be profoundly disturbing to all physicians who have relied on the coronary arteriogram to provide accurate information regarding the physiologic consequences of individual coronary stenosis (*obstruction.*)*[17]

Yet, the fact that most of these tests were published in the "learned" journals failed to make much of a dent in their widespread use — and the medical media (that is, reporters and commentators wined and dined by medical orthodoxy) simply failed to pick up what amounted to a major story: a primary heart-disease diagnostic tool is inaccurate at best, a scam at worst.

And of course there is the corollary problem that the diagnostic technique may be dangerous in and of itself — since, as of 1993, it was known that for every thousand angiograms performed, about one person dies from a complication related to the angiogram. Even a possibly fatal heart rhythm may be sparked simply by the presence of the dye-like tracing substance in the artery.[18]

A Department of Veterans Affairs (DVA) study released in 1997 suggested that early angiogram use could be harmful to survivors of "non-Q-wave" heart attacks or about half of heart attacks.[142]

The coronary angiogram is not the only expensive diagnostic toy which has come under a cloud of suspicion.

In 1991, a San Francisco Veterans Administration (VA) hospital study found[19] that a heart-scan technique utilizing drugs and radioactive isotopes (estimated to be performed on 500,000 patients a year at an annual cost of $500 million and costing between $700 and $1500 per test) was probably "useful" only a third of the time, "questionable" another third, and "not warranted" another third. Yet it had become a "standard presurgical test" since the Food and Drug Administration (FDA), the corrupted arbiter of "safety" and "efficacy" in medical diagnostics and therapeutics, had approved it earlier that year.

The controversy over diagnostics (whether they are useful, accurate or necessary, let alone their contribution to the total costs of healthcare in the United States) immediately dovetails with the controversy over therapeutics.

Of cabbages and things

The major heart disease therapies have consisted of the resurrected coronary bypass procedure, the insertion of inflatable balloons in blood vessels (balloon angioplasties — also called by the prodigiously cumbersome term PTCA, or percutaneous transluminal coronary angioplasty), and a shelf full of expensive drugs variously aimed at lowering cholesterol (this based on the notion — ever more in doubt — that cholesterol is the major contributor to heart disease), lowering high blood pressure, combatting irregular heartbeat (arrhythmia), dissolving clots, opening blocked vessels (vasodilators) and/or "channel blockers," each of which has constituted a spinoff mini-cardiovascular industry — and/or, for maintenance, inserting battery-driven heart stimulators (Pacemakers), another mini-industry.

Hyped to the public with virtually the same intensity and lack of balancing commentary as the coronary arteriogram and the need to assess cholesterol levels, the coronary bypass had, by the 1980s, become a multi-billion-dollar moneymaker all by itself, the Cadillac surgical procedure of cardiovascular medicine, the technique to which most advanced "coronary" patients were turned over in the belief that they were soon to be in the best medical hands possible. And in some advanced cases the procedure — and later, the "minimally invasive direct coronary artery bypass" or MIDCAB — truly saved lives.

The regular coronary artery bypass graft surgery (perhaps puckishly referred to from its acronym CABG as "cabbage") consists of removing veins from elsewhere in the body (usually the legs), connecting one end of the vein to a fresh blood supply from the aorta and connecting the other end to a blocked or obstructed artery at a point somewhere beyond the blockage — hence the term "bypass."

It is essential to realize that heart disease fatality rates were already falling consistently before the advent of the "cabbage" or, quickly thereafter, the balloon angioplasty, so that cardiovascular surgeons taking much credit for helping reduce heart disease deaths because of these expensive procedures are on a par with the promoters of certain vaccinations who take credit for the reduction in the incidence of an infection through the immunization process *after* the infection or disease is beginning to die out on its own.

Medicine loves high technology — and cardiovascular medicine positively fell in love with the coronary artery bypass graft approach (cabbage). Some 75,000 of the surgeries were done in 1975. This number increased to 230,000 in 1987, 392,000 in 1990, 407,000 in 1991, and slipped to 331,000 in 1993, while estimated at about 400,000 in 1996.[20,21,22,23] Since the technique, including a "heart-lung" machine to stop and re-start the heart, may cost anywhere from $25,000 to $60,000 and several may be done in one patient, the dimensions of the "cabbage" business are considerable. The total hospital bill for CABG operations in 1993 was set at $13.5 billion.[24]

Medical critic Charles McGee MD noted in 1993 that "the operating surgeon may charge between $3,000 and $6,000 for a cabbage. Multiply that by over 200 cabbages per year and it begins to add up to a respectable income. It is common for successful cabbage surgeons to bank over $1.5 million a year."[25]

Clearly, such techniques are for more affluent societies, whether they are paid for privately, through group private insurance plans or by the public. McGee observed that the incidence of coronary bypasses is 75 percent less in Europe, where medicine in general is far less expensive, and also far less in America's government-run Veterans Administration (VA) hospitals, where doctors are paid a salary.

But what did "qualified experts," by the 1990s, really think of the CABG?

In July 1992, the American Heart Assn. publication *Circulation* released results of an 18-year survey of about 700 veterans and found that whatever benefits there might be for the cabbage fade within five years and disappear within 11. The authors were primarily interested in the procedure's effects on stable *angina pectoris*, a severe heart disease-connected chest pain which some other studies had long suggested might be minimized by the complex surgery.[26]

In 1991, the *Journal of the American Medical Assn. (JAMA)*, observing fatality statistics from bypasses, reported[27] that heart disease patients might be up to four times more likely to die from a cabbage by one surgeon than by another, and that fatality levels varied from hospital to hospital. Hospital death rates for the bypass varied from 3.1 percent to 6.3 percent; the rate among surgeons caromed between 1.9 percent and 9.2 percent.

In 1996, British medical journalist Lynne McTaggart noted that heart surgeons "had known since the 1970s" that the bypass does not improve survival except for patients with severe left ventricle coronary diease — and that US government statistics showed that about 90 percent of patients received no benefit.[143]

But such fairly tepid studies were actually old-hat:

A Veterans Administration study in 1977 had found[28] that the 11-year survivals of coronary byass patients as contrasted with those who had been managed "medically" (essentially, by drugs) showed a statistically insignificant difference of 58 percent for the former against 57 percent for the latter. This was the first comparison study on the subject, and while it allegedly shocked cardiologists it did not dim establishment enthusiasm for the procedure.

In the Coronary Artery Surgery Study (CASS), released in 1990, a 10-year followup showed that the survival rate was 82 percent among those who had had the operation vs. 79 percent for those "medically" managed.[29]

As early as 1978, Dr. Henry McIntosh of Baylor College of Medicine's Methodist Hospital provided one of the first followup critiques of the CABG. According to his 10-year review:

> *Available data in the literature do not indicate that myocardial infarctions, arrhythmias, or congestive heart failure will be prevented, or that life will be prolonged in the vast majority of patients.*[30]

McGee noted that following publication of this first major negative criticism of the coronary bypass "McIntosh was forced to leave his position at Baylor."[31]

'Ballooning' profits, dilating for dollars

When cardiological experts are not deviating blood flow around a blocked artery they often turn to, or suggest, the alternative to the coronary bypass — the balloon angioplasty, introduced in the 1970s. This was a mechanical application of the theory of stretching or widening (dilating) arteries — in this case through insertion of a small balloon.

In 1990, cardiologists performed about 285,000 balloon angioplasties as contrasted with between 380,000 and 392,000 coronary bypasses, and some of these procedures were done on the same patients. About 303,000 were done in 1991.[32,33] The 1996 composite figure for both procedures was estimated at 550,000.[144] About $6.5 billion was spent on 380,000 angioplasties in 1993, evidence of a major industry by itself.[34]

But the "heart balloon," while less expensive ($16,000 and up) than the bypass, comes with risks. It was reported in 1988[35] that about 1 percent of angioplasty patients died, 4.3 percent suffered heart attacks, 3.4 percent required emergency surgery, and that in about a third of cases the blocked arteries reopened through the procedure would close again in several months and need to be reopened again. Earlier, Harvard Medical School had warned that "a coronary artery may be torn during the procedure, or a clot can form in the dilated area."[36]

The 1994 annual meeting of the American Heart Assn. was told that between bypasses and angioplasties about 16,000 patients were dying annually.[37]

In 1997 the anti-clotting drug ReoPro was shown to reduce the life-threatening complications of angioplasties — at a cost of $1,400 per dose.[154]

The problem of keeping artificially widened clogged coronary arteries open led to a flurry of interest in Europe and the United States for the "intravenous stent." This was a tiny tube formed of woven stainless-steel mesh designed to be inserted into a previously clogged artery after it had been reopened by surgery or after a balloon angioplasty had been performed.

The approach was first tested in Europe in 1988, but by 1991 it had become clear that "stent" patients were not faring any better than patients who had not received it. This led one American heart specialist to comment on this and similar artery-opening devices that

> *. . . (the process) has resembled the mating of elephants — carried out on a high level . . . with much noise and trumpeting, with the results not evident for two years and the product not perfect.*[38]

Even so, it was estimated that 100,000 of the $1,600-per-unit stents were placed in 1995 and that the figure would double by 1997.

Even the perhaps more promising laser recanalization (LR) technique (a catheter with a laser beam which burns out a hole in arterial deposits), which may often accompany a balloon angioplasty, is, according to one study,[39] only indicated in 10 to 15 percent of patients with blocked arteries, primarily due to age considerations.

We have already seen (*III*) that inserting battery-driven Pacemakers, at about $9,000 per implant, may be unnecessary or questionable in upwards of 50 percent of cases (in some surveys), but electronic technology as applied to faltering hearts keeps on ticking:

In 1993 the FDA approved a cigarette case-sized "defibrillator," an abdomen implant which sends "mild electrical impulses" to the heart both to prevent cardiac arrest and correct abnormally fast heart rhythms. The retail cost: $18,200.[40]

The allopathic fraternity, aware of cost differentials, continually debates whether the cabbage or the PTCA (balloon angioplasty) is "better," and all the data are not in.

But some are. A review of the first 2½ years of a 10-year comparative trial in the United Kingdom of one thousand randomized angina patients to determine long-term effects of one procedure against the other measured non-fatal heart attacks as the "primary endpoint." In data reported in 1994, or at 2½ years, the heart attack rates were 8.6 percent for the cabbage and 9.8 percent for balloons — or, as Robert Henderson MD, cardiologist of Manchester's Wynthenshaw Hospital, put it: ". . . The data suggest that the risk of death or MI [myocardial infarction] is the same whichever treatment strategy you use."[41]

And in another 1994 study — this on 200,000 Medicare patients who had suffered a heart attack in 1987 — it was found that some 25 percent of bypasses, angioplasties and catheterizations on older patients could be eliminated at a substantial cost savings with a negligible impact on mortality — simply because they do not do much good. Said Harvard's Dr. Mark McClellan, lead author of the report: "Virtually all medical technologies are useful in some patients. The question is, where do you draw the line?'"[42]

The same year, more studies, which contrasted cabbages with balloon angioplasties, added fuel to the fire, sometimes cloaking the controversy in considerable medical gobbledegook:

An Emory University-University of Washington survey of 132 individuals randomly assigned to various treatment groups found[43] that neither the coronary bypass nor balloon angioplasty differed "significantly with respect to the occurrence of the composite primary endpoint" and that "consequently, the selection of one procedure over the other should be guided by patients' preferences regarding the quality of life and the possible need for subsequent procedures."

The "primary endpoint" was "a composite of death, Q-wave myocardial infarction, and a large ischemic defect identified on thallium scanning at three years." The translation of all this seemed to be that since the pathological and/or mortal outcomes were essentially the same with either approach the best advice to patients should be, "take your pick."

To be sure, at the same time a German study[44] confirmed improvements in chest pain (angina) with both approaches, yet summarized negatively that "in order to achieve similar clinical outcomes, the patients treated with PTCA (angioplasties) were more likely to require further intervention and antianginal drugs, whereas the patients treated with CABG (coronary bypass) were more likely to sustain an acute myocardial infarction at the time of the procedure."

Inconclusive results of a multinational European study comparing the two procedures released in 1995 further muddied the waters,[45] as did a major comparative study by the National Heart, Lung and Blood Institute. In 1996 and 1997 the Bypass Angioplasty Revascularization Investigation (BARI) program's data from a five-hospital study found the five-year survival rate about the same for both procedures.[46]

But cabbages have an additional downside — 24,000 patients who undergo bypasses each year may be seriously impaired by stroke-causing blood clots in the brain, a 1996 study of patients at 24 medical centers showed.[146]

When in doubt, prescribe a drug

When cardiological orthodoxy is not "bypassing" arteries with veins removed from one part of the body and "harvested" elsewhere, or inflating clogged arteries with balloons, or reaming out arteries with a particular device (the atherectomy, held to be more fatality-prone than balloon insertions), or inserting various electrical devices into the body to stimulate or normalize flagging hearts, it is relying on ever-more-expensive synthetic compounds (drugs).

These, such as diuretics and "calcium channel blockers" or "calcium antagonists," are prescribed to combat high blood pressure (hypertension), considered a strong contributor to heart disease and estimated to afflict somewhere between 60 to 70 million Americans who spend more than $11 billion annually on this condition alone; or to lower cholesterol, a naturally occurring fatty substance which cardiology believes is the biggest single culprit in overall heart disease; or to combat irregular heartbeat (arrhythmia); or to break up clots in the circulatory system, since the latter can lead directly to fatalities; or to help control other aspects of the multiplicity of conditions and pathologies which directly or indirectly are involved in "heart disease."

Each class of drugs constitutes a spinoff or mini-industry on its own, and, of course, each has fallen under critical review and suspicion.

In her masterful roundup of medical ignorance, Jane Heimlich noted[47] both that "doctors don't know what causes 90 percent of high blood pressure" (itself an astounding reality, given the multi-billion-dollar, long-term research investment of medical and governmental orthodoxy in trying to find out) and that non-drug approaches to hypertension have been overlooked or ignored. However, so panicked are hypertensives over their mystery condition, and so generally successful are certain high blood pressure drugs at keeping the "numbers" down that increasing numbers of Americans are now lifelong consumers of drugs without which, they truly believe — or have been made to believe by their doctors — they cannot survive.

And, though this may be true in some cases, various lines of research have confirmed the ability to treat high blood pressure without drugs and/or for patients to be able to go off the drugs.[48,49,50]

As early as 1979, the National Heart, Lung and Blood Institute's Hypertension Detection and Followup Program found[51] that death rates among hypertensives could be reduced by almost 20 percent *without* drug treatment. Most convincing, multi-center research that a low-fat fruit-and-vitamin-rich diet might bypass the need for anti-hypertensive drugs altogether was presented in 1996.[137]

Then, the cleverly acronymed MRFIT (for Multiple Risk Factor Intervention Trial) found[52] in a one-year study on coronary heart disease prevention that patients who had been treated intensively with thiazide diuretics (the classic standby of high blood pressure treatment and aimed at ridding the body of excess fluids and salts) had *higher* death rates than those who either took other drugs or no drugs at all. This led to speculation that such drugs might themselves be toxic — but their use continued.

Other studies have shown that lowering blood pressure with diuretics may indeed reduce the risk of stroke — the most feared endpoint of hypertension — but does not prevent heart attacks. Also, noted Heimlich,[53] such drugs can cause biochemical changes which increase susceptibility to heart attacks.

That is, the classic drugs used to treat high blood pressure, a presumed key role player in overall "heart disease," may actually enhance the chances *for* "heart disease" and may be toxic in and of themselves.

In the late 1980s, the dangers in drugs developed to treat irregular heartbeat (arrhythmias) came to light, particularly with the flaps over Riker Laboratories' Tambocor and Bristol Laboratories' Enkaid, FDA-approved modalities both (*IX*), since a National Heart, Lung, and Blood Institute clinical trial had shown that they *increased* the risk of heart attack and death among the 200,000 or so Americans estimated to have the problem.[54]

"Calcium channel blockers," another class of drugs, have hardly fared any better.

Once the latest popular breakthroughs, it now seems clear that such products may help the patient feel better after a heart attack or a round of severe angina pain, but they will not save the patient's life.

A trio of US investigators concluded the above in 1989 after reviewing 28 controlled studies involving 19,000 patients. Their data, in the *British Medical Journal,* found both that channel blockers not only failed to protect cardiac patients against a heart attack or death but that "the data suggest a somewhat higher probability of harm than benefit."[55] And separate 1995 studies showed increased heart attack risks from the use of calcium channel blockers, beta blockers and "non-potassium-sparing" diuretics, hypertension drugs all.[56,57]

That year, some experts were beginning to warn that the calcium channel blockers Procardia and Adalat — taken by six million patients for whom 87.8 million prescriptions were written that year — might *cause* heart attacks.[155]

In 1996, a US-Italy study of 750 elderly hypertensives found a sobering new correlation with "calcium antagonists" — a doubling of *cancer* cases as contrasted with the use of other anti-hypertensive agents.[58] Boston University research a year later was said to have cast doubt on the study.[151]

In 1994, trials sponsored (even) by drug companies of the common anticoagulant drug heparin were halted because of what the *New York Times* called "an unexpectedly high risk of paralyzing and fatal strokes."[59]

The surprise finding in three studies concerning a common heart-attack drug was that high doses of it are unacceptably dangerous. A similar risk of strokes was found among individuals receiving hirudin.[60]

The above are umpteenth demonstrations of the classical medical dilemma in which the cure may be worse than the disease.

We mention elsewhere (*VIII*) the turf wars in the development and marketing of clot-dissolving drugs, during which, by 1993, the vastly more expensive T-PA (tissue plasminogen activator), at roughly $2,200 per treatment, had slightly edged out the much cheaper ($200 to $300 per treatment) Streptokinase for first place.

The 2½-year, $65 million study (largely financed by biotech giant Genentech, T-PA's producer) of 40,000 patients in 15 countries seemed at best a pyrrhic victory for T-PA, with health economists noting that when all was said and done treatment with T-PA rather than streptokinase would cost about $200,000 for each life saved. Since only about 20 percent of heart patients are treated with either drug (both of which must be injected within the first few hours of a heart attack to be effective), the question nagged: is it worth it?[61]

The answer may have been a qualified "yes," if results of a multi-university-monitored National Registry of Myocardial Infarction study announced in 1994 meant much — they showed a decline in hospital heart-related deaths coinciding with increased use of blood clot-dissolving drugs. The registry, though, was reportedly funded by Genentech.[62]

And, by 1997, Merk's "super aspirin" Aggrastat, in some research, was described as more effective than T-PA.[152]

T-PA has since come into its own as a *stroke* treatment if provided within the right timeframe — and out of which brain hemorrhage can result.[63]

Clot-busters or balloons (primary angioplasties)? In 1996, results of a 3,000 heart-attack patient study showed that there was no essential difference in death rates between the two treatments.[134]

Then, there is the huge industry in cholesterol-lowering drugs, keystone of the AIC's heart disease division. By 1996, it was estimated that US doctors were writing 45 million prescriptions for such drugs, generating more than $2 billion in sales for manufacturers.[140]

In 1991, American heart specialists were up in arms over a Finnish study criticized for its low numbers (though 1,222 patients followed over 15 years hardly qualifies as unduly low) that men who used drugs to lower cholesterol or high blood pressure died more often from *heart disease*, violence, accidents and suicide than did men who did nothing to cut the risk.[64]

What may be one of the last few nails being pounded into the coffin of the cholesterol theory of heart disease was a four-year survey of 997 patients studied by Yale and University of Connecticut cardiologists and released in 1994:

This review of cholesterol levels, coronary heart disease mortality and morbidity, and indeed "all-cause" mortality, led to a firm conclusion:

> *Our findings do not support the hypothesis that hypercholesterolemia or low HDL-C are important risk factors for all-cause mortality, coronary heart disease mortality, or hospitalization for myocardial infarction or unstable angina in this cohort of persons older than 70 years.*[103]

The question remained: how important are they for persons *younger* than 70 years?

And, noted physicians Stephen B. Hulley and Thomas B. Newman: "Treatment of cholesterol may produce harmful effects specific to older age. Adverse drug reactions become more common as drugs are used in combination and have less predictable excretion patterns."

They feared that "the most important harm is the possibility that cholesterol-lowering intervention could actually increase, rather than decrease, the overall death rate." Adding to the basic mysteries:

> *In elderly people, this inverse association extends over a wider range of cholesterol levels, and in women* total mortality rates appear to be lower in those with high blood cholesterol than those with moderate levels *[author's emphasis.] We do not understand the causal basis for this finding, and until we do, it is not safe to assume that lowering blood cholesterol in the elderly will have a net beneficial effect. A larger concern is the separate body of evidence revealing increased mortality from cancers and injuries in primary prevention trials* of middle-aged men *[author's emphasis].*[65]

In what the ever-creative drug industry might consider to be a "save" following such bad news, the 1994 meeting of the American Heart Assn. (AHA) was informed of a large Scandinavian study of the cholesterol-lowering drug simvastatin (Zocor), described as a "powerful" compound: in a five-year followup it was said to have "sharply" reduced the risk of death in people who had earlier been treated for heart attacks and angina pain. The data showed that the "need" for either a CABG or an angioplasty was thus lower in the treated group. However interesting the results (and there was no evidence the drug actually helps people live longer, nor are its long-term effects known), the study of 4,444 men and women at 94 hospitals was financed by . . . Merck & Co., a heavy hitter in cholesterol drug development.[66]

As the *Wall Street Journal* noted, the results also set the stage for a major market battle between Merck and Bristol-Myers Squibb, which claimed similar results with a competing drug, Pravachol.[67] A new class of cholesterol-lowering drugs — reductase inhibitors, or "statins" — thought to be safer than their predecessors, thus entered the picture.[68,69]

Pravachol was said in a 1996 study of 4,159 heart attack survivors with seemingly normal cholesterol levels (!) to have provided a 24 percent reduction in the risk of suffering another heart attack. Bristol-Myers Squibb paid for the test.[136]

With statins said to be effective both in preventing heart attacks and death from heart disease, a new healthcare dimension — replete with industrial considerations — has arisen: by 1996 there was a potential market of 50 million Americans, 4 to 6 million of whom were already on the drugs for life — potentially adding billions to healthcare costs.[147]

AIC cardiological orthodoxy, of course, was not cheered by 1996 research connecting the common anti-cholesterol drug families (fibrates and statins) with *cancer* risks in laboratory rodents.[70]

The above are elements of a gathering accumulation of data and observations from wary researchers beginning to question some of the central premises of American orthodoxy in "heart disease" — particularly that the excess of cholesterol is the major contributor to the problem, and that drugs to lower cholesterol therefore represent the best approach to solving it.

The great cholesterol conundrums

In fact, the cholesterol mania is probably the biggest false premise in cardiology, and has so colored this subdivision of the medical arts that it is roughly akin to the central, probably false, premise in oncology (*XI*) which holds that there are many separately caused kinds of cancerous tumors each requiring its own special treatment.

The heart disease division of the AIC split down the middle in 1996 over if and when to screen people for cholesterol levels, as we shall shortly see.

The passion over cholesterol in the 1970s-1990s led to confusion on a mass scale, as housewives were told first one thing and then another about the dangers of cholesterol-laden foods, what adequate cholesterol levels were or are, and, right along with the cholesterol concern, which kinds of fats (saturated, unsaturated, polyunsaturated) should be used or not used in the diet, and which cooking oils had how much of which.

In the meantime, as the cardiology industry and government joined forces to alert the public to the presumed dangers of excess cholesterol, let alone of fatty diets — forgetting that the American diet has *always* been fatty and that American "heart disease" was essentially an unknown entity before 1878 — food producers and processors also were driven into an intense round of labeling and re-labeling products to make sure that the correct amounts of cholesterol and other fats were noted. The situation reached *reductio ad absurdum* in the 1980s/1990s as distributors of foods which by their very nature could *never contain* any cholesterol began affixing on their products labels stating "does not contain cholesterol," an activity roughly akin to a paper clip manufacturer affirming that his product "absolutely contains no sugar."

The assumption that cholesterol is the central villain in heart disease (more culpable, indeed, than genetic predispositions, cigarette smoking, high blood pressure and diabetes, all known contributors thereto) was naturally, inexorably matched by the scramble to develop synthetic compounds (drugs) aimed at *lowering* cholesterol. Indeed, to excuse this whole series of unfortunate linear thoughts, the AIC orthodoxy needed to come up with a whole new disease — *hypercholesterolemia* (too much cholesterol) — as a rationale. (This may be different from the genetically influenced "familial hypercholesterolemia," which allegedly "runs in families.") Finding that civilized (rather than primitive) societies were afflicted with this disease was the semantical equivalent, at an earlier time when the benzodiazepines were drugs of choice as tranquilizers and sedatives, of believing that people had somehow been born with a Valium deficiency.

There is probably no area of medicine as fraught with contradiction, controversy, 180-degree-angle turns in concepts and outright confusion as the cholesterol theory of heart disease which, did it not have such potentially lethal and life-altering dimensions, would better be dismissed as a highly expensive comic opera.

In setting the stage for the cholesterol wars, two background realities should be made clear:

1. There are obvious connections between heart disease and the dietary practices of the "civilized" West. Since high-fat foods, *among other dietary things*, are factors in such connections, and since a measurable primary blood fat is in fact cholesterol, it does not require too great a leap of faith to assume, even inappropriately, as it may turn out, that there is some link between cholesterol and heart disease. Unfortunately, what seems to have happened is that the leap of faith was a jump to the wrong conclusion — or at least mostly so.

2. Cholesterol is an absolutely essential body compound, comprising a high concentration of normal brain tissue and serving as a basic building material for the manufacture of cortisone, sex hormones, Vitamin D and other essential body substances. *Too little* cholesterol could result in what medicine oftens calls a "negative outcome" — death.

The cholesterol theory — as part of the broader lipid (blood fat) theory — developed through research over time which seemed to show that certain groups of people who consumed large amounts of "saturated" (hard) fats also had higher rates of cholesterol and higher rates of "heart disease." It was known that cholesterol is a major contributor — but not the only one — to the buildup of materials which clog the circulatory system and which thus might lead to heart attack, stroke and other calamities. The corollary reality was that animal fats are high in cholesterol (which is of animal origin anyway), and that high-animal fat diets lead to higher cholesterol levels which lead to heart problems.

The trouble with this seemingly logical sequence of events is, as usual, in the multiple exceptions thereto. As Charles T. McGee MD and other researchers have pointed out, there are numerous *primitive* societies whose food patterns were or are high in saturated fats but among whose members heart disease is rare or unknown. There are examples of countries where fat consumption went down — but "heart disease" rates went up.[71,72]

As we shall see (*XVI*) no small part of these odd disparities may very well have to do not with how much but rather what *kind* of fat in general, and cholesterol in particular, is being consumed. "Primitives" are apt to be consuming "natural" rather than industrially altered "oxidized" cholesterol — a very likely crucial distinction.

More strikingly, information in the 1980s and 1990s developed which increasingly showed that heart disease might exist in people without noticeable elevations in cholesterol, that some very high-risk (from a cholesterol point of view) individuals were without heart disease — and, more astonishingly, that despite widespread efforts to lower cholesterol through dietary manipulation, levels often mostly remained about the same in the broadest sectors of the population.[73]

In other words, the combined research on dietary fats as related to cholesterol as related to atherosclerosis/arteriosclerosis (the buildup of fatty composite tissue in blood vessels leading eventually to hardening of the arteries) as related to "heart disease" is only somewhat better than thin and, at the very least, confusing.

But it has led to wholesale attacks on parts of the food-processing industry (by any measure a major contributor, albeit unknowingly, to the plague of Western chronic disease), particularly meat and dairy products producers. It has stimulated flipflops in domestic decision-making as to whether butter (saturated fat) is worse or ultimately better than margarine ("plastic" fat to some extent) and which kind of cooking oil to use, or how many eggs — if any — should be eaten.

A torpedo attack in the **Atlantic**

Although voices of dissent cropped up occasionally as the United States fell prey to a veritable frenzy of cholesterol-counting and label-changing, a roundhouse attack on the new national enterprise of reducing the fatty substance was not effectively mounted until 1989, when science writer Thomas J. Moore published *Heart Failure*,[74] with a preliminary chapter hitting the pages of the *Atlantic Monthly*[75] with the force of a well-guided torpedo.

In essence, reported Moore, the decades-long, multi-billion-dollar national campaign against high cholesterol was in fact an over-funded, hype-ridden exercise which had swollen the profits of drug manufacturers and even certain food processors while failing to show any real improvements in the longevity of "heart disease"-conscious Americans. Moore was instantly backed by a small group of heart specialists, and roundly assailed by the cardiologically orthodox.

Moore assessed years of studies and statistics on the cholesterol approach:

— *Lower* cholesterol levels may be related to *higher risks* for both cancer and stroke. (Not much later, it would also be found that lower cholesterol levels often also accompanied the development of AIDS conditions).

— The surest way to lower cholesterol, assuming such is a worthwhile activity, is to take alcoholic drinks — an observation backed, throughout the 1990s, by several lines of unrelated research.

— Neither long-term safety nor the ability to prevent heart attacks had been demonstrated for either of the major FDA-approved cholesterol-lowering drugs at the time (cholestyramine and lovastatin), and "if experience with animals is included, the potential long-and short-time hazards of lovastatin include heart attacks, cancer, stroke, liver damage, cataracts and severe muscle pain and damage."

— The promotion of lovastatin had turned into an industry itself, with Merck reporting in 1988 that 350,000 people were already taking the drug on a constant basis and an estimate of the profits from cholestryamine for some five million people estimated at about $10 billion per year.

— The National Cholesterol Education Program (NCEP), at the time underway full-bore in hospitals, schools, television stations, health fairs and in mobile cholesterol-checking vans, was at the time estimated to be costing between $10 to $20 billion a year.

Moore traced the evolution of the national preoccupation with cholesterol levels from 1951, described the extensive studies and federal involvement of the National Heart, Lung and Blood Institute and such private organizations as the American Heart Assn. in programs which attempted to show that dietary change could lower levels of the essential fatty acid substance and that somehow this would be a good thing to do.[76]

But long-term studies such as the ongoing Framingham Heart Study, the Heart-Diet Pilot Program, MRFIT, the Coronary Primary Prevention Trial (CPPT) and the Coronary Drug Project had mostly failed to connect dietary change with alterations in cholesterol levels or cholesterol-lowering drugs with the prevention of heart disease and the extension of life.

The data did not demolish the statistical connection between the so-called "bad" form of cholesterol — LDL (low-density lipoprotein) — and elevated heart disease risks for younger and middle-aged people: they simply failed to show, he analyzed, much relevance one way or the other for older Americans in whom "heart disease" risks were presumably higher.

Moore reported that 1988 had been the pivotal year when "the heart institute acquired powerful new allies." He wrote:

> *The American Medical Association, a major drug manufacturer and two huge drug companies joined forces to "declare war on cholesterol . . ."*
>
> *Although the effort appeared to be a public-service campaign, it was in reality a business scheme to sell products and physicians' services . . .*
>
> *The drug company Merck Sharpe & Dohme was already aggressively marketing its new cholesterol-lowering drug, lovastatin, under the name Mevacor. Kellogg was preparing to launch a new oat-bran cereal (Common Sense), and American Home Products to promote a cooking-oil spray (Pam) that, like almost every other vegetable oil, contains no cholesterol . . .*
>
> *Thus a progam that may have begun in sincere but*

misguided zeal for the public good became intertwined with greed. The world was learning how much money could be made scaring people about cholesterol. And the mainstream organizations were being joined by thousands of less responsible profiteers offering miracle treatments, wonder diets, instant cholesterol checkups, and a variety of other services and goods whose effects were non-existent, unproved or hazardous.[77]

Moore hardly had the last word. The cholesterol-fighting industry and national campaign, costing well over $20 billion dollars a year by the 1990s, relentlessly produced new evidence to attempt to link cholesterol with "heart disease," and some of which research certainly did suggest such connections — that is, it showed strong correlations between heart problems and dietary factors, among which high fat consumption seemed to be a major element.

In 1996, the AIC's heart disease division establishment in the USA split wide open over the issue of the cholesterol screening industry:

— The 85,000-member American College of Physicians (ACP), breaking with the American Heart Assn. (AHA), the National Heart, Lung and Blood Institute and the NCEP, said cholesterol screening should be limited to men aged 35 to 65 and women aged 45 to 65, the groups said to be at highest risk for heart disease, although screening might be done in those with "other factors."

Researchers Alan Garber and Stephen Hulley noted[78] that although there is strong evidence that people can get atherosclerosis at any age it is not clear that treating it at an early age has any benefit over treating it later in life.

The ACP added that routine screening for "seniors" 75 and older had failed to turn up any evidence that high cholesterol treatment saved lives in that age group.[79]

We suggest that much of the cholesterol mania has been focused, at least in part, on the wrong thing or things, primarily because of "paradigm capture" (attitudinal bias to support a pre-held conclusion — in this case, prove cholesterol to be the villain at all costs).

Cholesterol is a many-splintered thing

In American medical semantical manipulation — an intricate problem in an essentially free, rather than an authoritarian, society — shifts in premises and attitudes are only hinted at, and come slowly, as if the social-collective mental terrain should first be irrigated with new words and thoughts. Hence the semantical (as well as scientific) cholesterol capers:

The puzzled American public was first informed that cholesterol *itself* was the suspect villain, and standard blood chemistry tests would indeed spit out gross numbers indicating levels of the substance. A "high" — assessment of which tended to vary over the years — was contrasted with a "low" in terms of total cholesterol.

Just when this quantification exercise was more or less understood by doctors and patients alike, it started surfacing that actually it wasn't total cholesterol overall that made the difference — it was the contrasting amounts of the "bad" cholesterol, or LDL (low-density lipoprotein), and the "good" cholesterol (HDL — high-density lipoprotein). Then we learned there was VLDL (*very* low-density lipoprotein) and "small" LDL, smallness of the LDL particles correlating with coronary artery disease in a "statistically significant" manner.[135] And it was found there were at least two LDLs — "native" LDL and "oxidized" LDL. There is even an *IDL* — intermediate-density lipoprotein.

This gradually-induced attitude shift stirred confusion over counts, numbers, products and labels. Was a food dangerous because of "total" cholesterol? Was a blood test which did not discriminate between the two major cholesterols worth anything? Should one give up beefsteaks and Big Macs because of the first set of numbers or the second? Puzzlement galore.

Several new dimensions have expanded the cholesterol

conundrum:

• A UCLA study in 1993 indicated that actually HDL is not totally a "good" cholesterol after all, but that there is — among its five subdivisions — a "bad" version of it, and that tests might have to be refined in order to distinguish between various forms of HDL, quite aside from the established need to distinguish between LDL and HDL.[(80)]

• Stanford and Cambridge University studies, as well as the observations of some independent researchers, found[(81)] how a recently described mysterious form of cholesterol called Lp(a) — lipoprotein (a) — might clog arteries. This research suggested that Lp(a) could permit cells that make up arterial walls to proliferate unchecked — hence accounting, at least in part, for "occluded" arteries.[(82)]

A 1996 study by Dr. Andrew Bostom of the National Heart, Lung and Blood Institute on 2,191 men showed that excess levels of Lp(a) accounted for 10 percent of cases of "premature" heart disease (those occurring before age 55).[(83)]

(Both Vitamin C champions Linus Pauling PhD and Matthias Rath MD, a Hamburg University heart specialist, were primary groundbreakers in advancing the Lp(a) cholesterol theory, and both asserted that the best nutritional route to arterial/circulatory health is Vitamin C.

(Rath, particularly, has outlined how Vitamins C and E and the amino acids lysine and proline constitute the more natural ways to prevent and reverse atherosclerosis,[(84)] a nod to the "oxidation theory of coronary artery disease." Such research not only continues to strengthen the case for ascorbic acid [Vitamin C] in overall health but to vindicate the decades-old notions of the pioneering Shute brothers in advancing Vitamin E for heart health in general.

(Too, as Rath has pointed out,[(85)] the Vitamin C deficiency connection to heart disease is *not* new:

(— In 1941, Canadian cardiologist J.C. Patterson reported that more than 80 percent of his heart disease patients had an ascorbate deficiency as a significant risk factor.

(— In 1948, American physicians R.W. Trimmer and C.J. Lundy reported that 70 percent of their coronary artery disease patients had very low Vitamin C serum levels.

(It should be emphasized that the Shute brothers were viciously assailed by US-led Western medicine for their views of Vitamin E at an earlier time, just as Pauling, Irwin Stone and the Vitamin C champions were later when insisting that ascorbates played a role in health in general, and cancer, the common cold, and arterial disease prevention in particular.)

Further confusing the issue, several studies suggested that the widespread bacterium *Chlamydia pneumoniae* might be playing a very big role in everything from atherosclerosis (since Finnish studies suggested it might be a "causative agent" in 60 to 70 percent of cases) to clogged arteries in general to heart attacks.[86]

To say nothing of several lines of 1997 research speculating that the bacterial infections of periodontal disease might also be contributing to clogged arteries.[153]

To say nothing of increasing evidence linking elevated levels of the amino acid homocysteine to hardening of the arteries, with a claim made that some 21 percent of Americans have such higher levels and that they correlate to threefold higher heart disease risks.[87,88]

In 1996 the *Washington Post,* reporting on studies of patients with coronary disease in which some 50 percent had higher levels of homocysteine than those without artery disease, commented on a seemingly sudden splurge of interest by the Heart, Lung and Blood Institute in three B vitamins — B6, B12 and folic acid. All are considered useful in lowering homocysteine. A European nine-center, 28-researcher study published in 1997 confirmed earlier work and called for "controlled randomized trials of the effect of vitamins" on homocysteine levels.[156]

A 1996 study of 5,000 Canadians showed that those with the greatest folic acid intake had 96 percent less fatal coronary heart disease than those with the lowest intake.[89]

The interest in B vitamins against homocysteine was in no small way a vindication of the research of former Harvard pathologist Kilmer McCully, who had made the links between homocysteine/coronary artery disease and homocysteine/folic acid in 1969.[157]

And, further, some research has suggested that — as certain arterial blockages "resemble" cancerous tumors — they might arise from the uncontrolled growth of smooth-muscle cells in arteries injured by plaques (or even by angioplasties). Enough blockages turned up the presence of mutated p53 genes (as in cancer) and even of cytomegalovirus (CMV), a virus among whose many negative aspects seems to be involvement in heart disease, to somehow implicate the latter two elements in arterial problems.[90]

University of California-Irvine investigators reported in 1996 that destructive inflammatory procedures due to the body's own macrophages might be more important than plaque buildup in setting the stage for arterial disease.[138] This was at least a partial bow to the "oxidative" theory of heart disease (*XVI*).

Total cholesterol? LDL but not HDL? Small particle LDL in "pattern B" men? A version of HDL? IDL? Lipoprotein (a)? Any or all of the above plus chlamydia? Periodontal disease? Homocysteine? Gene p53? CMV? Macrophage activity? Was "medical science" truly closer in the 1990s to unraveling the cause or causes of occluded arteries, coronary artery disease and heart attack? (Let alone of hypertension?)

As early as 1981, foreign blood fat (lipid) experts were questioning both whether cholesterol or dietary fat in general caused atherosclerosis or if elevated cholesterol levels were related to higher death rates.[91]

Typical of their opinions was that of Peter Skrabanek, professor of community health, Trinity College, Dublin, who argued that

Lowering cholesterol does not lower overall mortality. None of these studies have shown people live any longer. It

is a fascinating sociological phenomenon that some experts, in the face of massive evidence to the contrary, have come up with recommendations based on wishful thinking and dogmatic beliefs. They are guilty of unethical behavior.[92]

In 1984, the Lipid Research Clinics Coronary Primary Prevention Trial was said to have the first hard evidence that a cholesterol-lowering drug, cholestyramine, was associated with a lower rate of heart attacks.

This study has been subjected to criticism for statistical prestidigitation, but perhaps the most important parallel element to come out of it was the startling reality that in this survey of 3,806 men at "high risk" for a heart attack there were three times more deaths from suicide, homicide and trauma in the drug-treated group than in the control group. When this difference was taken into account, the difference in death rates essentially vanished.[93] This, and other studies, have led some to wonder whether certain heart disease drugs might be causally related to violence.

McGee has also described[94] how the so-called Consensus Development Conference of "cholesterol experts" meeting in Bethesda MD in December of that year (1984) was actually rigged to promote the cholesterol hypothesis in advance of the meeting.

The past president of the American Heart Assn. (AHA) in 1990 greeted a recently published study in the *New England Journal of Medicine* as "the smoking pistol" while the director of the National Heart, Lung and Blood Institute called it research which would "knock down the critics of the cholesterol hypothesis."[95]

What stimulated the glee was a 10-year followup study on 863 patients which seemed to show that by lowering blood cholesterol levels the need for invasive procedures against "heart disease" could be greatly reduced, and that lowering cholesterol seemed to be connected to a reduction of plaque in the arteries and thus a reduced risk of heart attack. It was said that this study of people with normally functioning hearts — and not all of the elements of whose lifestyles were taken into account — should "put everything to rest except die-hard critics whom nothing will satisfy."[96]

The fight over fat

But the critics kept right on coming. In the Summer 1992 *The Choice*, we reported on the following recent studies:

— While dieting is good, it is not good enough to have much of a cholesterol-lowering effect and, in some people, may do more harm than good. (*Stanford University*)

— "Several large studies" in the US and Europe indicated that although lowering cholesterol reduced the risk of fatal heart attacks, "through mechanisms that scientists do not understand, the decrease in deaths from heart attacks has been offset by an increased risk of death from suicides, violence and accidents." (*Los Angeles Times*)

— Experiments in monkeys showed that lowering cholesterol reduced levels of the brain "neurotransmitter" serotonin. Low levels of serotonin in humans had previously been linked to an increased risk of suicide and aggressive behavior. (*Same*)

— Dietary manipulation by changing from (ostensibly high-cholesterol) saturated fats to unsaturated fats "can cause more health problems than it solves." (*New England Journal of Medicine*)

Dr. Hyman Engleberg, internist at Cedars-Sinai Medical Center, set the issue squarely:

> *These studies knock into a cocked hat the whole proposition that every American should lower cholesterol levels. People who have had a heart attack, stroke or a very bad early history have everything to gain than to lose by lowering their cholesterol, but for a healthy population, they have as much to lose as to gain.*[97]

But the campaign droned on, with the cardiological/federal establishments arguing that everybody should be aware of his cholesterol levels — with some groups even arguing that this awareness should begin at age 2! Such ideas, of course, provided a virtually open-ended market for cholesterol tests and, in an anticipated millions of cases, the lifelong need for drugs.

In 1992, two impressively large reports hit the cholesterol hypothesis with what should have been a mortal blow.

First, a report in the *British Medical Journal* evaluated 22 studies in which efforts had been made to see if lowering blood cholesterol rates would mean a concomitant fall in heart attack deaths. In roughly half the studies death rates rose — in the other half they fell. The author stressed that since 1970 only articles backing the cholesterol hypothesis had been cited in medical references. He added:

> *Lowering serum cholesterol concentrations does not reduce mortality and is unlikely to prevent coronary heart disease. Claims of the opposite are based on preferential citation of supportive trials.*[(98)]

But that was Great Britain.

In the USA, the AHA journal *Circulation* released a huge review (525,737 men and 124,814 women in the United States, Japan, Europe and Israel). The general conclusion: dropping cholesterol levels might have little value for healthy people, low-cholesterol diets for healthy children could be dangerous, and cholesterol levels in women in general had little connection with death rates.

Though the 13 authors of the 19 studies admitted uncertainty as to how to evaluate the raw data, they nonetheless pointed out that in men the only groups who died more often were those whose cholesterol levels were either very high or very low. For the other 64 percent, there was simply no meaningful correlation between levels of the substance and death rates.[(99)]

At the same time, a growing number of heart experts were questioning the recent recommendations that low-fat diets be implemented for all children 2 and over. Dr. Thomas B. Newman, University of California-San Francisco, found such recommendations to be a "national scandal."[(100)]

In 1993, research in the *Journal of the American Medical Assn. (JAMA)* argued[(101)] that national guidelines calling for screening of the nation's 80 million young adults could cost the country billions of dollars a year and end up doing more harm than good to those screened.

There simply is no justification for routine cholesterol tests before age 35 in men and 45 in women, the authors argued. The study pointed out that the long-term effects of cholesterol-lowering drugs were not known and that studies touting the benefits of lowering cholesterol levels were tipped more toward the middle-to-old age bracket than any other. Leaders of the Heart, Lung and Blood Institute and the NCEP program were "appalled" at the information.

Also in 1993, yet another study, this by the National Health and Nutrition Survey, tracking 13,000 Americans between 20 to 74, found[(102)] that average blood cholesterol levels as well as heart disease deaths in general had declined over the prior 12 years, again suggesting a possible relationship between the two. The survey had the benign effect, at least, of arguing for dietary change, weight loss and exercise as treatments of choice for those with high cholesterol.

By the 1990s, Merck's lovastatin (Mevacor) had become the top cholesterol-lowering drug and had captured 50 percent of the market in this class of drugs. Yet, as Moore had speculated in the *Atlantic Monthly* from animal-study data, Mevacor's principal adverse reaction is liver damage, reported to occur in some 1.9 percent of its users. Liver function tests were recommended at monthly intervals and then periodically.[(103)]

The trouble with cholesterol-lowering medications, as is so often the case with other drugs, has been that their effects are temporary. Cholesterol-drug treatment only, then, has usually meant that suspension of the drug signals the return of higher cholesterol levels. The result is, as usual, the option of lifelong use of the medication.

By the 1990s, the total costs of taking cholesterol-reducing drugs along with lab tests and doctor visits was estimated at $3,000 per year per patient the first year, then $2,000 annually forever. Hence, it was not unexpected for Merck to announce wholesale profits of lovastatin at $1 billion annually.[104]

Enter the triglycerides

Just as the cholesterol-counts-most school of American cardiovascular thought seemed sufficiently riddled with contradictions to lead any honest researcher to look elsewhere for blood-fat connections to heart disease, the matter of "the other" major lipid, triglyceride, entered the picture.

The American Heart Association's annual meeting in 1991 was spiced with hints that maybe the cardiovascular establishment might have it if not all wrong then quite a bit wrong by its concern over the ever-more-dismembered cholesterol (that is, HDL, LDL, VLDL, other lipoproteins, subdivisions and particles of the same).

It was pointed out that triglycerides are important as heart-disease risk factors particularly when combined with high levels of certain cholesterols. And a review of the voluminous and ongoing Framingham Heart Study noted that people with high triglyceride levels have the highest blood-sugar levels and twice the risk of developing diabetes as people with normal triglyceride levels. This becomes doubly important since it is broadly assumed that diabetes itself is an important risk factor for heart disease.[106]

In January 1992, Helsinki University's Dr. M. Heiki Frick reported[107] that people with *normal* cholesterol levels but with high triglycerides were four times as likely to suffer heart attacks and might wrongly be given a clean bill of health by cholesterol-conscious doctors.

In 1994, a US team showed that even when drug therapy aggressively lowered LDL cholesterol, triglycerides continued to contribute to the growth of heart vessel blockages.[108]

In 1995 Tufts research showed that a low-fat diet alone could promote weight loss and lower LDL cholesterol "without adverse effects" on triglycerides in the middle-aged to elderly.[109]

Two 1996 studies suggested that currently acceptable blood

levels of triglycerides are too high and that the fat does more damage than thought.

The good news was that triglycerides are more responsive than cholesterol is to exercise and a low-fat diet. The "Omega-3" fatty acids, found in numerous fish, lower triglyceride levels.[139]

Bringing home the groceries

Lurking behind such research are of course several issues — including the fact that, assuming fats of one kind or another are indeed linked to heart disease, which seems a fair assumption, a multi-billion-dollar industry has been looking at the wrong one or ones and at the very least developing potentially damaging drugs to be used against these wrong targets.

This would be a common error in allopathic thinking — the wrong cause of a condition is attacked by the wrong weapon, while attempting to prevent the condition in the first place remains a vaguely understandable concept.

(The earliest pharmaceutical attempt to find a drug way to treat atherosclerosis dangled from the same false linear logic. In the early 1960s, as Dr. Edward L. Lambert noted,[110] researchers who realized that patients who died prematurely of heart attacks usually had increased amounts of cholesterol in their blood [though increased amounts of whatever else were not clarified], and assuming a diet low in animal fats would reduce cholesterol, but also aware that it was difficult to get meat-happy Americans to change their diets, looked for the typical "quick fix" to do the trick. What they came up with was the William S. Merrell Company's drug triparanol.

(The FDA, naturally, approved the drug — on the basis of animal tests and a single clinical [human] trial. Thousands of patients received the drug, but a thousand of them developed cataracts from doing so. After it was later found the drug had little effect in reducing atherosclerosis, it was removed from the market. That is to say, American patients were *presumed* to have a disease

— too much cholesterol — and they were given a drug to treat the "disease." But many of them developed a *real* condition from taking the drug. Another bright moment in allopathic logic.)

What is in play in all the above considerations is the fact that, for the Allopathic Industrial Complex (AIC), heart disease is *big business*, no sin in and of itself, but that very business provides an impetus for the industry and its subsidiaries *not* to look for cheaper, better approaches — including the best one of all, of course, which would be prevention of heart disease as an overall aspect of promotive health. This is not to say that many cardiologists, researchers and physicians are *not* legitimately interested in finding ways to prevent heart disease — it simply means that the economic mechanism favors expensive drugs and high technology in diagnostics and therapeutics, as is true in virtually all other areas of allopathic medicine. Treatment, not prevention, "brings home the groceries."

The parallel reality is that standard medical (that is, allopathic) thinking as it involves heart disease is simplistic in that it looks for that "quick fix" — a single orderly solution to a complicated medical problem. The allopathic paradigm (*IV*) needs "things to treat" and treatments. It is allopathic in essence to see a breakdown of the heart/circulatory system as a mechanical breakdown which needs, in essence, a plumbing job. Something needs to be re-routed, or widened, or cut or burned out.

Yet, as in every other area of medicine, clues and information abound that heart disease calamities are mostly if not entirely preventable (as many heart specialists themselves are beginning to sense, and as some have argued), and that dietary and other lifestyle factors are pre-eminent in its prevention. We discuss the nutritional/metabolic/alternative therapy revolution both in this section and elsewhere (*see Introduction, XVI*) as it applies to heart problems and health promotion in general.

Because, in the heart disease subdivision of the AIC, there are sufficient existing data available, should anyone seek them out, not only to establish the utility of nutrients against heart/circulatory problems and for overall cardiovascular health (notably diet programs, very much including the challenging one put together by Dean Ornish MD in seemingly outright defiance of the heart disease industry) and enough information on nutritional aspects (deficiencies/excesses) in *all* disease states for even the minimally curious to wonder why such things are not more generally known about.

The exercise/diet teeter-totters

By the mid-1990s it was also becoming increasingly evident that two of the pillars of non-drug heart disease prevention — over-exercising and over-dieting — not only could not be relied upon to cut meaningfully into heart disease statistics but might also be making the problem worse.

A 45-hospital, 1,228 heart attack-survivor study conducted by Boston's Deaconess Hospital stressed that out-of-shape individuals who suddenly undertake strenuous activity face 100 times the risk of a heart attack, particularly if they never exercise at all. Analysts claimed this meant that about 4 percent — or 60,000 — heart attacks in any given year were provoked by a sudden outburst of strenuous activity (splitting firewood, moving the furniture, suddenly exercising). The risk was said to be less for those who worked out regularly, but even those who exercised five times a week doubled their risk of a heart attack if they suddenly did something strenuous beyond the usual workout.[111]

And several studies showed that "yo-yo" dieting — making intermittent efforts to "eat right" followed by gaps in the program — and/or constantly trying diets showed a higher correlation to heart disease and diabetes than never dieting at all (!)

In what epidemiologist Steven N. Blair described to the American Heart Association as a "paradox", results of a study of 12,025 Harvard University graduates also showed that men who kept their weight steady — even if overweight — had less risk of heart disease than men with very fluctuating weights.[112]

Out of such studies come increasing emphasis on prudence rather than faddism — suggestions that rational eating habits (more fruits and vegetables, fewer fats) rather than crash diets, and reasonable exercise rather than sudden involvement in extreme physical activity, equate with better coronary health.

The EDTA chelation saga

And, incredibly, within the precincts of allopathic thought there exists in heart disease prevention and management a time-honored, well-tested technique which deals mechanically with the very problem which orthodox cardiology insists is at the root of so much cardiovascular distress — the "occluded" blood vessel.

And, also incredibly, this technique or procedure, about which thousands of research articles have appeared worldwide in appropriately "peer-reviewed" medical literature, and which is currently practiced by a thousand or more credentialed US medical practitioners, is virtually unknown to the American medical consumer whether he assiduously views television news programs and reads news magazines and newspapers or not. This technique or procedure has already saved hundreds of thousands of lives, is itself essentially non-toxic and only minimally "invasive" and — at the real root of its being unknown to the public at large — is far less expensive than standard surgical and drug therapies in heart disease. Too, its proponents would add, it is all that much more effective.

The fact the American public is basically oblivious to it and that heart disease victims are routinely not even informed about it, while some of its most credentialed and otherwise allopathically educated proponents have usually been unable to publish about it in "learned journals," is a casebook example of the AIC at work, and of how all parts of the AIC can coalesce to jam the information-processing apparatus even of an ostensibly free society.

The technique/procedure in question is chelation therapy — usually meaning EDTA chelation therapy — and, to compound the irony, it is largely a product of American research and original application whose central element, EDTA itself, is both a recognized treatment for lead poisoning and a preservative widely used in medicine.

For proponents and researchers it is the best, if not the only, way to unclog blood vessels, the best way to return flexibility to the rubbery system of capillaries, veins and arteries through which the body's life-sustaining blood is pumped from its master organ, the heart. And, it seems to have many positive ancillary effects as well.

It is not the province of this book to elucidate the technique in detail. This has been done by a battery of both credentialed researchers and lay medical writers. (The author includes himself in the latter category as co-author with the late Harold Harper MD, one of chelation therapy's pioneers, of a 1977 book on this subject,[(113)] and journalistic treatment of it in another.[(114)]) In the modern era, significant contributions in the United States to the chelation literature have been made by Drs. Harper, E.W. McDonagh, Bruce W. Halstead, Garry F. Gordon, Elmer Cranton, Morton Walker, Richard Casdorph, James P. Carter, L. Terry Chappell and John P. Stahl, and such informed lay medical writers as Harold and Arline Brecher and Jane Heimlich, among the more prominent.

Chelation therapy (from the Greek word *chela*, meaning "claw"), is the administration of a substance (usually intravenously, although natural "chelators," such as certain vitamins and other nutrients consumed orally, exert some of the same action) which has the ability to rid the body of heavy metals and minerals, substances usually thought of as toxic, and decidedly so when they are in excess. The primary substance used is the synthetic amino acid ethylene-diamine-tetraacetic acid (EDTA), known under other names, and similar compounds.

Understanding the way in which EDTA and similar compounds "bind to" toxic metals or minerals involves a knowledge of physics. The empirical reality is that such "binding"occurs, and the result is that certain heavy, potentially toxic metals and minerals may be made soluble so they may be excreted through the kidneys, depending on the integrity of the same and other factors. Because some necessary minerals may also be removed in the process, a standard EDTA "drip" includes replacement minerals.

While synthesized in Germany in 1931, it was an American — Dr. Norman E. Clarke Sr. MD, cardiologist at Providence Hospital, Detroit — who discovered the multiple uses of the compound ranging well beyond its utility in curing lead poisoning.

There is some conflicting information about the early days of EDTA chelation therapy, including the scattered research on it which produced anything negative (and which is parroted today by the medical establishment), since scores of favorable papers were published at home and abroad (primarily during the 1950s) as to its effectiveness against several conditions, particularly arteriosclerosis. Indeed, as late as 1970 even the FDA referred to calcium EDTA or disodium EDTA this way:

> *This drug is possibly effective in occlusive vascular disorders and the treatment of pathologic conditions to which calcium tissue deposits of hypercalcemia may contribute . . .*[(115)]

As late as the early 1960s, Abbott Laboratories' "package insert" for EDTA contained arteriosclerosis as an "indication" for its use.

But it was also in the early 1960s that the Food, Drug, and Cosmetic Act was once again amended, with the FDA securing the power to oversee both the "safety" and "efficacy" of drugs — an event which vastly expanded FDA clout and also allowed the federal agency to be used as a weapon by gigantic companies to block competitors (*IX*). It was also time for Abbott's patent on EDTA to run out. To attempt to re-license an "old drug" for a new purpose meant in effect investing millions of dollars in a generic drug it could not control. For this and other reasons EDTA was left — in terms of its demonstrated utility in various forms of heart disease — in a kind of regulatory limbo.

Worse for the compound, though, it represented a monumental challenge to the rapidly developing heart disease industry — an essentially far-less-expensive alternative to complicated, expensive surgery and medications.

But research concerning its use went on throughout the world. Dr. Clarke was hailed as a chelation pioneer in the Soviet Union, which elevated EDTA chelation therapy to the second most common treatment for artery disease. It became the preferred method of heart disease treatment in Communist-era Czechoslovakia and throughout many countries was administered successfully against all kinds of blood vessel diseases, gangrene, stroke, senility, diabetes, kidney disorders and other degenerative conditions. Our own research group found that it seemed to "potentiate" another form of US-"unapproved" medicine — "live cell" or "cellular" therapy.

While research went on around the world, with the ultimate publication of literally thousands of articles in scientific and medical journals extolling the multiple benefits of EDTA, the US heart disease industry was growing by leaps and bounds. Just as, at about the same time, the cancer industry was not about to be sidetracked by laetrile, megavitamins or any other nutritional form of treatment, the heart disease industry looked askance at the use of an old, potentially inexpensive compound cutting into the growing surgical/heart drug business.

Joining the 'alternative' revolution

Worse, for the American medical orthodoxy, EDTA chelation therapy largely fell into the hands of medical mavericks who began to utilize multifactorial nutritional protocols against degenerative disease. Shunned as an outsider, it now became part of American outlaw medicine, at least in the eyes of the AMA, FDA and the American Heart Assn. (AHA). It became that most despicable of medical entities in the USA — an "alternative" medicine. It thus fell under the same kind of legal/judicial attack that all other aspects of "alternative" therapy faced in the United States.

Yet unlike so many of these, EDTA chelation therapy was among the best-documented, most provable of therapies both domestically and around the world. An organization of allopathically trained American physicians who believed in and practiced EDTA chelation therapy was formed. The organization developed more research and protocols for use of the compound and fought for its acceptance and authorization. Even so, EDTA ran up against the same sorts of stone walls the AIC hurled against non-toxic cancer treatments.

By 1993, it could be reported that over the years EDTA chelation therapy had had a tremendous track record for safety and that some 500,000 Americans had been treated with it with no reported fatalities as long as the protocol advanced by the chelating doctors' group, now called the American College for the Advancement of Medicine (ACAM), was used.[(116)]

In their 1996 survey of EDTA chelation therapy effectiveness in 19 studies on 22,765 cardiovascular patients, Drs. Terry Chappell and John P. Stahl found a "clinical improvement" rate of 87 percent — and that 58 out of 65 bypass surgery candidates and 24 out of 27 patients scheduled for limb amputation were able to cancel their surgeries.[(148)]

The lengthy battle of EDTA chelation therapy for recognition in the United States, particularly well described by such modern-day writers as the Brechers,[(117)] and Drs. McGee and James Carter,[(118)] has followed a path similar to that of laetrile against cancer. It has been subjected to media and institutional bias and literally rigged or bias-riddled research aimed at finding it "unproven," and was the only item listed as "quackery" by the FDA's publication *FDA Consumer* which we are aware of that ever won both a retraction and an apology from the agency publication.

While more than a thousand American physicians practice EDTA chelation therapy, most of the publications in which they are forced to report their research and successes are not "cross-indexed" into medical computer banks. Articles favorable to or simply open-minded about chelation hence mostly appear in "alternative" and foreign medical journals. The mainstream American public simply does not know, in the main, that this relatively simple approach to numerous heart and circulatory problems, costing so little in comparison with "accepted" procedures, exists.

Chelation therapy, while officially "unapproved" at the federal level, has been officially sanctioned by several states, and in others has been "legalized" by court action. But at this writing securing public and private medical insurance coverage for the technique usually ranged from the difficult to the impossible — another key way in which "unwanted" therapies are harassed in the United States.

Because of its cold-shouldering by US orthodoxy and its necessary flirtation with "unorthodoxy," EDTA chelation therapy has won a distinctive place in "alternative" treatments and thus will form part of the medicine of the future.

Not always successful by itself as a single modality (as so few things are when arrayed against multifactorial degenerative diseases), EDTA chelation therapy takes its place within individualized, integrated protocols along with diet, detoxification and nutritional support as an extremely valuable therapeutic tool.

In the meantime, its struggle for recognition and vindication against the massed forces of the AIC epitomizes what the fight for medical freedom of choice in America is all about.

The dietary heart of the matter

In parallel fashion, the new dimensions in the therapy and management of cardiovascular calamities — in totality the current major medical threat to "civilization" as we know it — point to *promotive health* as a guidepost for the 21st century.

Within promotive health is the fullscale retooling of eating habits and dietary programs (*see XV*) as they relate to the promotion of health overall and the prevention of chronic disease in general.

Even in a world of chemically tampered-with foods it is already within our grasp to identify those dietary elements which help lead to cardiovascular good health.

Among the more recent developments have been those which strongly point to the so-called "Mediterranean diet" as among the heart-healthiest of the Western world.

In 1994, the Lyon Diet Heart Study (Michel de Lorgeril *et al.*) concluded from a study of patients who had had initial heart attacks that a "Mediterranean diet" seemed to be "more efficient than presently used diets in the prevention of secondary coronary events and death."(119)

The strongest correlative feature in such a diet, the study noted, was the high presence therein of alpha-linolenic acid, an essential *fatty* acid which — again, as metabolic and other outside-the-pale medics and researchers had long argued — is useful in overall cardiovascular health (and may also contribute to better immunological health). But as the authors were quick to note, the diet — being high in vegetables and fruits together with olive oil — is also high in antioxidants, which are increasingly coming into their own as protective against chronic diseases (*XVI*).

In the Lyon study, rapeseed margarine substituted for olive oil and was the chief source of alpha-linolenic acid. The study, assessed *The Lancet*, "raises the question of whether [alpha-linolenic acid] could have effects similar to those of eicosapentaenoic acid [*another fatty acid long suspected of overall health benefits*] and other long-chain n-3 fatty acids derived from fish." Moreover

> . . . *[I]f high intakes of [alpha-linolenic acid] are as effective as oily fish in reducing the risk of coronary heart disease, there are considerable implications for preventive strategies, since it is easier to substitute vegetable oils rich in [alpha-linolenic acid] for other sources of dietary fat than to increase consumption of oily fish on a mass scale. Few vegetable oils contain much [alpha-linolenic acid], the most readily available in western countries being soya oil and rapeseed oil . . .*(120)

The Lyon study followed by about five years the earlier "diet and reinfarction trial" (DART), in which eating only "oily" fish was associated with a 29 percent reduction in total mortality in the first two years following an initial heart attack.(121)

The Lyon study preceded a 1994 report by Boston University School of Medicine which noted that advice then in place which touted the advantages of a low-fat diet was off-base — at least insofar as certain essential fatty acids are concerned — and in so doing again vindicated the beliefs and practices of many metabolic therapists.[122]

The Boston research pointed out that a major risk factor in atherosclerosis is an insufficiency of the EFAs (essential fatty acids) linoleic and linolenic acid. Since they cannot be manufactured by the human body they need to be consumed from outside sources — particularly soybeans, green leafy vegetables and various nuts and seeds in which they are plentiful.

Linoleic acid, an "omega-6" fatty acid, is particularly abundant in safflower oil, corn oil, cottonseed oil and soybean oil. Linolenic acid, as found in fish oils, also is prominent in soybean and canola oils, flaxseed and purslane.

All of which might help explain why a 10-year, 24-country, 55-population study by epidemiologist Dr. Yukio Yamori and colleagues at Kyoto University found that the low incidence of heart disease in Japan (and among other selected populations) is likely the result of the seafood-rich diet of its residents. "Oily" fish, shrimps and octopus, the researchers found, contain substances which may prevent the clogging of arteries.[123]

In 1995, University of Washington research into the "n-3" polyunsaturated fatty acids found that one serving of "fatty" fish per week could reduce the risk of cardiac arrest by 50 to 70 percent.[124]

In 1993, the Dutch "Zutphen Elderly Study" had found yet another factor — flavonoids — as useful in reducing the risk of death from coronary heart disease in elderly men.[125]

Flavonoids also fall within the ever-broadening confines of the "antioxidants" and are present in vegetables, fruits and such beverages as tea and wine. They are known to inhibit the oxidation process of the so-called "bad" cholesterol, LDL, at least in the test tube.

By mid-decade information on vitamin supplements as being useful in preventing heart disease continued to be noticeable in studies and surveys both large and small.

At the Second International Conference on Antioxidant Vitamins in Disease Prevention in Berlin (1994), Canadian researchers, reporting on a seven-year followup of 2,226 men aged 45 to 76, showed that those who used vitamin supplements — particularly Vitamin E — were less likely to develop or die from heart disease than those who did not. Laval University epidemiologist Francois Meyer's work showed that vitamin pill-popping men have about a fifth the risk of developing heart disease than those who are not.[126]

In 1995, University of Southern California studies showed[127] that moderate amounts of Vitamin E reduced the development of fatty arterial deposits in 156 men with heart disease followed over two years.

While some thought they could hear a roar of spiritual laughter from the Shute brothers, 1996 research seemed to clench the Vitamin E/heart disease connection:

- Cambridge University scientists who studied 2,000 heart patients announced that Vitamin E supplementation reduced the risk of heart attack by a "massive" 75 percent, outperforming cholesterol-reducing drugs and even aspirin by several lengths.[128]
- University of Minnesota scientists who studied 34,486 older women with no outward signs of heart disease over seven years showed that those who ate lots of Vitamin E-rich foods had cut their chances of heart disease by about two-thirds.[129]

Little wonder that Harvard School of Public Health's Walter Willett exclaimed that Vitamin E "is the most exciting, interesting area in diet and heart disease at the moment."[130]

In 1996, the federal government's own National Institute of Aging reported on tracking regular Vitamin C and E supplementation in 11,000 citizens aged 67 to 105 over a 6-to-9-year period. Results:

Vitamin E use was correlated with a 33 to 50 percent reduced risk of dying from coronary heart disease and a 33 percent reduced risk from dying of any cause.

When the two were taken together the risk of all-cause mortality dropped by 50 percent. Researchers found that E protects the heart by preventing the oxidation of LDL cholesterol.[149]

And North Carolina School of Medicine research showed that carotenids, of which Vitamin A-providing carotene is the best-known member, were associated with 36 percent fewer heart attacks and deaths over 13 years among men with higher as compared to lower levels.[131]

A 1995 spinoff of the Framingham Heart Study also weighed in with important new research: middle-aged men who ate a lot of fruits and vegetables were significantly less likely to suffer strokes over a 20-year period than other men.[132]

The same year, University of California-San Francisco researchers found that even a few walnuts and/or small amounts of soybeans or canola oil in the diet provided a source of alpha-linolenic acid which in turn was linked to a lower risk of stroke in middle-aged men considered to be at high risk for cardiovascular disease.[133]

And animal research — enhanced considerably by a study on 200 monkeys presented in 1997 — continues to show that restricting calories (eating less) adds to longevity and reduces total blood fats while raising HDL ("good") cholesterol.[150] The message for *Homo sapiens*: eat less, live longer.

All such research is pointing, one seemingly trivial study at a time, as the allopathic thought-process tediously struggles to see the forest rather than the trees, to the overriding importance of proper diet not only in enhancing overall cardiovascular health but helping improve health in general.

In this general view, more fish, fish oils, and certain vegetable oils, together with a diet high in fruits and vegetables, would seem to be rational eating options, along with vitamin supplementation. Together with the "poor people's diet," emphasizing less animal fat and protein, no or fewer refined carbohydrates and stimulants, we are nearing the metabolically logical dietary program.

That such a diet correlates increasingly with the absence of advanced chronic disease — and hence the reliance on drastic measures to manage the same — helps explain the lukewarm enthusiasm for such research on the part of significant sectors of the AIC.

The continuing tragedy is that while so many billions of research dollars have been pumped into the AIC for diagnostics and drug development against the human-created diseases of civilization, so little has gone into adequate nutritional science which, more than any other factor, would provide ironclad evidence of how to prevent or at least mitigate them.

References

1. American Heart Assn., January 1993.
2. Scripps-Howard News Service, Feb. 18, 1997.
3. *The Choice*, XXII:1, 1996.
4. "New statistics show increasing prevalence of diabetes." *American Medical News*, Nov. 6, 1995.
5. American Heart Assn., January 1992.
6. *The Choice*, XIX: 1, 1993.
7. The Associated Press, Nov. 15, 1995.
8. The Associated Press, January 1994.
9. Ubell, Earl, "When is heart surgery really called for?" *Parade*, March 13, 1994.
10. *Ibid.*
11. McGee, CT, *Heart Frauds*. Coeur d' Alene ID: MediPress, 1993.
12. *J. Am. Med. Assn.*, Nov. 11, 1992.
13. Grodin, CM, *Circulation* 49, 1974.
14. Zir, LM, *et al.*, *Circulation* 53, 1976.
15. *Medical World News*, Dec. 24, 1979.
16. White, CW, *et al.*, *New Eng. J. Med.* 310, 1984.
17. Cited in McGee, *op. cit.*
18. McGee, *op. cit.*
19. *The Choice*, XVII: 3,4, 1991.
20. McGee, *op. cit.*
21. *The Choice*, XVIII: 2, 1992.
22. The Associated Press, Jan. 18, 1984.
23. de Lisser, Eleena, "Number of major cardiac surgeries was nearly flat in 1993, survey finds." *Wall Street Journal*, Oct. 3, 1994.
24. *Ibid.*
25. McGee, *op. cit.*

26. *The Choice,* XVIII: 2, 1992.
27. *J. Am. Med. Assn.,* August 1991.
28. *New Eng. J. Med.* 311, 1977.
29. Alderman, EL, *et al., Circulation* 82, 1990.
30. McIntosh, HD, *et al., Circulation* 57, 1978.
31. McGee, *op. cit.*
32. Natl. Center for Health Statistics and Commission of Professional Hospital Activities, Washington DC, 1992.
33. *The Choice,* XVIII: 2, 1992.
34. de Lisser, Eleena, *op. cit.*
35. "New caution on the heart balloon," *US News & World Report,* July 25, 1988.
36. "Hearts and balloons," *Harvard Medical School Health Letter,* November 1986.
37. Raeburn, Paul, *The Associated Press,* Nov. 16, 1994.
38. *The Choice,* XVII: 1, 1991.
39. Seeger, JM, *et al.,* "Initial results of laser recanalization in lower extremity arterial reconstruction." *J. Vasc. Surg.* 1, 1989.
40. *The Choice,* XIX: 2, 1993.
41. Goldsmith, MF, "Once again, CABG vs. PTCA — trial results today." *J. Am. Med. Assn.,* Jan. 26, 1994.
42. Winslow, Ron, *The Wall Street Journal,* Sept. 21, 1994. Also: McClellan, Mark, *et al., J. Am. Med. Assn.,* Sept. 21, 1994.
43. King, SB, *et al.,* "A randomized trial comparing coronary angioplasty with coronary bypass surgery." *New Eng. J. Med.,* Oct. 20, 1994.
44. Hamm, CW, *et al.,* "A randomized study of coronary angioplasty compared with bypass surgery in patients with symptomatic multivessel coronary disease." *New Eng. J. Med.,* Oct. 20, 1994.
45. "First-year results of CABRI (coronary angioplasty versus bypass revascularisation investigation)." *Lancet,* Nov. 4, 1995.
46. *The Choice,* XXII: 3, 1996.
47. Heimlich, Jane, *What Your Doctor Won't Tell You.* New York: HarperCollins, 1990.
48. *Ibid.*
49. Langford, HG, *et al.,* "Dietary therapy slows the return of hypertension after stopping prolonged medication." *J. Am. Med. Assn.,* Feb. 1, 1985.
50. Stamler, Rose, *et al.,* "Nutritional therapy for high blood pressure." *J. Am. Med. Assn.,* March 20, 1987.
51. "Five-year findings of the hypertension detection and follow-up program." *J. Am. Med. Assn.,* Dec. 7, 1979.
52. "Multiple risk factor intervention trial." *J. Am. Med. Assn.,* Sept. 24, 1982.
53. Heimlich, *op. cit.*
54. *Ibid.*
55. *The Choice,* XVI: 1, 1990.
56. Psaty, Bruce, American Heart Assn. annual meeting 1995, cited in *The Choice.* XXI:2, 1995.
57. *Ann. Int. Med.,* Oct. 1, 1995.
58. Pahor, Marco, *Am. J. Hypertens.* 9, 1996.
59. Altman, LK, *New York Times,* Oct. 17, 1994.
60. *Circulation,* October 1994.
61. *The Choice,* XIX: 2, 1993.
62. Bishop, JE, "Drugs to dissolve blood clots save lives, study shows." *Wall Street Journal,* Nov. 16, 1994.
63. *New Eng. J. Med.,* Dec. 14, 1995.
64. *The Choice,* XVII: 3,4, 1991.
65. Hulley, SB, and TB Newman, "Cholesterol in the elderly: is it important?" *J. Am. Med.*

Assn., Nov. 2, 1994.
66. Haney, *loc. cit.*
67. Bishop, JE, "Class of anticholesterol drugs cuts risk of death, researchers find." *Wall Street Journal*, Nov. 17, 1994.
68. Shepherd, James, *et al.*. "Prevention of coronary heart disease with provastatin in men with hypercholesterolemia." *New Eng. J. Med.*, Nov. 16, 1995.
69. "Statins prevent coronary heart disease." *Lancet*, Nov. 25, 1995.
70. Newman, TB, and SB Hulley, "Carcinogenicity of lipid-lowering drugs." *J. Am. Med. Assn.*, Jan. 3, 1996.
71. McGee, *op. cit.*
72. *Medical World News*, June 7, 1982.
73. McGee, *op. cit.*
74. Moore, TJ, *Heart Failure*. New York: Random House, 1989.
75. Moore, TJ, "The cholesterol myth." *Atlantic Monthly*, September 1989.
76. *Ibid.*
77. *Ibid.*
78. Garber, A, and S Hulley, *Annals Int. Med.*, March 1, 1996.
79. *The Choice*, XXII:2, 1996.
80. *The Choice*, XIX: 2, 1993.
81. *Ibid.*
82. Schaefer, EJ, *et al.*, "Lipoprotein (a) levels and risk of coronary heart disease in men." *J. Am. Med. Assn.*, April 6, 1991.
83. Bostom, A, *J. Am. Med. Assn.*, Aug. 25, 1996.
84. Rath, Matthias, *Eradicating Heart Disease*. San Francisco CA: Health Now, 1993.
85. Rath, Matthias, "Vitamin C deficiency: the primary cause of cardiovascular disease." *Body & Soul*, IX: 2, 1994.
86. The Associated Press, May 1993, cited in *The Choice*, XIX: 2, 1993.
87. Lee, Arthur, in *Proc. Natl. Aca. Sci.*, cited in *USA Today*, July 5, 1994.
88. Perry, IJ, *et al.*, "Prospective study of serum total homocysteine concentration and risk of stroke in middle-aged British men." *Lancet*, Nov. 25, 1995.
89. *J. Am. Med. Assn.*, June 26, 1996. See also *The Choice* XXII:2, 1996.
90. Speir, Edith, *Science*, July 15, 1994, and cited in *USA Today*, July 15, 1994.
91. McGee, *op. cit.*
92. Brisson, GJ, *Lipids in Human Nutrition*. Englewood NJ: JK Burgess, 1982.
93. Moore, TJ, "The cholesterol myth." *Op. cit.*
94. McGee, *op. cit.*
95. *The New York Times*,, cited in *The Choice*, XVI: 4, 1990.
96. *Ibid.*
97. *The Choice*, XVIII:2, 1992.
98. Ravenskov, U, *Brit. Med. J.* 305, 1992.
99. Jacobs, D, *et al.*, and SB Hulley, editorial, *Circulation* 86, 1992.
100. San Jose *Mercury News*, cited in *The Choice*, XVIII:3, 1992.
101. Hulley, SB, *et. al.*, *J. Am. Med. Assn.*, March 17, 1993.
102. *J. Am. Med. Assn.*, cited in *The Choice*, XIX: 2, 1993.
103. Krumholz, HM, "Lack of association between cholesterol and coronary heart disease mortality and morbidity and all-cause mortality in persons older than 70 years." *J. Am. Med. Assn.*, Nov. 2, 1994.
104. McGee, *op. cit.*
105. *Ibid.*
106. *The Choice*, XVIII: 1, 1992.
107. *Ibid.*
108. Hodis, HN, *et al.*, *Circulation*, July 1994.

109. Schaefer, EJ, *et al.*, "Body weight and low-density lipoprotein cholesterol changes after consumption of a low-fat ad libitum diet." *J. Am. Med. Assn.*, Nov. 8, 1995.
110. Lambert, EC, *Modern Medical Mistakes*. Bloomington IN: Indiana University Press, 1978.
111. The Associated Press/*New Eng. J. Med.*, December 1993.
112. The Associated Press, March 20, 1994.
113. Harper, Harold, and ML Culbert, *How You Can Beat the Killer Diseases*. New Rochelle NY: Arlington House, 1977.
114. Culbert, ML, *What The Medical Establishment Won't Tell You that Could Save Your Life*. Norfolk VA: Donning, 1983.
115. McDonagh, EW, *Chelation Can Cure*. Kansas City MO: Platinum Pen, 1983.
116. McGee, *op. cit.*
117. Brecher, A, and H Brecher, *Forty Something Forever*. Herndon VA: Healthsavers Press, 1992.
118. Carter, JP, *Racketeering in Medicine*. Norfolk VA: Hampton Roads, 1992.
119. de Lorgeril, Michael, *et al.*, "Mediterranean alpha-linolenic acid-rich diet in secondary prevention of coronary heart disease." *Lancet*, June 11, 1994.
120. "Commentary," *Lancet*, June 11, 1994.
121. Burr, ML, *et al.*, "Effects of changes in fat, fish and fibre intakes on death and myocardial reinfarction: diet and reinfarction trial (DART)." *Lancet II*, 1989.
122. Siguel, EN, and RH Lerman, *Metabolism*, September 1994, cited in Brody, JE, *The New York Times*, Aug. 24, 1994.
123. Scott, Susan, "Healthy ocean fisheries healthy for human hearts." Honolulu *Star Bulletin*, June 13, 1994.
124. Siscovick, DS, *et al.*, "Dietary intake and cell membrane levels of long-chain n-3 polyunsaturated fatty acids and the risk of primary cardiac arrest." *J. Am. Med. Assn.*, Nov. 1, 1995.
125. Hertog, MGL, *et al.*, "Dietary antioxidant flavonoids and risk of coronary heart disease: the Zutphen Elderly Study." *Lancet*, Oct. 23, 1993.
126. "Vitamins might help to fight heart disease." *Orange County Register*, Oct. 8, 1994.
127. Hodis, Howard, *et al.*, *J. Am. Med. Assn.*, June 21, 1995.
128. Stephens, NG, *et al.*, "Randomised controlled trial of vitamin E in patients with coronary heart disease: Cambridge Heart Antioxidant Study (CHAOS)." *Lancet*, 347: 1996.
129. Kushi, LH, *et al.*, "Dietary antioxidant vitamins and death from coronary heart disease in postmenopausal women." *New Eng. J. Med.* 334: 1996.
130. *The Choice*, XXII:2, 1996.
131. Morris, Dexter, *J. Am. Med. Assn.*, Nov. 9, 1994.
132. *J. Am. Med. Assn.*, April 12, 1995.
133. Cited in *The Choice*, XXL:2, 1995.
134. Every, NR, *et al.*, *New Eng. J. Med.*, Oct. 24, 1996.
135. Gardner, CD, *et al.*, *J. Am. Med. Assn.*, Sept. 18, 1996.
136. Sacks, FM, *et al.*, "The effect of prevastatin on coronary events after myocardial infarction in patients with average cholesterol levels." *New Eng. J. Med.*, 335: 14, 1996.
137. American Heart Assn., annual meeting, New Orleans, 1996. Brody, JR, *New York Times*, Nov. 14, 1996.
138. Marquis, Julie, "Doctors offer explanation of heart attacks." *Los Angeles Times*. Nov. 13, 1996.
139. "Triglyceride studies see greater risk to heart." *New York Times*, Nov. 12, 1996.
140. Philp, Tom, "Vitamin therapy for heart disease?" *Sacramento* (CA) *Bee*, Nov. 24, 1996.
141. Coleman, Brenda, The Associated Press, Feb. 19, 1997.
142. Hilchey, Tim, "Angiograph use questioned." *New York Times*, March 19, 1997.
143. McTaggart, Lynne, *What Doctors Don't Tell You*. San Francisco: Thorsons/HarperCollins, 1996.

144. The Associated Press, March 5, 1997.
145. "Five-year clinical and functional outcome comparing bypass surgery and angioplasty in patients with multivessel coronary disease." *J. Am. Med. Assn.* 227: 9, March 5, 1997.
146. Mangano, Dennis, *et al.*, *New Eng. J. Med.*, Dec. 9, 1996.
147. Winslow, Ron, *The Wall Street Journal,* December 1996.
148. Chappell, LT, and JP Stahl, *Questions from the Heart.* Norfolk VA: Hampton Roads, 1996.
149. Losonzy, KG, "Vitamin E and Vitamin C supplement use and risk of all-cause and coronary heart disease in older persons." *Am. J. Clin. Nutr.* 64:2, August 1996.
150. Roth, George, report to *Am. Assn. for Advancement in Science,* Seattle WA, February 1997.
151. Jick, Hershel, *et al.*, *Lancet,* Feb. 21, 1997.
152. Haney, DQ, The Associated Press, March 18, 1997.
153. Haney, DQ, The Associated Press, June 8, 1997.
154. *New Eng. J. Med.*, June 12, 1997.
155. Editorial ("First Do No Harm"), *Townsend Letter for Doctors and Patients,* October 1996.
156. Graham, IM, *et al.*, "Plasma homocysteine as a risk factor for vascular disease." *J. Am. Med. Assn.* 277: 22, June 11, 1997.
157. McCully, KS, *The Homocysteine Revolution: Medicine for the New Millennium.* New Canaan CT: Keats, 1997.

XI
CANCER CON: Of mice, men, money and malignancy

"We've poured in many billions of dollars in an effort to find improved cancer treatments, we've given it our very best scientific talent, and it just hasn't worked. It's time to recognize it hasn't worked."

— John C. Bailar III, University of Chicago Department of Health Studies, 1997

"For too long we've made false promises . . . We don't know when we're going to cure cancer . . . But we cannot confuse the frustration with not curing it with the conclusion we're not making progress."

— National Cancer Institute Director Richard Klausner, 1996

". . . The prognosis for the patient who is diagnosed with advanced invasive and metastatic disease remains little better than it was 25 years ago. As we approach a 25th year of this immense war to find a cure for cancer, we need to re-evaluate our triumphs and failures . . . I start with the assumption . . . that cancer is a preventable rather than a treatable disease, and that much of our frustration with the 'cancer problem' stems from our inability to bring this concept to fruition."

— Dr. Michael B. Sporn, Dartmouth Medical School, 1996

"Although it is shielded from the public by high-minded pronouncements and scientific jargon, the cancer establishment is afflicted with a mental and moral malaise. It is more interested in maintaining the status quo than in finding the answers to the cancer riddle, and will defend that status quo against all comers. Its struggle to retain credibility and power may well last decades and cost millions of lives, unless the source of its funding — the taxpaying public — demands reform."

— Gerald B. Dermer PhD (*The Immortal Cell*), 1994

"This 'cancer establishment' pushes highly toxic and expensive drugs, patented by major pharmaceutical firms which also have close links to cancer centers. Is it any wonder they refuse to investigate innovative approaches developed outside their own institutions? . . . We clearly need a complete restructuring of the losing war against cancer. Prevention must get the highest priority. Industrial carcinogens must be phased out or banned. Innovative non-toxic therapies must get independent evaluation."

— Dr. Samuel Epstein (*USA Today*), 1992

The unkindest cuts

In 1991, the *Honolulu Star-Bulletin* reported the case of the 46-year-old woman who "didn't want to wait for ovarian cancer to kill her." [1]

Her grandmother, aunt and cousin had died of ovarian cancer in their 40s, hence giving the woman — according to the "best" medical minds — a "fifty percent chance of getting the disease," noted the newspaper.

So, "I got up the courage to ask my doctor if he could remove my ovaries, uterus and fallopian tubes as a preventative measure." Apparently, he obliged. She now believed her chances of getting ovarian cancer had dropped to "zilch." The newspaper reported the woman had spent the foregoing nine months getting grass-roots support in seven states for similar research efforts.

In 1992, the *Wall Street Journal* reported[2] that about 20 percent of 800 mastectomies (breast removals) per year at the famed Memorial Sloan-Kettering Hospital, New York, were "prophylactic" — that is, they had been carried out to *prevent* breast cancer under the oncological theory that if cancer "runs in families" and if the location of a tumor mass at a single site represents cancer as defined by that site, organ or tissue, then it made sense to remove the site, organ or tissue.

By that time, reported the *WSJ*, the "prophylactic" mastectomy was also being carried out at other well-known cancer research hospitals.

That same year the British medical journal *Lancet* reported[3] that in a worldwide analysis of breast cancer it was found that removal of a woman's healthy ovaries following breast surgery (a total mastectomy or simple lumpectomy — removal of the lump only) improved the 10-year survival rates of cancer-stricken women under 50 by 11 percent.

Still and all, *USA Today* quoted[4] Memorial Sloan-Kettering's Larry Norton as saying that such a double-whammy surgical approach was not without "major disadvantages" — including osteoporosis, increased cholesterol, and higher risks of heart attack and stroke.

Between the earlier "bilateral prophylactic mastectomies" performed on a few dozen women to those done on hundreds, if not thousands, now (the true figures may never be known), something had happened:

First one, then two, then three genes said to be "correlated" with breast cancer (BRCA1, BRCA2 and CHK) were discovered as the nation's cancer industry swerved vertiginously from the viral theory of cancer to the genetic theory.

With the new notion of genes predisposing to various "kinds" of cancer and the development of tests to detect such mutated or aberrant replicatory packages interest in "pre-emptive strikes" grew accordingly.

New data presented in 1997 at an American Assn. for Cancer Research convention could thus be described as either chilling or optimistic depending on one's frame of mind (paradigm):

A Mayo Clinic study of 950 women who had had "prophylactic mastectomies," mostly because of a familial history of breast cancer, were said to have reduced their risk of the mammary malignancy by 91 percent (the remaining 9 percent attributed to the fact that surgeons may leave small amounts of cancerous tissue on the chest wall.)

But because the same genes said to increase the risk of breast cancer also have a small but seemingly genuine correlation with ovarian cancer, one researcher found that *75 percent* of women who had learned from blood tests that they carried the "cancer genes" believed that removal of their ovaries was a "reasonable choice."

Which is to say, a small but significant percentage of healthy women who have had tests to detect genes which *may* predispose to cancer are perfectly willing to remove both breasts and their ovaries to prevent cancer![(132)]

By 1997, with the discovery of a genetic predisposition to "hereditary nonpolyposis" — some 3 to 5 percent of colorectal cancer — the removal of healthy *colons* in "carriers" was suggested.[(141)]

Within weeks of the earlier data, *The New England Journal of Medicine* presented a series of research papers which should have come under the heading "Whoops, have we made a mistake?"

In the 1997 research, including a study of more than 5,000 US Ashkenazi Jews, the connection between mutated genes and either breast or ovarian cancer, while still high, was significantly lower than earlier predictions, as was that for men with an alleged predisposition for prostate cancer.

Said Dr. Jeffrey Struewing, lead investigator for the study by the National Cancer Institute's Genetic Epidemiology Branch:

"While the average risk is still high, it's below most previous estimates." He added that such statistical connections cannot be applied to an individual woman with any precision because "we don't know what factors modify cancer risk."[142]

This frank admission may fall on the deaf ears of women who have gone through prophylactic surgeries at the suggestion of their doctors and wonder if they did the right thing after all.

While an incredulous public found it difficult to believe that there could be such a thing as selective, authorized self-mutilation to prevent cancer even in the absence of any signs and symptoms of the disease (Faulkner Breast Center surgeon Susan Love in Boston was quoted as saying, "I think the idea of removing a body part preventively is really crazy") it unfortunately was a natural result of the linear thought processes of standard or allopathic medicine's cancer subdivision — oncology (whose name, from the Greek *onkos*, really means "the study of bumps.")

The falsest premises

Since American oncology still believes, indeed insists on, the notion that there are hundreds of "forms" or "kinds" of cancer (definable by tumor and tissue type), then there is a kind of primeval logic in the notion that a cancerous tumor in a mammary gland is "breast cancer," that a cancerous tumor in the lower digestive tract is "colon cancer," that a cancerous tumor mass in the cerebrum is "brain cancer" . . . etc.

The fact that there *are* some localized tumors which essentially do not spread, or at least do not seem to spread to distant sites, and whose removal may equate with at least five years without symptoms or recurrence ("cures") helps strengthen the core notion in oncology that somehow the tumor *is* the disease.

The concept that there is a single, underlying, subclinical *malignant process* (the unitarian theory) is still held by only a handful, though growing, number of researchers. If unitarianists are right, of course, then most tumors are not the disease process itself — they are only symptoms, albeit in many cases life-threatening ones, and therefore the basic thrust of oncology, which years ago some of us baptized "cut, burn and poison" (surgery, radiation and chemotherapy), is not only conceptually wrong — it is lethally, fatally wrong. If unitarianists are anywhere near the mark, removing a tumor in the breast is no more a "cure" of cancer than, more than a hundred years ago, was poisoning an ulcerating skin lesion with gold or arsenic a "cure" of syphilis, even though such approaches might "buy time."

A modified unitarian view is that malignancies arising in epithelial tissue — the majority of "kinds" of cancer — are at point of origin one and the same. This would leave the door open to a few "tumor types" possibly "caused" by viruses or other factors.

To most unitarianists, cancer is not an outside invader (since at its earliest manifestation no immune response is mounted against it) and every day cancer cells — described as normal cells whose genetic machinery has somehow gone awry — are produced in otherwise healthy bodies, a process which may never result in clinical — that is, visible or diagnosable — cancer.

The widespread presence of such factors as mutated gene p53, the "immortalizing enzyme" telomerase, human chorionic gonadotropin (hCG), the "switch-off" enzyme Rce1, and "antimalignin antibody" in a majority of "cancer types" helps make the case for unitarianism.

An endless carnage

However, unitarianists or crypto-unitarianists do not have to be either right or wrong in the American debate over cancer:

Despite a sudden flurry of statistics in 1996 which on the one hand revealed an actual decline in cancer mortality between 1990 and

1995 — following nine decades of relentless increase — cancer *incidence* was shown to be climbing and was about 2½ times greater than the death rate.

Following earlier assessments that same year on just how gloomy the quarter-century national anti-cancer effort had been, a joint statement of the National Cancer Institute (NCI), American Cancer Society and the Centers for Disease Control and Prevention (CDC) dramatically announced[(5)] the decline in mortality rates (from a high of 135 per 100,000 in 1990 to 130 in 1995) which was at least a ray of good news.

As we shall see, and the experts were careful to note, declines in death rates almost certainly had more to do with improved diagnostics than treatments, even though a gradual awareness on the part of Americans as to the importance of diet and cancer, and decades of propagandizing against cigarette smoking, must also be taken into account.

Even so, epidemiologist John Bailar III, chairman of the University of Chicago's Department of Health Studies, and long-time puncturer of Cancer Inc.'s optimism balloons, once again begged to differ:

Death rates from all cancers were actually 6 percent higher in 1994 than in 1970, noted Bailar in a cold-water report in a major journal. Said he:

> *"I wouldn't want to say we're losing the war on cancer, but boy, it would be hard to argue that we're winning . . .*
>
> *"We've poured in many billions of dollars in an effort to find improved cancer treatments, we've given it our very best scientific talent, and it just hasn't worked. It's time to recognize it hasn't worked."*[(145)]

Despite the presumptive good news in a slight decrease in cancer mortality rates, these realities remain:

Cancer is the fastest-growing, most life-threatening disaster of all the disasters of the plague of chronic, systemic, metabolic disorders sweeping not only the United States and North America but indeed of the "civilized" Western world. It does not take a doctorate in logic, philosophy or statistics to figure out that the basic premises on which American oncology has mounted its disastrously failing campaign against "the big C" not only are wrong, but are *very* wrong.

For, any way one measures the statistics, and from any angle, there is more cancer, both in terms of incidence and fatalities, and more people are dying from it at ever earlier ages than ever before in the history of our planet. Given the conservative mid-decade projections of an estimated 600,000 to 700,000 new American fatalities annually from the malignant process, following the earlier half-million which had been reported for several years (and understanding that official figures are usually at least two to four years old), then even the analogy we used for several years had become passé:

Going into the decade of the 1990s, it was appropriate to assess a new cancer death every minute (60 seconds) in the USA, with *two* new diagnoses roughly in the same period, meaning that in any 24-hour period there would be upwards of 1,500 cancer deaths or 3,000 diagnoses of the disease. This added up to the approximately 550,000 annual deaths and more than 1 million new diagnoses being reported or estimated by "the experts."

Even by 1990, the analogy our own Committee for Freedom of Choice in Medicine Inc., had used through the foregoing decade — daily American cancer deaths were the approximate equivalent of what would be occurring if two jumbo jets collided every day, killing all aboard on both airplanes — was somewhat conservative. If such a thing were happening, the American people would demand a full-scale investigation. That was then.

By 1993, the officious if not official American Cancer Society (ACS), which has heavily dominated what Americans know, think and believe about cancer and which has done such yeoman work in broadly disseminating the very likely false premises on which US oncology is built and nurtured, projected almost 1,900,000 cancer cases for the year — a catastrophically high figure, even though 700,000 were thought to be what the oncological establishment calls "curable," that is, non-melanoma skin cancer, non-spreading lesions in the cervix, and a few others. The remaining 1.2 million were of the "metastatic" (that is, spread-capable) "forms" of the disease.[6]

Projections from available data are that by the century's end, cancer deaths may be in the range of 1 every 45 seconds, or 1,900 per day or worse.

There are various ways to describe what all this means:

Cancer is now striking 1 out of every 3 Americans, at least statistically, up from 1 out of 4, which had been the level for many years, but is expected to be killing 1 out of 5, or down from 1 out of 4. This means, in oncological parlance, a slight improvement in "cure" rates. It is still occurring in two out of three families. Other ways to assess the mid-decade figures were that as many Americans died monthly from cancer as died during the entire Vietnam War, and that the disease was the biggest killer of the middle-aged, the second biggest killer of the elderly, and the major "natural" killer of children through age 14.

There is no stretch of semantics by which American medicine can truly deflect the central reality — failure — either by arguing that there is more cancer because people are living longer (which indeed explains a small amount of new cases) or even, more appropriately, that improvements in diagnostic techniques (the major bright star in cancer "progress" in the USA) are detecting more cancer than would have been detected earlier (which also is true for a small part of the rise).

Giving the devil his oncological due, it is also not specifically the guilt of organized medicine or organized oncology that cancer incidence ballooned in the USA, other than — as we will see — those areas in which cancer *treatments* actually helped cause "secondary cancer" years later. The reasons for the mass explosion of cancer incidence and fatalities are societal and collective in nature and far transcend even the medical miasma.

Year by year, the incidence of cancer, quite aside from the fatalities therefrom, has long risen inexorably in terms of cases per 100,000 and this has been true since reliable cancer statistics began being tracked earlier in this century, or at about the time the

American Cancer Society (ACS) was established as a fairly unimportant fund-raising group for what was at the time a fairly unimportant medical problem. Neither the rise in population nor the fact more Americans are living (that is, surviving) longer can account for this increase.

Indeed, in 1994, Assistant Secretary for Health Devra Lee Davis and statistician/epidemiological colleagues reported that increases in cancer in white people between 1973 and 1987 could not be explained either on the basis of age or smoking patterns.

"In light of these results and similar studies in Sweden, changes in carcinogenic hazards in addition to smoking are likely to have occurred and need to be studied further," Davis *et al.* concluded.[7]

They were not long in being criticized by other elements of the cancer research establishment for the "models" used, but there still was no "positive spin" on the fact ever more Americans were developing and dying from cancer than ever before.

In 1991, the American Hospital Assn. predicted[8] that by 2000 cancer would bypass the constellation of pathologies called "heart disease" as the leading cause of death in the USA (as it had already done in Japan), so that by the millennium's end oncology would replace cardiology as the number-one medical specialty and cancer incidence might well be 1 out of 2.

The Association publication *Meditrends* was even being conservative: it estimated that 1.6 million Americans would be diagnosed with cancer throughout each year of the 1990s, and that cancer would soon be gobbling up to 20 percent of the nation's healthcare costs. That would now conservatively mean that cancer currently constitutes approximately $200 billion a year of the nation's healthcare cost crisis. This would take into account the 1992 estimate (Dr. Samuel Epstein) of $110 billion in direct costs, and add on billions more in lost productivity and indirect costs. The 1992 estimate was that cancer (industrially described) was about 2 percent of the entire gross national product (GNP). It had, said a group of experts questioning progress against the disease, increased in incidence a frightening 44 percent since 1950, with breast cancer having increased 60 percent during that time, and cancers of the testis, prostate and kidney up by 100 percent.[9]

In 1994, a 15-member panel made up of representatives of the cancer industry — asked by Congress to explain why cancer was still on the rise after the expenditure of $23 billion since 1971 on the "war on cancer" — called for a sweeping overhaul of the entire anti-cancer effort (shades of 1971) including, of course, additional monetary outlays. The panel did seem convinced about the necessity of encouraging "translational research" — that is, actually putting some worthwhile scientific leads into practice more quickly — and emphasizing preventive aspects more.[10]

A ministry of misinformation

While cancer incidence and fatality levels have tended to rise year by year with no real end in sight, the constellation of elements we style "Cancer Inc." has constantly and with gnat-like tenacity spoonfed the American public an endless battery of statements, statistics and projections. These have attempted to put what Washington politicians would describe as the best possible "spin" on an otherwise disastrous situation.

This has been done through the ministry of propaganda and anti-"alternatives" misinformation which the ACS so often simply has been — despite the charitable instincts of its many volunteers, the objectives of its original founders, the undoubtedly good intentions of its well-paid executives and lesser officials and also the good intentions of the great majority of researchers, doctors and analysts within the American oncological paradigm or belief system. It also has been carried forth through the federally funded National Cancer Institute (NCI), conduit of tax-supported research into cancer yet second in societal impact to the private ACS. From both we have heard an endless symphony of optimism.

Cancer has been variously described as "among the most curable of diseases" (true if we mean five years without symptoms constituting "cures," and most of these related to non-melanoma skin lesions or small local "primary" tumors which have not yet spread and have been surgically or otherwise removed). It has also been called a disease condition susceptible of a fifty-percent cure rate, and the disease for which the "light at the end of the tunnel," the "turnaround" or "breakthrough" have been predicted annually, sometimes monthly.

Though more Americans than ever are developing cancer, Cancer Inc. — the ACS, the NCI, the industries which turn out the latest weapons (viral/genetic vaccines), toxic chemotherapeutic drugs, major research and treatment centers, the medical discipline of radiology, oncological surgery, the multi-billion-dollar cancer detection and diagnosing business, the animal research industry, special cancer insurance plans, and on and on — has kept assuring the citizenry that the nation's commitment to high technology (gene splicing, monoclonal antibodies, recombinant DNA, etc.) will lead to the super-tech knockout of the disease. And perhaps it or they will.

But in the meantime, such high-handed rhetoric and bombast are redolent not of any solid achievement in cancer but more of the Vietnam War — with the troops to be home by Christmas, lights constantly appearing at the ends of tunnels, a turnaround in body counts, and all that went with it, before the negative realities set in.

In fact, the oncological revolution is occurring as much from within as without — credentialed "experts" from within the entrails of allopathic medicine can no longer remain silent or passively acquiesce to the propaganda bilge. They are speaking out and breaking ranks, as we shall see.

A quarter-century bummer

The oncological subdivision of the Allopathic Industrial Complex (AIC) greeted the 25th anniversary of the "War on Cancer" in 1996 with data and projections best synthesized by the words of Ellen Stovall of the National Coalition for Cancer Survivorship:

"The war on cancer got stuck and there's no way

to unglue it."[11]

This was a fair assessment of the first 25 years after President Nixon's 1971 launching of the "Conquest of Cancer" program, which had eaten up $29 billion in federal funding alone.

Summarizing the situation for *The Lancet*, Dartmouth's Dr. Michael Sporn observed:

> "*[T]he prognosis for the patient who is diagnosed with advanced invasive and metastatic disease remains little better than it was 25 years ago . . . We need to re-evaluate our triumphs and failures . . .*"[12]

The latest director of the National Cancer Institute (NCI), Dr. Richard Klausner, frankly opined:

> "*For too long we've made false promises. we don't know when we're going to cure cancer . . . But we cannot confuse the frustration with not curing it with the conclusion we're not making progress.*"[13]

"Progress" would mean much more information on the genetic origin of how natural cells become malignant and the fact that, proportionally, cancer deaths per 100,000 have somewhat dropped with the glaring exception of lung cancer, whose rates keep rising.

Yet, the hype and hoopla of it aside, there *have been* tiny advances against cancer, though hardly matching the billions of dollars committed to the federal "Conquest of Cancer" program let alone the many more billions spent in private research. Diagnostics and monitoring have improved, though they mostly confirm just how much more cancer there is, and how little it basically responds to therapeutic oncological orthodoxy. The touted gains in five-year survival rates are noticeable in childhood leukemia and Hodgkin's disease, yet these "forms" of cancer hardly comprise more than 2 to 3 percent of total cancer.

The drop in some other "forms" of cancer has been attributed to a payoff for the anti-cigarette campaign.

Some "forms" of cancer, such as stomach malignancy, seem to have dropped all by themselves (or, some would say, due to the unexpected anti-cancer effects of certain food preservatives in the otherwise highly carcinogenic Western diet), and some "forms" remain highly "curable" if, again, by "cure" one means five years free of symptoms. Such is the case, for example, with most non-melanoma skin cancer, testicular cancer in teenage males, and even early primary breast cancer.

It is the *metastatic*, or easily spread-capable, "forms" of cancer, the killer cancers, which are devastating the Western population, where so little progress has been seen despite however semantics are twisted or rhetoric deployed.

Malignant truth-twisting

As we see throughout the Allopathic Industrial Complex (AIC), the deft manipulation of semantics — tortured language to hide a simple truth — is employed time and time again either consciously (deceit) or, more often, unconsciously (paradigm capture/cognitive dissonance) to obscure realities.

Ah, semantics, semantics — how its twists and turns can be used to obfuscate.

In cancer, we are presented both with the only case of a disease in which "cure" usually means five years free of symptoms and one in which the most notable symptom is usually confused with the disease itself. The fact a patient drops dead on the first day of the sixth year leads to the dumbfounding reality that, by this kind of logic, a person can be listed as both "cured" of, yet dead of, cancer at the same time! It is also true that the five-year gold standard has been altered somewhat — in certain "forms" of the disease (particularly among the elderly, whose overall life expectancy is much less anyway) it has been argued that even two or three years without symptoms might be "cures," thus inflating "cure rates."

And, for decades, Cancer Inc. has played fast and loose with arithmetic, giving support to the notion of "rubber" numbers:

By including non-melanoma skin cancers and localized primary tumors whose surgical removal might indeed correlate to five years or more without a recurrence of cancer-related symptoms, and perhaps forgetting that such "forms" of cancer have been "curable" since the days of Hippocrates, Cancer Inc. can, virtually at will, inflate its "cure rate" to lead the American Cancer Society and others to talk about the possibility or even likelihood of "curing" at least "half " of all cancer.

(In the laetrile wars of the 1970s, court testimony by my friend and long-time cancer statistician and physiologist, the late Dr. Hardin B. Jones of the University of California-Berkeley, was introduced which showed that, incredibly enough, if cancer patients were placed into two categories — the treated and the untreated — the latter lived longer and felt better![(14)])

But such realities have seemingly had little impact on the cancer establishment.

Ponder, for example, the outright gobbledegook issued to explain the perpetual rise in, and failure in the therapeutic control of, adenocarcinoma of the lower gastrointestinal tract — that is, "colorectal cancer," one of the major killers in the United States:

A "consensus conference" of the National Institutes of Health (NIH), the sprawling federal bureaucracy which oversees the NCI, informed one and all in 1990 that "despite the high resectability [*that is, surgical removal*] rate and a general improvement in therapy, nearly half of all patients with colorectal cancer will die of metastatic tumor."[(15)]

The "general improvement" referred to seemed to be a slight increase in efficacy from toxic chemotherapy, burning radiation and the new component in oncology, immunotherapy, together with improved longevity rates of those who survived initial surgery of a "Stage I" tumor and lived out their normal lifespans. The quality-of-life level of such patients was apparently not measured.

Yet in an intriguing use of linear logic the experts summarized that "patients with Stage III colon cancer or Stage II/III rectal cancer are at a high risk for recurrence and warrant adjuvant therapy."

But, we are informed in the second breath, "optimal adjuvant therapy for Stage II and III colon cancer has not yet been devised" (!) so that "continued clinical trials in this disease are essential to discover more active adjuvant therapies."

In an introduction to the analysis, the experts frankly opined that

> *[O]ver the past three decades, many clinical studies have failed to demonstrate benefits from adjuvant therapy. Claims of efficacy have been viewed with skepticism* [although] *recently, new data from several studies have demonstrated delays in tumor recurrence and increases in survival for specific groups of patients.*[16]

Translating all the extensive verbiage, one is left with a simple overview: orthodox oncology is mostly failing most of the time in metastatic (spread) colorectal cancer. Simply expressing this crude fact in plain English seems to be extremely problematical for the experts.

Lies, damned lies, and statistics

In the past few years, Cancer Inc. has made much of the probably correct statistic (though, as Benjamin Disraeli observed, falsehoods come in three forms — "lies, damned lies, and statistics") that slightly more than 50 percent of cancer victims are surviving their disease more than five years, the odd number by which oncology defines "cure."

The 1991 figure indicating this first important crossover event (50.9% five-year survivals vs. 49.1% years prior) was said to be an indication — however irrelevant — of some kind of payoff for the vast investment in private and public funds to rein in cancer.[17]

Yet, as probing experts have long argued, the increase in five-year survival rates may be viewed as a "statistical artifact" — not as a proof of any real improvement in therapeutics.

This is because improved diagnostics simply move the

survival clock backward — a tumor or pre-cancerous condition discovered *earlier* will lengthen the time between diagnosis and death *despite* whatever therapies are employed. Earlier detection hence artificially inflates five-year survival rates which thus artificially sustains Cancer Inc.'s dubious claims to impressive progress against cancer.

In 1993 the President's Cancer Panel, a top-drawer, blue-ribbon group of individuals supposedly set up as a kind of presidential palace guard to report on "progress" against cancer, convened once again. The mood was — as *Scientific American* reporter Tim Beardsley put it — one of "euphoria" since so many new research breakthroughs and experimental therapies were being talked about (as they had been each year prior).

Then entered the room the aforementioned John C. Bailar III, at the time professor of epidemiology and biostatistics at Canada's McGill University.

Bailar, who seemed constantly unfazed by both cancer euphoria and propaganda, had created a major stir in 1986 by publishing a report on the "Conquest of Cancer" program and finding an utter lack of progress in the pull-out-the-stops effort unleashed in 1971 the American way: hurl enough money at the problem and it will be solved.

This time, he was back for another assessment of the American cancer program. Beardsley recorded it:

> *"In the end, any claim of major success against cancer must be reconciled with this figure,"* [Bailar] *said, pointing to a simple graph that showed a stark continuing increase in US death rates from cancer between 1950 and 1990. "I do not think such reconciliation is possible and again conclude, as I did seven years ago, that our decades of war against cancer have been a qualified failure. Thank you."*[18]

His numbers had been provided by the NCI itself and they had been adjusted to account for the changing size and age composition of the population, so they could not be blamed on Americans' dying less from other diseases. The statistical extrapolation was chilling: US cancer death rates went up 7 percent between 1975 and 1990 despite all efforts at control and therapy, all statistical and semantical legerdemain, and all the $25 billion expended on the "war on cancer" so far. Dr. Bailar was simply as candid and logically direct in 1993 as he had been in 1986: the "war on cancer" was — is — a "qualified failure."

As we have seen, he made essentially the same analysis in 1997.

He and other experts have argued whether nationwide campaigns to detect possible precancerous conditions earlier (mammography for breast, Pap smear for cervical, PSA for prostate) can be said to have precipitated or, paradoxically, *caused* a decline in the reported numbers of such "forms" of cancer.

If one is oncologically oriented — that is, considering cancer to be hundreds of different kinds of tumors — then by 1993 (NCI figures monitored between 1973 and 1990) it could be said that cancer death rates were impressively down for testicular cancer, Hodgkin's disease, cervical and uterine cancer; that they were drastically up in lung cancer (so drastic, in fact, as to offset the combination statistical progress in all other "forms" of cancer), melanoma and other skin cancers, non-Hodgkin's lymphoma, and brain cancer; rates were moderately up for liver, prostate, esophageal, kidney and brain cancer; holding their own in breast and leukemia; and were moderately down in colorectal, mouth and pharynx, thyroid and stomach cancer.[19]

It should be pointed out that these figures antedated estimates of an allegedly mass increase in prostate cancer (primarily because of the PSA test) and sudden surges in breast cancer (the mammography controversy reaching white-hot proportions by mid-decade), two examples in which it could not truly be determined whether there was vastly more cancer of these "kinds" or simply that they were being detected earlier and in greater numbers.

Shaking up The Club

By any measure, the oncological division of allopathic medicine is that which most reflects the scientific bankruptcy of the allopathic paradigm or mind-set. While the "heart disease" calamity has lessened, at least in terms of falling death rates (*X*), and still constitutes, for a time, the number-one killer in the United States and the Western world, it is cancer which is growing either geometrically or exponentially and hence dimming the optimism for standard medicine against chronic disease in general. We will see (*XIII*) that this is even truer, on a so far lesser numerical scale, for the calamity of AIDS.

Yet, ironically, it is precisely because of the failure of oncology, more than any other element, that the entire apparatus of the AIC has been profoundly shaken. It is because of the failure of orthodox oncology that so-called "alternative" medicine, sparked primarily by the laetrile revolution of the 1970s (*XII*), became a major challenge to organized medicine itself and began to work its way into the mind-set of orthodoxy, so much so that by 1993, incredibly enough, there actually was an Office of Alternative Medicine (OAM) established within the federal NIH — something utterly unthinkable a decade prior.

It is because of oncology's manifest failure in the West's most rapidly advancing killer chronic condition that physicians, researchers and observers from within the ranks of the AIC itself have strongly questioned key elements of the American health paradigm, have actually argued that prevention of disease should take priority over treatment, and have observed that promotion of health should be the central target of medicine. In questioning the existing establishment apparatus, such doctors, researchers and observers have unavoidably begun to vindicate, validate and justify decades of practices and observations made by outside-the-pale practitioners and others dismissed by so many for so long as eccentrics at best, quacks at worst.

It is thanks to the cancer disaster and the laetrile revolution it spawned that more interest in dietary aspects of health and disease are now being seriously looked at both from within and without orthodoxy in just a few years' time than ever before in the history of American medicine.

In parallel fashion, the elephantine awkwardness of Cancer Inc. in attempting, often viciously, to suppress the ever-growing list of "alternative" cancer treatments, and to lie, cheat and obfuscate on the utility of dozens of worthwhile (if often non-allopathic) modalities and techniques against cancer, has helped generate a political freedom-of-choice backlash which is entirely salutary to the health of the republic.

Even so, Cancer Inc. still remains committed to its central premises, probably all of them false, mostly false, or misleading. It is committed because the greed factor is so enmeshed therewith — far more money is made off treating cancer than preventing it, far more people have profited from "looking for the answer" than from finding it, and a cancer patient with metastatic disease (the majority of cancer) may conservatively be said to represent a $100,000 profit — minimally — for organized medicine. Long-term cancer bills into the high six-figure and even low seven-figure range are by no means rare, and in state after state the "oncological surgeon" is often the best paid (sometimes the most egregiously paid) of the "healthcare delivery team." He is trained to cut, wants to cut — so he cuts.

The big business of Cancer Inc.

By any aspect, cancer is big business — and probably bigger by now than the total cardiovascular industry, with no signs of letting up.

A big part of its 20 percent take of the trillion-dollar "healthcare delivery cost crisis" still resides in the use and promotion of toxic drugs (chemotherapy) despite an avalanche of credible research questioning just how useful such chemicals are.

Former Sloan-Kettering public affairs officer Ralph Moss

PhD, a hero of the laetrile era and since that time an author of three major books exposing the economic side of Cancer Inc., has written and testified that as recently as 1991 cancer drugs brought in $3 billion in profits in the USA annually and that such compounds had a 22 percent growth in "profitability" in a year's time.[20]

We discuss here and elsewhere (*VIII*) the sudden advent of PSA (prostate-specific antigen) screening for prostate cancer, the linchpin of an estimated $28-billion-a-year new industry in this "form" of cancer alone, with little evidence that earlier detection (if in fact that is what the PSA provides) leads to a meaningful decline in death rates.

In 1990, a private market research analysis primarily brought to light by Moss in his newsletter[21] gave some indication of just how big the big business of cancer is:

The profit in cancer treatments and devices was estimated in 1989 at $1.03 billion in 1989 with a projection of $1.74 billion in 1993.

Many of the facts and figures were from market researchers Frost & Sullivan and published in an incredibly expensive 641-page report called *Market for Cancer Therapy Products*.

After noting how cancer products and devices had topped $1 billion for the first time in 1989, Frost & Sullivan added that chemotherapy at the time currently had three-quarters of the market share, with radiation second at 17.1 percent. In descending order were hyperthermia techniques, "immunoproteins" and various experimental items. Chemotherapy's share of the cancer pie was projected to drop to 52.3 percent by 1993 and radiation's to 12.3 percent.

These figures suggested astute observation or inside information or both and took into account the rapid rise of immunotherapy through high technology, just beginning to be highly noticeable in the cancer armamentarium:

The market for such synthetic immune boosters as alpha-, beta-, and gamma-interferon, as well as interleukin-2 and tumor necrosis factor (TNF), was expected to jump from a 5.8 percent share of the 1989 market (or $60 million) to a 24.6 percent share (or $428 million) by 1993. "Monoclonal antibody conjugates" were expected to be marketable by 1991 and to command a 9.1 percent market share (or $158 million).

Moss observed:

> *[T]he market report, not intended for public consumption, is refreshingly candid about radiation and chemotherapy's drawbacks, such as "lack of specificity, with adverse side effects caused by damage to normal cells and tissue." Radiation equipment is "extremely expensive, and sales at present are suffering from cost containment pressure," the study says.*[22]

It should be recalled that various interleukins and interferons were rushed onto the market in the late 1980s and early 1990s with great fanfare amid hopes that each would constitute the breakthrough, the big payoff in biomedical high technology which would win the "war on cancer." As of this writing, all had failed to do so.

In terms of breast cancer, a 1993 US Office of Technology Assessment (OTA)/*Washington Post* survey found[23] that annual manual breast cancer screening for all women between 55 and 65 meant a $15,500 "net cost" per woman for every one-year extension of life, and that if mammograms (specialized X-rays of the breast) were added to the same age group, the "incremental cost" per year of life extension per woman was $84,000 — and this, based on 1988 data.

It should be pointed out that mammograms are at the root of a decades-old controversy pitting various parts of Cancer Inc. against each other. Early suggestions were that mammograms might cause as many cancers as they detected, and that their track record in detecting early cancers was not all that confidence-building to start with.

By 1993, the NCI, long dominated by the ACS, had split with the latter on the need for annual mammograms in women between age 40 and 50.[24] The schism continued, unresolved, in 1997, after a goverment panel was unable to agree on guidelines for women in their forties. The American Cancer Society had for years made the pushing of mammograms one of its major public relations campaigns, on a par with its attack on the tobacco industry.

(A central ACS/NCI excuse for runaway increases in lung cancer, particularly among women, has been laid at the door of the American tobacco industry, with the implied argument that if all cigarettes could be banned lung cancer rates would plummet and this would greatly enhance cancer survival statistics. Usually not discussed is the nettling reality that in some other countries, higher rates of cigarette smoking — as in Japan — do not necessarily correlate with higher rates of lung cancer. This is not a defense of cigarette smoking, so replete with pathological perils, but it is a suggestion that Cancer Inc. has often used the tobacco industry as a convenient scapegoat to excuse its own failures.)

And more test traps

The same 1993 *Post/OTA* survey also found that Pap smears for cervical cancer conducted every three years for women aged 20 to 75 cost about $13,300 for every year of life saved and that if done annually resulted in an "incremental cost" of $1 million per each additional "life-year" saved.[25]

In 1993, a medical journal report of a six-year observation of 1,017 post-surgical colorectal cancer patients found[26] that monitoring through the CEA (carcinoembryonic antigen) test not only had identified only 39 percent of recurrences (that is, a failure rate of 61 percent) while finding "elevated CEA levels" in 16 percent of cases in whom *no* recurrence was found — but that the financial costs were significant.

In an editorial note in the *Journal of the American Medical Assn. (JAMA)*, Robert H. Fletcher MD observed that the financial costs of CEA monitoring are "considerable — almost $500,000 per possible cure . . . and perhaps much higher."[27]

There remains, thus, a huge business in cancer screening programs let alone the costs of "managing" cancer once the unlucky victim enters the "medical loop," from which he will be fortunate to escape without coming out feet first, particularly if he has "metastatic disease" (spread cancer).

For it is in the "spread cancer" cases where so little meaningful progress has been made, and which has led to an all-out attack on standard cancer therapies even by allopathic experts themselves, many of whom have no truck with "alternatives" and would not be caught —er—dead using or recommending apricot seed extract (laetrile) or Vitamin C.

The roots of illogic

Currently, the "big three" — some call it the Terrible Triad — of American (and therefore, Western) oncological treatments remain "cut, burn, poison" — surgery, radiation, chemotherapy. These three are based on the ancient observation that the tumor *is* the disease. In fact, the spread of surface tumors over the body in a shape approximating that of the crab led to the Latin definition of the disease — *cancrum*, or crab. It was an understandable mistake to believe that if the "crab" could be cut off or burned away by fire (the actual conceptual basis of surgery and radiation in the twentieth century), and if the patient seemed to survive either treatment for a credible amount of time, then this was the way to "cure" the disease.

This physical observation was enhanced by the 17th-century guiding notions of allopathy (the Cartesian-Newtonian postulates) as they related to what would later become "the scientific method" and to the overall paradigm of allopathy itself — cancer, whether conceived of as a single wayward cell or a tumor or a swollen spleen or any number of aberrations in elements of serum — is an externally produced disease "caused" by a thing or things; therefore the answer is to kill or block those things. If the disease is mistaken for its most notorious symptom, the tumor, as it usually is, the "cure" means getting rid of the tumor. After microbiology and high-resolution microscopy entered the field in the twentieth century, a parallel goal became somehow getting rid of every last cancer cell in the body — a feat more likely to be accomplished with a Smith and Wesson (through total extinction of the host) than through the ministrations of cut-burn-and-poison.

By the middle of the decade, as theories of cancer origin rapidly switched from viral to genetic causes, the development of genetic therapy as the latest great hope broke out on all sides.

Treatments worse than the disease

Perhaps the factors which most militate against the "big three" cancer treatments are their ancillary effects — they range from being painfully disfiguring to producing nausea, hair loss, skin lesions, liver and other internal damage, and at one point or another depress immune functions, sometimes profoundly so. It has long been a common observation that while toxic chemicals might indeed attack or slow down the advance of cancer cells, the corollary damage done to host defense is such that simple infections which might otherwise have been held in check or stopped outright are now killing the patient, despite the condition of his tumor or tumors.

As an information officer for a south-of-the-border hospital specializing in cancer, I was visually exposed to hundreds of cases in which it was horribly clear that the damage done to the patient (internal organs literally cooked with radiation, for example; botched surgeries which had done irreparable harm to the body) in the name of "treatment" had been worse than the disease process itself. I heard to the point of exhaustion horror stories of patients sickened and terrified even by the prospect of one more round of "chemo" or one more assault by X-rays, and I could assess by the 1990s that I had heard literally hundreds of patients state that they preferred death or no more treatment to being further subjected to medical orthodoxy.

As a California pathologist friend told me (and I have heard similar estimates elsewhere): "Half the bodies I autopsy are of cancer patients. And half of these were killed by chemotherapy." When I inquired, "Will you go public with that?" the response was, "Of course not. I'm in the AMA."

Death due to the *treatment* of cancer is not routinely mentioned on a death certificate, even though death due to "complications of " cancer may be.

Until the 1990s, hardly any meaningful method had been devised — or could be, due to the lack of randomized, cross-over, placebo-controlled, double-blinded studies demanded in the interest of "the scientific method" — to attempt to measure the *subjective* effects on the patient of cancer therapy. *Objective* evaluations could indeed measure shrinking tumor masses, more normalizing white-cell counts, better ranges of platelets and hemoglobin, more normalizing spleens. But since there was no way (though the advent of the Karnofsy Scale has helped) to truly measure how the patient was faring subjectively, the question of greatest importance to the multiply assaulted cancer patient remained that held to be the least "scientific" of all — *how do you feel?*

The rapid growth of so-called nutritional/metabolic approaches to cancer was due as much to the fact that, as a group, cancer patients simply *felt better* under such therapies as it was to claimed miracle successes of such treatments or even the ever-more-noticeable failures of orthodoxy.

"Quality of life" became a very real, very palpable element for consideration among cancer patients. I am personally aware of hundreds of cases in which, even though the advanced cancer patients eventually expired due to some complication of their disease, they felt their involvement with "alternative" therapies of a nutritional nature, so intrinsically benign, had literally made all the difference in the world. For the first time they had less or no pain, had recovered much of their appetite, had more energy; some had been able to go back to school or work for extended periods of time. But these were "non-quantifiable" elements to Cancer Inc., "subjective responses" somehow hypnotized into the unwitting cancer patient by "quacks" who were applying "unproven" or "dubious" or "unscientific" modalities.

From microbes to viruses to genes

As cancer incidence exploded in the USA and the Western world, allopathy's obsession with "causes" shifted from the more generic "microbes" to the "new kids on the block" — viruses — and it was preached for a long time, and in some cases still is, that viruses "cause" cancer. Part of this allopathic assumption lies in the confusion between correlation and causation — because certain viruses *do* seem to correlate with certain "kinds" of cancer, it is a linear allopathic leap of faith to conclude that this correlation implies a causation. (A Texas medic puckishly put this line of thinking to me this way, as it related to the obsessive notion that a single virus "causes" all of AIDS: broken twigs in the barnyard absolutely correlate 100 percent with a tornado, but only virologists might argue that the broken twigs actually *caused* the tornado. But such is the allopathic thought process.)

Unquestionably, certain viruses have been correlated with various "kinds" of cancer — Epstein-Barr Virus (EBV) with a number of "tumor types" ostensibly connected with immune depression as well as Burkitt's lymphoma and some nasal/pharynx cancer, HTLV-1 with adult T-cell leukemia, KSHV with Kaposi's sarcoma (and, indirectly, with multiple myeloma), hepatitis B and C with liver cancer, various human papilloma viruses (HPV) with genital, cervical and anogenital cancers. Some animal "cancers" have also been linked to viruses.

Yet a sobering review of viruses and cancer in 1995 stressed both that "the incidence of such [virus-'caused'] cancers is much lower than the frequency of virus infection, suggesting either that infection alone does not result in cancer and that cellular events in addition to the presence of the virus must occur, or that cancer occurs only if viral proteins are expressed in an inappropriate cell type or in an immunocompromised host," and that "it is now clear that acquisition of a malignant phenotype usually requires accumulation of multiple genetic changes by the cell."[28]

Translation: viruses might help "organize" a malignant process, but they are less likely to be single or direct "causes." (We will explore in *XIV* the possibly sinister origins and roles of certain "new" viruses developed during cancer research which may have been used for biological warfare/immune-depressing endeavors.)

By the late 1980s and early 1990s, while viruses still headed the list of suspects in cancer causation, advances in genetic research began to accord genes — these "tiniest" of all little sacks of replicatory information and even "tinier" than viruses (though at the submicroscopic level, actual mass recedes in importance) — an increasing role in "causing" cancer, either on their own or through mutation, absence or inheritability of the same. Hence the rise of *oncogenes* (literally, bump-genes).

Under current genetic theory, an unknown number of genetic events is implicated in causing a normal cell to turn into a cancer cell. Involved are 30 to 40 genes which may seemingly induce, or another group which may suppress, the chain of events leading to the conversion of a cell to its primitive cancerous state. Some initiating event or events will somehow alter a gene in a chromosome within the nucleus of a normal cell as step one in the process.

From here on, ideas become somewhat murky: some of these "altered" or "mutated" genes are the real culprits; in some cases, the *absence* of certain genes is considered to be key.

By 1994, as highly funded genetic research blossomed across the biomedical horizon with the same rapidity that had marked viral research earlier, two different research teams claimed to find that a loss of a "suppressor" gene variously called p16 and MTS1 was "detected" in 60 percent of breast cancer cases, 82 percent of one "type" of brain cancer, and might play a role in many other "forms" and "types" of the disease. Thus, they seemed to be replacing in importance the recently discovered p53 gene which had been thought by some to be the genetic *sine qua non* of cancer induction.[29] A "cousin," p73, was reported in 1997.

Experts were not of one mind in claiming that the absence of "suppressor" genes directly causes cancer (though some believe they do) but they, and other newly found genes (for example, BRCA1 and RB1), seemed to be proof of why at least hereditary cancers — cancers that "run in families" — might occur.

The discovery of a gene called FHIT, correlated to (the "cause" of, oncologists claimed) some esophagus, colon and various other tumors, was hailed as "the Rosetta stone of cancer study" by the NCI and enthusiastic champions of the genes-are-behind-everything school of thought.[30]

Just as decades earlier biomedical high technology pursued the viral cause, ever-more-expanded biomedical high technology now pursues the genetic cause — and that is where the lion's share of cancer research has been directed, at least as of the late 1990s.

But, as usual, the devil is in the details, exceptions — and defectors from the research establishment.

First, one of the "fathers" of retrovirology and "discoverer" of oncogenes, Berkeley molecular biologist Peter H. Duesberg PhD — perhaps better known as a heretic against the theory of AIDS causation by a "new" retrovirus (*XIII*) — has stated flatly:

> *There is still no proof that activated proto-oncogenes are sufficient or even necessary to cause cancer.*[31]

It is Duesberg who, more than any other, has forced the AIC to ponder the chasm between correlations and causes — be it of viruses in AIDS or oncogenes in cancer.

In 1994, Gerald B. Dermer PhD, long-time cancer researcher (cell biologist turned cancer pathologist), ripped into the high-technology American cancer research establishment on many fronts in a book. He wrote:

> *There is absolutely no evidence from observations of human tumors to indicate that the mutation of any proto-oncogene is essential for any cancer . . . The evolution of the viral theory of cancer into the oncogene theory of cancer is a classic example of how the cancer establishment manages*

to preserve its image even in the face of evidence that refutes its doctrines and favorite models.[32]

Dr. Dermer was not saying there is no role for genes in cancer (particularly in the seemingly "inherited" childhood cancers), but he argued strongly that the research establishment was pinning its hopes for the conquest of cancer on a series of catastrophic scientific miscues — one of the most notorious being reliance on "immortal cell lines" synthetically developed in petri dishes. He found such reliance essentially devoid of honest-to-God science, but nonetheless a fad (along with the earlier obsession with viruses and various forms of high-tech immunotherapy) helping to keep nourishing a $100 billion governmental-academic-medical-industrial complex which has developed around cancer research and treatment and whose hub is the National Cancer Institute (NCI).

Reliance on petri dish-produced "unnatural cells as a model for the human disease has been directly responsible for our ongoing defeat," he wrote. "These cultures . . . give incorrect and clinically useless information about cancer."

As a victim of the system itself, he noted that

> *Research proposals that do not conform to the status quo are deemed invalid and left unfunded. Papers that openly criticize the reigning model rarely see the light of day on journal pages. By controlling the purse strings, the cancer establishment also controls the direction of all cancer research, crowding out innovation and real advancement in favor of the status quo. In essence, the system rewards mediocrity instead of excellence.*[33]

The biomedical high-technology pursuit of genes as underlying disease itself was in full flower by the middle of the decade, and several had been found to be possible "causes" of several diseases.

With ethics now entering the picture (if refined new tests can detect aberrant genes which are expected to *cause* a disease, should the carrier be treated even in the absence of symptoms and/or should couples sharing the trait be denied marriage or procreation because they will surely "pass it on"?) some sober minds must be heard.

One of them belongs to University of Michigan geneticist Dr. Charles Sing, who told *Newsweek*:

> "*What is a good gene and what is a bad gene depend on how you treat it. Genes don't wake up until they are exposed to some environmental factor . . . We're overselling. We're not going to be able to deliver* [on promises to predict and prevent disease]. *We're being dishonest.*"[34]

As one gene after another appears in research labs as the "cause" of something, the same unanswered question about viruses continues to be raised a decibel or two: is correlation causation? Inquiring medical integrationists want to know.

In 1994, the National Institutes of Health's National Advisory Council for Human Genome Research — overseer of an ambitious project aimed at "mapping" each and every gene in the body — warned against going overboard about genetic testing.

In a statement, the council noted that "it is premature to offer testing of either high-risk families or the general population as part of general medical practice until a series of crucial questions has been addressed."[35]

This was a sobering recommendation to stop and look before leaping and to bring some sanity to the obsession.

Without a doubt, genes have a role to play in disease induction — but are they central causes or machinery through which true causes are mediated?

The Bradford Research Institute (BRI) proposed "the primordial thesis of cancer" as a unitarian concept of malignancy — that is, cancer can be described more than anything as the reversion of a normal, aerobic (oxygen-using) cell to the most primitive, genetically "remembered" life form on the planet, an *anaerobic* (non-oxygen-using, acid-oriented) cell. This process assuredly involves a series of repressing and de-repressing genetic events. A true *cause* of cancer would be that which sets this chain of events into play; a true *cure* of it would be that which prevents such a chain of events.[36]

In this particular view, the "environmental factor" — or factors — which might directly or indirectly influence a cell to begin its genetic reversion are the culprits. And there are many of these *organizers* — carcinogenic chemicals (allegedly through "phase 1" enzymes), viruses, radiation, stress for example — but, as we shall see, the central element is almost certainly nutrition (excesses and deficiencies).

As we shall also see, even cancer orthodoxy itself is now according vastly more importance to lifestyle and diet as "causes" of cancer, the most salutary developments to come out of the oncological disaster.

Indeed, in 1996 a major "orthodox" study correlated genes to only 10 percent of cancer, with smoking and diet each accounting for 30 percent. The Harvard School of Public Health showed that smoking, poor diet and a lack of exercise contributed to 65 percent of cancer.[127] Other estimates have placed the dietary element at anywhere from 50 to 70 percent.

But in the meantime, American oncology, by its nature, training and persuasion, remains committed to the Terrible Triad in attempting to "cure" the disorder. In the last decade or so, the advent of immunology/immunotherapy has provided oncology with a fourth leg and experimental gene therapy with a fifth one. Up to now it has largely meant highly expensive and potentially toxic manufactured proteins aimed at manipulating human immunity since most of organized allopathy, blinders on, does not like to admit the flood-proportion biochemical research data and massive empiricism attributing immune-boosting and immune-modulating properties, let alone anti-carcinogenic effects, to an ever-growing range of naturally-occurring nutrients.

Indeed, nothing seems to be more viscerally terrifying to Cancer Inc. than the concept that cancer can be treated by unpatentable, natural nutrients — unless it is the more sweeping concept that cancer can largely be *prevented* by the same, thus bringing to an end a $200 billion element in the nation's "healthcare delivery cost crisis."

A litany of failure and disaster

But what of the "standard" or "accepted" or "scientifically proven" therapies?

— In 1989 and 1990, information gathered or published by the medical establishment itself was so negative for chemotherapy (including synthetic hormones) and radiation that in some quarters there was raised the question of just how much longer chemotherapy would still be around. This was not only because of the lack of very much efficacy from such toxic compounds but the ever-more-obvious fact they helped *increase* the likelihood of cancer.

A *New England Journal of Medicine* study, for example, found[37] that the administration of chemotherapy for Hodgkin's disease and ovarian cancer enhanced the chances of leukemia developing later. The same learned journal had reported a year earlier that the use of X-rays during infancy significantly increased women's chances of developing breast cancer when they reached their 30s.

— The General Accounting Office (GAO) found in 1989 that despite an increase in the US of chemotherapy since 1975 there had been no detectable increase in survival rates in breast cancer and that "the benefits of chemotherapy are small and therefore difficult to detect."[38]

— Leading surgeons, sharply challenging the NCI, argued[39] in 1989 that women with breast cancer should not necessarily undergo chemotherapy, with one stating that for many cancer patients "high costs and side effects probably outweigh the benefits" of the toxic drugs.

— An NCI study published in 1997 found that bone-marrow transplants (BMTs) used to "cure" cancer could cause more cancer years later. The research was on 20,000 BMTs done between 1964 and 1992 and pointed an accusing finger at the high doses of radiation used in such procedures.[133]

(It should be pointed out that, despite the appearance of a united front of surgeons, chemotherapists and radiologists against the "cancer quacks," many of whom believe cancer can largely be prevented let alone managed by nutritional factors, the three schools in private often detest each other with the vigor of Yale vs. Harvard. Surgeons, who were first on the scene as virtually the sole managers of cancer — even engaging in a ghastly technique called the "hemicorporectomy" [cutting the body in half to halt advancing tumors] in the 19th century — felt threatened first by the radium industry early in this century [with its insistence on burning out, rather than cutting off, tumors] and, decades later, by the chemotherapists, who believed cancer could be poisoned away.)

— A Swedish/NCI study concluded[40] that long-term treatment with estrogen (female hormones or their artificial analogues) seemed to be associated with an increased risk of breast cancer although subsequent research has tended to play down the connection.

By 1990, the "war on cancer" had yet another skipper, Dr. Samuel Broder, and at a cancer treatment conference in Tucson he was blunt about the campaign: since declaration of the "war" in 1971, overall cancer incidence had risen by 14 percent and the death rate had gone up by more than 5 percent, he said.

"There are several [cancer] diseases [in which] by any measure there has been inadequate or no progress — areas where we have gotten nowhere," he forthrightly stated.[41]

A Bristol-Myers Co. cancer researcher was equally on-target: "The process of drug discovery and drug development over the past 20 years has had very little effect on the evolution of drug treatments. The progress has been very slow, and our strategies may need re-evaluation," he said.[42]

By 1991, the utility of chemotherapy was attacked head-on in *The Lancet* by Albert S. Braverman MD, division of hematology-oncology, Division of Medicine, Health Sciences Center of the University of New York at Brooklyn, who wrote:

> *[T]he time has come to cut back on the clinical investigation of new chemotherapeutic regimens for cancer*

and to cast a critical eye on the way chemotherapeutic treatment is now administered . . . No disseminated neoplasm [cancer] *incurable in 1975 is curable today . . . Many medical oncologists recommend chemotherapy for virtually any tumor, with a hopefulness undiscouraged by almost invariable failure . . . The oncology community should respond to the data of the past decade by scaling back the whole chemotherapeutic enterprise. Chemotherapy should be prescribed only when there is a reasonable prospect either of cure or benefit in quantity and quality of life.*[43]

Earlier that year, an *Annals of Internal Medicine* had reported[44] Italian studies showing that three chemotherapeutic drugs given in breast cancer might lead to esophageal cancer later, and American research on leukemia therapy published in the *New England Journal of Medicine* showed that treatments with the chemotherapy agent doxorubicin could result in "clinically important heart disease in later years" through "progressive increase in left ventricular afterload."[45]

The same year, Heidelberg cancer biostatistician Ulrich Abel unleashed through the widely distributed German magazine *Der Spiegel* another roundhouse attack on chemotherapy.[46]

Abstracted from his 1990 data, Abel insisted:

[T]here is no evidence for the majority of cancers that treatment with these [chemotherapeutic] *drugs exerts any positive influence on survival or quality of life in patients with advanced disease . . . The almost dogmatic belief in the efficacy of* [chemotherapy] *is usually based on false conclusions and inappropriate data . . . Ten years of activity as a statistician in clinical oncology . . . and a . . . sobering and unprejudiced analysis of the literature have rarely revealed any therapeutic success by the regimens in question. . .*[47]

He also hit oncology in its tenderest of concepts:

Contrary to standard oncological thought, he added, "reduction of tumor mass does not prolong expected survival."

(Here was an appropriately credentialed attack on a concept at least off-handedly suggested by oncologists to their patients — that somehow there is a correlation between what happens to the tumor [did it go "up" or "down"?] and their life expectancy. The major proponent of laetrile long called this, correctly, "the false criterion of tumefaction.")

1991 was also the year when the NCI released the startling news that "secondary" cancer was on the rise, primarily because of the success of "cures" for "primary" cancer — again, a twist of semantics that left honest minds groping to make sense of it all:

An NCI survey showed[48] that 1 out of 8 cancer-stricken, orthodoxy-treated children would develop "secondary" cancer within 25 years, and that for Hodgkin's patients the risk of developing a "secondary" cancer in 15 years was greater than 1 in 6. It hence argued that chemotherapy and radiation, "treatments of choice," increased the risks of cancer later.

This was not a surprise to many researchers, since virtually every toxic chemotherapy drug on the market had been shown, or suggested, as a cause of cancer in animal tests (assays of dubious validity, to be sure) and, even in humans, were suspected of inducing cancer unless carefully monitored.

In 1993, the NCI had new data on a five-year followup of 1,100 cancer survivors:[49]

While more children were surviving the disease, many faced learning disabilities, memory loss and even stunted growth and possibly heart failure because of the aggressive chemotherapy and radiation which had ostensibly "cured" their malignancies.

Radiation came in for some of the worst criticism since, as Dr. Paula Lemper, director of the Late Effects Clinic at Children's Hospital, Orange CA, put it: "we used to radiate everyone" as a precautionary measure but "now we radiate the heads of only 20 to 25 percent of child cancer patients."[50]

The most damaged survivors are those who had radiation to

the brain.

The NCI data also parenthetically raised the issue: *is* there "secondary" cancer, or simply a continuation of the underlying malignant process which has either been slowed — or exacerbated — by aggressive treatment of childhood tumors?

Even so, the fact that children who might have died faster in an earlier era were surviving long enough to develop "secondary" cancer later was, in its own strange way, a net plus for cancer orthodoxy.

Belling the cat

By 1992, unquestionably the cancer establishment's primary failure-baiter was Dr. Samuel Epstein, professor at the University of Illinois School of Public Health and author of a major book *(The Politics of Cancer)*, which belled the cat, at least partially.

In a 1992 press conference in Washington, Dr. Epstein and 65 other American cancer experts in an open statement denounced the US cancer establishment, claiming that it had "misled and confused the public and congress" by continually claiming significant progress against the disease.[(51)]

Epstein told the media that "the public has been hoodwinked" and that "Congress was sold a bill of goods by the cancer establishment. 'Give us the money,' they said, 'and we'll cure cancer.' Congress was bulldozed into funding massive amounts for supposed 'cancer cures.'"

Earlier, in *USA Today*, Dr. Epstein was even more explicit:

> *This "cancer establishment" pushes highly toxic and expensive drugs, patented by major pharmaceutical firms which also have close links to cancer centers. Is it any wonder they refuse to investigate innovative approaches developed outside their own institutions? . . . We clearly need a complete restructuring of the losing war against cancer. Prevention must get the highest priority . . . Until then, Congress must refuse to fund NCI and the public should boycott the bloated American Cancer Society.*[(52)]

Dr. Epstein's long-time battle has been to convince the public that it is cancer-causing industrial and agricultural chemicals (carcinogens) far more than smoking and dietary fat which are linked to rapidly rising cancer rates in the West.

(Which of course pits two branches of the cancer research community against each other: those who generally downplay the role of industrial, synthetic chemicals in the environment and those who, like Epstein, believe they may be paramount.

(The widespread chemicalization of not only the food supply but practically everything else in the environment strongly correlates to the plague of man-made or man-altered "modern" disease conditions which have in common profound dysregulation of the immune system(s) [*see XV*]. Whether chemicalization leads to cancer is a less important question than is the reality that such chemicals, to which we are continually, consistently, and *cumulatively* exposed, *do* correlate with chronic disease conditions across the board. The record is clear: industry absolutely does not want to have such connections looked at too closely, and therefore is happier with the conclusion that dietary problems and too many cigarettes are more to be blamed.

(When researchers many of whose grants directly or indirectly come from one or more wings of vested interests — be they the food industry, the drug industry, the chemical industry, the power industry — pontificate on any of these connections to, say, cancer, it is always appropriate to wonder how objective the data really are. The interplay between vested interests does *not*, however, necessarily mean that research with which such interests are somehow involved is bereft of meaningful contributions to our knowledge about cancer.)

In the *Washington Post*, Epstein added:

> *While explaining away soaring cancer rates, the establishment, abetted by cheerleading science journalists, grossly exaggerates treatment successes. Periodic announcements of dramatic advances are based on initial reduction in tumor size rather than on prolonged survival.*

For most cancers, survival has not changed for decades. Contrary claims are based on rubber numbers.

Furthermore, the establishment is financially interlocked with giant pharmaceutical companies (grossing $1 billion annually in cancer drug sales), with inherent conflicts of interest . . .[53]

Word games and cognitive dissonance

None of the above should suggest that American cancer orthodoxy always fails: there *are* cases of long-term survival through the cut-burn-poison approach to advanced cancer, just as there increasingly are cases of long-term survival *without* such approaches — the institutional difference is that the former successes are called "statistics" and the latter are dismissed as "anecdotes."

This has been a standard technique for downplaying seeming cancer victories by an ever-growing list of "unproven" or "unscientific" modalities, and it has always run this way:

If a patient with advanced cancer (meaning spread from one site to another) seems to be doing very well on an "unorthodox" program, and is approaching, or bypassing, the five-year survival rate ("cure"), then one of three things must be true —

• He was either misdiagnosed (lack of a "histopathologically confirmed" tumor) by his standard or orthodox physician, let alone by the "quack" now claiming victory or

• He was somehow belatedly responding to earlier "orthodox" therapy even though the failure on same is what probably led him to the "unorthodox" practitioner in the first place; or

• Should he be a "virgin case" — that is, cancer confirmed by an "accepted" cancer research facility but *no* orthodox therapy having been done — it must be a clear case of "spontaneous remission." This is a religious term which would normally have no place in "science" except for orthodoxy's urgent need to sweep away every last crumb of doubt.

As we argue throughout, the "spontaneous remission"

argument is generally not deceitful or of malicious intent but rather a reflection of what psychologically may be called *negative cognitive dissonance* — inability or unwillingness of the observer to process unwanted or startling new information. The new information in this case would be, for example, that laetrile, proteolytic enzymes, various vitamins and diet seemed to have clinically eradicated an obvious case of cancer. The mental mechanism is: since what seems to have occurred cannot possibly have occurred (because "quack" therapies do not work), then what did occur really did not occur — the answer must lie elsewhere.

(I am reminded of a case south of the border in which an American gentleman from an Eastern city seemed to be doing spectacularly well on an all-natural program with an advanced "form" of cancer [mesothelioma] which medical orthodoxy has never "cured." He came to the Mexican hospital with a confirmed diagnosis by a well-known cancer expert. His prognosis, by orthodoxy, was a few weeks to live at most. Upon his return home, his original doctor was so startled to see him in such seemingly good condition that he pondered the most self-deprecating reality of all for a physician — perhaps he had made a diagnostic mistake. Searching through medical tomes to find some pathology which seemed to match the symptomatology of advanced mesothelioma, he hit upon a rare tropical disease, and announced that this might very well have been what the man had had. The fact the gentleman had never been in the tropics was only an irritant to this workout in a form of cognitive dissonance.)

When any of the above arguments do not work, then it is easy for orthodoxy to point to some orthodox component of a total integrative program (for example, a synthetic hormone suppressor administered along with vitamins, minerals, enzymes, fatty acids, laetrile and diet in prostatic cancer) and explain the good success thanks exclusively to the hormone suppressor. Conversely, should the patient *not* be doing well on the same program, hormone suppressor and all, failure can then be attributed to the "useless" metabolic therapy.

This form of brain-scrubbing is of course more successful when those who control the information and research channels in the cancer industry have the greater access — as they do — to the media.

As we explore in the discussion on heart disease (*X*), among cardiology's various failings have not only been inappropriate or even dangerous therapies which frequently either fail or otherwise harm the patient — the diagnostics alone leave a great deal to be desired.

So it is for cancer.

Keeping abreast of a scandal

The General Accounting Office (GAO) was back in the news in 1992 with a cold assessment that "there have been no gains in preventing breast cancer over the past two decades, and its relentless rise, primarily among American women, cannot be explained on the basis of earlier diagnostics."[(54)]

The decades-old controversy over mammograms for breast cancer reached critical mass in 1993, when the NCI, splitting with the ACS, declined to advise women in their 40s to have mammograms every year, as recommended by the Society.

The split occurred again in 1997, when the National Cancer Advisory Board was unable to come up with definitive guidelines for women in that age group. At an earlier time, there were suggestions that women even younger have annual or biannual trips to the mammogram specialist — the only "sure" way to find the tiniest of mammary malignancies before they became problematical. The ACS had made promotion of the same (at between $50 and $150 per imaging) a major public relations effort for decades.

In 1992, a Canadian study of 90,000 women at 15 hospitals conducted by the University of Toronto failed to find that women between 40 and 49 received any benefit from the technique.[(55)] By 1993, analyses of new data from around the world supported the Canadian findings.

The *Lancet* editorialized:

There are no reliable data to suggest that screening [mammograms] *reduces mortality in the youngest or* oldest [author's emphasis] *age groups, so this leaves us with a 30 percent or so reduction in breast cancer specific mortality for the middle group.*

Even a 30 percent reduction in the relative risk of relapse or death following local treatment of breast cancer, important though this may be in public health terms for so common a disease, still means that most patients with clinically overt breast cancer still will die of their metastases if followed for long enough. . .

So, if we acknowledge the failures of primary therapy and secondary intervention, our frustrated attempts at primary intervention, and the true increasing incidence of the disease, we should not be surprised by the static overall mortality from carcinoma of the breast.(56)

In 1994, the Canadians were back in cancer news again with research indicating that the mammogram procedure itself — the painful squeezing of the breast into a kind of vise whereby it can be properly "scanned" — is so traumatic to the mammary tissues that it can induce the spread of cancer on its own.(57)

(As we shall shortly see, the mammogram element in breast cancer is but the tiniest tip of a massive iceberg involving radiation scandals galore, and the controversy is far from over.

(We also note that some maverick research indicates that the fashion-enforced ritual of the tight brassiere — unnaturally over time traumatizing breasts — is a possible contributory factor.)

More worthless tests

In 1993, Mayo Clinic researchers were reported that the widely used screening test for colon cancer, the Hemoccult test (which checks for cancer in the stool), was practically worthless: a three-year study of 13,000 patients showed it missed more than 70 percent of colorectal cancers that were later diagnosed through X-rays or colonoscopic examination. Blood in the stool equated with cancer less than 10 percent of the time.[58] Two months later, a 13-year University of Minnesota survey of 46,000 people reached contrary conclusions and said the test had reduced colon cancer deaths by 33 percent.[59]

And the earlier-mentioned 1993 Moertel study on CEA monitoring of post-surgical colorectal cancer not only found this long-used assay to be mostly irrelevant, as well as expensive, but in an editorial which accompanied the study's release, Robert H. Fletcher MD noted:

> *But it is not just a matter of money. There is also the inconvenience and discomfort of repeated blood tests, worry over what the result may be, extra surgery, and knowing about recurrence of cancer earlier than one would ordinarily, even though many of these patients cannot be cured. I am skeptical that the benefits outweigh the costs, all things considered.*[60]

The great PSA caper

The taker of the cake in terms of relevance of screening, however, was the launching with fanfare (*VIII*) of the PSA (prostate-specific antigen) test to detect prostate cancer in men.

Since the age levels of men thought to be incubating possible or probable prostate cancer keeps ranging downward — to around age 50 — the use of a test which could detect the tiniest "marker protein" for the disease should ideally alert middle-aged men to what might be upcoming. (It naturally also increases the market for PSA tests). It was already generally known, at least in North America, Australia, New Zealand and much of northern and western Europe, that if a man lived long enough, he almost certainly would develop prostate cancer. This was not true, of course, for males in many other societies, many of whom lived as long or longer than Western males.

But the development of yet another new test with a new number to be worried about posed the most serious of dilemmas:

Since there had been no meaningful improvements in prostate cancer therapies, and they ranged from the more mutilating orchiectomies, castration and complete prostatectomies to the less destructive but unpredictable and far from risk-free TURP (trans-urethral resection of the prostate), as well as radiation and application of female hormones, or selective freezing,and often would be followed by impotence, incontinence or both, the question remained:

Why would a middle-aged to elderly man really want to know if he had the problem when its "management" was so devastating and results so uncertain, and when it was also not at all clear that simply "having" prostate CA would necessarily be much of a problem, particularly if the growth were confined to the prostate?

By 1992, the *Sacramento Bee* could synthesize the prostate cancer mishmash thus:

> *Physicians treating prostate cancer face an unusual medical problem: 40 percent of [American men] have prostate cancer but only 10 percent are diagnosed. And while 3 percent of American men will die of prostate cancer, most of those who have the disease never know it and are not affected by it.*[61]

Some studies had already shown that, particularly due to the advanced age of men with diagnosed prostatic cancer, survival outcomes were not influenced much, if at all, by therapy. And some research showed no treatment at all to be just as good.

In a key study, Swedish researchers following a group of 200 men whose prostate cancer remained localized in the prostate gland, which was initially left untreated, found[62] that (a) only 8.5 percent had died of prostate cancer after 10 years while (b) almost half died of some other cause during the time of the study, and (c) of a subset of men who 10 years earlier had met current standards for radical prostate surgery but did not receive it, the survival rate was an impressive *88 percent.*

Five years later, the Swedish researchers had followed up to 642 patients for five more years — to 15 — and reached some intriguing conclusions:

• "Patients with localized prostate cancer have a favorable outlook following watchful waiting" (essentially meaning, doing nothing.)

• Not providing "radical initial treatment" to such patients limits deaths.

• "An aggressive approach to all patients with early disease would entail substantial overtreatment" but

• "Patients with locally advanced or metastatic disease need trials of aggressive therapy to improve their poor prognosis."

The Swedes warned about the widespread use of screening and aggressive treatment, "a development that will escalate the risk of overdiagnosis and overtreatment."[134]

H. Ballantine Carter, author of a Johns Hopkins study, opined:

> *The bottom line is, we don't know which patients are going to get into trouble from the disease. It's very, very difficult to tell a patient he may do just as well without any treatment, but we can't assure him of that.*[63]

And, added Dr. John Wasson, who participated in two studies whose results were published in 1993: "We have, in essence, an epidemic of treatment and no scientific proof that it's valid."[64]

In yet another report, this one a survey of six separate studies of early-stage prostate CA in 828 men, University of Chicago surgeon Gerald Chodak claimed[65] that the analysis "shows that watchful waiting is a reasonable option."

Seemingly throwing up their hands over all of this, some researchers were ready, by mid-decade, to suggest the Swedes' "watchful waiting" (also known as "expectant observation") in men with diagnosed prostate cancer.

In 1994 the FDA licensed Eli Lilly's Hybritech unit to make PSA prostate cancer screening tests available. The federal agency thus approved the test kits for the actual detection of cancer (they had been accepted as monitors of the disease and as detectors of benign prostatic hypertrophy or hyperplasia [BPH] before.) Approval followed on the heels of the FDA's agreeing that PSAs could be used for detection — but only in combination with the vintage digital examination. Despite the fanfare, the FDA's Susan Alpert noted that both tests had a "combination predictive value" of about 50 percent — meaning they could miss prostate cancer half the time![66]

No sooner had the FDA approvals been announced than a University of Toronto study claimed that "screening for prostate cancer cannot be justified as a rational health policy" and that mass PSA screening would cost anywhere from $113,000 to $729,000 in doctor, hospital and other bills simply to gain one year of life-expectancy from early treatment, while lowering the quality of life for many men.[67]

And in 1997 research reviews commissioned by the United Kingdom's National Health Service (NHS) advised against routine screening for prostate cancer.

One scientist noted that "two out of three men with a positive PSA will turn out not to have a cancer but will have to undergo further investigation and anxiety."[135]

But, since in the US the PSA had already been estimated (*VIII*) as the keystone of a new $28 billion per year industry, the new figures seemed unlikely to deter Cancer Inc.

Mass availability of PSA tests by 1997 had led to a sixfold increase in surgical removals of the prostate, itself a growing industry.[143]

The PSA detection business has thus added hundreds of thousands of prospective clients to the cancer-treatment pool. I am aware of numerous cases of elderly asymptomatic men who spent small fortunes on therapy whether it was necessary or not — lured into the medical loop by a "suspicious" PSA and delighted to see its numbers drop whether this had anything to do with cancer or not.

I also became aware of an iatrogenic problem involved with the PSA obsession — a "suspicious" PSA number is usually followed by a biopsy of the prostate, the only authentic confirmation of cancer. In some cases, the massive spread of prostate cancer occurred *after* the biopsy. This chain of events would almost certainly not have begun if there had been no PSA test in the first place.

Hence, as in the case of breast cancer screening, the jury is out on whether mass screening of males for PSA will account for more lives lost or saved.

In 1995, Washington University-St. Louis researchers told the American Urological Assn. that detection of a "free" PSA fragment could detect 90 percent of prostate cancers and thus greatly lower the guesswork and reduce the number of unnecessary biopsies. The news was timely in that *USA Today* was reporting at about the same time that the standard PSA test was falsely diagnosing the disease in an amazing two out of three cases, which the UK confirmed later.[68]

Yielding to such data, the 100,000-member American College of Physicians (ACP) in 1997 broke with Cancer Inc. and recommended against routine prostate cancer screening for all men.[144]

And now, drugs as preventives!

True to allopathic linear logic, the oncological establishment through the NCI in 1993 launched two programs involving synthetic drugs (neither free of possible side effects) in order to *prevent* breast cancer and prostate cancer in otherwise healthy people.

Tamoxifen, considered useful in breast cancer, was being tested for five years on 16,000 randomly selected healthy women thought to be at some kind of higher risk for the disease, to see if the synthetic hormone would prevent the disease. Should the tests check out, women would be advised to stay on tamoxifen (at $3.60 per day) *for the rest of their lives*. The Women's Health Network found the effort "a perversion of women's health."[69,70]

And the NCI began a 10-year, $60 million assessment of finasteride (Proscar), which had already shown some utility against the most common (and non-malignant) form of male prostate problems, BPH (benign prostatic hypertrophy or hyperplasia), to see if it could prevent prostate cancer.[71]

Both notions are allopathic thinking writ large.

It is essential to bear in mind that even as orthodox oncology was running up the white flag in breast cancer and was baffled over what to do about prostate and to some extent colon cancer, and while the use of potentially toxic synthetic drugs as preventives was being catapulted into taxpayer-subsidized research, information was pouring in linking fatty diets to cancer in general and to various vitamins as well as (of all things) aspirin to prevention of various "forms" of the disease. A race between biological wisdom and drug company profits had thus broken out, with the cancer-stricken public caught in between.

Tamoxifen ran into trouble almost from the start — as plans for its preventive use moved ahead in the USA and Canada and as similar trials were about to begin in the United Kingdom, Australia and Italy, a thorough review of the extant literature by Adriane Fugh-Berman and Samuel Epstein found links between the drug, a synthetic steroid, and endometrial cancer, retinopathy, clot-forming events, liver problems and menopausal symptoms.[72,73]

Claiming widespread use of the compound constituted not so much disease prevention as disease substitution, they argued:

> *Tamoxifen is too dangerous to use in healthy women. The Breast Cancer Prevention Trial, by accepting the concept of disease substitution in place of disease prevention, sets a dangerous precedent in public health research. The priorities of the cancer establishment need fundamental reform . . .* [74]

British researchers also found cause for concern.[75]

Perhaps even more ominously, it became clear in 1994 (as Cox News Service reported[76]) that in 1992 the Food and Drug Administration (FDA) had dismissed warnings from one of its own safety officers that women taking part in the tamoxifen trial were being misled about the risks of taking daily doses of the stuff.

In fact, Cox reported, by Oct. 28, 1992, the very day that safety officer Paul Goebel wrote a memorandum claiming that a consent form female volunteers were required to sign downplayed the risks and overstated potential benefits of the drug, four uterine cancer victims from an earlier tamoxifen trial had already died of the disease.

In 1996, long-term studies came in with pluses and minuses for tamoxifen — it has seemed to increase better survival times for breast cancer patients treated with earlier surgery but its use beyond five years confers no such advantage and — confirming earlier warnings — is linked with increased risks of endometrial cancer and blood clots.[124]

The carcinogen-of-the-month club

In the meantime, in terms of "causes" of cancer, what we began to call "the carcinogen of the month club" continued to terrify the American (and in general the Western) population with every new disclosure that this chemical or that was linked to cancer development, usually based on animal studies.

To some extent, the hunt for carcinogenic chemicals had reached *reductio ad absurdum* proportions by the 1980s, for data derived from using proportionally gross amounts of potentially harmful chemicals on animals was being extrapolated from the infinitesimally small amounts of the same that humans might be receiving.

This did not, of course, undercut the possible dangers of continual, *accumulated* buildup of chemicals and synthetic hormones dumped into the nation's food chain (see *XV*) nor mitigate the real possibility of overexposure to all manner of industrial chemicals, pesticides, herbicides and insecticides.

The span of opinion ranged from that of Dr. Epstein, who spent a lot of time alerting the public to the understated dangers about and links between cancer and industrial chemicals, and chemical company-backed researchers and apologists who liked to pooh-pooh such attacks and were happier to blame cancer almost exclusively on tobacco. Added to both was scattered research over several years suggesting correlations between certain "forms" of cancer and exposure to electric power lines, extremely low electromagnetic fields (ELFs) in general, and to everything from television sets and electric curlers to cellular telephones, in addition to the increasingly obvious connection between cancer and prior exposure to nuclear radiation.

In 1996, a 23-member National Research Council (NRC) panel, assessing 17 years of controversy, found no "convincing evidence" of a cancer-EMF connection. But three members dissented, citing "a reliable, though low, statistical association between power lines" and leukemia.[128]

The issue had long pitted power and utility companies against independent scientists.

The radiation holocaust — 'security' and coverup

By the mid-1990s the nuclear radiation exposure/cancer connection matter was assuming research dimensions which implied a much vaster problem and was becoming far too great to be considered other than as a series of nationwide scandals.

The scandals had a whiff of political agenda since they bore on women's issues — particularly breast cancer (though, in fact, a small and even more aggressive "form" of breast cancer occurs in men) — and, as a subdivision, on higher breast cancer rates in "minority" women. But the scandals implicated the perils of radiation and cancer *in general*, a point often missed in the political hoopla.

As we noted in *II*, the dangers of radiation via X-rays and through the touted mammography program were noted years ago, although not too much attention was paid to them at the time. But subsequent research went on, and it produced worrisome questions: *is* there a "safe" dose of radiation? How long does it take for the accumulated effects of radiation to show up? How much radiation can one absorb in what amount of time before serious problems occur?

John W. Gofman MD PhD, professor emeritus of molecular and cell biology, University of California-Berkeley and former associate director of California's Livermore National Laboratory, has relentlessly crusaded to warn of the downside of "medical exposure to ionizing radiation" — one, he noted, that "is barely ever mentioned as a prime explanation for the current high rate of breast cancer."[77]

By mid-decade, the ever-quotable Dr. Epstein was on hand to warn of "mammoscam" — his assessment of "national breast cancer awareness day" for women — and to argue forcefully that there simply had not been demonstrated, as late as 1994, any benefit from mammography in premenopausal women even as the radiation industry and hawkers of radiological products were plumbing the "pre-menopausal market."[78]

Even more ominously, data released in 1993 by Ernest J. Sternglass, professor emeritus of radiology, University of Pittsburgh, and Jay M. Gould, of the Radiation and Public Health Project, New York, found "highly significant rises" in breast cancer over time among women who lived near nuclear reactors. Breast cancer mortality rates in 268 counties within 50 miles of reactors were studied.[79]

At a San Diego meeting, Dr. Sternglass asserted:

> *For the period between 1950 and 1989, the age-adjusted breast cancer mortality rate rose 10 percent near the reactors and only 4 percent for the average in the US. Of the 51 sites involved that began operation before 1982, the five oldest operated by the Department of Energy such as Hanford and Oak Ridge known to have had the largest releases registered an even greater increase of breast cancer mortality of 41 percent, from 20.7 deaths per 100,000 women in the five-year period 1950-54 to 29.2 in 1985-89.*[80]

The scientists pointed out that in the case of Oak Ridge TN, one of the oldest sites of atomic bomb development,

> *[F]or the downwind counties within 40 miles, the breast cancer mortality increased by 39 percent, in striking contrast to a 4 percent decline for women living in four nearby upwind counties.* The same pattern exists for all cancers combined (*emphasis mine*).[81]

The Sternglass-Gould research — admittedly "in response to

the call by the National Breast Cancer Coalition for an increase in investigator-initiated research to find the cause for the recent sharp rise in breast cancer" — used official data from the Nuclear Regulatory Commission (NRC) and the National Cancer Institute (NCI) to reach its sobering conclusions and cannot be said to have juggled figures to prove a point.

The work bore a great deal on "very low concentrations of radioactivity in milk, meat and drinking water" and the nuclear fission products strontium-90 and iodine-131. Such "tiny emissions are almost as dangerous as the Hiroshima explosion and nobody wanted to believe it," said Dr. Sternglass.[82] ***(See NOTE, Page 485)***

Abstracting from copious data before them, Drs. Sternglass and Gould summarized that nuclear fission products in diet and drinking water constituted "the previously neglected factor in the rise of breast and other types of cancer that has accelerated since the operation of large nuclear reactors began" and that

> *Tragically, the desire to build and test ever larger numbers of nuclear weapons and therefore to suppress all research and epidemiological studies of very low dose effects of nuclear fallout . . . because of fear that serious health effects of nuclear fallout would lead to a demand for an end to nuclear weapons testing . . . led to the premature construction of nuclear plants near large population areas before the seriousness of free-radical damage to the cells of the immune system produced by strontium-90 and other bone-seeking fission products was recognized . . .*
>
> *Failure to face these mistakes of the cold war will not only cause further increases in human suffering, but it will also prevent us from slowing the enormous rise in health-care costs brought about by the combination of costly medical technology and the rising incidence of cancer and other chronic diseases now known to be caused by the action of free radicals that are produced by the fission products, often acting synergistically with other toxic agents and*

hormones that we are continuing to release into our milk, our drinking water and our diet.[83]

(One of the synthetic hormones added to milk, gonadotropin-releasing hormone [GRH], may, according to Dr. Epstein, induce osteoporosis, and its advocacy among California scientists to counteract the "incessant ovulation" that some argue is a "cause" of increased breast cancer "promotes the interests of Imperial Chemical [a United Kingdom-based pharmaceutical giant]."[84])

The charges made by various investigators looking into the hidden-radiation peril are that as early as 1943, or even before the first atomic bomb was exploded, American scientists knew that there were extreme dangers involving nuclear fallout — and that the US government secretly experimented in hundreds (and probably thousands) of tests on humans to attempt to determine what the dangers were.

In a "preliminary report" released in 1994, the 14-member Advisory Committee on Human Radiation Experiments, a group of investigators reviewing the history of government-sponsored atomic experiments, found that

> *Cold War secrecy and bureaucratic sprawl created a patchwork of policies that unwittingly exposed many humans to potentially dangerous radiation [and] government officials extensively debated the need for human experimentation and the policies that should govern it. But because that debate was often secret, many contractors and university researchers apparently were unaware of the legal and ethical concerns surrounding the experiments they were paid to conduct.*[85]

Johns Hopkins University medical ethicist Ruth Faden, a panel member, claimed that the group had documented 400 government-sponsored radiation experiments that exposed humans to radiation between 1947 and 1977 but that by the time the huge data-gathering effort was to be completed the number of experiments probably would turn out to be "in the thousands."

In a "final tally" released in 1995, the Department of Energy (DOE) acknowledged that 16,000 Americans had been used in radiation experiments from World War II to 1970. It claimed many such experiments were for "heroic" medical purposes."[86] By 1997, the federal government was beginning to reimburse survivors with millions of dollars in compensation for admittedly "unethical" behavior.

The radiation-exposure problem may explain in part the unusually high rates not only of cancer in general but also elements of immune dysregulation (*XIV*) in such areas as New Mexico, home of Los Alamos and many other experimental nuclear outlets — a state where, I was staggered to learn in 1994, more than a tenth of the entire adult population was on the federal payroll, particularly that of the Department of Energy (DOE).

It is in vintage nuclear-experiment New Mexico where, quite aside from above-normal levels of breast and other "forms" of cancer, so many victims of alleged "e.i." (environmental illness) cluster that it may become increasingly difficult to find a truly healthy resident of the state. It is also true that clusters of "e.i." patients moved there from other polluted areas of the USA seeking open spaces and better air in a quest for improved health. To a great extent, they have not found it.

Intriguingly, the onrush of information as to radiation (obvious, low-dose or occult) and its connection to cancer and to immunological disarray in general points to the increasing validity of oxidology (*XVI*) as a vital medical subspecialty — both in explaining the nature of many chronic disorders and their resolution.

There is also increased information to suggest that various toxic chemicals, as well as synthetic hormones, particularly estrogens — and of various substances the human immune system(s) may "scan" *as* estrogens — may interact with radiation. Given the frequent disturbance of a woman's hormone pool by steroids and "the pill," quite aside from enforced life-long dependence on estrogens and/or progesterone following hysterectomies or other medical events, and the interplay of substances the body may detect *as* estrogens let alone alterations already underway due to accumulated low-dose or other radiation, there can be little wonder that breast cancer rates are so stratospheric that the actual incidence may soon be closer to 1 out of 8 rather than the (as of 1995) officially recognized 1 out of 9 in the USA.

In the meantime, the chemical industry itself is not too entranced with research which may indicate a malignancy-"organizing" role for the multiple substances of industry and agriculture — yet testing them for possible carcinogenicity has itself become a major industry in the hunt for "causes" of cancer.

Suffer the little animals

The animal research industry, itself a multi-billion-dollar undertaking involving the breeding and mutation of animals, typically mice, rats and rabbits, and also of chimpanzees and monkeys, has usually been the conduit through which information on alleged carcinogenic dangers developed.

In the oncological industry, in alignment with allopathic thinking and the dictates of the Food and Drug Administration (FDA), there arose an imperative to test both suspected cancer-blocking drugs as well as suspected cancer-causing agents on animals — which, when one thinks of it for more than five seconds, is frankly irrational.

The extremes of oncological inanity occur as tumors taken from another species are transplanted into animals already bred to have no significant immune response. Then potential anti-cancer drugs are used on such animals (that is, against their transplanted tumors) to see "what will happen." If there seems to be tumor reduction, this result is then transferred to the human species — an allopathically sound, FDA-approved chain of linear thought. A major reason for testing cancer drugs on animals, of course, is that, given their inherent toxicity, it somehow would be immoral to try out a suspected toxic drug on humans willy-nilly — so why not force it on animals, however far removed by species they might be from *Homo sapiens*, to establish an "LD50" (code for "dose at which 50 percent of a given lot of test animals will die of lethal effects")?

A similar cascade of linear thought has occurred in testing compounds thought to be cancer-causing (carcinogenic): use amounts of the substance at biologically unreasonable levels in animals to test their possible carcinogenicity. If found to be carcinogenic, announce this fact to the world.

There certainly are *some* reasons to follow both lines of reasoning — but they pale alongside the central consideration: the only appropriate test model for a human being as it relates to that which might "cause" or "cure" cancer or anything else is man himself. This simple truth dislodges much of the underpinning of the heavily funded "vivisectionist" industry (experiments on sentient animals for either drug or cosmetic development, sometimes reaching levels of horrific cruelty).

But in the medical/pharmaceutical world of cancer — since virtually *every* alleged cancer-blocking drug *is* toxic or potentially toxic, even at a relatively modest level — there is no escaping a certain amount of animal tests before a compound may be "cleared" for human use.

(The same system, parenthetically, makes it frankly either impossible or unreasonable to test non-toxic, natural, nutritional factors on animals. How measure the anti-cancer or antioxidant effects of exogenous Vitamin C, for example, on test animals, most of which already produce their *own* Vitamin C? How *really* test for "toxicity" in naturally-occurring laetrile in a test rat, let alone determine what the "useful dose" of apricot-seed extract is on a human while injecting it into a hybrid animal in which a tumor has been transplanted?)

In *Science* in 1990, research scientists not known for being unfriendly to industry dismissed as "bankrupt" the idea that cramming test animals with carcinogenic compounds and issuing the results, thus "scaring the country sick," is a rational thing to do.

University of California biochemist Bruce Ames, who has long argued there are as many or more "natural" carcinogens in plants and the pristine environment than produced by the chemical industry, said in new research that there was a growing body of biological evidence to suggest that often it was not the chemical makeup of a substance, but the high dose of it, which produced cancer in laboratory animals.[87]

And in 1991, the federal Environmental Protection Agency (EPA) came up with research showing that male rats have a special protein (alpha-2U-globulin, not found in humans) that makes them particularly *prone* to cancer — a disclosure which, it was thought, might very well invalidate literally millions of tests of chemicals, herbicides, pesticides, preservatives and additives which have been banned because of their cancer-causing potential in rats.

In its own peculiar language, the EPA stated that cancer found in laboratory rats is a "species-specific effect inapplicable to human risk assessment."[88]

The ACS: propaganda central

The great amount of what Americans know or think about cancer is heavily influenced by the American Cancer Society (ACS), whose name suggests a degree of officialness which it does not have. Hardly any literate American is unaware of ACS smokeouts, celebrity yacht cruises, elegant fund-raising events of all kinds, and the noisy campaigns against cigarette smoking and in favor of mammograms. Most news media are well aware of the annual "science writers' conferences" at which the ACS wines, dines and "informs" science writers and assorted journalists so they can be kept "updated" on the latest breakthroughs in cancer research and application.

The vision of selfless volunteers going door to door soliciting coins for the endless war on cancer constantly comes to mind. And, truth to tell, the marching troops of the ACS are indeed well-meaning volunteers — just as the marching troops of the originally anti-polio March of Dimes, American Heart Assn.

(AHA) and American Lung Assn. (ALA), plus lesser charities, were and are well-meaning volunteers.

But time, vested interests, the establishment of bureaucratic monoliths and, naturally, the management of money, take their toll on *any* organization, be it charitable or not (see *III*).

In 1990, charities critic and economics professor James T. Bennett reported that the ACS held land valued at $14 million, $42 million worth of buildings and leasehold improvements, and $6 million in buildings under construction."[89]

In 1992, the ACS — whose influence over the smaller, federally funded NCI has long been described as the classic example of the tail wagging the dog — was kept scrambling to explain away a piercing article by University of Tennessee-Chattanooga economics professor Thomas J. DiLorenzo.

In the *Wall Street Journal*, DiLorenzo charged that "ACS affiliates have diverted substantial sums away from providing cancer service in order to accumulate large holdings of cash, securities, land and buildings."[90]

He claimed that "the typical affiliate spends more than 52 percent of its budget on salaries, pensions, fringe benefits and overhead" and that "chief executive officers earn six-figure salaries in a number of states."

He added:

> *For every $1 spent on direct service, approximately $6.40 is spent on compensation and overhead . . . The financial statements . . . reveal that Cancer Society affiliates are wealthy organizations, despite their fund-raising appeals, which stress an urgent and critical need for donations to provide cancer services.*
>
> *As of 1990 the California affiliate . . . had accumulated $36 million in cash, certificates of deposit and securities; Florida had set aside $20 million; Texas, Ohio and Colorado held about $10 million each. The average affiliate in this sample of 10 held $10.8 million in cash reserves.*[91]

He reported that, in terms of land and buildings, the Texas ACS affiliate had $11.3 million in such assets, and the California and Florida affiliates more than $3 million in property.

The then-current ACS president, responding in the *WSJ*, called ACS financial statements a "snapshot in time" which reflected both program expenses of a current year and funds accumulated for the following year's programs and made much of the fact the Society was the "first non-profit health organization to use an independent auditor and issue a combined national financial annual report."[92]

The Society, he said, "does not spend money it does not have," although how this could be used to "categorically refute each of the allegations by Thomas J. DiLorenzo" was not clear.

In 1994, DiLorenzo and Dr. Bennett noted that for every $1 spent by the ACS for research, Americans paid $15 — and that the National Cancer Institute was spending more on cancer research each year than the ACS had in the past half century. They added that at the end of 1993 the ACS had a net worth of $520.3 million — and owned more than $61 million in real estate.[93]

The ACS had earlier been looked at with a critical eye by investigative reporter Peter Barry Chowka, who wrote in 1978 that in fiscal 1976 the Society had spent $114 million while its assets totalled $181 million and that between 1970 and 1973 ACS' net profit doubled.

Moreover, he noted:

> *With so many millions of dollars invested and deposited in checking and savings accounts, ACS is a prime banking customer. At least eighteen members of the ACS Board of Directors and House of Delegates are executive officers or directors of banks. As of August 31, 1976, 42 percent of ACS' cash and investments, totalling $75 million, were maintained in banks with which these eighteen men were affiliated.*[94]

In 1977, as part of its ongoing review of the national "Conquest of Cancer" effort, the House Committee on

Governmental Operations, while investigating the NCI, found that the federal agency and the ACS in effect had interlocking directorates — though neither side had taken particular pains to hide this fact, and it was not a crime.

As this writer noted in 1983:

> *The most obvious example of the comfortable relationship between the NCI as a spender of taxpayer monies in the cancer war and the major lobby for conducting that war in the first place was the hiring of former NCI Director Frank Rauscher as an ACS senior vice president — at a doubling of his annual salary.*[95]

The spectacular fund-raising successes of the American Cancer Society (ACS) and its strong influence over how research funds are ultimately used is due to the fact it has long been dominated by experts in advertising, public relations and business.

Indeed, the PR volleys which the ACS annually fires off in a most professional way can largely be attributed to the virtual takeover of an otherwise lackluster charity (founded in 1913) by Albert Lasker, "father of modern advertising," and his socially well connected wife, Mary, and Elmer Bobst, "father of the modern drug industry."[96]

Some rays of hope

In defense of the ACS, it can be said that the Society, for all its excesses, took cancer — once a whispered-about malady rarely mentioned in polite society — out of the closet. As cancer rates climbed, it was infinitely better to draw attention to it than to try to obscure the reality. And the ACS campaign against cigarette smoking — over-done in that ACS has been too quick to blame cancer in general on tobacco, hence providing the oncological industry with a partial excuse for failure (people just won't stop smoking) — has been salutary to the extent that there are a lot of health problems connected with lighting up and nicotine addiction appears to be the toughest of all to overcome.

It is also true that, despite the fact that the Society has been a heavy hitter against "alternative" cancer therapies and a major voice of disinformation against such "unapproved" approaches as laetrile, it has nonetheless been more open to integrating new information than certain other elements of Cancer Inc.

After arguing for years that anybody who connected cancer with diet was deluded at best, a charlatan at worst (the Cancer Inc. general "line" for decades), the ACS, yielding to a torrent of epidemiological, biochemical and empirical research to the contrary, gradually switched its position.

While in the 1950s it had actually lobbied Congress to hold hearings to investigate what it considered to be false claims that there was a connection between nutrition and cancer, by 1989 the Society had zig-zagged by about 180 degrees and could baldfacedly state:

> *There is strong evidence that perhaps people can be protected from cancer by what they eat or drink, or by other substances or lifestyles that serve as defense mechanisms . . . This is a new and important area which needs further research so that recommendations can be developed on how people should change their lifestyles to reduce their chances of getting cancer.*[97]

By the 1990s, the Society was running ads and television spots *in defense* of the concept that a more vegetarian, more fruit-oriented, lower-refined carbohydrate, lower-animal fat and protein, higher-natural fiber diet might be associated with the prevention of cancer!

For long-time ACS watchers and observers of Cancer Inc., this campaign represented a quantum leap away from earlier established doctrine that it was just plain insane to make any connection between cancer and diet. It also, of course, strongly validated what numerous physicians and researchers long derided as "cancer quacks" had been saying for decades.

By this writing, the ACS was not quite ready to take the next leap (bearing in mind the aphorism that "that which prevents, also cures") to actually *suggest* elements in the cancer-prevention diet might also be used to *treat* it, despite growing evidence to that effect from biochemistry — a discipline always a decade or more ahead of medicine itself. But it *was* "studying" the idea. Hope springs eternal . . .

The fact that major executives of the ACS, AHA or ALA have large salaries, or that such operations as the ACS have bulging bank accounts and heavy investments in real estate and buildings implies neither criminal nor immoral behavior — it simply points to one of the ambivalent elements in the American healthcare mess:

There is a lot of money to be made in "charity" fund-raising, and organizations aimed at solving a problem, no matter how noble the cause or effort, will, when exposed to hard cash, tend to self-perpetuate.

By mid-decade, Cancer Inc.'s continuing attack on "alternative therapies" — the vast majority of them involving nutritional approaches to cancer — was beginning to ring hollow, despite the enthusiasm and barbarity with which the FDA and other federal state and local agencies continued to raid nutritional-therapy clinics, arrest offending doctors and terrify patients (*I*).

It was simply clear that a wide range of nutrients, including some veteran standbys (Vitamins A,C,E, beta-carotene, selenium, certain B vitamins) and some "non-nutritive food factors" and "phytochemicals" in the plant kingdom (phenols, indoles, isothiocyanates, monoterpenes) by themselves and/or within whole foods, where they were joined by other ingredients, and even some spices and condiments,[(98)] were associated with the prevention of cancer.

Research around the world said so and, most importantly, research at home said so.

Sometimes research came up with unexpected findings and bolstered unpopular theories:

In 1996, the Nutritional Prevention of Cancer Study Group, studying the effects of 200 mcg per day of selenium or placebo in 1,312 patients seen at seven dermatology clinics in the Eastern US, was looking for effects of the mineral on skin "cancers" — basal and squamous cell carcinoma.

The investigators found that selenium treatment did not seem to protect against the skin cancer "types" — yet seemed to reduce the incidence of "carcinomas of several sites," particularly lung, colorectal and prostate. Unitarianism?[136] An "independent trial of appropriate design" was called for before "new public health recommendations regarding selenium can be made."

By 1997, information on anti-cancer factors within grapes and wine was growing too fast to be ignored. A food research group at the University of Illinois-Chicago found that the substance *resveratrol* in grapes can help keep healthy cells from turning malignant and inhibit the spread of malignant cells.[137] Such research, and that of other lines of investigation on grapes from which red and white wines are made, would seem to be a back-handed defense of the "grape cure" of cancer promoted in "alternative" circles decades ago.

University of Nevada research published in 1997 enhanced claims made for the effects of the "omega" fatty acids as found in fish oil — that fish oil fed to mice shrinks breast tumors while reducing the wasting syndrome (cachexia) and other toxic effects often associated with cancer chemotherapy treatments.[138]

Such research, including findings that lycopene, a carotenid antioxidant found only in tomatoes, seems to reduce the risk of prostate cancer, helped strengthen claims for the "Mediterranean diet" (including wine, tomato sauce, pastas) already said to help reduce "heart disease (*see X*).

With ever-conflictive information both damning and condoning coffee consumption over the years, champions of the black brew were cheered in 1997 with University of California chemist Takayuki Shibamato's research showing that freshly brewed coffee forms potent antioxidants (volatile heterocyclics) which may help prevent cancer — which researchers of *in vitro* studies called "an exciting start."[139]

Research from many areas points to cancer-fighting properties in green tea to anti-cancer "liminoids" in numerous fruits to a synthetic form of vitamin D and even to pasta and other complex — but not simple — carbohydrates.[(140)]

In 1992, on the heels of an assessment by the NCI of strong links between cancer prevention and dietary factors in an impressive 156 studies, a national survey to examine eating habits was launched by the Cancer Society (*XV*).[(99)]

And, in 1994, nutritional aspects in cancer constituted a major theme at the annual convention of the American Assn. for the Advancement of Science (AAAS).

There, the aforementioned Dr. Ames was on hand to note that of 172 studies in the orthodox scientific (that is, "Club") literature examining the role of fruits and vegetables in cancer prevention, 129 had shown a "significant protective effect." He and others noted that while the general overview is that one can cut one's risk in half "for every major cancer" by eating far more fruits and vegetables, virtually no research money was going in to bolster such stupendous conclusions.[(100)]

In 1995, a 400-scientist meeting called by the American Institute for Cancer Research revealed that more than 200 studies had been done on the relationship between cancer, fruits and vegetables, the vast majority showing correlations.[(101)]

In 1996, Daniel Nixon MD, Medical University of South Carolina, claiming that recent reseach connected diet with the prevention of "nearly seventy percent" of cancers, observed that science knew of nearly "one thousand possible chemotherapeutic compounds in plants" useful against cancer.[(125)]

Diet and malignancy

How diet and nutrition might affect cancer causatively let alone therapeutically falls into several areas:

— Ways in which refined carbohydrates or other aspects of a chemically altered food supply may directly influence cellular integrity so that a cell, in allegiance to the implied primary directive of life itself — adapt or die — may adapt by reverting to its primitive (that is, cancer-like) stage.

— Ways in which toxic chemicals used to treat or process food may, by accumulation, lead to a possible cancer-organizing cascade, including factors which the body may scan as hormone-like and hence respond to by altering its own "pool" of such messenger substances, leading to "hormone-dependent" expressions of cancer, particularly breast and ovarian in women and prostate in men.

— Ways in which overly fatty diets may help provide reservoirs for toxic synthetic chemicals which in turn can initiate the cancer process.

— Ways in which specific dietary and nutritive deficiencies deplete the body's store of natural scavengers of toxic oxygen ("free radicals"), allowing the latter to proliferate and damage every system in the body (cancer itself utilizing the "free radical cascade" as a way to spread) and possibly to induce the malignant process itself via genetic damage (*see XVI*).

— Ways in which certain "phytochemicals" inhibit "phase 1" enzymes or induce "phase 2" enzymes, said to be of key importance in carcinogen exposure.

— Ways in which various nutrients may enhance host defense and aspects of immunity indirectly against the malignant process.

— Ways in which excesses (for example, of animal protein) may interfere with a natural defense system (proteolytic enzymes) against cancer, enhancing the malignant process.

(As we shall see [*XII*], the "laetrile theory" has much going for it since a class of compounds described as *nitrilosides* or "Vitamin B17" seems strongly linked to the prevention of clinical cancer and, in the form of laetrile, to be useful in its management — the heart of one of this century's major medical controversies).

Each of these areas presents a world of biochemical possibilities which in their totality add up to the importance of diet in the induction and/or suppression of the malignant process, with some relevance at every step of the process.

The dietary element — by this reckoning — would be

involved regardless of all other aspects — presumed hereditary predispositions (genetics), possible "organizing" events such as viruses and radiation, inadequate wound healing, and even mental stress, the effects of a universe of manmade synthetic chemicals affecting both the internal and external ecology of human beings, and alterations in the hormone pool, part of which may be directly related either to dietary or chemical factors.

For 'control' rather than 'cure'

For decades, practitioners who usually call themselves "metabolic therapists," whether their view of cancer is unitarian or not, have been more likely to seek the "control" of cancer than the "cure" — for, as we have seen, "cure" is at its best a supremely deceptive and tricky word which, to many people, means the entire eradication of a disease and the likelihood it will never occur again.

Many of the views of metabolic doctors have focused on the reality that cancer is itself not an interloper, not a foreign invader (the probable reason why an immune response is *not* mounted against it, at least in the early phase) — and hence not "curable" in the classical sense of the word.

Such physicians — and metabolically oriented writers, including the present author — have stated that the maximum goal in cancer management, therefore, should be *control* and that the most common analogy is diabetes. The latter is a chronic, systemic condition which is not basically "curable" (though it has reportedly been reversed through diet) but which can be controlled for the whole of an individual's genetically predisposed span of life by diet alone or diet plus insulin. A diabetic may thus live a life that is within 90 percent of "normal". Most metabolic physicians argue that the same is true for cancer.

Cancer should be controllable and manageable for the whole of a person's life. This is the strong suggestion from long-term survivors of even very advanced malignancies who have been on nutritionally-oriented, essentially natural, metabolic treatment regimens.

Such doctors and researchers, for so long denounced as quacks, could only express some satisfaction when the Western cancer establishment began, in this decade, actually to start speaking in the same terms.

In a 1994 *Journal of the American Medical Assn. (JAMA),* a "commentary" by Alan B. Jastrow, St. Vincent's Hospital and Medical Center, New York, was called "Rethinking Cancer." In it, Dr. Jastrow further expanded on arguments made by a Canadian research group in 1993 — namely, that the goal of cancer therapy might better be "controlling" rather than "curing" malignancy.[102]

In a spring 1994 *Time*, Dr. Lance Liotta, described as "the [NCI's] leading metastasis expert," stated something oncologically unthinkable just a few years before:

> "*After all, we don't cure diseases like diabetes and hypertension. We control them. Why can't we look at cancer that way?*"[103]

This was conceptual progress by any definition.

Later the same year, a Canadian investigator (and Canadian and British cancer experts seemed to take the lead in arguing for the new paradigm[126]), assessing the calamity of breast cancer in women, seemed to be undergoing virtual holistic catharsis in a "viewpoint" editorial in *The Lancet*. Dr. James E. Devitt observed:

> *In focusing on the breast lesion, the tree, have we failed to see the forest, the whole patient with her plethora of growth-restraining factors, both systemic and local, and of the growth potential directed by the chromosomes in each cell? If the breast lesion is not the cause of the disease but merely the local expression of a combination of changes in both local and systemic growth-restraining factors, and if such a combination was more or less specific for producing breast-tissue-like growths, they would be more easily induced and occur earlier in breast tissues. . .*[104]

And Canadian cancer specialists in 1996 made it even clearer:

"... [R]ather than trying to cure cancer by killing off every last cell, it would make more sense to control the disease, and extend latent disease-free periods ..."[130]

The same year, one Establishment view of the US "war on cancer" was that "obsession with cure of advanced disease rather than the prevention of early disease, and the need to arrest preneoplastic lesions ... have served to make victory elusive."[105]

In grappling with the nature of the cancer cell itself — now much more understood through the revolution in basic molecular and cell biology in recent years — Dr. Michael Sporn observed:

[T]he process of carcinogenesis, which is driven by multiple interactive factors, including genetic mutation, excessive cell proliferation, and changes in the extracellular milieu, entails a prolonged series of many failures in the reciprocal interactions between epithelium and its underlying stroma.[106]

A free translation would be that there are many elements involved in the malignant process, not just genetic ones.

Breakthroughs in understanding the nature of the cancer cell have, perhaps unintentionally, helped bolster the "oxidation," "primordial" and "trophoblastic" theories of cancer origin.

In 1996, Stanford University researchers —closing in on gene p53 and the failure of various anti-cancer drugs — developed a model to explain how utilization of oxygen is influenced by the size of an incipient malignancy and how advancing hypoxia (absence of oxygen) will help trigger the genetic changes ("p53-mediated apoptosis") which will help surviving cells multiply more rapidly into more aggressive cancer.[107]

In 1995, research by Hernan F. Acevedo *et al.* strengthened a cancer unitarian approach by noting that portions of the hormone human chorionic gonadotropin (hCG), already known to be a common feature both of embryonic *and* cancer cells (ostensibly for protection against immune response), could be recovered from 78 "malignant cell lines" and that genes governing hCG production were "active in every sample" in 28 of them.[108]

While the more recent Acevedo research might lead to vaccine development it again strengthened both a unitarian concept of cancer and the older "trophoblastic" theory (*see XII*) which found so many connections between the birth-related tissue and cancer that it considered them one and the same.

In 1996, a Seattle biochemist presented evidence that cancer is more the result of free-radical attack on genes than it is of dysfunctional genes. Such evidence strongly supported the idea of consuming antioxidant nutrients. (*See also XVI*)[131]

But research is one thing. Politics and economics is another.

While dramatic new ideas of cancer were developing, Cancer Inc. was not about to let "natural" therapies go unchallenged.

More tigers in the jungle

The new tigers in the jungle that Cancer Inc. was seeking — depending on the situation — to exterminate, co-opt or control going into the end of this decade, believing (incorrectly) that it had gotten rid of laetrile, include these:

• 714X, essentially a camphor-based product promoted in Canada and finding numerous adherents, particularly in the USA, where FDA "regulatory action" — naturally — swung into high gear against it in mid-decade.

• The late Canadian nurse Rene Caisse's Essiac herbal tea, which had been around for many decades and is now produced by several companies while gathering supporters particularly from the cancer and AIDS communities.[110]

• Both bovine and shark cartilage, the center of a major controversy in the 1990s largely due to the success of an insightful book by William Lane[111] but largely building on earlier research by Dr. John Prudden.[112] Cuban research had sustained in part some of the claims made for shark cartilage (particularly its apparent ability to block *angiogenesis*, whereby cancer tumors create their own circulatory systems) and NCI trials on the substance began in 1995.

• The various natural products developed over decades by the brilliant Rumanian-born physician/scientist Emanuel Revici MD of New York, who turned 100 in 1996 and, despite many years of harassment by New York state authorities, had to his credit some of the best-documented long-term survivors of cancer and AIDS.[113]

• The antineoplaston therapy of Polish-born physician/biochemist Stanislaw Burzynski (*see I*), a long-running controversy which reached nationwide and global dimensions as Burzynski and his patients fought for their right to use a widely researched and essentially non-toxic substance that even the NCI licensed for investigation.

Cancer Inc. seemed exceedingly slow to respond to the presence of several well-documented or long-used modalities internationally known but either blocked or ignored in the US. These include, among the better known:

• Medical ozone, with which thousands of Europeans have been treated for cancer, AIDS and numerous other conditions; as well as other oxidative agents, including hydrogen peroxide, Dioxychlor and similar products (s*ee XVI*).

• MTH-68, a modified attenuated strain of the Newcastle disease virus in chickens.

• Iscador, a liquid extract of *Viscum album*, the mistletoe plant, used experimentally for much of this century against specific tumors.

• Ukrain, a drug derived from the folk-remedy herb greater celandine (*Chelidonium majus*), which itself had been in medical use for more than 3,500 years. European research and some in the USA found the semisynthetic derivative highly beneficial both as a non-toxic cancer treatment and an immune booster.[114,115]

• Hydrazine sulfate, the rocket fuel-derived therapy researched and promoted by Dr. Joseph Gold with some credible research and application internationally.[116,117]

• Carnivora (as drops for oral or inhalation use and as the injectable product Carnivorain), Dr. Helmut Keller's well-researched extract of the Venus flytrap (*Dionaea muscipula*). Rave reviews over more than a decade have brought almost a "magic-bullet cure" status for cancer, AIDS and other conditions to this product, rather similar to claims made for "cures" by ozone. It clearly has a lot going for it but has been ignored by US orthodoxy.[118,119]

• The butyrates, certain fatty acids on which a surprisingly significant amount of research as to anti-cancer value has been done.[120,121]

• Or the never-convincingly-described CanCell, which has its own share of living and breathing true believers and which the FDA has tried desperately to stamp out as an "unproven new drug."

• Or the late Dr. Lawrence Burton's IAT (immunoaugmentative therapy), driven to the Bahamas from New York, and to which some patients believe they owe their lives.[122]

• Or meaningful followup on Dr. Chisato Maruyama's anti-cancer vaccine in Japan, which has aided tens of thousands of patients in many countries.[123]

• Or the placenta-based VG-1000 therapy of Russian immunologist Valentin I. Govallo, carrying a reported 64 percent 20-year survival rate, a striking figure by anybody's calculations.

Or, in what may turn out to be major egg-on-your-face results for America's IQ-challenged "quackbusters," who long derided blue-green algae as "pond scum," cryptophycin, a promising NCI research-backed algae compound, and *Spirulina fusiformis*, a beta carotene-rich algae, eliminated preneoplastic lesions in WHO-and US Department of Agriculture-supported research in India. In 1996 the former was on the way to being developed for market in its synthetic (and thus far more expensive) form by a major pharmaceutical company.[129]

• Or "Rife machines," speaking to lines of bioelectrical and magnetic therapy which have a highly interesting pedigree (*see XVII*).

• To say nothing of the closely-guarded "Greek treatment" (a combination of apparently non-toxic compounds for intravenous use) of the late Dr. Hariton Alivizatos; metallurgy-derived "chondriana" or "life crystals"; and a special herb combination designed to wipe out intestinal flukes said by one proponent to be, when in the presence of isopropyl alcohol, a "universal cause" of cancer.

True, patients threatened by death from cancer often — and understandably — carom from one off-the-wall "cure" to another. However silly some of the ideas and however many opportunists have crowded the field, the real guilty party (in suppressing many cancer alternatives while promoting so many that do not work) remains made-in-America Cancer Inc., through its abject inability to stop much cancer.

As some have noted, most of the better-known "alternatives" which Cancer Inc. has so viciously suppressed have one or more things in common:

They are usually (a) natural, (b) non-toxic, (c) essentially inexpensive, (d) not patentable as new drugs, (e) researched abroad even if developed originally in the US, and (f) highly effective in one or more aspects of the disease.

But perhaps the proudest old tiger still growling in Cancer Inc.'s jungle remains laetrile — which, more than any other single factor, had so shaken Cancer Inc. and the whole AIC that neither would ever fully recover.

References

1. *The Choice*, XVII:2, 1991.
2. Cited in *The Choice*, XVIII:1, 1992.
3. Cited in *The Choice*, XVIII:1, 1992.
4. Cited in *The Choice*, XVIII:1, 1992.
5. McCullough, Marie, Knight-Ridder News Service, Nov. 14, 1996.
6. American Cancer Society, January 1993.
7. Davis, DL, *et al.*, *J. Am. Med. Assn.*, Feb. 9, 1994.
8. *Meditrends 1991-1992*, American Hospital Assn., May 1991.
9. *The Choice*, XVIII:1, 1992.
10. Cimons, Marlene, *Los Angeles Times*, Sept. 30, 1994.
11. Neergaard, Lauran, Associated Press, July 4, 1996.
12. Sporn, MB, "The war on cancer." *Lancet*, May 8, 1996.
13. Neergaard, *op. cit.*
14. Culbert, ML. *What The Medical Establishment Won't Tell You That Could Save Your Life.*

Norfolk VA: Donning, 1983.
15. *J. Am. Med. Assn.*, cited in *The Choice*, XVI:4, 1990.
16. *Ibid.*
17. National Cancer Institute national cancer survey, August 1991.
18. Beardsley, Tim, "A war not won." *Scientific American*, January 1994.
19. National Cancer Institute chart, in Beardsley, *loc. sit.*
20. Testimony before "Cancer treatment: new directions for the 1990s" seminar, convened by Staten Island Borough President Guy V. Molinari, New York, September 1993.
21. *Cancer Chronicles*, cited in *The Choice*, XVI:2,3, 1990.
22. *Ibid.*
23. *The Choice*, XIX: 3,4, 1993.
24. *Ibid.*
25. *Ibid.*
26. Moertel, Charles, in *J. Am. Med. Assn.*, Aug. 25, 1993.
27. Fletcher, RH, in *J. Am. Med. Assn.*, Aug. 25, 1993.
28. Morris, JDH, *et. al.*, "Viral infection and cancer." *Lancet*, Sept. 6, 1995.
29. *The Choice*, XX:1, 1994.
30. "The Rosetta stone of cancer study." *US News & World Report*, March 4, 1996.
31. Dermer, GB, *The Immortal Cell*. Garden City Park NY: Avery, 1994.
32. *Ibid.*
33. *Ibid.*
34. "When DNA isn't destiny." *Newsweek*, Dec. 6, 1993.
35. Lehrman, Sally, *San Francisco Examiner*, March 6, 1994.
36. Bradford, RW, and HW Allen, *The Primordial Thesis of Cancer*. Chula Vista CA: Bradford Research Institute, 1990.
37. *New Eng. J. Med.*, Jan. 4, 1990.
38. *The Choice*, XVI:1, 1990.
39. *Ibid.*
40. *Ibid.*
41. *The Choice*, XVI: 2,3, 1990.
42. *Ibid.*
43. *Lancet*, April 13, 1991.
44. Sartori, Sergio, *et al.*, *Ann. Int. Med.*, February 1991.
45. Lipschultz, SE, *et al.*, *New Eng. J. Med.*, March 21, 1991.
46. *The Choice*, XVII:1, 1991.
47. *Ibid.*
48. *The Choice*, XVII: 3,4, 1991.
49. *The Choice*, XIX:2, 1993.
50. *Ibid.*
51. *The Choice*, XVIII: 1, 1992.
52. *USA Today*, Dec. 23, 1991.
53. *The Washington Post*. Feb. 5, 1992.
54. General Accounting Office (GAO), January 1992.
55. Canadian National Breast Cancer Screening Study, Nov. 13, 1992, cited in *The Choice*, XVIII: 3, 1992.
56. "Breast cancer: have we lost our way?" *Lancet*, Feb. 6, 1993.
57. *The Choice*, XX: 1, 1994.
58. *The Choice*, XIX: 1, 1993.
59. *The Choice*, XIX: 2, 1993.
60. Fletcher, *loc. cit.*
61. The *Sacramento Bee*, Nov. 8, 1992.
62. *J. Am. Med. Assn.*. cited in *The Choice*. XVIII: 2. 1992.

63. *Ibid.*
64. *J. Am. Med. Assn.*. May 26, 1993.
65. Chodak, Gerald. *New Eng. J. Med.*. Jan. 27, 1994.
66. *The Choice*, XX: 2-3, 1994.
67. Winslow, Ron. "Prostate-cancer test may be more costly than beneficial." *Wall Street Journal*, Sept. 14, 1994.
68. *The Choice*, XXI:2, 1995.
69. *The Choice*, XVIII: 2, 1992.
70. *The Choice*, XX: 1, 1994.
71. *The Choice*, XIX: 3,4, 1993.
72. Fugh-Berman, Adriane, and Samuel Epstein, "Tamoxifen: disease prevention or disease substitution?" *Lancet*, Nov. 7, 1992.
73. Fugh-Berman, Adriane, and Samuel Epstein, "Tamoxifen for breast cancer prevention: a cautionary review." *Reviews on Endocrine-Related Cancer* 43, 1993.
74. *Ibid.*
75. Kedar, RP, *et al.*, "Effects of tamoxifen on uterus and ovaries of postmenopausal women in a randomized breast cancer prevention trial." *Lancet*, May 28, 1994.
76. Cox News Service, Aug. 18, 1994.
77. Gofman, JW, "A prime cause of breast cancer: what did we know, and when did we know it?" Presentation, the American Assn. for the Advancement of Science (AAAS), San Francisco CA, Feb. 22, 1994.
78. Epstein, Samuel, presentation, Women's Health & the Environment: Action for Cancer Prevention, Albuquerque NM, Oct. 15, 1994.
79. Sternglass, EJ, and JM Gould, "Summary of study on the relation between breast cancer and nuclear fission products in the diet and drinking water." *Int. J. Health Serv.*, Oct. 1993.
80. Sternglass, EJ, "Breast cancer linked to nuclear releases." Presentation, American Assn. of Naturopathic Physicians, San Diego, CA, Sept. 8, 1994.
81. *Ibid.*
82. *The Choice*, XX: 2-3, 1994.
83. *Ibid.*
84. Epstein, presentation, *loc.cit.*
85. Healy, Melissa, "Cold war secrecy tied to radiation peril." *Los Angeles Times*, Oct. 22, 1994.
86. The Associated Press, Aug. 18, 1995.
87. *Science*, Aug. 31, 1990.
88. *The Choice*, XVII: 3,4 1991.
89. Bennett, JT, *Health Research Charities: Image and Realities*. Cited in *Pittsburgh Courier* and *The Choice*, XVI: 4, 1990.
90. *Wall Street Journal*, March 13, 1992.
91. *Ibid.*
92. *Wall Street Journal*, April 6, 1992.
93. "Uncharitable charities." *USA Today*, July 19, 1994.
94. Chowka, PB, "The cancer charity ripoff." *East-West Journal*, July 1978.
95. Culbert, *op. cit.*
96. *Ibid.*
97. *Cancer Facts and Figures 1989*, American Cancer Society, 1989.
98. Bradford, RW, and HW Allen, "The significance of diet in cancer prevention." Chula Vista CA: Bradford Research Institute. Abstracted in *The Choice*. XIX: 3-4, 1993, and XX: 1, 1994.
99. *The Choice*. XVIII: 3, 1992.
100. *The Choice*. XIX: 1, 1994.
101. Marwick, Charles. "Learning how phytochemicals help fight disease." *J. Am. Med. Assn.*,

Nov. 1, 1995.
102. Jastrow, AR, "Commentary," *J. Am. Med. Assn.* Feb. 26, 1994.
103. Nash, Madeleine, "Stopping cancer in its tracks." *Time*, April 25, 1994.
104. Devitt, JE, "Breast cancer: have we missed the forest because of the tree?" *Lancet*, Sept. 10, 1994.
105. Sporn, MB, *op. cit.*
106. *Ibid.*
107. Seachrist, Lisa, "Only the strong survive." *Science News*, April 6, 1996.
108. Cowley, Geoffrey, "A clue to cancer." *Newsweek,* Oct. 23, 1995.
109. Acevedo, HF, *et al.*, "Human chorionic gonadotropin-beta subunit gene expression in cultured human fetal and cancer cells of different types and origins." *Cancer* 76, 1995.
110. Culbert, ML, *What the . . . , op. cit.*
111. Lane, IW, and L Comac, *Sharks Don't Get Cancer.* Garden City Park NY: Avery, 1992.
112. Lerner, M, and D Flint, *Does Cartilage Cure Cancer? The Shark and Bovine cartilage Controversy: an Independent Assessment.* Bolinas CA: Commonweal, 1995.
113. Eidem, WK, *The Man Who Cures Cancer.* Bethesda MD: Be Well Books, 1996.
114. Nowicky, JW, *et al.*, "Evaluation of thiophosphoric acid alkaloid derivatives from *Chelidonium majus L.* ('Ukrain') as an immunostimulant in patients with various carcinomas." Vienna: *Drug Exp. Clin. Res.* 17, 1991.
115. Culbert, ML, *Ukrain.* Publication of American Biologics-Mexico SA Medical Center, Tijuana, BC, Mexico, and Bradford Research Institute, Chula Vista CA, 1995.
116. Gold, J, "Use of hydrazine sulfate in terminal and pre-terminal cancer patients; results of IND study in 84 evaluable patients." *Oncol.* 32, 1975.
117. Culbert, ML, *What the. . ., op. cit.*
118. Keller, HC, "Carnivora: immunomodulator and cytostatic. Study of treatment of Carnivora in patients with advanced malignant disease." Nordhalben, Germany: *Carnivora Forshungs Gmbh,* 1994.
119. Walker, M, "The carnivora cure for cancer, AIDS and other pathologies." *Townsend Letter for Doctors.* Part I: June, 1991. Part II: May, 1992.
120. Prasad, K, "Butyric acid: a small fatty acid with diverse biological functions." *Life Sciences* 27, 1980.
121. Nordenberg, J, *et al.*, "Biochemical and ultrastructural alterations accompany the anti-proliferative effect of butyrate on melanoma cells." *Br. J. Ca.* 55, 1987.
122. Culbert, ML, *What the . . . ,op. cit.*
123. *Ibid.*
124. *J. Natl. Ca. Inst.,* Nov. 6, 1996.
125. *Natural Health,* July/August 1996.
126. Schipper, Harvey, *et al.*, "A new biological framework for cancer research." *Lancet*, Oct. 26, 1996.
127. "Cancers tied to diet and way of life." *New York Times,* Nov. 20, 1996.
128. Davidson, Keay, "Power lines cleared as cause of cancer." *San Francisco Examiner,* Oct. 31, 1996.
129. *The Choice*, XXII: 2, 1996.
130. Schipper, *op. cit.*
131. Malins, Donald, *Proc. Natl. Aca. Sci.*, Nov. 26, 1996.
132. Haney, DQ, The Associated Press, April 14, 1997.
133. Curtis, RE, *et al.*, *New Eng. J. Med.*, March 27, 1997.
134. Johansson, JE, *et al.*, "Fifteen-year survival in prostate cancer." *J. Am. Med. Assn.*, Feb. 12, 1997.
135. Morris, Kelly, "UK experts advise against prostate cancer screening." *Lancet* 349, Feb. 15, 1997.
136. Clark, RC, "Effects of selenium supplementation for cancer prevention in patients with

carcinoma of the skin." *J. Am. Med. Assn.* 276:24, Dec. 25, 1996.
137. Pezzuto, John, *et al., Science,* Jan. 10, 1997.
138. "Fish oil recommended to fight cancer." *Las Vegas Sun,* Feb. 10, 1997.
139. The Associated Press, April 15, 1997.
140. Duerksen, Susan, "Cancer-fighting nutrients studied." *San Diego Union,* April 17, 1997
141. "A cancer gene makes colon removal an option." *New York Times,* March 19, 1997.
142. *New Eng. J. Med.,* May 14, 1997; Scripps Howard News Service, May 15, 1997.
143. Suplee, Curt, "Prostate cancer exam benefits are questioned." *The Washington Post,* March 15, 1997.
144. *Ibid.*
145. Bailar, JC, and HL Gornick, "Cancer undefeated." *New Eng. J. Med.,* May 29, 1997; *The Boston Globe,* May 29, 1997.

NOTE

The National Cancer Institute (NCI) in August 1997 announced that radioactive iodine (iodine-131) fallout from atomic bomb tests might "cause" between 10,000 and 75,000 cases of thyroid cancer in people who were living in the USA in the 1950s and 1960s.

The NCI study noted that for 160 million Americans living in the 48 contiguous states at the time of the tests the average radiation dose to the thyroid was 2 rads per person, or well above the 0.1 rad per person the average American receives annually from naturally occurring radioactivity.

In some counties east and north of the nuclear test sites exposures were estimated to be as high as 9 to 16 rads, the NCI added.

XII
APRICOT POWER:
Laetrile as the Marine Corps of the 'alternative' revolution

"At no time in American history has there been a more effective challenge to medical expertise and authority than that mounted by the contemporary laetrile movement. Despite opposition from the FDA, the American Medical Association, the American Cancer Society, and virtually all of the American medical community, support for this purported cancer cure [sic] *continues to grow. . ."*

— Sociologists G.E. Markle and J.C. Peterson, to the American Association for the Advancement of Science (AAAS), 1979

"Laetrile completely eclipsed any other unorthodox therapy ever used for any disease in our time."

— Charles G. Moertel MD, The Mayo Clinic, 1982

"Although . . . Laetrile utilization in this country is proceeding . . . in spite of FDA prohibitions, it is even more so because of unwarranted FDA procedures, and lack of FDA scientific and medical justification for its stand, extending to probable unconstitutionality . . . I have hundreds of letters sent to me enclosing FDA information sheets and pronouncements, in which the senders of these letters point to the extensive falsification, duplicity, deviousness, red herrings and literal lies . . . promulgated by the FDA with respect to Laetrile, as well as similarly on the part of certain high officials . . . of the American Medical Association, the American Cancer Society, the US Department of Health, Education and Welfare, and state agencies . . ."

— Dean Burk PhD, National Cancer Institute, to Rep. Louis Frey Jr., 1972

"You may wonder, Congressman Roe, why anyone should go to such pains and mendacity to avoid conceding what happened to the NCI-directed experiment [involving laetrile on a tumor system.] *Such an admission is crucially relevant. Once any of the FDA-NCI-AMA-ACS hierarchy so much as concedes that Laetrile anti-tumor efficacy was indeed even once observed in NCI experimentation, a permanent crack in the bureaucratic armor has taken place that can widen indefinitely . . ."*

— Dean Burk PhD, National Cancer Institute, to Rep. Robert A. Roe, 1973

An apricot kernel shakes things up

There was a strangely dominant theme in the 1979 convention of the prestigious American Association for the Advancement of Science (AAAS):

Laetrile.

Not if, how, why or why not laetrile, the most recent "unproven" remedy found "anecdotally" useful against cancer while opposed by the totality of the forces we call Cancer Inc. actually "worked."

But why so many people could be led to believe that it did — when medical orthodoxy and oncological expertise insisted it did not.

No less than five papers on "the laetrile phenomenon" were presented at the AAAS convention that year — and they came not from physicians, biochemists or oncologists but from Western Michigan University sociologists. The latter abstracted:

> *At no time in American history has there been a more effective challenge to medical expertise and authority than that mounted by the contemporary laetrile movement. Despite opposition from the FDA, the American Medical Association, the American Cancer Society, and virtually all of the American medical community, support for this purported cancer cure* [sic] *continues to grow. . .*
>
> *The first paper takes a case-study approach and focuses on the recent laetrile controversy at the Memorial Sloan-Kettering Cancer Center illustrating the richness and complexity of the dispute. The next paper provides an historical context to the recent success of the movement. The third paper examines the conceptualization of the laetrile problem and attempts to explain a variety of legal issues, including the right of privacy; the rights of physicians, informed consent, and government control, are considered. The final paper examines the social context of the controversy and attempts to answer the following question: Why has the laetrile movement been so*

successful in the late 1970s?[1]

Even Mayo Clinic cancer researcher Charles Moertel (dead of cancer himself in 1994), who led the team in the federal "amygdalin (laetrile) clinical trial" in 1980-81 which was used to wreck the laetrile movement, observed that "Laetrile completely eclipsed any other unorthodox therapy ever used for any disease in our time."[2]

The issue: freedom of choice

The sociological savants could have saved themselves an enormous amount of research hours had they simply switched their paradigm meter over to "common sense":

Laetrile was fast becoming a dominant issue because, for the first time in the long and tortured history of suppressed cancer "alternatives" in the United States, it had, unlike its predecessors, "gone political."

A personal note here: I began my involvement as a science writer and health-rights activist on the laetrile issue, which I entered as a trained — and skeptical — journalist. As the primary writer/journalist of what became the Committee for Freedom of Choice in Cancer Therapy Inc. (later, Committee for Freedom of Choice in Medicine, Inc.) I decided very early that the issue was neither scientific nor medical but political. And that issue was — is — simple:

What right does the state have, or should it have, to intervene in medical decisions between a patient and his doctor, particularly if that patient is dying of a "terminal" disease for which there is no known, or guaranteed, cure?

The marching slogan of the CFCCT became, as agreed by the rough-hewn self-taught visionary who founded the organization, Robert W. Bradford, several collaborators and myself, a simple one:

Freedom of choice, with informed consent, for physician and patient.

It was *this* issue, the freedom of choice concept, which so captivated the public and which led to many regional public opinion polls and, more impressively, such national samplings by those of the Harris (1977) and Roper (1978) organizations in which clear majorities of Americans believed at the very least in the *right* to have laetrile.

It was this basic, horse-sense approach, so consonant with the public at large, which lofted laetrile into the most impressive anti-establishmentarian phenomenon of a medical nature in this century and which set off what many would later call "the metabolic revolution" — the forcing, from the grass roots, of the Allopathic Industrial Complex (AIC) to begin to look at dietary elements in the prevention and management not only of cancer but of chronic disease in general.

What opponents styled "the political success of a scientific failure" — for the AIC would bestir itself to attempt to thwart the upstart laetrile movement with prostituted "science" of a high order — was the catalyst for increasing interest at all levels in nutrients against disease.

Laetrile captures 24 states

By the time of the 1979 AAAS convention, and usually led by the Committee for Freedom of Choice, pro-laetrile forces had "captured" one statehouse after another and were causing state legislatures to write into law various statutes either to protect doctors from punishment should they prescribe laetrile, or to protect patient access to the substance, or simply to make it an available option in cancer treatment and prevention.

Between 1976 and 1981, in a series of frequently stunning political events which shook the AIC and the nation at large, some 24 states containing more than half the population of the United States approved legislation which in one way or another either "decriminalized" or "legalized" laetrile. In others, such as New York, pro-laetrile laws passed the legislature only to be vetoed by state governors, actions which, as in the Empire State, were sometimes impossible to overturn.

Actually, those of us in "the laetrile movement" more or less stealthfully planned it that way — we decided *against* federal legislation (for what the federal government enacts on Wednesday it can repeal on Thursday, while also strengthening that very level of government) and decided on "legal guerrilla warfare" at the state-by-state level, beginning with Alaska in 1975/1976.

Uniting Left and Right

The movement was also a populist revolution and strongly ideological, because much of the early leadership of the Committee was drawn from the conservative John Birch Society (JBS), many of whose members took the freedom of choice issue to heart and, already experienced in lobbying and politicking, provided an unofficial support mechanism for the Committee.

Yet, much to the chagrin of some of the major media and various apologists of the AIC, neither the laetrile movement in general nor the Committee in particular were "Birch fronts" — support for individual freedom of choice in medical matters spanned all shades of the political landscape, all religions, races and socioeconomic levels.

As a journalist, I was drawn from the early days to the broad spectrum of the controversy, and was uniquely positioned to become informed:

It was the arrest of my *own* physician and friend, the late John A. Richardson MD, of Albany CA, on State of California charges involving laetrile, which was the actual catalyst for the formation of the original Committee for Freedom of Choice in Cancer Therapy Inc. "Dr. John" was a long-time Birch Society member. Yet at his initial hearings and trials within the Berkeley-Albany municipal jurisdiction — perhaps the most *left*-leaning in the country at the time — it was common to see youthful student radicals and hippies with McGovern-for-President buttons showing up *in support of* an outspoken Birch Society physician. Hence, from its ancestral origin in 1972, the Committee confounded the AIC just as the laetrile movement confused the scientific intelligentsia of the AAAS who so desperately wanted to know just how or why the American public could be "for" laetrile when the massed forces of institutional expertise so opposed it.

Laetrile, of course, had been kicking around long before the Richardson arrest and the advent of the Committee.

An ancient background

The history of the laetrile concept and the use and application of the substance were covered by myself in two books[3,4] as well as by Kittler,[5] Griffin[6] and Halstead.[7]

Permit me to synthesize:

In modern times, the word "laetrile" (apparently concocted by the major modern-day proponents, the late Ernst T. Krebs Sr. MD and his biochemist son, Ernst T. Krebs Jr. DSc, from the biochemical terminology "*lae*vo-mandeloni*trile*") has usually referred to the chemical amygdalin, first isolated and studied in the 19th century. The term also covers a manufactured, refined injectable product developed in the 1950s and which has not been duplicated since. The term "laetriles" has also been used to cover what the State of California calls "substantially similar compounds," particularly prunasin, linamarin, dhurrin, and several others.

These, plus sambunigrin, lotaustralin and more exotic compounds, have variously been described as "cyanogenetic glucosides," "cyanophoric glycosides" and, particularly as championed by the late Krebs Jr., "nitrilosides." They are impressively abundant in nature, as in all the black and brown bitter fruit seeds in North America, and are in many other seeds as well, and are found in many varieties of beans, peas, berries, tubers and grasses throughout the world — a ubiquity virtually unmatched among nutrients other than by Vitamin C.

Whatever their names, the compounds have in common one or more sugars attached to benzene or acetone "rings" and carry a "cyanide radical" — that is, they are cyanide-bearing sugar compounds. They are so widespread in nature that the Krebses, the earlier McNaughton Foundation (first in Canada, then in California, as a research apparatus for the development of laetrile) and the late Dean Burk PhD, the peppery biochemist who for years headed the cytochemistry division of the National Cancer Institute (NCI), decided that altogether they constituted one or a complex of B vitamins — which they agreed should be the 17th in order of definition: Vitamin B17.

They argued that ubiquity in nature of such compounds was a proof, but not the only proof, of their vitamin nature. Their essential non-toxicity and solubility in water are other characteristics, Dean Burk always argued,[8] that added to their B-vitamin status. But the crux of the vitamin argument was whether or not their absence or depletion led to a pathological condition. For the laetrilists, their absence or depletion did indeed lead to a pathological condition: cancer. Not only that, but laetrile and its breakdown products are involved in a host of other metabolic processes.

Beyond that, amygdalin was known in medical history as both a poison, as implemented by the Egyptians, and as an elixir, as utilized by the Romans, and had been first successfully used on its own against cancer by the Russians even though amygdalin-laden black and brown bitter fruit seeds were described as anti-tumor agents in the herbal pharmacopeia of ancient China.[9]

We know that ancient Sumerians used a poultice made of laetrile-rich juniper berries, prune kernels and dried wine dregs for a skin condition which today seems reminiscent of mela-noma.[10]

The Assyrians used fruit seed-derived medications for conditions whose symptoms remind modern-day scholars of cancer.[11]

By the 17th century AD John Gerarde, an English herbalist, used peach kernels for "stoppings of the liver and spleen (and) those who have the Apoplexy."[12]

The medical use of fruit kernels, mostly of the laetrile-rich *Rosaceae* and *Prunasae* families, was advanced in the US in the 19th century primarily by the Confederate side of the Civil War.

Confederate surgeon Francis Peyre Porcher was among the first to suspect that the hydrocyanic acid (cyanide) within peach kernels was the agent most likely of medical benefit.[13]

It was within the same century and in Europe that the active principles in the various seeds which seemed to have such medical merit were determined to be the cyanide-bearing sugar compound amygdalin and similar structures.

Proofs from epidemiology

The notion of nitrilosidic prevention of cancer had enough adequate study in the current century to stand on its own and not simply be construable as a pretext for developing a product.

Whether assembled by the Krebses, the McNaughton Foundation, or various independent researchers, the epidemiological aspects of "Vitamin B17" — correlations with much lower rates of cancer to no appreciable cancer at all in studied populations — are impressive:

Essentially cancer-free or minimally cancer-afflicted populations have been studied, including, in South America, the Ecuadorian Vilcabamba Indians in particular (though numerous peoples of the Andean highlands and the Amazon Basin have been known to be either without cancer or to be minimally afflicted with it), the apricot kernel-popping Hunzakuts of Pakistan (observed by several investigators over decades), various tribes and peoples of Southeast Asia (including at least one group in the southern Philippines which, I found on-site, had no word for the disease itself but, when explained what it was, called it "the Christian disease" — of meat-eaters), the Abkhasians of the former Soviet Union, Arctic Circle Eskimos prior to their "civilizing" by the Dutch Reformed Church and other entities; and various American Indian tribes in the Southwest and in Mexico.

Krebs Jr. and the McNaughton Foundation gathered data on the essential absence or modest presence of cancer in other groups and in wild animals of many species (contrasting them with domesticated animals in the civilized West, among which cancer is highly present and growing.[14,15]) They and others have pointed out that Western eating habits and the food processing industry have essentially eliminated nitrilosides from the common dietary — historically, the change from consuming nitriloside-rich millet for higher consumption of wheat in the making of bread and the Western habit of depriving North Temperate peoples of high sources of nitrilosides (as in fruit seeds) by spitting out or throwing away the same are milestones in the history of dietary nitriloside depletion. At the same time, the continuing high presence of "B17" compounds in grazing grasses (sudan, arrow, etc.) on which range animals feed may explain why these animals are cancer-free while their human handlers are often cancer-stricken.

The existing data can be construed several ways: laetrile compounds consumed in the natural diets of "primitive" peoples (as certain tribes in Southeast Asia for which B17-rich cassava is a staple food — "the poor man's bread") are part of a total eating regime which is best encompassed by the term "the poor people's diet." It consists not only of natural laetriles, but dozens of other natural-state nutrients in a diet largely built around non-chemically-treated fresh vegetables, unrefined grains, fresh fruits and berries, and a much lower prevalence of animal meats and proteins, the virtual non-existence of refined carbohydrates and few or no stimulants.

This *entire* dietary lifestyle in general terms highly correlates to the absence not only of cancer but of the chronic, metabolic diseases of the "civilized" Western world in general.

The foods bearing "B17" compounds also usually contain a treasure trove of many other useful nutrients — including the apricot kernel itself, the usual source in the Americas for the extraction and manufacture of laetrile. It has become clearer with time that various of the factors in these foods, perhaps captained by the nitrilosides, are specific against malignancy, and are even more effective in combination.

The earlier developers of laetrile were as beholden to the pharmacologically-inclined allopathic thought process as anyone else in attempting to find "the" anti-cancer element. Perhaps not one, but many, were found — and an entire complex of compounds, some clearly within the nitriloside category and others simply similar to it, may work synergistically either to prevent the establishment of an incipient subclinical malignant process or, at the very least, to thwart or slow down one already in place.

Prevention, of course, is one thing — a nutrient construed as a "drug" is quite another.

For Cancer Inc. laetrile — almost always defined as the better-known chemical amygdalin, occurring in virtually all black and brown bitter fruit seeds in North America — is everything a cancer treatment should not be:

It is a natural nutrient, not a patented drug (though American and British patents have defined various refined and/or synthesized amygdalins which have never been marketed and may not even be producible), it is allegedly effective both in cancer prevention and therapy, it is not toxic at least in the doses long recommended and utilized, and it is usually provided as a central part of a "metabolic" program involving dietary change, protein-digesting enzymes, and other natural components.

Cancer as a nutritional deficiency

The rationale of laetrile against cancer also strikes at the very root of oncological wisdom:

It suggests that cancer is, more than anything else, a dietary deficiency disease (the deficiency being "Vitamin B17"), that cancer is unitarian in nature (there are not hundreds of "kinds" of cancer), that cancer is not "tumor disease" *per se* and that thus what happens or does not happen to tumors is not a fair determinant of the efficacy of an anti-cancer program, that cancer is easily preventable, that cancer treatments should be natural.

It is, hence, too simple, too "unscientific" and — worst of all — far too inexpensive for the AIC, let alone the orthodox oncological establishment, which now lays claim to an incredible $200 billion per year of the nation's trillion-dollar "healthcare delivery" bill (*III*).

Adding insult to injury, Ernst T. Krebs Jr., the biochemist, was a major proponent of another fruit seed derivative, which he and others baptized "pangamic acid" or Vitamin B15, which has a shorter, but equally controversial, history in against-the-grain unorthodoxy, and of the "trophoblastic thesis of cancer."

A lifelong scientific innovator in a family of scientists, Krebs Jr. died in 1996 at age 85 — free of cancer.

His physician/father had died in the 1970s at age 93. Brother Byron Krebs MD and another Krebs, Otto, had also devoted much of their lives to researching cancer and laetrile.

John Beard and the trophoblasts

The trophoblastic thesis, Krebs Jr.'s major scientific obsession outside laetrile, as an updated version of an idea put forward at the turn of the century by Scots embryologist John Beard, states[16] that cancer is nothing more or less than misplaced trophoblast, an invasive birth cycle-related tissue essential to the fetal development of mammalian life. Under "Beardian" thinking, whatever naturally inhibits the natural trophoblast tissue in the birth cycle should also inhibit cancer. Since pancreatic enzymes are apparently involved in the inhibition of trophoblast, they should be useful against human cancer — hence the German/American and modern-day twin theories espoused by the Krebses and, for a long time, by the modern laetrilists: proteolytic enzymes and the body's host defense system constitute the "endogenous" first line of defense against cancer; the nitrilosidic food compounds, "Vitamin B17," serving as a second team or backup, constitute the "exogenous" second line of defense.

The AIC detested Vitamin B15 (probable active factor: N,N dimethylglycine), which received rave notices in Europe and the ex-Soviet Union, where much research on it was conducted and where it has been widely used. And, of course, Cancer Inc. seemed terrorized by the trophoblastic, vitamin-nature and/or any other unitarian explanation of cancer. Simple economics alone ultimately explains the institutional aversion, particularly to the vitamin theory of cancer.

There is increasing evidence to support a unitarian — if not necessarily trophoblastic — understanding of cancer (including the discovery of the "immortalizing enzyme" telomerase, the nearly-ubiquitous presence of hCG hormone and a whole host of mutated defective or missing genes [*see XI*] in most "tumor types") and abundant evidence that either laetrile or laetrile-like compounds, and other natural nutrients, are protective against cancer and hence useful in its management.

It is not the province of this study to explicate the multiple controversies of laetrile, which we have done elsewhere. What we demonstrate here is that laetrile became a major challenge not only to the scientific claims of oncology in general but, far more importantly, to the authority of the Allopathic Industrial Complex (AIC) or The Club, wounding the AIC in its tenderest of tissues — the economic one — and hence had to be destroyed scientifically, conceptually, legally, administratively, and every other way.

The Laetrile War, then, is a template for the AIC vs. its challengers — be they homeopathy, as in the last century, or chiropractic, as in the present.

Cancer Inc.'s war on 'unprovens'

Historical background is essential:

The primary "red flag" in "alternative" medicine in the United States during most of this century has been *cancer*. While "unproven" or "dubious" methods have been developed against other chronic diseases, nothing has seemed to excite such a storm of institutional, ideological and legal responses as the open advocacy of a "cancer cure" developed outside the parameters of the AIC.

Hence, the history of what the medical establishment derides as everything from "quackery" to "unproven remedies" in cancer is tangled, extensive and disgusting. Medical and research careers have been ruined and innocent people prosecuted and persecuted in an allegedly free society for involvement with, or the purveying of, "unapproved" "cancer cures."

There seems almost a visceral reaction from within the AIC to strike out at the same, probably because cancer (even before AIDS) was the most noticeable failure of American (and Western) "scientific medicine" and was growing exponentially through Western society. There seemed to be an unstated fear that any attack on the basic tenets of oncology (cancer as tumors — hence the destruction of tumors equating to the "curing" of the disease) somehow meant an attack on the doctrines of allopathic medicine itself. Worse, since the greater amount of the "unproven" remedies usually involves natural substances or ultimately simple and inexpensive techniques, the enormous profitability of Cancer Inc., under construction for many decades, has sensed in the non-toxic "unprovens" the greatest of threats.

In an excellent recounting of the cancer industry, Ralph Moss PhD — who was fired from his public affairs position at Memorial Sloan-Kettering Cancer Center in New York over the laetrile affair — summarized the American Cancer Society's list of "unproven remedies" (commonly called the "quack list").[17]

(The concept of "unproven" therapies suggests that there are "proven" ones — that is, chemotherapy, radiation, surgery and a few high-tech immunology boosters. With well over 1,500 Americans dying per day from cancer by mid-decade, with more than 4,000 being diagnosed with the disease at the same time and with historic highs in both the fatalities from and incidence of cancer, the notion of a "proven" cancer remedy provokes as much funereal humor in the unbiased observer as does the hoary Cancer Society concept of "unproven" methods.)

Moss found that of 63 ACS-listed "unproven techniques," by the 1990s an incredible 44.4 percent had undergone no investigation by the ACS or any other agency, public or private, before having been condemned as "unproven" — which is to say, "quack."

Moreover, among some 70 advocates of "unorthodox therapies" — often described by Cancer Inc. as "snake-oil salesmen" (a phrase which needs some rethinking inasmuch as some Asian research has demonstrated actual anti-cancer efficacy *from* "snake oil") — Moss noted that over 77 percent were or are medical doctors or doctors of philosophy in various scientific disciplines.

And, further, as he has noted with some humor, when at the National Cancer Institute (NCI) — the federally funded government research unit largely brought into being by the private ACS and long dominated by it — a researcher seeks a new lead into cancer management he is apt to reach first for the "unprovens" list.[(18)]

Cancer was grist for the mill of genuine quackery in centuries gone by — when cancer rates were tiny compared to those of today — simply because it was then, as today, mostly incurable. As I discovered while researching my first book on the laetrile affair, even in the 19th century there was an American Indian anti-cancer remedy with the suspiciously familiar name *Leotrill*.[(19)]

To be sure, the mysterious nature of cancer and its seeming incurability made it a target for con men and opportunists, so we are not here making the case that all suppressed would-be cancer "cures" were indeed legitimate research efforts: *of course* there truly was charlatanry involved in some of them. Yet, given the dismal record of the "scientifically proven" cancer remedies it has often been appropriate to draw a fine line between "unapproved quackery" and "approved quackery."

We note elsewhere (*V*) the triumph of the allopathic paradigm in medicine, backed by solid financial considerations, toward the end of the 19th century. In terms of cancer, allopathy's victory meant the institutionalization of the notion that cancer is tumors, and that there are hundreds of different kinds of tumors, each requiring its own "cure," and that the latter surely would be found in surgery, and then radiation, and then toxic chemicals. That is, mechanical assaults on the tumor mass were understood to be "scientific" approaches to a disease whose Greek-derived specialty name (oncology), as we have seen, means "the study of bumps."

The notion that homeopathics, fever therapy, special serums, let alone plant and other natural nutrients, might "shrink tumors" met with shrill opposition.

The beginnings: Coley, Warburg, Gerson

In the US, from the advent of Coley's toxins, one of the first "unprovens" — and later removed from that category in modern times for further research since it belatedly became obvious that the theory and practice of the same had some genuine value — "unproven" remedies against cancer grew parallel to the geometric rise in cancer incidence and deaths.

Both cancer rates and "unproven remedies" boomed in the immediate post-World War II years.

Dietary theories concerning cancer and how to manage it are not new: Otto Warburg in Germany described a dietary connection to malignancy decades ago. Straddling Germany and the United States, the late Max Gerson MD probably did more than any single physician/researcher to bring dietary and nutritional elements to light in the management of the disease, and was among the major challengers to the allopathic paradigm.

Despite widespread evidence of efficacy against cancer through Gerson methods of detoxification and dietary manipulation, the German physician in the 1940s underwent an all-out attack by the then-fledgling Cancer Inc.: neutralization, isolation, and professional elimination. So "Gersonism" was one of the first of the widely used "unprovens" to abandon the United States and reappear in Mexico as well as in other countries around the world.

An "unproven" method called the Lincoln bacteriophage therapy helped the cancer-stricken son of Senator Charles Tobey recover in the 1950s, leading the legislator to attempt a full-scale investigation into the American cancer industry — one definable as that even as early as 1953. Just years prior, in 1946, American Medical Assn.-influenced legislators had blocked a proposal by

Senator Claude Pepper for a $100 million research effort into *all aspects* of cancer therapy.

As chairman of the Senate Interstate and Foreign Commerce Committee it was Tobey who hired attorney Benedict F. Fitzgerald Jr. of the Justice Department as special counsel. Senator Tobey died of a heart attack before his cancer-probe project could get underway, and his successor, Senator John Bricker, proved to be far more favorable to the AMA. Even so, Special Counsel Fitzgerald's investigation of cancer treatments in the United States resulted in the first general "official" overview of what was going on, and it was the first time the word "conspiracy" was used to describe the activities of Cancer Inc. in an official forum.

By the time Fitzgerald's report was published in the *Congressional Record* in 1953, several "alternative" cancer therapies had had or were in the process of having an appreciable impact on United States medicine aside from the Gerson controversy. The major ones:

— Dr. William F. Koch's Glyoxylide, one of the first examples of an "alternative" therapy hounded into near-extinction internationally and which we now recognize as an early precursor of oxidative treatments.

— Krebiozen, an animal blood serum-derived therapy pioneered in the United States by physiologist Dr. Andrew C. Ivy, vice president of the University of Illinois, after having been introduced to it by Yugoslav physician Stephan Durovic.

— The Hoxsey herbals, perhaps — second only to laetrile — the best-known, long-running controversy pitting Cancer Inc. vs. a natural method.

The campaign against Glyoxylide

Dr. Koch's treatment had such support earlier in this century that by 1921-22 the AMA was, of course, lobbying against it. No one at that time had any inkling of either "free radicals" or oxidative treatments. Koch's work had continued through the

1930s and 1940s with major research and use of this modality occurring in Canada, whose Ontario Cancer Commission in 1939 and 1940 provided objective forums in which to indicate Glyoxylide efficacy.

Dr. Koch worked in Mexico and Brazil in 1940 and 1941, using the substance also for treating mental conditions. He was arrested in Florida in 1942 on a charge of false labelling, with a district attorney noting that his (for the time) high bail of $10,000 was set at that level in order to keep him from returning to Brazil to finish research work.

Despite thousands of case histories in support of Glyoxylide — "anecdotes," as Cancer Inc. calls such testimonials — Dr. Koch was subjected to Food and Drug Administration (FDA)-triggered trials in 1942 and 1946 which led to a permanent injunction against the treatment in 1950. Nobody could understand his ahead-of-his-time approach, out of which the kindred product Rodaquin (later available in Mexico) was developed. Harassment, legal fees and the lack of any political savvy on the part of Glyoxylide's supporters spelled the essential demise of what had been a promising avenue of research.(20)

Taking on Harry Hoxsey

Between the 1920s and 1940s thousands of Americans were successfully treated with many "forms" of cancer with the herbal preparations originally developed in the 19th century by John Hoxsey and promoted in the United States by his descendant, Harry Hoxsey.

Because of early support by several physicians of the Hoxsey method, and also because the flamboyant Harry Hoxsey refused to turn over the herbal formulations to another doctor, American medical officials began a lengthy persecution of the maverick in Illinois, Pennsylvania and Texas, all of which at one time or another had Hoxsey clinics to which thousands of Americans turned for at least partial remedies of their cancer cases.(21)

While the Krebiozen controversy was just beginning and as Fitzgerald was investigating cancer in general, laetrile was also being quietly looked at by various physicians in several countries. Dr. Krebs Sr. had pioneered it in the 1920s when it was developed as an unexpected byproduct in efforts of the San Francisco innovator to make Prohibition Era whiskey taste better. Compounds, of which amygdalin may have only been one, and later compounds which turned out to be refined amygdalin, were seriously studied in several countries, as the laetrile research-sponsoring McNaughton Foundation pointed out. But by the 1950s laetrile was not the "news" that the Koch compounds, Krebiozen and the Hoxsey herbals were.

Dr. Ivy and Krebiozen

Dr. Ivy, one of America's most prestigious scientists and scholars, found Krebiozen to be useful in terminal cancer patients and went on to promote its use as a major anticancer medicine, one which reportedly was sought by two major drug companies whose takeover offers he spurned. Despite some 20,000 cases attesting to Krebiozen usefulness, including 530 described by Fitzgerald, the US government, equipped with an amended Food, Drug and Cosmetic Act, took Dr. Ivy to court in 1964.[22]

Even though he was cleared of all the counts against him in an expensive, 289-day showcase trial, the negative publicity from Cancer Inc. virtually ended Krebiozen in the USA.

By the time Fitzgerald issued his *Congressional Record* assessment of cancer research in 1953, there had been considerable hoopla generated by the Hoxsey, Krebiozen, and Glyoxylide controversies. They were larger challenges to Cancer Inc., which also had to fend off many other unwanted approaches, compounds and techniques.

The pattern was ever similar: a lone researcher or doctor would stumble upon an apparently useful anticancer compound, test it, then attempt to gain federal licensing and recognition.

Suddenly the representative of a drug company would appear bearing sufficient gold and would attempt to induce the inventor to turn over the formula or share in the profits. Failure to do so would often mean actual harassment of the inventors and compounds.

Occasionally, unpleasant truths slipped out. In the 1980s I was intermittently researching and writing a still-unpublished account of the incredible story of the development of anti-cancer compounds derived from the head-shrinking process of the Jivaro Indians of South America, as researched over many years by the late "white medicine man" Wilburn Ferguson.

In the not-commercially-available recounting of his professional life among the Jivaro (or Shuara)[23] and in many interviews with me, he described how an officer of a major drug company in the USA had actually told him that to legalize the Jivaro compounds would put cancer drug development out of business. This was why, Ferguson felt, that despite years of effort and a bureaucratic runaround, he had received little federal support to follow up on highly promising cancer research which at one point had been supported by the Ecuadorian government.

Fitzgerald lets a cat out of the bag

This is the kind of backdrop against which Benedict F. Fitzgerald's report should be read, and the laetrile controversy understood.

The attorney summarized in the August 28, 1953, *Congressional Record* that:

> *There is reason to believe that the AMA has been hasty, capricious, arbitrary and outright dishonest* [in its statements against various "unapproved" therapies] *and could involve the AMA and others in a conspiracy of alarming proportions . . .*
>
> *Behind and over all this* [apparently successful response to Krebiozen in hundreds of cases] *is the weirdest conglomeration of corrupt motives, intrigues, selfishness,*

jealousy, obstruction and conspiracy that I have ever seen . . .

Should we sit idly by and count the number of physicians, surgeons and cancerologists who are not only divided but who, because of fear or favor, are forced to line up with the so-called accepted view of the American Medical Association, or should this Committee make a full-scale investigation of the organized effort to hinder, suppress and restrict the free flow of drugs which allegedly have proven successful in cases where clinical reports, case history, pathological reports and X-ray photographic proof, together with the alleged cured patients, are available?

Accordingly, we should determine whether existing agencies, both public and private, are engaged in and have pursued a policy of harassment, ridicule, slander and libelous attacks on others sincerely engaged in stamping out this curse of mankind . . . My investigation to date should convince this Committee that a conspiracy does exist to stop the free flow and use of drugs in interstate commerce which allegedly (have) solid therapeutic value. Public and private funds have been thrown around like confetti at a country fair to close up and destroy clinics, hospitals, and scientific research laboratories which do not conform to the viewpoint of medical associations. How long will the American people take this?[24]

The answer was: at least several more decades.

Between the Fitzgerald report and the laetrile outbreak of the 1970s, the Food, Drug and Cosmetic Act was amended (see *IX*), a move which, among many things, made it extremely difficult for a natural substance to be federally licensed as a "new drug" — unless a proponent group had many millions of unrecoverable dollars to spend on the effort.

Even so, the McNaughton Foundation made an effort to secure

FDA licensing for laetrile, only to be sandbagged at the last moment.[25]

Enter Dr. Dean Burk

The entry into the laetrile field of National Cancer Institute (NCI) cytochemistry chief Dean Burk, PhD, a biochemist, added a variety of clout to laetrile that its predecessors and contemporary challengers to the medical orthodoxy never had:

"The Dean" was uniquely credentialed and positioned to defend laetrile from within the very bowels of the American research establishment, and he did so repeatedly and incisively.

While scattered laetrile research in the United States and other countries had been strongly favorable for what was in essence a derivative of apricot kernels, the compound was receiving a major boost with the opening of an anti-cancer clinic in Tijuana, Mexico, and official interest by the Mexican government.

On May 30, 1972, Dr. Burk wrote to Congressman Louis Frey Jr. that

> *Although . . . Laetrile utilization in this country is proceeding . . . in spite of FDA prohibitions, it is even more so because of unwarranted FDA procedures, and lack of FDA scientific and medical justification for its stand, extending to probable unconstitutionality, concerning which many thousands of cancer-afflicted persons and their relatives and physicians are rapidly becoming aware.*
>
> *. . . I have hundreds of letters sent to me enclosing FDA information sheets and pronouncements, in which the senders of these letters point to the extensive falsification, duplicity, deviousness, red herrings and literal lies . . . promulgated by the FDA with respect to Laetrile, as well as similarly on the part of certain high officials . . . of the American Medical Association, the American Cancer Society, the US Department of Health, Education and Welfare, and state agencies . . .*

It is becoming evident that the current generation of cancer sufferers is coming to regard the intransigence and palpable lies of the FDA and the above-indicated related organizations with a marked measure of contempt on the basis of prima facie evidence provided by these organizations themselves as to their integrity and credibility and that something of a Boston Tea Party mode of action is being undertaken by an increasing number of cancer sufferers in this country, who intend to be hoodwinked no longer; in short, an active backlash is developing even at the grass-roots level . . .[26]

My friend and mentor (who died in 1989) was quite prescient — for just a few days later, in June 1972, an event occurred in Northern California which would change the American medical landscape forever.

A newspaper editor gets hooked

As a checkup patient of Dr. John A. Richardson and as editor of the *Berkeley Daily Gazette*, I was suddenly thrust into an awkward position when a friend in the Alameda County (California) district attorney's office called to inform me, just as he had other media, that a "cancer-quack bust" was in the works for tomorrow.

When I inquired just who the cancer quack to be "busted" was, and he told me, "that Dr. Richardson out in Albany, the one using the laetrile," I gulped. I had a moral quandary: I was given privileged information in my role as a journalist, yet the information directly bore on my own physician, who was also a friend.

I agonized over what to do and decided that it was not my role to interfere with the "bust." It took place — police swarmed into the Albany clinic to arrest Dr. Richardson on various counts involving violation of specific California codes aimed at laetrile.

True enough, Dr. Richardson had ballooned into prominence (together with the pioneering Ernesto Contreras Sr. MD in Tijuana) as a major laetrile-using doctor with a rapidly growing caseload of essentially satisfied patients.

It was the arrest of Dr. Richardson, a John Bircher, which ignited the firestorm of national agitation not so much over laetrile as over the issue of freedom of medical choice, a concept not only near and dear to Birchism but to Americans of many political persuasions. When fellow medics in the San Francisco Bay area, Stanford University scientist Robert Bradford, Birch writer G. Edward Griffin, and various patients and businessmen rallied to the legal-defense cause of Dr. Richardson the first Committee for Freedom of Choice in Cancer Therapy Inc. was set up.

Dr. Richardson ultimately went through three trials involving laetrile, losing one and tieing two, litigations which sparked the explosive growth of the original committee into a nationwide movement. Eventually, there would be committees for freedom of choice in all 50 states with an activist membership variously estimated at anywhere from 20,000 to 50,000.

On July 3, 1973, more than a year after the Richardson raid and as the committee was congealing as a national movement, Dr. Burk wrote to Congressman Robert A. Roe that laetrile had been successful in NCI-directed studies of the compound against Lewis mouse lung cancer even while the federal agency, Dr. Burk's employer, was consistently denying overall efficacy from the substance. Wrote Dr. Burk:

> *You may wonder, Congressman Roe, why anyone should go to such pains and mendacity to avoid conceding what happened to the NCI-directed experiment. Such an admission and concession is crucially relevant. Once any of the FDA-NCI-AMA-ACS hierarchy so much as concedes that Laetrile anti-tumor efficacy was indeed even once observed in NCI experimentation, a permanent crack in the bureaucratic*

armor has taken place that can widen indefinitely by further appropriate experimentation.[27]

By this time, more and more "anecdotal case histories" of Americans responding to the "laetrile program" of oral and intravenous laetrile, proteolytic enzymes and special diet were coming forward and gaining media attention. Initially as a skeptic, I also was interviewing several dozen laetrile users, most of them Richardson and Contreras patients, for my first book, being consistently amazed by what I found, heard and saw.

When I asked state authorities for the official version of what was wrong with laetrile, I was referred to an aging 1953 report on some 44 dying, terminal cancer patients who had received tiny doses of experimental laetrile in the early 1950s. Since the patients died this was taken as a sure sign of a lack of efficacy. Yet I was bewildered to read that improvements in overall well-being and cessation of pain had occurred in many of these terminal patients. Even as a non-MD journalist, it seemed clear to me that this obviously harmless substance should be further studied if only for its apparent ability to reduce pain and enhance subjective feelings of improvement.

The laetrile juggernaut

From 1973, the laetrile juggernaut began to roll with an intensity which had never been experienced by any other anti-establishmentarian medical movement in America:

It was learned that collaborative trials between the Mexican government and the prestigious Memorial Sloan-Kettering Cancer Center (MSKCC) in New York were in the offing and that more physicians were coming forward admitting they were finding merit in laetrile in their cancer patients. The "guru" of the movement, indefatigable San Francisco biochemist Ernst T. Krebs Jr., was joining Committee national chairman Robert Bradford and laetrile-using doctors on speakers' platforms around the country.

The rapid proliferation of Committees for Freedom of

Choice became a phenomenon in its own right, and it was matched by politicking — the very thing in which proponents of earlier cancer unorthodoxy in the United States had not engaged.

In 1975, three events galvanized the movement:

First, US District Court Judge Luther Bohanon, Oklahoma City, ruled that the FDA had no right to keep US patients from being able to secure their own supplies of foreign laetrile and that "the FDA has abdicated its duty to make a clear determination as to whether Laetrile should or should not be placed in commerce since the drug has been in use for many years." The legal move entered by attorney Clyde Watts on behalf of terminal cancer patients as a class instantly allowed Kansan Glen L. Rutherford (described as "cured" of bowel cancer by Dr. Contreras' laetrile program) "legal" access to Mexican laetrile. The legal fight would go on for years, twice reaching the Supreme Court, allowing American cancer patients an affidavit system through which foreign laetrile could be procured.

Then, an underground research group at Sloan-Kettering revealed a "coverup" of seven series of animal tests of laetrile which had shown efficacy even as the New York research center was denying that its testing program had shown any benefits. (In my 1974 book, a Sloan-Kettering vice president had confirmed to me that there had in fact been beneficial results, so much so that further trials were planned.[28]) I was one of the newspapermen to whom the data were anonymously "leaked." I immediately confirmed (by speaking with Sloan-Kettering's veteran biochemical researcher, Dr. Kanematsu Sugiura) that the results were valid and were his.

That the nation's foremost cancer research facility would fudge on positive test results with an essentially non-toxic cancer compound provided a major piece of evidence that Cancer Inc. was alive and well. Not long afterward, the "underground" at Sloan-Kettering would emerge as disgruntled staff members openly opposed what they saw as a front-office effort to suppress positive test results with "Vitamin B17." It worked out that Ralph Moss PhD, assistant public affairs director at MSKCC, was a key element in the "underground." In a bold move, Dr. Moss — sent by MSKCC to a press conference in part sponsored by the Committee for Freedom of Choice in Cancer Therapy — took advantage of the conference to announce his disagreement with MSKCC's laetrile coverup. He was promptly fired.

The MSKCC disclosures also galvanized me personally and radicalized me on the subject: no longer was this simply a journalistic exercise — life-and-death issues revolved around the fight over freedom of choice let alone the possible efficacy of laetrile. 1975 was the year of my moving from "straight" journalism into the advocacy camp of the Committee.

The 'great laetrile smuggling trial'

The third major event occurred in Christmas Week, 1975, when federal officials conducted a nationwide crackdown on the incipient laetrile movement: former Standford University scientist Robert W. Bradford was among 16 individuals ultimately arrested and/or indicted on charges of smuggling Mexican laetrile into the United States. The police deployment was considerable: at least 20 federal agents in a dozen vehicles were involved in a surveillance operation stretching from the Mexican border to the San Francisco Bay Area in the effort to nab Bradford. In Minnesota, an entrapment scheme involving US-ordered, US government-dispatched, US government-seized and US government-followed laetrile was used to raid two private residences and set up the arrests of presumed laetrile distributors there.

The "international laetrile smuggling ring" trial was to become the lengthiest federal conspiracy case ever tried in a San Diego federal court. While the principals were ultimately found guilty, no prison time was meted out, and the court record was replete with the scandalous efforts of US federal authorities to induce, entrap and set up presumed laetrile distributors as if they were heroin importers or vicious criminals. Court testimony brought out that the federal side paid Mexican "mules" (professional smugglers) to bring clandestine laetrile (apricot seed extract) into the United States in order to aid in the entrapment of members of the "ring."

In the seeming acting out of a Greek drama, each new element of the controversy simply set the stage for an even greater element later.

A revolt starts in Alaska

In 1976, the next major element dramatically occurred in Alaska:

The state legislature passed a law protecting physician/patient freedom of choice in cancer therapy, with laetrile clearly the target. The American Cancer Society, the American Medical Assn. and the FDA, all of which opposed the bill, did not fully realize that the Alaska action, spurred by Committee chapters, was only a shot fired across the bow. Cancer Inc. and American medical orthodoxy failed to assess the symbolic importance of the Anchorage legislation and for that reason unexpectedly ceded so much terrain to the laetrile movement that the Allopathic Industrial Complex (AIC) would ultimately have to go to the greatest — and dirtiest — lengths in its history to suppress what became the stiffest-ever challenge to its power and authority.

For, as noted, between 1976 and 1981 bills either "decriminalizing" laetrile (that is, barring the state from punishing a physician for administering, or a patient from having, laetrile) or outright "legalizing" it (accepting it as a useful medication, allowing its distribution and, occasionally, its manufacture) were approved in 24 states, which encompassed more than half the population of the United States. In some states, laetrile legislation was simply appended to existing medical statutes; in others, whole new statutes were written and passed. Following the rapid-fire approval of laetrile-connected legislation in Indiana, Florida and Texas, Cancer Inc. and the AIC began to note that they had a considerable problem on their hands.

The Committee-spearheaded efforts at taking one statehouse after another, activities also backed by other health-freedoms groups, captured media attention and popular interest. The Committee stuck to a single sweeping principle — that the issue was not so much freedom for laetrile as it was freedom of informed consent in cancer therapy in general for physician and patient. In virtually every professional opinion-sampling poll taken, be it national, state or local — and including Roper, Harris and Gallup — the concept of freedom of choice won by margins ranging from 2 to 1 to 12 to 1. The revolt drew scorn and shock from the AIC, fresh rounds of police action by the FDA (which even circulated Post Office "wanted"-style posters called "Laetrile Warnings" across the country), and such reflections of academic concerns as the laetrile-dominated AAAS meeting of 1979.

Since I was an eyewitness to, and frequent participant in, these state-by-state campaigns, I am fully aware — as the opposition slowly came to recognize — that we had a considerable populist tiger by the tail: an upsurge of grassroots rejection of the institutional, scientific and academic forces of the American establishment not so much over the issue of laetrile efficacy or lack of same but over the burning, central issue of freedom of choice. One observer after another joined the conceptual battle and usually remained clear on the separation of the issues of freedom of choice in medicine vs. the efficacy of laetrile: by what stroke of logic or presumed vested interest does the state have the right to intervene in life-and-death decisions between a physician and a patient, particularly when the patient is said to be "terminal," as with cancer? The AIC and the establishment in general never could offer a sound, coherent answer to that question. It still cannot. Hence, the tactics of the opposition changed.

From the scientific side, famed Mayo Clinic researcher Charles Moertel MD opined publicly that even though there was no proof of laetrile efficacy, at least in "accepted" circles, neither was there sweeping evidence *against* the compound. He and other front-rank researchers suggested there might be sufficient "biochemical background noise" to suggest the "valid sign of efficacy," the "shred of evidence" which Cancer Inc. kept arguing did not exist for laetrile — increasingly recognized as amygdalin and often described as "Vitamin B17." There were too many doctors stepping forward with case histories, some published in book form, too many dissident scientists claiming there was some merit in the notion of anti-cancer efficacy from glycosidic compounds, and far, far too many "anecdotes" from patients treated in Mexico or even within the USA to be able to make the claim the apricot kernel extract was totally without value.

With a US district court protecting citizen access at least to foreign laetrile, with one state after another either legalizing or decriminalizing the use of laetrile products in total disregard of the official positions of the FDA, AMA and American Cancer Society, with doctors and patients in ever greater numbers saying good things about the substance, and with cancer death rates ever worsening even after the Nixon Administration declaration of a "war on cancer," it became obvious that Cancer Inc. had to take another position.

The Establishment counterattack

In the earlier years of the controversy, the general establishment "line" on laetrile had been that it was worthless yet essentially harmless and that its only real danger lay in diverting cancer patients from "useful" treatments — a dodge argument inasmuch as the great majority of laetrile treatment seekers were advanced cases whose likelihood of being "cured" by "useful" therapies was quite low.

But given the political successes of the laetrile movement, the worthless-but-harmless argument needed to be amended. The new position was that it was not only useless but harm*ful* — the harm primarily attributable, to nobody's surprise, to the fact that an excess amount of the oral product could indeed produce a low-grade cyanide toxicity. Even though virtually no laetrile-using physician prescribed oral doses above the presumed therapeutically useful maximum oral amount (1.5 grams daily), and intravenous laetrile was regarded as so essentially non-toxic at even huge levels (one Mexican hospital once slow-dripped a breathtaking 97,000 milligrams — 97 grams — into one patient over 24 hours), the cyanide component of laetrile became the cornerstone argument.

I have recounted[29] how Cancer Inc. scoured world literature ("anecdotes" by any measure) to find scattered accounts of seeming "laetrile poisoning." These included the intoxication of garbage-plundering Turkish waifs years before who might have eaten too many fruit seeds, and the intoxication of a "hippie" couple in California who became ill after drinking a slurry of ground-up apricot kernels kept in a glass of water left standing in an open window the night before. Even the case of a woman who, averse to injections, broke open several vials of injectable laetrile and drank the contents before becoming fatally ill, made the news. While accounts of several hundred babies per year dying of aspirin intoxication was clearly not news, the mere suggestion that laetrile overdoses *might* be dangerous *became* news.

Major research centers turned to celebrated animal tests to attempt to alert the people to the "dangers" of laetrile.

In 1978 studies in Ohio, toxicity from oral amygdalin was said to have occurred in test animals when up to 1.3 grams *per kilogram of body weight* was provided for monkeys and up to 6.4 grams *per kilogram of body weight* for dogs. These enormous levels, extrapolated to humans, meant that from *five to 300 times* the normal oral doses of amygdalin for a 150-pound man were provided to the test animals. No doubt about it: toxicity occurred.[30]

Results of the incredible "laetrile toxicity study" at the University of California-Davis in 1978 were provided to the press and public at large as evidence that the consumption of certain vegetables together with oral laetrile could kill, and that even the "laetrile diet" recommended to laetrile patients was dangerous.

But the test was actually a sophisticated effort to produce

cyanide intoxication in animals: dogs were starved, drugged (to suppress vomiting), and then administered by inserted gastric tube a mash of sweet almonds mixed in a plastic blood bag with amygdalin at a temperature sufficient to allow an enzyme within the almonds to "hydrolyze" the amygdalin, causing cyanide release. This tactic did indeed intoxicate several dogs — but it had nothing to do with the ways in which either dogs or man eat or how they consume "B17" compounds.[31]

By the time of the laetrile trials, American orthodoxy had taken a belated interest in potentially toxic chemicals in the plant kingdom, very much including the nitrilosides, and no effort was spared to serve up frightening new evidence that overdosing on such compounds could indeed be life-threatening. Scattered research also suggested that inappropriate uses of such compounds might be *mutagenic* — that is, change-causing and hence predisposing to cancer — as if such information constituted important new discoveries.

Most of these findings, of course, were already well-known to chemists and biochemists who were fully aware that too much of anything, including air and water, and/or the misuse of virtually any compound, herb or medication could lead to serious problems, even death. Yet the AIC was forced, by sheer weight of laetrile's political successes, to overkill the issues of danger from cyanide-bearing compounds and to track down, and extrapolate from, every isolated datum that could be found which might produce a negative for laetrile. No such campaign of any such dimension had ever been mounted before in American medical history.

The medical establishment continued to write off laetrile case histories pointing to seeming successes the time-honored way — such cases were either misdiagnoses, belated responses to earlier orthodox therapy or, when all else failed, "spontaneous remissions," the line of defense used consistently throughout this century against the "unprovens" (*XI*).

It also made certain that notable failures of laetrile-centered therapy got plenty of press attention, particularly if the failures came from the growing caseloads of Drs. Contreras and Richardson. Such negatives were indeed reported in gruesome detail — yet it was only an occasional journalist who dared contrast failures on laetrile therapy with failures on vincristine, 5-FU, adriamycin, radiation and surgery, since somehow a failure on an orthodox modality was somehow less a failure than one on unorthodox therapy.

The Establishment also chose most of the time to overlook the fact that modern-day laetrilists absolutely denied that amygdalin was a "cure" of cancer (even if the original proponents of laetrile seemed to have believed it was), and that the maximum claim being made for its use by the great majority of doctors and researchers was that laetrile, as part of a total "metabolic program," might lead to the lifelong "control" of the disease.

But for every Establishment setback of laetrile research there were countermoves by "unorthodoxy" — even when well-credentialed. Cancer Inc. seemed particularly enraged when Loyola University (Chicago) biochemist Harold Manner PhD and a team of graduate students released data in a "non-standard" publication on tumor shrinkage in laboratory rats with a combination of amygdalin, proteolytic enzymes and vitamins.[32] Tests conducted at Salisbury State College in Maryland suggesting cancer prevention by *ad libitum* consumption of apricot kernels by test rats not only were not followed up on but got the key researcher in hot water.[33]

The late Harold Manner would fall under heavier attack after he started inducing foreign cancer clinics to utilize his "Manner cocktail" (not very divergent from the laetrile "metabolic therapy" already in place) against human cancer, in which he claimed striking success against breast cancer in particular.

Independent-minded researchers frequently tried to bring reason out of the war. University of California-Berkeley chemist James Cason PhD, who found merit in the "B17" theory, wrote in a scientific publication in 1978:

If I believe that eating 100 mg of nitriloside and 2

g of vitamin C per day will prevent me from becoming a cancer victim, and I live according to my stated convictions, and I am wrong, *I suffer no penalty for my poor judgment, because I am doing nothing other than eating food that is commonly regarded as nutritionally beneficial.*

If one who believes that all this stuff about cancer resulting from nutritional deficiencies is nonsense, lives by his convictions, and he is wrong, *that individual stands a very good chance of paying an awesome penalty for his faulty judgment.*[34]

This was just the kind of argument, as advanced by a properly credentialed American scientist writing in a properly credentialed scientific journal, that Cancer Inc. did not wish to hear — but could do little about.

Attempted KO: the 'laetrile clinical trial'

The laetrile controversy, simmering both politically and scientifically, had a final denouement in the scientific arena with the federal 1980-81 "laetrile clinical trial," an outgrowth of Senate subcommittee hearings in 1977 (another landmark event for an "unapproved" remedy). With the trial, the Committee for Freedom of Choice took a calculated risk: providing the government with the tools to test a compound already found anecdotally useful for thousands of patients could either vindicate or destroy it.

Even so, as I reasoned, the mere fact that such a trial had to be done in the first place was an unprecedented event by itself, and it seemed unlikely that such a study would be uniformly negative.

The laetrile movement wandered into the trial quicksand poorly prepared: there were arguments about the proper manufacturing procedures for intravenous laetrile, there remained differences of opinion even over the definition of the word "laetrile," and too often laetrile proponents had explained theories as to how amygdalin "worked" as facts rather than as educated speculations.

And, too, as in any orthodoxy-denied activity (prostitution, alcohol consumption at an earlier time), there were commercial pimps and criminal elements ready to take advantage of a legally unserviceable market: there were indeed phony laetriles, cases of fifty-dollar vials of bootleg laetrile, and some manufacturers of both vials and tablets were not always honest in reporting true weights and contents of tablets and vials.

The presence in the contraband market of numerous laetriles of uncertain origin both compounded the fight for acceptance and provided the AIC with propaganda targets.

Yet such presence bespoke a greater reality: there was a growing popular clamor for access to laetrile, whose legal availability — and therefore the nature and purity of which — could not be guaranteed *because of* state-sanctioned interference with the availability. Such a situation was a most well-fertilized breeding ground for con men, opportunists, and criminals. Yet these were exploiters rather than causers of the situation, the true creator of which was the Allopathic Industrial Complex (AIC).

The "laetrile clinical trial" was conducted on 178 patients at four major research centers after a "retrospective analysis" conducted by the National Cancer Institute (NCI) turned up evidence of laetrile efficacy (as understood by orthodoxy) in nine of a mere 93 case records submitted, somewhat timorously, by US physicians.

American Biologics, a California company which in no small part was an outgrowth of the Committee for Freedom of Choice in Cancer Therapy Inc., had offered to provide for free a Mexican-manufactured supply of laetrile — certainly a risky maneuver if in fact the company, as a major proponent of amygdalin, knew the material to be worthless. The government refused the offer, only later admitting the material to be used was a reproduction of Mexican laetrile seized during a confiscation and that the injectable form was not pure amygdalin but in fact a "racemic" form of it. Our group attempted unsuccessfully to block the trial in court when evidence surfaced that the material originally planned for use would not release cyanide. It is not clear exactly which material was ultimately used, or if the same material was consistently used.

The "laetrile clinical trial" was wholly unprecedented in American medical history and — as our group noted in a point-by-point rebuttal of its findings[35] — wound up being in essence a US government-sponsored test of an uncertain laetrile product whose application was in the hands of doctors and scientists known to be or assumed to be hostile to laetrile, whose patients were anonymous, and the test results of which, being coded, could not be individually released or cross-checked. Worse, the patients accepted for entry into the program were variously described as "terminal" or beyond the hope of cure by conventional means, yet not at the "final stage."

The government also saw fit to release data on the test before the trial results were published — itself an unprecedented move — before a special audience as a kind of slide presentation. But a Committee observer at the event was able to photograph the relevant slide which showed that a significant amount of test patients had remained "stable" while on the injectable part of a program whose oral protocol, we had every reason to believe, was not very strongly adhered to (and parts of which, as in suggested Vitamin A levels, seemed not to have been followed at all.)

By the time the results were published, in the *New England Journal of Medicine*,[36] an abstract of them summarized that the clinical trial had shown laetrile to be ineffective as a cancer treatment — yet the fine print did not truly substantiate the analysis. For, depending on how the numbers were read, either a small majority or a large plurality of patients had remained "stable" while on the injectable part of the program, and only advanced into further disease after the 21 days of injections ceased. It later surfaced "anecdotally" that at least one patient was urged not to continue on the program (claiming he had "done too well"[37]). As a corollary, a preliminary test found amygdalin not to be toxic, at least in the ranges suggested for therapeutic use.

In all, the results, far from putting laetrile to rest, raised far more questions than they answered. Yet the press was provided with an abstract-based account which had the desired effect: "LAETRILE FAILS" and similar headlines greeted the release of the findings. The *New England Journal of Medicine* subsequently allowed brief dissents by cancer researcher Edwin Bross, acclaimed scientist Linus Pauling, and myself, but the damage was done, and it was extensive.

Laetrile's real victories

Despite the fact that for the first time ever the AIC and Cancer Inc. had had to play unusually rough to quench an unwanted competitor, and despite the fact that for a time the Mayo Clinic-centered "laetrile clinical trial" had a chilling effect on use of the substance itself, it had all been a matter of too little, too late:

Just as plans for the trial were getting underway, Rutgers University, in diabetes-oriented research, came up with a finding it seemed almost too flustered to report — that amygdalin is a useful natural "scavenger" of the deadliest of the "free radicals," hydroxyl radical.[38] This finding substantiated laetrile's role as an antioxidant (scavenger of free radicals), an activity being seen of increasing importance in the way cancer spreads (metastasizes). Then, just as the test furor was hottest, the National Academy of Sciences (NAS) published an incredible, federally funded study appropriately called *Diet, Nutrition and Cancer*.[39]

In it, essentially American research (most of it from the University of Minnesota) found a wide spectrum of plant kingdom factors apparently useful in the *prevention* of cancer, including Vitamin C. Among the more prominent, widely dispersed plant compounds was a class of what researchers called "non-nutritive food factors" and among these a key family was referred to as "benzyl-aromatic-isothiocyanates" — or, as we reported it, BAITs, for short. However much anti-laetrilists wished to gloss over the fact, BAITs refer to compounds which at the very least are structurally similar to "Vitamin B17" even though their mode of action against cancer has not been well elucidated. It seemed a kind of hollow scientific victory for our side in the propaganda war, and of course went essentially unnoticed by the media and certainly by the major organs of the AIC: laetrile might be a "dirty" but a benzyl-aromatic-isothiocyanate was a "clean."

While the NCI laetrile trial was widely reported to have "put laetrile to rest," use of products said to be laetrile, in natural or manufactured form, continued apace — and still do. It was up to such entities as the Bradford Research Institute (BRI) to place the use of the cyanide-bearing sugar compounds (natural laetriles) into their proper slot within a total metabolic program and to publish by far the most definitive study on how amygdalin might or might not work against cancer, which occurred in 1981 in a research paper which helped to demystify "Vitamin B17" but remained essentially unknown.[40]

For years, German researcher/physician Hans Nieper MD has developed laetrile-based or laetrile-related medications showing great promise.[41]

Research in the 1980s, primarily in Japan,[42,43] indicated that benzaldehyde — usually a considerable portion of "B17" compounds — has anti-cancer properties on its own. The institutional observation that BAITs, "benzaldehyde inclusion compounds" — and indeed *aldehydes* in general as natural "genetic repair" compounds and/or other natural factors which tend to metabolize in the body to laetrile-like substances — has only helped strengthen the overall concept of a dietary-deficiency theory of cancer.

That oral "B17" compounds convert to *thiocyanate*, a chemical useful in almost two dozen natural body functions, including regulation of blood pressure, has also bolstered the notion of a natural "surveillant, antineoplastic" mechanism against cancer. It may be that the "real" Vitamin B17 is in fact thiocyanate, and that the cyanogenetic glucosides or nitrilosides are "pro-vitamins."

Before his death in 1996, I received what was apparently the last of the famous "Krebs memos" (undated, and sent in July) to the various researchers and writers Ernst T. Krebs Jr. considered to be his "laetrile family."

Never in all his professional life with laetrile and the trophoblastic theory had "ET" budged an inch from both concepts, but at least as regards to laetrile he was willing to make a scientific concession (which, aside from reflecting a certain openness of mind, in a sense strengthened the case *for* laetrile). He wrote:

> *"[T]o the fact of extrinsic or dietary control of [cancer] we have the extrinsic or dietary control of non-toxic nitrilosides. Amygdalin is one of such closely related nitrilosides. The presence of the free benzaldehyde derivable by the enzymatic hydrolysis of such is the antineoplastic power of them all.*
>
> *"The-CN [cyanide] moiety of Laetrile itself is important to the molecule. I was in error in giving antineoplastic priority to the -CN of the nitriloside* . . . [44]"

Here, Krebs was saying that the benzaldehyde segment within nitrilosides is probably more important as an anti-cancer agent than the cyanide, with which it virtually always occurs in such compounds.

It is great men, scientists or others, who are able to admit to error.

Whatever the research outcome, the case for laetriles and laetrile-like compounds as useful against the malignant process — and useful in numerous *other* processes — has been enhanced over time.

Scientifically, laetrile's victories have thus been confined to a kind of pyrrhicness: the substance itself remains a Cinderella compound, yet the plant families in which it and similar substances are often found (as in the *Brassica, Rosaceae, Prunasae*) are those families in which modern-day research has isolated indoles, flavones, phenols and many other compounds in addition to BAITs as useful anticarcinogenic agents.

Too, what for years laetrile doctors called the "laetrile diet" is, broadly speaking, the diet now promoted by, of all things, the American Cancer Society and Cancer Inc. in general: less animal fat, less animal protein, fewer stimulants, fewer refined carbohydrates, more natural fruits and vegetables in as natural, raw or sprouting a stage as possible, and more fiber and unrefined grains. And aspects of the metabolic program of which laetrile is usually a part — as beta-carotene and Vitamin C — have come under close scrutiny for increasing evidence they are useful against cancer.

It is as if laetrile gave a party it was not allowed to attend — or, as one long-time "laetrilist" put it, "modern, establishment-accepted nutritional therapy against cancer and without laetrile is rather like Christianity without the Virgin Birth."

Even so, long-term "laetrile/cancer survivors" — people with advanced malignant states who used laetrile as a central part of a total metabolic program — abound. Some have written books about their experience with the apricot-kernel derivative, including long-term survivor Helen Curran of Laguna Hills CA, whose inspiring book carries the same name as this chapter.

And there was Kansas' Glen Rutherford — the man for whom the original US Supreme Court case involving freedom of access to laetrile in the 1970s — is named.

In 1996, Rutherford was a self-described "eighty years young," and a quarter century away from the prognosis of fatal colorectal cancer that had sent him to Mexico in the first place. Along with his oral laetrile, Rutherford daily consumed upwards of 80 supplements a day and was a stickler on the "cancer diet." Not only had colorectal cancer not returned in more than two decades — neither had he had the flu in all that time, he was pleased to report.[45]

But perhaps laetrile's major victory was, as our group

analyzed, at the political level.

The fight for freedom of choice for laetrile ballooned into a much broader fight for freedom of choice in medicine itself. The attempt by Cancer Inc. to suppress the growing "anecdotal" efficacy of Vitamin C against cancer followed on the heels of the Laetrile Revolution, and paralleling both was a substantial increase in the use by physicians of natural nutrients in both the prevention and management of chronic diseases, including cancer. Laetrile had let a major cat out of the bag, and it would never go back in.

The apricot kernel extract had become the Marine Corps of the integrative medical revolution — first on the beach, first to be bloodied, first to open the door to what would come after.

References

1. Markle, GE, and JC Petersen, five papers, American Assn. for the Advancement of Science, January 1979.
2. Moertel, CG, *et al.*, "A clinical trial of amygdalin (laetrile) in the treatment of human cancer." *New Eng. J. Med.*, Jan. 28, 1982.
3. Culbert, ML, *Vitamin B17: Forbidden Weapon Against Cancer.* New Rochelle NY: Arlington House, 1974.
4. Culbert, ML, *Freedom from Cancer.* New York: Pocketbooks (Simon & Schuster), 1977.
5. Kittler, GD, *Laetrile — Control for Cancer.* New York: Paperback Library, 1963.
6. Griffin, GE, *World Without Cancer.* Westlake Village CA: American Media, 1974.
7. Halstead, BW, *Amygdalin (Laetrile) Therapy for the Nutritional Support and Control of Cancer.* Colton CA: Golden Quill, 1977/78.
8. Burk, Dean, *A Brief on Foods and Vitamins.* Sausalito CA: McNaughton Foundation, 1975.
9. Halstead, Bruce, *Amygdalin (Laetrile) Therapy.* Los Altos CA: Choice Publications, 1978.
10. Civil, M, "Prescriptions medicales sumeriennes." France: *Rev.d' Assyriologie* 54, 1960.
11. *Ibid.*
12. Gerarde, J, *The Herball or Generall Historie of Plantes.* London: 1633. Cited in Heinerman, J, *The Treatment of Cancer with Herbs.* Orem UT: Biworld Publisher, 1984.
13. Porcher, FF, *Resources of the Southern Fields and Forests.* Charleston: 1863. Cited in Heinerman, *op. cit.*
14. Krebs, ET, Jr, "The nitrilosides in plants and animals." In *The Laetriles — Nitrilosides in the Prevention and Control of Cancer.* Sausalito CA: McNaughton Foundation, 1967.
15. Krebs, ET, Jr, "The nitrilosides (Vitamin B-17) — their native occurrence and metabolic significance." *J. Appl. Nutr.* 22, 1970.
16. Beard, John, *The Enzyme Treatment of Cancer and its Scientific Basis.* London: Chatto and Windus, 1911.
17. Moss, RW, *The Cancer Industry.* New York: Paragon House, 1991.
18. Testimony, Cancer treatments seminar, sponsored by Staten Island Borough President Guy Molinari, New York, September 1993.
19. Culbert, ML, *Vitamin B17, op. cit.*
20. Culbert, ML, *What the Medical Establishment Won't Tell You that Could Save Your Life.* Norfolk VA: Donning, 1983.
21. *Ibid.*
22. *A Complaint Against Medical Tyranny as Practiced in the United States of America: American Medical Genocide.* San Francisco CA: Committee for Freedom of Choice in Medicine, Inc., June 1984.
23. Ferguson, Wilburn, *Tsanza,* unpublished memoirs, 1982. Also, Ferguson, Wilburn, *The Jivaro and His Drugs.* Quito, Ecuador: Editorial Casa de la Cultura Ecuatoriana, 1957. And extensive private communications.
24. Fitzgerald, BF, *Congressional Record,* August 28, 1953.
25. Culbert, ML, *Freedom, op. cit.*
26. Culbert, ML, *Vitamin, op. cit.*
27. *Ibid.*
28. *Ibid.*
29. Culbert, ML, *What the.. op. cit.*
30. *Ibid.*
31. *Ibid.*
32. *The Choice,* IV:2, March 1978.
33. Culbert, ML, *What the.. op. cit.*
34. Cason, James, in *Vortex,* American Chemical Society, June 1978.
35. *Response of the Committee for Freedom of Choice in Cancer Therapy, Inc., to the Publication of the National Cancer*

Institute 'Amygdalin (Laetrile) Clinical Trial' Los Altos CA: Committee for Freedom of Choice in Cancer Therapy, Inc., Jan. 29, 1982.
36. Moertel, *op. cit.*
37. "Dr. Nieper assails the NCI 'laetrile trial.'" Rochester MN *Post-Bulletin*, Feb. 8, 1982.
38. Heikkila, RE, and FS Cabbat, "The prevention of Alloxan-induced diabetes by amygdalin." Pergamon Press Ltd., *Life Sciences* 27, 1980.
39. *Diet, Nutrition and Cancer.* Washington DC: National Academy Press, 1982.
40. Bradford, RW, *et al.*, *Amygdalin: Its Nature, Biological Interactions, Implications for Therapeutic Use in Cancer, and Quality Control.* Los Altos CA: Bradford Research Institute, 1981.
41. Nieper, HA, "Modern medical cancer therapy following the decline of toxic chemotherapy." *Townsend Letter for Doctors and Patients*, November 1996.
42. Tatsumura, T, *et al.*, "4, 6-0-benzylidene-D-glucopyranose (BG) in the treatment of solid malignant tumors." *Br. J. Cancer* 62, 1990.
43. Kochi, Matsuyuki, *et al.*, "Antitumor activity of benzaldehyde." *Cancer Ther. Reports.* (N.I.H.), 64: 1, 1980.
44. Personal communication, July 1996.
45. *The Choice*, XX: 2-3, 1994.

XIII
AIDS SCAMS AND SCHEMES:
End of humanity or end of allopathy?

"There is hope, but let's not exaggerate. Let's not switch from very dark pessimism to hype and overoptimism so we will all have a hangover within six months or a year."

— UN AIDS Program Director Dr. Peter Piot, 1996

"Cure is a dangerous word . . . This won't be a magic bullet. This virus has surprised us before . . ."

— Dr. Martin Markowitz, Aaron Diamond AIDS Research Center, 1996

"Even if you accommodate [HIV] virus with all sorts of absurd and paradoxical hypotheses that doesn't get you around the solid number of 4,621 HIV-free AIDS cases. Here we have a real cover-up."

— Molecular biologist Peter H. Duesberg PhD, 1993

"Our national pride is at stake. We claimed that the US discovered the cause of AIDS, and we would develop a vaccine and some antiretroviral drugs. The government has literally funded nothing but HIV research for years, and it's very difficult for any bureaucracy, especially the federal government, to admit that they were wrong. I suspect what's going to happen is they will continue to say that HIV is the cause of AIDS, but the entire rest of the chapter will be about how 'co-factors' are necessary, and so forth."

— Michigan State medical researcher
Dr. Robert S. Root-Bernstein, 1993

"The mystery of that damn virus has been generated by the $2 billion they spend on it. You take any other virus, and you spend $2 billion, and you can make up some great mysteries about it, too."

— Kary Mullis PhD, Nobel Prize for Chemistry, 1993

"Although HIV is universally accepted as the cause of AIDS, the evidence is still not all that compelling. In fact, HIV infection is not even required for a diagnosis of AIDS, according to the Centers for Disease Control and Prevention. The current definition of AIDS is any one of 27 different diseases accompanied by low numbers of CD4 cells in the immune system. Thus the causal agent (HIV) of a disease (AIDS) is not required to cause the disease. Is this a bit of scientific legerdemain or what?"

— Dr. Gordon Edlin, professor of biochemistry and biophysics,
University of Hawaii, 1993

AIDS as apocalypse

Only superlatives have been used to define the pandemic of AIDS:

It is variously described as an unprecedented threat to world health, a Black Death of the late-20th century, even as an end of civilization provoked by nature, manmade errors or biological warfare.

Never before in medical history has such a massive global effort been mounted in such a short time, and never before has so much money in research funds been raised in such a short time, to stop or at least slow down a menace which in its first 16 years (1981-1997) had thwarted every effort at cure — if agreement is reached on the meaning of the word "cure" (let alone agreement on the word "AIDS.")

In 1994, repeating earlier official statements of gloom and doom, Michael Merson, director of the "Global Program on AIDS" of the World Health Organization (WHO), synthesized: "The end is nowhere in sight. The pandemic is certain to continue well into the 21st century. There is no breakthrough and I do not think one is imminent. We will not have a magic potion for AIDS before the year 2000."[1]

This had been WHO's message of gloom at virtually every international AIDS meeting at least until the Eleventh International Conference on AIDS in Vancouver, Canada, in 1996.

Then, for the second time (the first had been a decade prior) the drug company-dominated, worldwide but US-led AIDS research establishment came up with a modicum of good news — a new class of potentially toxic (and expensive) antiviral drugs, offered as "cocktails" with older antivirals, in a small group of patients seemed capable of greatly lowering (and possibly banishing) from the body detectable levels of the putative "AIDS virus," HIV, for more than a year, while bolstering immunity.[2,3]

The technique was dubbed HAART (for "highly active antiretroviral therapy") and led to 1997 assessments of lower death rates from AIDS for the first time since 1981.

Offsetting virtually a decade and a half of near-hopelessness in AIDS, the latest thrust from AIDS Inc., the ever-growing amalgamation of research grants, virological endeavors, and public-private scientific investigation, provided a ray of hope that somehow, perhaps, AIDS could finally be beaten down by a combination of synthetic drugs, a goal which had eluded science for so long.

Despite the initial enthusiasm, by the end of 1996 the first reports of AIDS patients "crashing" — that is, returning to advanced pathological conditions following their earlier, often dramatic, upswings — began to come in, and some elements of AIDS Inc. doubted whether such "cocktails" would do much for individuals who had been infected for HIV for more than a year.

And a California newspaper survey in 1997 found the HAART combinations failing in 10 to 40 percent of patients as reported by physicians with various caseloads.[3a]

A 1997 Italian survey of 300 patients suggested growing multidrug resistance,[114] and the Food and Drug Administration (FDA) reported the same year that some patients on the drugs developed diabetes.[115] (***See NOTE, Page 594***)

But the new "protease inhibitor" drugs — with yet another category ("integrase inhibitors") waiting in the wings — had provided some solid optimism that in at least some people the drug-centered approach could change lives at least temporarily to nearly normal.

Should this turn out to be true, it would be occurring in the nick of time:

By 1996, according to WHO, the United Nations and epidemiologists, perhaps as many as 27.9 million people (including 2.4 million children) were "living with HIV infection" with 10,000 being infected daily, and between 5.8 million and 6.4 million people were said to have died of AIDS — or, rather, of any of the 30 or so opportunistic infections and "forms" of cancer said to be part of the syndrome — with another 11 or 12 million more projected infections by 2000.[4,5,5a,5b,5c] Some 21.4 million or 94 percent were said to be in the "developing world."

By 1997, AIDS had been diagnosed in over 580,000 Americans and had killed over 300,000 of them. In descending order of AIDS cases, as of 1997, were the US, Brazil, Tanzania, Thailand and France, among the top five countries, though reporting from 191 WHO member states ranged from responsible to spotty.[(5d)]

Geopolitically, AIDS is thus said to be far more devastatingly affecting that part of the world (the "third world") which can least afford to pay for any of the expensive new antivirals, with ominous messages constantly beamed which point to a virtual wipeout of the population of central Africa and enormous fatalities-to-come in India and Southeast Asia.

Before Vancouver, most international meetings had simply been recitations of just how bad the problem was, and how little progress had been made.

As in all previous conferences, actual rates of infection and caseloads were thought to be severely underreported due to poor statistics-gathering in many countries. Some estimates have it that the HIV infection rate could reach or surpass 50 million by the end of the decade, with the actual number of AIDS cases continuing to balloon exponentially by then.

It was estimated by mid-decade that "full-blown" AIDS had killed or would be killing at least 60 percent of AIDS cases. By then the United States accounted for 40 percent of reported cases (though only 13 percent of the estimated total), down from 50 percent a few years earlier. It was assumed — based on projections of HIV incidence — that a wide swath of central Africa and a substantial portion of Asia would eventually succumb to AIDS. There was no truly useful drug — or vaccine — to stop the slaughter.

In fact, as the message of doom developed over the years — following the headier days of the early 1980s when the alleged "cause" of the syndrome was said to have been described and antibody tests developed to find it — international AIDS conferences had become biennial rather than annual events as an embarrassing paucity of research progress was turning up every 12 months.

In the United States, the AIDS-monitoring Centers for Disease Control and Prevention (CDC) in 1994 reported[6] a doubling of AIDS cases primarily based on yet another broader definition of just what AIDS is. It was also estimated that somewhere between 650,000 and one million Americans were "carrying" HIV, consistently reported in the United States as "the AIDS virus" (although this ironclad description for a long time had been less definitive, particularly in Europe.)

The million-infectee figure had been holding steady for several years, and was actually a compromise between some estimates which placed infection levels as considerably smaller or even greater. The infection level was "downsized" by 1996 (to 750,000, at least according to *AIDS Clinical Care* figures in fall of that year) in a rejuggling of AIDS data some found suspicious at best. No one knew for sure just how many people were infected with "the AIDS virus," let alone what it really meant to be infected with it.

Static to declining numbers of HIV infectees made it clear that an "AIDS pandemic" had *not* hit the American population in general — if the HIV/AIDS theory holds up. That is, the pandemic had failed to affect the majority (heterosexual, non-drug-using, non-hemophiliac) population in pandemic proportions despite having allegedly done so in Africa and Asia.

AIDS had also become a political and social phenomenon in the US, frequently enmeshed with and tainted by the politics of organized homosexuality and civil rights. By being incorrectly described since the outset as a "gay disease," it had provoked as much sociological as medical concern and had lulled the non-gay world into a protracted period of feeling somehow immune to a multifactorial disorder which, as it turned out, might take many years to appear (if it appeared at all) and then could kill in a combination of gruesome ways.

AIDS also became a gigantic new industry, rapidly gaining on cancer, and by mid-decade as much federal research funding was being dumped into the hunt for an "AIDS cure" as for a "cancer cure," even though cancer was still killing far more Americans than was AIDS (and, of course, almost a quarter of AIDS is, by definition, cancer). This was a result of political organizing and deft media manipulation. The federal AIDS bill for 1994, involving research, "education" and prevention, was $6.2 billion — but even that was only an estimated 35 to 45 percent of total HIV-related spending,[7] and only a portion of the estimated $40 billion spent since the syndrome's outbreak in 1981.

For by the 1990s, both domestically and worldwide, AIDS had become a major moneymaker: billions of potential dollars loomed in the ownership and use of "AIDS tests" (primarily antibody tests but also various higher-tech methods to capture HIV or parts of it) and, more important, there was enormous profitability in developing either drugs designed to trick, thwart or inhibit "the AIDS virus" or to attempt to manage any of the multitude of "opportunistic diseases" which came about *because* of the alleged "AIDS virus" and actually did the killing and crippling. It was obvious even after the first few years of AIDS that insurance policies, and even some whole insurance plans, were being wiped out simply by patients' attempting to pay for one or more "AIDS drugs" — none of which "worked" in the sense of completely eliminating a 30-plus-disease syndrome.

The demographic aspect of AIDS was also dramatically changing by the latter part of the decade:

Worldwide, AIDS is *far more* a heterosexual disorder than it is a "gay disease" and, as some had argued for a decade, in the Western world more related to drug abuse than to sexual habits even though sexual promiscuity remains highly correlated with AIDS. In areas of the world allegedly facing mass extermination because of presumed widespread infection by HIV, which in turn is presumed to develop at some point into "full-blown" AIDS for a majority of people, the sexual deployment of the syndrome is almost equally between men and women, with an apparently easier likelihood of transmission *to* women.

Even in the United States, whose CDC first characterized the "gay" nature of the original infectees (though many printed lines down from the first paragraph it was also revealed that these same five infectees also were drug abusers[8]), new infections among homosexual males were beginning to level off with the highest increases noticeable among women (primarily "minority"), intravenous drug abusers of both sexes and children born to infected women. At least half of America's hemophiliacs were thought to be infected by "the AIDS virus," yet — intriguingly — nowhere near a majority of these had "died of AIDS."

(The HIV/AIDS/hemophilia connection in the US involves several possible scandals: the first is that the plasma from which the hemophiliac-using anticlotting elements, particularly Factor VIII, are made, preferably came from promiscuous male homosexuals, many of them drug users, in the early 1980s, the high levels of hepatitis among such donors seen as biologically beneficial for clotting-factor raw material. That such factors came from pooled blood, most of it from homosexuals, at a time when blood products and drug companies knew, suspected, or *should have known* that the agent or agents "behind" AIDS were blood-borne, is shocking.

(That these companies did not inform hemophiliacs of the mostly-gay, and often gay/drug-abuser origin of pooled blood — the factors actually being elements from *thousands* of donors — when an epidemic was breaking out among that very population is a parallel scandal. Only recently has it become known how such companies actively recruited male homosexuals as blood donors for the "plasma fractionation" business which could bring a half-million dollars per lot of clotting factors. That the FDA was overseeing the process is yet another black mark against this most notorious of federal agencies [*see IX*].[8a]

(That perhaps 10,000 American hemophiliacs — continuing recipients of tainted blood from the early 1980s — were expected to die at some point from AIDS-related conditions does not necessarily depend on the HIV theory of AIDS: it is impossible to tell *how many other* agents may have been — and might still be — in such clotting factors, made from the pooled blood of *thousands* of donors and the continual use of which is somewhat immunosuppressive to begin with.)

There also were increases in "no identifiable risk" cases of HIV infection where there simply was no clear reason (some of the victims, including children, were of course not practicing male homosexuals, some "practiced" no sex at all, had had no blood transfusions or blood products, were not hemophiliacs, were not intravenous drug users, and were not the sexual partners of any of the above). Such cases called into question the reliability of HIV antibody tests in general, the nature of HIV itself — and the entire HIV theory of AIDS causation.

The course of the syndrome also seemed to be changing:

While there still were "fast" AIDS cases where death seemed to ensue a few months to a few years following diagnosis, the syndrome was increasingly seen as a long, lingering, up-and-down affair, almost an Allopathic Industrial Complex (AIC) delight since it meant extensive periods of ultimately unsuccessful therapies which seemed to be prolonging death rather than extending life. Since a variety of its various opportunistic diseases and cancers could be temporarily "managed," the syndrome became more chronic than acute. The parallel reality was that just as many hospitals were emptying the endless assortment of lingering "AIDS" conditions appeared in time to fill some of them up again.

Common sense vs. panic

With the world facing what seems to be an imminent catastrophe of mind-numbing proportions over AIDS, it is necessary to bring some doses of common sense to the fore while by no means denigrating the reality that AIDS is and will continue to be a significant medical problem. But there is this startling reality:

Almost everything originally said about AIDS (including its mostly being a "gay disease") has turned out either to be all wrong, mostly wrong, or misleading.

On the ever-growing bill of particulars:

— The word itself: *a*cquired *i*mmune *d*eficiency *s*yndrome (AIDS) is a syndrome — that is, a combination of symptoms, diseases and disorders — and not *itself* a disease. Hence, nobody has truly "died of AIDS."

— The definition of elements of this syndrome has been both "officially" and "unofficially" altered both domestically and internationally so many times that AIDS is not easy to define. As this was written (1997), an individual "presenting with" any one or a combination of (by my count) 34 ("officially," 29) "opportunistic" fungal, parasitical, bacterial, mycoplasmic or viral infections and/or "forms" of cancer and who had a "count" of 200 or fewer "helper" (that is, CD4 or T4) cells per cubic millimeter of blood, and who was positive for antibodies to the HIV (human immunodeficiency virus types 1 or 2 or their subtypes), was an "AIDS case."

— As I pointed out in an earlier book,[9] definitions of AIDS are now allowable even in the absence of blood tests — that is, simply from clinical signs and symptoms and a physician's merely guessing at the patient's presumed "lifestyle." What this may mean, some of the dissidents to the key theories of AIDS and HIV have stressed, is that a significant amount of diagnosed "AIDS cases" might not be AIDS cases at all!

— Even if the linchpin theory that a "new" virus, HIV, is the single "cause" of AIDS, and that antibody tests (and, more recently "viral load" assays) somehow remain the gold standards in spotting presence of the pesky virus, there exists the irritating reality that an individual with virtually *any* disorder may be classified as "AIDS" simply on the basis of a positive antibody test. What this means, for example, is that a tuberculosis patient who is antibody-positive for HIV automatically becomes an *AIDS* case. The list of conditions gathered under the AIDS umbrella has grown so swiftly that it became a funereal joke among some researchers in the mid-1990s to wonder if a big toe infected by a rusty nail on which it stepped should be classified as an opportunistic AIDS symptom if the stepper should turn out to be HIV antibody-positive.

— By 1997, or some 14 years after the alleged "cause" of the syndrome had been breathtakingly announced to the world, despite billions of dollars of research it was still not clear just exactly how HIV "works" — that is, how it actually "causes" AIDS, although the research had come up with some fascinating possibilities. And at least two HIVs — 1, 2, and nine "genetic subtypes" of the former (among some eight "clades" or families of ever-mutating HIV) — were thought to be threatening the human population.

(AIDS reseacher Max Essex of the Harvard AIDS Institute in Boston noted that globally as of 1996 there seemingly were *two* "simultaneous epidemics" of HIV — the more familiar American/European strain known as subtype B, and subtypes known as A,C,D and E, said to be responsible for some 20 million infections, mostly in the "developing countries."[10]

(The above have been designed "Group M" viruses. By 1996 yet another strain, called Group O, originally concentrated in central and Western Africa and said to have "extensive genetic divergence" from the Group M viruses, began showing up in the USA. This virus was said not to be "consistently detected" by the usual antibody tests.[11]

(If the rapidly developing HIV epidemiology is to be believed some strains or subtypes are more correlated with heterosexual than with homosexual sex [something new all by itself in medical history] and yet all are ostensibly blood-borne. With the vast amount of AIDS cases in the world now infected with subtypes other than B and mostly involving heterosexuals, and with AIDS-associated tuberculosis now the top killer in the syndrome,[12] the natural history of AIDS — if in fact there is only one syndrome — has become extremely confusing, to say the very least. And it was becoming clearer that HIV was not likely causing AIDS all by itself.)

— The notion that there was a "latency period" between HIV infection and disease was all but abandoned by 1996. The new view is a life-and-death struggle between HIV and the immune system from the outset.[13,14]

— In the earlier days of AIDS, the most common deadly sequelae were *Pneumocystis carinii pneumonia* (PCP), variously described as a fungal or protozoal infection primarily of the lungs, and Kaposi's sarcoma, an often hideous skin cancer — or cancer-like condition — which, like melanoma, can become lethal, particularly if it internalizes. (Tuberculosis became the major AIDS killer worldwide by 1996.) For a time, PCP alone was accounting for approximately 60 percent of the deaths of American AIDS patients. Yet, PCP — as is true for all the 33 (28?) other presentations and forms of AIDS — is not a new disease, and was last encountered *en masse* among immune system-depressed German children and infants at the end of World War II. And the medical establishment had a hard time figuring out whether KS, thought to be a "form" of cancer, was truly a part of AIDS, a parallel infection, or an expression of the syndrome occurring toward the beginning, rather than the end, of it.

— Research by mid-decade was linking KS to a separate virus.

(Our BRI research group suggested in 1986 that KS might be a parallel viral infection, particularly since on an experimental blood test "AIDS" patients presenting only with KS were exhibiting a viral-infection pattern, not a cancer one, at least in earlier stages.

(A year earlier, research in *Human Pathology* strangely not followed up on with much vigor indicated[15] that KS was much more widely distributed in patients than earlier suspected. Such investigations drew a distinction between "typical" KS and "inflammatory" KS. When aspects of "inflammatory" KS were considered in an "autopsy series" involving Haitians of both sexes,

IV drug users of both sexes, gay males, hemophiliacs and three with "unknown risks," the disease was found to be widespread.

(The view that Kaposi's might be a parallel viral infection was strengthened in late 1994 when a Columbia-Presbyterian Medical Center team announced the controversial discovery of yet another human herpesvirus which it found highly correlated with KS.[16] While other research cast doubt on its causative role,[17] and other research made strong correlations,[17a] the terms KSHV (Kaposi's sarcoma herpesvirus) and HHV-8 (human herpesvirus 8) have now entered the medical lexicon. How it (they) might "cause" KS remained unknown in 1997[17b] even though some research has suggested that the HIV "transactivator" gene *tat* might "activate" HHV-8.[17c])

— As information developed that increasing numbers of KS patients even in the United States [it has long been common in North Africa and parts of the Mediterranean as a relatively unimportant skin cancer] were *negative* for HIV antibodies [as was also true for a small but growing number of PCP patients — the PCP having been *induced* in some cases by chemotherapy drugs for cancer![18]] — then it became obvious: neither PCP nor KS alone should always be considered to be AIDS. If, of course, PCP and KS were removed from the combination of AIDS diseases, then the *true incidence* of AIDS deflates on a monumental scale.

— Data continued to surface that the vaunted HIV "antibody tests" — earlier the primary ways to detect the alleged "AIDS virus" — were not always reliable.[19] While the standard ELISA (enzyme-linked immunosorbent assay) and the allegedly "confirmatory" Western Blot tests were conceivably error-prone themselves, information developed that *other* infections and conditions could cause "false positives" on such antibody tests.[20]

(In fact, HIV antibody test dissidents by 1996 had catalogued almost 60 conditions, infections and immune responses which might be "cross-reactive" with the standard HIV antibody tests — that is, cause a patient to be "seropositve." Such an avalanche of information, from suitably "peer-reviewed literature," may have been a primary reason why AIDS Inc. had to turn to expensive, and equally controversial, tests which attempted to find the actual virus, or parts of it, in patient blood and tissues — by no means a closed book by the time this was written.[20a] After all, some people were committing suicide based on a single HIV antibody-positive test.)

It also became increasingly clear, particularly among healthcare workers exposed to possible HIV infections, that there could be actual infection, however transient, which the antibody tests would not "pick up."[21]

Adding these realities to the continually disturbing ones concerning difficulties both in isolating whole viruses or parts of whole viruses, let alone how to interpret such findings, it is now obvious that there *is* no single guaranteed blood test which actually tells an individual he or she *has* AIDS. There simply are tests (including, by 1994, a saliva test) to indicate exposure to HIV, and the expensive "viral load" assay to indicate the presence of active virus.

— The advent of "viral load" tests, as stressed again and again at the Vancouver meeting, together with the "cocktail" antiviral drug approach, gave AIDS Inc. yet another "buzzword." While some research[22] has called into question just *how* definitively "viral loads" of HIV are detected, how they are counted, and what they mean, it is relatively clear that high "loads" of HIV correlate with AIDS-related disease. But such tests are new, expensive and of difficult access to most of the world. Their presence does indicate a watershed of sorts — downplaying the far-less-reliable antibody tests for determinants of actual virus in the body.

— Accompanying the appearance of the "viral load" has been, almost overnight, the abandonment of the longest-held of the orthodox AIDS-related theories — namely, that falling numbers of CD4 ("helper") cells in the immune system, HIV's apparent main target, equate absolutely with staging the various aspects of AIDS.[23] Under this thinking (and it *was* often observed) after CD4 levels reached a certain low plateau (200 or less per cubic millimeter of blood is part of the definition of AIDS), the AIDS-related cancers, infections and other "opportunistic" infections which actually do the killing would break out and overwhelm the host.

It has since become clear that falling CD4s accompanied by rising CD8s ("suppressor T-cells") do not always relate to AIDS but may indicate various forms of immune dysregulation, so that the long-ballyhooed "inverted ratio" between CD4 and CD8 cells might turn out to be essentially meaningless in predicting who had, or would have, an AIDS-defining illness.

— The fact that CD4 counts alone did not necessarily mean much (in fact, their transient rise following antiviral therapy allegedly might be providing the "AIDS virus" with even more targets of opportunity) was also a small nod to "alternative" AIDS doctors, who, early in the epidemic, noticed that neither declining CD4s nor critically altered CD4/CD8 ratios always equated with disease.

The American Biologics-Mexico group of research doctors was among those who found that significantly high rises in CD8 cells often equated with the clinical absence of disease for very long periods of time, even *if* CD4s were critically low. We reported that long-term HIV-infected survivors often remained clinically free of disease, or only moderately diseased, as long as CD8s remained high, regardless of CD4 levels. These patients, just as those often reported elsewhere, were usually on some form of "unorthodox" therapy.[24]

Several ranking American AIDS researchers also observed this phenomenon and one of them, San Francisco's Jay Levy, long proposed a possible viral-killing or other control factor from a subset of CD8/T8 cells.[25,26] By 1995, it was determined that CD8s secreted various anti-viral substances and might constitute a second line of defense against AIDS,[27,28] though CD8s are also infected by HIV and their roles in disease progression are by no means fully understood.[29]

— The social ramifications of AIDS remained equally muddled.

With *most* of the worldwide AIDS pandemic not related to homosexuality, some voices in the US raised the spectre that the reverse was true somehow in the Western world — that most of AIDS in the West is no particular threat to heterosexuals. There is even some evidence that the US medical establishment, at least in the early days, might have overplayed the dangers of "heterosexual AIDS"[(29a)] — yet the growing presence of HIV/AIDS in heterosexual women and children in the Western world, however modest alongside cases among drug abusers and promiscuous male homosexuals, may yet vindicate the earlier warnings concerning AIDS and "unsafe sex."

Questions began to surface which could not effectively be answered: How many AIDS syndromes are there? Why is the clinical picture so staggeringly different between Nashville and Nairobi? Are there really sex practice-specific viruses? How can some people be incubating "AIDS viruses" so long without becoming ill? How could some be constantly exposed to them and not "get" AIDS? And, if one, two or more viruses are the causes of AIDS, *just where did they come from and why hadn't we known about them before 1981? How could they just suddenly "emerge"?*

— It was obvious enough so that I could recount the data in two AIDS studies in the 1980s that the following observations could be made concerning the conventional wisdom about AIDS: increasing numbers of patients with immune disturbances and HIV antibody positivity were either only minimally ill or not ill at all and had remained that way for years; and increasing numbers of patients ill with one or more AIDS-related illnesses had little or no immune perturbation and some were negative for HIV antibodies.

— By the 1990s, these earlier observations were now becoming far more commonplace, and they led to three startling sets of data which, together, influenced increasing numbers of well-credentialed independent AIDS researchers (about 500 in the USA by mid-decade, including two Nobel Laureates) to question the key premise put forth by the orthodoxy about the syndrome (namely, it is singly caused by HIV):

• First, it had become ever clearer, primarily from studies of long-followed "cohorts" of potential AIDS patients tracked for their HIV "seropositivity," as well as a rising wave of anecdotal data and some from statistical extrapolations, that a significant number of HIV-infected individuals were living well over a decade — perhaps a *third* up to 14 to 15 years (based on backtracking their blood tests) — without developing even significant immune disturbances or any clinical signs and symptoms of AIDS.[30] (Many, but by no means all [and there was no way to determine this fully] were on "unorthodox" preventive therapies).

• Second, information developed that there might somehow be "milder" strains of ever-mutating HIV which, while infecting a given group of people, provoked no significant disease. Australian research was particularly precise on this point.[31] And surveys of healthcare workers who had had known exposures to HIV through needlestick injuries and other treatment accidents pointed both to very low infection rates of HIV and cases in which there was "transient" infection — that is, the virus "hit," but it was overcome by body defenses before antibodies formed.

• Third, and more astounding for defenders of the HIV theory, it was increasingly being reported in both the "standard" literature and more widely in "unorthodox" circles that ever-growing numbers of patients were "presenting" with terminal, full-blown AIDS symptoms and their concomitant immune system disorders assessable in blood tests without *ever* having had either antigens (actual pieces of) HIV or antibodies to them! One controversial estimate by 1993 was that there were at least 4,621 "HIV-negative" AIDS cases in the world, with at least a third of those in the United States — and that even many US AIDS cases had been "presumptively" (rather than hematologically) diagnosed with HIV.[32]

But with HIV now constituting the most-studied virus in history, it may very well be that the ever-more-startlingly-unique features of this structure have allowed it to hide so well so long that it was really there but wasn't detected (the will-o'-the wisp argument.)

Or, that AIDS Inc. has gone to awesome lengths to retain control of the central theory: a syndrome with a single viral cause, and the billions of dollars in public/private research funds dependent on the theory.

Making the facts fit the theory

As we have seen, this nation's Allopathic Industrial Complex (AIC) is nothing if not adroit in manipulating semantics and making the facts fit the theory. We note in *X* how the AIC essentially invented a new disease — *hypercholesterolemia* (too much cholesterol) — as a pathology needing to be treated by cholesterol-lowering drugs, cornerstones of the cardiovascular industry.

In terms of AIDS, it became ever more obvious that numerous people — both from "risk groups" (that is, married to, or the sexual partners of, allegedly HIV-infected people) and, more importantly, those *not* from "risk groups," a reality which most damaged the paradigm — had either AIDS-related diseases and/or AIDS-like immune disturbances without ever having had any evidence of HIV. Hence, a new term was created, literally out of wholecloth, to explain what this new subset of individuals seemed to have:

"Idiopathic CD4 T-lymphocytopenia." The translation of this phrase: "helper T-cells falling for no known reason." ICL become the common abbreviation.

The questions nagged supremely: if, by mid-decade, there were at least hundreds (and probably thousands — maybe even millions throughout the world) of people infected with the HIV virus who had failed to come down with either pre-AIDS or AIDS conditions for a decade or more, and if, on the other hand, there were reportedly (and presumptively) hundreds to thousands of so-called AIDS patients without HIV, then:

How could it still be said that HIV is the cause, or at least the sole cause, of the admittedly devastating syndrome?

The observation that HIV is a *lentivirus* — that is, a slow developer — was insufficient as a total answer.

The American AIDS research network, originally funneled — strangely enough — through the failure-prone National Cancer Institute (NCI), continued to go to extravagant, elegant, byzantine and even outrageous lengths to explain all of this away.

The way HIV infects people and "causes" AIDS remained only partially understood as late as 1997, even though the retrovirus had been found in virtually every body fluid and numerous tissues. Abstruse theories were adduced as to how HIV still could "cause" AIDS even if various antibody and antigen tests cannot find it.

With literally billions of dollars at its disposal, AIDS Inc. attempted to answer each new HIV conundrum by posing yet another theory.

By 1996/1997 the latest good news about HIV — if in fact it and it alone is the "cause" of AIDS — was that some people might have a natural immunity to it, or at least have inherited genetic mutations (CCR2, CCR5) which could slow it down.

This was a bow both to the impact of the well-stocked coffers of AIDs Inc. and its utter tenacity in not turning loose of the HIV theory as well as a role for the rapidly advancing world of genetics.

And, yes, by any virological definition, HIV is an unusual, seemingly clever, escape-prone virus which "replicates" and mutates so fast no two isolates from the same person are ever the same. And HIV seems to be associated with, correlated with, somehow linked to, certain aspects of AIDS, including dementia, and is a possible cancer factor (lymphomas) — but again, there has been no smoking gun to prove the above.

Most intriguingly, almost from the moment HIV (originally baptized HTLV-III) was pronounced, in 1983, to be the "cause" of AIDS by an American medical establishment under heavy political pressure to explain the nature of the seemingly new syndrome, whose numbers had been growing exponentially since it was first delineated in 1981, a few key experts begged to disagree.

The most vocal dissenter was University of California-Berkeley molecular biologist Peter Duesberg PhD. Duesberg is not just a heretic: he is one of the fathers of retrovirology and a discover of "oncogenes" in cancer. Possessed of an innovative mind, Duesberg argued both that it had not been specifically proven that any so-called oncogene actually *causes* cancer (*XI*) — and he argued for years that it had not been proven anywhere that HIV actually *causes* AIDS. He has attributed AIDS more to drug abuse than anything else and has published repeatedly and convincingly on the reasons why, drawing both professional wrath and reductions in research funds for doing so. [33,34,35,36]

Too, however fiendish HIV seems to be — able even, it would seem, to mutate in a host more rapidly than other rapidly mutating viruses, and selectively targeting the quarterback of the immunological team (the CD4 cell) — "the AIDS virus" seems almost benign alongside some other quick killers.

By the mid-1990s, perhaps the most horrific of the "emerging viruses" was that causing the rapidly fatal Ebola hemorrhagic fever. And there was the hantavirus, said to infest deer mice, which led to alarming numbers of rapidly killed Americans beginning in 1993 (yet, interestingly, others allegedly infected recovered), and there were "new" — or newly discovered — viruses linked to other potentially fatal syndromes. Science was hard pressed to answer: where do these things come from?

And this question — where *have* the "emerging new viruses" come from? — is the central concern of a startling, even unnerving, answer from new research which, even if it is only partially correct, could explain just why HIV (and a growing number of other structures simply not known about before the 1970s) is so "different."

The multiple "differences" of HIV from so many other viruses may be due to a shocking reality the ramifications of which are sinister at best — and we will address them in the next chapter.

A "company line" has also developed to explain away dangerous seemingly "new" viruses, and it surely produces part of the answer — that the destruction of the planetary habitat by encroaching human population (let alone the possibility of easy transfer of bacterial, viral and parasitical diseases through jet airplane-enhanced international travel) has unleashed dangerous new organisms into the human race from their hidden or subsurface sanctuaries.

While it is not the aim of this account to become involved in all the multiple scientific aspects of the HIV debate, suffice it to say that by the mid-1990s some 500 American scientists, researchers and AIDS investigators were on record as dissenting from the HIV-as-single-cause theory, and the list included two Nobel Laureates. One of these was San Diego's Kary Mullis, inventor of the PCR (polymerase chain reaction) test, one of the precision assays used for isolating HIV. Some of the most compelling data gathered against the HIV theory was in print not only from Duesberg but also from Michigan State medical researcher Dr. Robert Root-Bernstein.(37)

A British journalist, recanting years of favorable reporting on the HIV theory, in 1996 did an about-face with the publication of a startling book.

Wrote Neville Hodgkinson:

> *Ten years of reporting on HIV and AIDS, and three years of deep involvement in the controversy over AIDS causation, have led me to the conclusion that a decade ago we became ensnared in a mass illusion surrounding the issue.*

Namely, that the "new" retrovirus HIV singly causes the syndrome.

But we should also point out that, long before it was fashionable, the maverick Bradford Research Institute (BRI) was the first international research organization to question the HIV-as-single cause theory, and I outlined the reasons why in a 1986 monograph and a 1990 book.[38,39]

With more than a decade of debate behind us, it seems likely that HIV surely has *some* role in AIDS, primarily through an attack on various cells of the immune system. It seems increasingly *un*likely that it is the single cause of AIDS.

HIV's role in AIDS, if any, may be categorized this way:

1. "Company line:" HIV is a slowly evolving animal-derived virus which "jumped species" into mankind sometime within the last century. It is the single cause of AIDS.

2. "Conspiracy theory:" HIV is a biological warfare weapon developed by "crossing" animal viruses and testing them in humans the research for which may have begun with the benign intention of studying viral and vaccine approaches to cancer. Whatever, it is the single cause of AIDS (*see next chapter*).

3. "Moderate position:" HIV, whatever it is or wherever it came from, has a role to play in AIDS but cannot be the single cause. It has one, two or more co-factors which will determine who "gets" AIDS or who doesn't.

4. "Radical dissent position:" HIV, whatever it is or wherever it came from, is an irrelevant structure which may not even exist (some question whether retroviruses are even real) and, even if it exists, is not causing a disease.

It should be noted that each of these positions has well-credentialed researchers with respectable credentials as disciples.

Dissidents to the HIV theory — just as in the case of dissidents to the broadly held cancer-cause theories — found it difficult to publish their ideas and impossible to secure research funds. The hermetically sealed mind of the AIDS research apparatus, growing faster even than the cancer one, has been no more enthusiastic about free thought or novel new ideas than the cancer industry, despite a seemingly all-out effort to study, explain and stop AIDS.

Yet the same central allopathic errors abound in AIDS:

The allopathic paradigm needs to find single causes for single diseases, and then to fashion "contraries" against the causes.

This 17th-century approach dominates Western —that is, American — medicine, as we see time and again throughout this study. It is neither greater nor lesser than in the case of AIDS.

But the result in AIDS has been, proportionally, even more devastating:

For, by 1997, the 16th year of the Plague, adherence to the notion that a single virus — new, old, mutated, manmade or whatever — is the single "cause" of the syndrome; and to the notion that only devastatingly toxic "nucleoside analogue," or "non-nucleoside reverse transcriptase inhibitor" or "protease inhibitor" or "integrase inhibitor" drugs can slow down or stop the virus had so far failed to "cure" a single case of AIDS.

Enter the 'co-factors'

By mid-decade the complex of public and private research institutes and renowned scientists (as well as fund-raising organizations) we style "AIDS Inc." was running out of excuses for what seemed the endless failure to find an AIDS "cure." Slowly, a trend of thought introduced from within the orthodoxy was gathering steam:

If HIV *alone* is not the cause of the syndrome, then it must have help, perhaps a lot of it. The term "co-factors" surfaced even by the middle 1980s among some scientists who were beginning to suspect that, however interesting HIV was, it could not be doing its devastation all by itself. Only a few on-line physicians (such as Joseph Sonnabend MD, New York, who was among the first to suggest "multifactoriality" both in AIDS causes and treatments[40]) had voiced their suspicions of the establishment "line."

So the HIV dissidents split into two general camps: a few, as headed by Duesberg, suggesting that HIV is a totally irrelevant retrovirus playing no meaningful role in AIDS at all, and the bigger group, believing that HIV might be a "sentinel" or "marker" virus for something else or at least be contributing in some way to the syndrome. (Widely disseminated photos from the scanning electron microscope did, in fact, display HIV seeming to invade its target of choice — the regulating CD4/T4 "helper" cells of the immune system, surveillant over viral infections and hence a vital target for a weapon which seemed aimed at provoking immune collapse.)

While numerous researchers found likely co-factor viruses from the better-known families (particularly the herpes family, headed by Epstein-Barr [EBV] and cytomegalovirus [CMV]), none seemed to fit the mold as probable "catalyst" or "trigger" viruses.

By the late 1980s, even researchers within the orthodox camp were beginning to talk about "co-factors" (the last redoubt, as one dissident scientist told me, when one cannot consistently fit the pathology with the etiology) to HIV. By then, even Robert Gallo, the National Cancer Institute (NCI) investigator who allegedly co-discovered HIV and originally claimed that any dissent from the notion that the retrovirus was the cause was "crazy," had begun to talk of "co-factors."

And the Pasteur Institute's Luc Montagnier, who actually was the first scientist to isolate the alleged "AIDS virus," broke ranks earlier — he insisted that although HIV must be involved, surely a tiny structure called a *mycoplasma* must be a "co-factor." Independent research by US Army Institute of Pathology scientist S-C Lo, virtually ignored at first, even showed that it was a kind of mycoplasma which, when injected into test animals, could sicken and kill them with AIDS-like diseases while HIV remained unable to do significant damage to any non-human species.[41,42] *(See XIV)*

(In October 1994, *Science* reported[43] that an "AIDS-like" condition had been induced in baboons by a strain of the "second AIDS virus," HIV-2. The fact that six test baboons had "sero-converted" following infection by this particular strain, that four developed swollen lymph nodes, while three had immunological features similar to "AIDS infection" and one was killed after developing significant disease, was broadly parroted by the media[44] as a sign that, finally, test animals had developed "full-blown AIDS" apparently from an HIV virus. Yet there was no way to know how the animals lived or were fed or what other infections they might have had — and the HIV-2-UC2 strain is not the virus commonly said to be infecting humans. And, as more test animals seemed susceptible to HIV infection it rarely caused symptoms, let alone deaths.)

As we shall shortly see, human herpesvirus 6 (HHV-6) has jumped to the top of the list of probable "co-factors" to HIV — and some believe it is more important in AIDS *than* HIV.

But by the time AIDS Inc. began talking "co-factors," at least in the United States, there were enormous industrial considerations at stake: HIV as the cause, and only toxic nucleoside drugs, led by Burroughs Wellcome's AZT (Retrovir, zidovudine, azidothymidine), and, later, "non-nucleoside reverse transcriptase inhibitors" and "protease inhibitors" or "cocktails" of them all, able somehow to "slow down" what was still widely called "the AIDS virus." The thinking was to hit HIV "early and hard" and in different viral regions before it could mutate — even though mutability and eventual tolerance to any drug seemed to be certain with this virus. Such an approach seemed at least able to "buy time," with long-term outcomes unknown.[45,46,47]

The HIV-as-single-cause theory was the central excuse for the entire federal (and interconnectedly private) research effort. The mass testing of the population (leading, in Cuba, to the actual quarantining of "AIDS carriers") with HIV antibody tests was itself a new industry. Between billions dumped into research on "the AIDS virus" and development of antibody tests as well as a spate of far more precise virus-isolating assays, and multi-billions more in toxic drugs, AIDS research and propaganda seemed to take off wildly on a course of their own; anyone who stood in the way would not be taken seriously.

For the medically (in distinction to the biochemically) minded, questions arose early over why so much research was directed at HIV when, by any valid assessment of the syndrome, it was *other* viruses, bacteria, parasites, yeasts, fungi, probably mycoplasmas — and cancer — that were doing the actual sickening and killing of patients.

At some point in the AIDS infection curve, rampant yeast infection, elevated "titers" of Epstein-Barr Virus (EBV) and cytomegalovirus (CMV) occurred, yet little was done to find ways to curb these pathogenic conditions in terms of fresh research. Some older drugs, essentially antibiotics, were found to slow down or even prevent PCP, but these often were also toxic and sagged in efficacy over time.

Intense diarrhea and a multiplicity of pulmonary disorders were killing AIDS patients, along with rare "forms" of cancer, but research seemed strangely not to concentrate on these truly lethal diseases. The AIDS research establishment remained obsessively focused on HIV, often concentrating such efforts in continually failing endeavors to fashion a useful vaccine..

As the second decade of the Plague Era began it was ever more obvious that allegiance to HIV as single cause and the hopes pinned on AZT as some kind of pharmaceutical white knight were probably misplaced. As we shall see, there also loomed nettling possibilities that, if in fact there is a single catalyst for AIDS and it is viral, orthodox research may have focused too much attention on the wrong virus.

Aside from ominous hints of conspiracies and coverups including everything from a global conspiracy to wipe out a segment of humanity to institutional efforts either to hide biological warfare research or simply to paper over a series of shocking laboratory blunders, there also arose the terrible consequence of misplaced faith in nucleoside analogue drugs — that they might be *causing* AIDS symptoms in and of themselves (a point made by Duesberg and a growing band of observers) and also killing patients. (As we have seen in cancer [*XI*], this would be nothing new — toxic chemotherapy [which AZT was originally developed to be] is a "cure" often worse than the disease and may kill directly or indirectly a significant portion of patients said to have died from "complications of cancer.")

Just as toxic AZT received a "breather" as a useful anti-HIV agent following years of failure and just as the only hope against AIDS seemed to lie outside the realm of standard medicine, the rush to market in 1995-1996 of both "non-nucleoside reverse transcriptase inhibitors" and "protease inhibitors" gave the drug approach a tremendous resuscitation, particularly after the Vancouver conference. Nine such drugs were available at this writing.

The fact that a small group of people who could tolerate a combination of such not only felt better and had rises in their CD4 cells, accompanied by the seeming vanishing of all signs of HIV from their blood ("viral load" tests), for a year or more, was hailed as a major breakthrough. The word "cure" began to be heard.

But, sober research minds were on hand who warned about over-optimism. They had seen how, a decade before, AZT had been rushed to the market with similar fanfare and how, largely, it had failed. (Some of the relevant warning quotes are lead-ins for this chapter.)[(48)]

The "downsides" of the drug-cocktail (HAART) approach in 1997 were these:

• If HIV is the true or major cause of AIDS, vastly falling numbers of HIV in the serum ("viral loads") still meant there could still be plenty of virus left over to return to overwhelm the host.

• There remained the uncertainty as to whether HIV would simply adapt to the new drugs (as it had to the older ones) and perhaps become even more virulent.

• The long-term side effects of the admittedly toxic new drugs were simply not known.

• It was assumed that AIDS patients would remain on such drugs for the rest of their lives.

• The sudden expansion in CD4 "helper" cells following administration of the drugs might mean not that more such useful cells were being newly produced but simply that they were being released from other (lymphoid) areas.

And what has been so far the abject failure of AIDS Inc. to solve mankind's fastest growing menace may turn out to be the final rapier thrust to finish off the allopathic paradigm in medicine, a key element in the revolution of medical paradigms now underway.

Some historical background is necessary if one is to attempt to make any kind of sense of the AIDS disaster.

Cancer Inc. joins AIDS Inc.

It should be remembered that the ever-more-funded National Cancer Institute (NCI) was the federal conduit through which, President Richard M. Nixon hoped, a hugely financed "Conquest of Cancer" program would wipe out this greatest of the diseases of civilization. Raise enough money, open enough labs, and cancer will be wiped out the American way, the citizenry was assured.

It should also be recalled that for decades of the post-WWII era, and in sound alignment with the linear, monofactorial allopathic paradigm which controls the chief concepts of American-led Western medicine, the "viral theory of cancer" was paramount. Billions of research dollars were spent publicly and privately to find cancer-causing human viruses let alone ways to "inhibit" (but not truly kill, since viruses are not actually "alive" in a biological sense) the same. Decades came and went, and though some viral activity might be inferred in some "tumor systems," rare was the virus that could be isolated which absolutely and irretrievably could be said to have "caused" a malignancy.

By the time the first few years of the "Conquest of Cancer" program were assessed, in the 1970s, it was clear that there were more cases of, and fatalities from, cancer in the United States than ever before in our history. The massive campaign to track down a cancer-causing virus and then stop it, thus vanquishing cancer, was plainly failing. If anything, the NCI, by the latter 1970s, was a good example of the institutionalization of error as funded and refunded by taxpayers and propped up by politicians. In the private sector, such bungling would have, and should have, led to enormous job layoffs. But federal employment, just as federal agencies, endures. And endures.

And, as we shall see, the fact that the NCI continually received swollen federal funds for research that seemed to be going nowhere may have a more sinister side (*Chapter XIV*).

Suddenly, in 1981, there was AIDS — a term settled on after some earlier unwieldy acronyms (even GRID, as "gay-related immune deficiency") were dropped. No doubt about it: something seemingly new and menacing had broken out along the socially-perceived pestilential soft underbelly of the population: promiscuous male gays and intravenous drug users were coming down in ever spiralling numbers with a variety of conditions and diseases previously seen only in chemically or nutritionally immune depressed people. They had somehow "acquired" an immune deficiency. Hence the evolution of the concept of the acquired immune deficiency syndrome.

For whatever reason, the major research effort to halt a rapidly developing new plague was handed to the NCI, the very same apparatus which had so miserably mismanaged the "war on cancer." And the NCI was still guided by 17th-century allopathic beliefs about single causes for diseases and still entranced with the endless hunt for viruses, around which so many other industries (particularly the development of "immortal cell lines," and several early waves of genetic technology) were already flourishing. The unstated mandate was *find the virus*.

By 1983, France's legendary Institut Pasteur and the American NCI seemed to be racing neck-and-neck to determine which would "find the virus." It is now clear — despite a rather childish, testy and expensive dispute between the Americans and French that took years to settle and involving patents on test kits which ultimately enriched both countries and several researchers, including the US' Robert Gallo to the tune of $100,000 a year[(49)] — that the French got there first, but close enough in time so that both could take credit for "co-discovering" what at first was more correctly called "the virus most often associated with AIDS." That is, a majority of persons who had developed full-blown AIDS were thought to be harboring this agent, and antibodies to it had been detected.

As we shall see [next chapter], if the biological warfare theory has merit, certain NCI scientists, and probably some at the Pasteur and other major research centers, may have known perfectly well what the "AIDS virus" was long before it was "discovered."

The hasty announcement by the US government that the AIDS "cause" had been found seemed to be a payoff for American research and sound scientific technology. With the "etiological agent" now identified, the next phase would be to research its structure and fashion weapons to knock it out or a vaccine to prevent it. Sound allopathic thinking.

Indeed, over the years more money was raised in a short time to study the HIV virus than had ever been raised as fast in medical history for any virus — and more is known about it than any other virus in history. All of which makes the lack of full evidence that it is *the* single cause of AIDS so triply frustrating and humiliating.

As more data continued to come in worldwide, it seemed that Africa might have been the source of the virus which the NCI's controversy-plagued Robert Gallo and associates originally called "HTLV virus type three" (from earlier descriptions of a presumed family of "human T-cell-lymphotropic" structures). Travel patterns between AIDS patients and Africa suggested such an origin, even though outbreaks of AIDS seemed spontaneously to have occurred in three separate geographical areas, all at the same time — central Africa, the Caribbean and the gay enclaves of New York and San Francisco.

Since HTLV-III, later to be rechristened HIV-1, seemed to be a blood-borne virus and so many American victims were male homosexuals or intravenous drug users or both, it seemed a safe assumption that HIV was essentially a blood-and-semen-carried virus and that AIDS, hence, must be a kind of venereal disease. The "gayness" of the syndrome dominated the American response, primarily due to the Centers for Disease Control's 1981 definition, a move which arguably set back AIDS research and muted effective social response to it for the better part of five years.

AIDS in Africa: horror and hoopla

But questions arose fairly early: the Africans said either to be infected by HIV or dying from AIDS or both were overwhelmingly heterosexual and were not IV drug users. In southern Europe and the Mediterranean, AIDS was considered — and by the mid-1990s was still considered — to be more an intravenous drug user's disease than anything else.

How research on AIDS got off on several wrong feet and ran smack into the vested interests of ego and misplaced research was recounted by the late Randy Shilts (himself an AIDS victim) in *And the Band Played On* (1987), one of the first popular works which helped to galvanize American awareness of the onrushing syndrome.

The international viral research community held to the notion— or was induced into believing — that somehow a mutated simian virus had "jumped species" into man some time in Africa as the origin of the syndrome, and it spread outward in a pattern similar to that of an allegedly related virus, HTLV-I. But was it new or old? Ultimately, it was postulated that AIDS-like conditions had killed at least one American and one Englishman in the 1960s and that HIV-like antibodies had been traced back to *healthy* Amazonian Indians in the 1960s and to Africans in the late 1950s. It turned out that at least one of the early British AIDS cases probably was not one after all. The research establishment was agreeing, by the 1990s, that HIV was new but not terribly new — no older than 100 years, maybe only a few decades. It must have mutated from lower animals, ran the thinking. Perhaps it did.

Throughout AIDS' first meteoric decade, AIDS Inc. kept informing the world that in the "AIDS belt" of central Africa (some nine countries in the sub-Saharan part of the continent) a whole population was about to be wiped out, and that HIV infection and AIDS cases there would dwarf anything seen in the USA. Even so, during most of that time at least half the world's reported AIDS cases were in the admittedly more statistics-and-quantification-obsessed USA than in Africa.

Nonetheless, since "the AIDS virus" was said to have originated there, had been incubating there longer, and had infected so many, droves of people should in fact be dying of AIDS in Africa. And, indeed, some television and even print media reports did find some terrible examples of people in AIDS-like death throes.

Even so, journalists who took the trouble to visit Africa in the 1980s began questioning just how many people were truly "dying of AIDS," whose clinical pattern was usually so utterly distinct to that in Europe and the USA. A media investigation in 1987 cast doubt on the main conclusions about African AIDS.[50] It has also been suggested[51] that the seeming sudden outbreak of HIV or AIDS in Africa in the mid-1970s may have been due to sociopolitical disruptions.

AZT-baiter John Lauritsen, one of the few cool journalistic heads in the AIDS catastrophe, quoted from Richard and Rosalina Chirimuuta (*AIDS, Africa and Racism*) about what may have really gone on in the "AIDS belt:"

> *"[Western doctors] conducted small and unreliable seroepidemiological surveys that 'proved' that millions of Africans were infected with the virus. (One Belgian team spent three weeks in Kinshasa, diagnosed 38 people as having AIDS), 'then figured out how many cases this would amount to in a year's time, divided that by the total population of Kinshasa and estimated an annual rate of developing AIDS in that country to be about 17 per 100,000.'"*[52]

Yet, when West German researchers examined thousands of serum samples from central Africa, they found only four contained HIV antibodies. Their findings, noted Lauritsen, were ignored because they did not fit the "AIDS plague myth."

And the "AIDS belt" countries involved contain roughly only about 10 percent of the population of Africa.

Seeming virtually to be fighting back to convince the world that there *is* a major AIDS plague in Africa, Centers for Disease Control (CDC) officers editorially described as "confirmed and quantified" in 1994 a rather strange report on "two-year HIV-1-associated mortality" in an area of rural Uganda. It was said to be "the largest prospective study of its kind in sub-Saharan Africa."[53,54]

True, Daan W. Mulder *et al.*, in assessing 9,389 individuals, found 89 deaths in individuals seropositive for HIV (as opposed to 198 who were seronegative), including 64 adults. Of these, five were said to have died of AIDS by a *pre*-1987 definition thereof called the "Bangui case definition"; 31 had "one or more major symptoms" and 28 "*no major symptoms.*" Overall, disease progression to death in general was higher among those infected with HIV. The highest mortality rates were for children under 5 and adults over 55 whether they were positive for HIV or not.

The report discussed "excess mortality" as a statistical correlate of those with HIV. It did not prove HIV causes AIDS. Since it is not clear exactly what these individuals died of, or whatever else they may have been "positive" for, such research raised more questions than answers.

By 1995, the Ivory Coast, in w*est* Africa, was reporting among the highest rates of HIV infection and AIDS cases, with prostitution considered a major "vector."[55]

But what also is true about Africa — where the main presenting feature of AIDS was long reported to be "slim disease," the gradual wasting away of the body accompanied by intense diarrhea?

The same "AIDS belt" countries said to be awash in AIDS are also countries which have long had galloping rates of amoebic dysentery, other protozoal diseases and parasites of all kinds, malnutrition, malaria, yellow fever, leprosy, tuberculosis, syphilis, yaws, pinta and a galaxy of other bacterial and viral infections. Blood samples from such chronically diseased people are "interesting," to say the least.

In 1993 and 1994, studies by well-credentialed scientists and researchers, in part based on African "AIDS," began to raise the question of usefulness of HIV antibody tests to ever higher octaves: Zairian officials, working with US AIDS expert Max Essex, found that certain bacterial infections (leprosy and tuberculosis among them) could cause up to an astounding 70 percent of "false positives" on HIV tests![56]

Earlier, an Australian research team, going so far as to argue that such tests might be "counterproductive," suggested that the assays, far from detecting the presence of a virus, might simply be reacting to cellular proteins — in which the blood of multiply infected people is noticeably aswarm. Such observations strengthened the thinking of others that retroviruses themselves might be artifacts — that is, results of, rather than causes of, disease.[57] (Retroviruses are viruses which must "replicate" by "transcribing" the reproduction-capable amino acid combination RNA to DNA, the catalyst of cellular growth in normal cells.)

The new attacks on HIV antibody tests, particularly those run on the blood of multiply infected people, of course throw into doubt all assessments based on generalizing just how much HIV is present in any population. Antibody tests, at best, measure responses to something, and not the *somethings* themselves.

In Africa, the possibility has thus been raised that one of two things or both might be occurring: that great numbers of diseased people (that is, diseased with tuberculosis, malaria, yellow fever, syphilis, amoebic dysentery, leprosy, gastrointestinal parasites), are being "transferred" to the AIDS column because either HIV antibodies are found or are *presumed* to be found in them (the cost of such tests in significant numbers is simply beyond economic reach for several countries); or that great numbers of people carrying proteins produced by disease states (tuberculosis, leprosy, for example, whether they have any clinical signs or symptoms of these diseases) are showing "false positive" on HIV tests.

Either reality greatly inflates both the AIDS and the AIDS-prone categories and nourishes the belief in the worldwide mass infestation of HIV as a global threat to the human population.

As of 1995, at least from reviewable records from admittedly backward countries, it could not be demonstrated that the population of central Africa was being wiped out by AIDS (birth rates were rising) even though — of course — the ever-lengthening incubation period of the all-purpose killer virus could indeed simply mean that the wipeout was taking far longer than expected. We cannot discount this possibility — only call it into question while noting an ongoing African AIDS problem.

Too, however bad the AIDS (or seeming AIDS) epidemic is in parts of Africa, a United Nations report in 1994 showed that even in the presence of a galloping HIV/AIDS juggernaut, the population growth in the 15 most affected countries would be 2.38 percent per year, as opposed to 3.13 percent without the syndrome.[(58)]

Natural immunity?

But even assuming the worst about African AIDS, there also developed a ray of optimism which, if extrapolated to humans as a whole, bodes well:

At the end of 1993, 25 Nairobi female prostitutes were under "intensive scientific study" because, although some of them had had repeated, unprotected sexual activity for up to 13 years, not only did none of them have AIDS conditions, neither were they "positive" for HIV. This group of sex workers in a high-AIDS area, together with groups of both promiscuous male homosexuals and hemophiliacs all of whom allegedly must have been exposed to HIV but developed neither antibodies nor any other reaction to it, seemed to provide, as *Time* put it, "the strongest evidence yet that people can have a natural immunity to AIDS."[(59)]

By 1996, 239 of 424 initially HIV-negative Nairobi prostitutes studied since 1985 had "seroconverted" — but investigators found that a certain proportion of "highly exposed" prostitutes remained "negative." This strongly suggested natural immunity.[(59a)]

From either the HIV theory point of view or the general assumption of the venereal-disease nature of AIDS, that was, at the very least, good news.

And, in 1995, scientists who studied prostitutes in Gambia reported that in at least three cases "killer cells" called "HIV-specific cytotoxic T-lymphocytes" had been able to kill HIV-infected cells, a possible reason the trio had not developed any sign of "HIV infection." The same cells have also been found in other AIDS-less HIV-infected people — another sign of a possible fail-safe element of immunity.[60]

Added to the disclosures in 1996/97 that some genetic factors might actually block HIV — meaning that some people are naturally immune to the virus 100 percent and others are partially immune — there seemed to be at least some good news on the prevention front — providing, of course, that HIV is the sole cause of AIDS.[61,62,63,63a]

The above would also demonstrate that somehow Mother Nature always finds a way to save at least part of a species from extinction by disease, even if it might be manmade.

An oriental conundrum

AIDS surveillance in other "third world" countries also undercut certain beliefs about the syndrome while strengthening others:

Two points in passing are Thailand and the Philippines.

In the former, AIDS has been traced since 1984.[64] Ten years later, it was estimated that the country had at least 700,000 HIV-infected people, proportionally the highest infection rate in the world, even though — while 1,600 had died from 8,000 cumulative cases of the syndrome — most people had still not developed symptoms and a "safe-sex" campaign seemed to be paying off by 1996.[65,66] (Some Thai estimates by 1997 were up to a million infections and up to 60,000 AIDS-related deaths.)

In the Philippines, AIDS has been traced since 1985 — beginning with outbreaks among "sex workers" at the American

Subic Bay Naval base (highly suggestive of a port of entry from US servicemen). Yet twelve years later, even though officials generally agreed the numbers were probably underestimated, only 916 AIDS cases and 159 deaths had been reported. Even projections for the syndrome for the year 2000 were far under anything estimated for nearby Thailand.[67,67a]

As a frequent traveller in both countries, I was fully aware of the intensely promiscuous, socially bisexual nature of both Thai and Filipino societies. Sex was, and is, easy, casual, and omnipresent. Prostitution of women *and* men is common, and, in both countries homosexual or bisexual sexual activity is far less shameful or restrained than in the Western countries, particularly the farther one moves away from the highest social classes. Hence, the statistical correlate of sexual promiscuity is significant in both countries.

Yet, as we have seen, for the incidence of both HIV infection and actual definable AIDS there is a chasm of difference. In both countries, claimed heterosexuality is a far greater correlate than claimed homosexuality (though part of this may be due to social convention and an obscuring in such societies of what is meant by such frankly idiotic words as "straight" and "gay"). In both, as of mid-decade AIDS cases were roughly divided equally between the sexes.

There is a difference, however, in one key factor between the two societies, particularly in the earlier years — drug abuse, particularly intravenous drug abuse, was far more common and of easier access, and remained so throughout the early AIDS years, in Thailand than in the Philippines. In the latter, the authoritarian regime of Ferdinand Marcos, ending in 1986 and overlapping the early years of AIDS' presumptive mass spread through a mostly unknowing population, had virtually, but not totally, eliminated drug abuse. It increased in the post-Marcos years.

If AIDS is primarily a venereal condition, incidence of infection and actual cases should at least be proportionally similar in both countries. But if — as some of us argued in the early AIDS years — drug abuse *of all kinds* has a higher correlation with AIDS than does sexual promiscuity, then such noticeable differences may be explained. (It also helps explain the AIDS/HIV pandemic in India, thought by 1997 to be the most infected country of all.)

This does not diminish the reality that sexual promiscuity and specific sexual acts (particularly insertive anal intercourse) are strongly related to AIDS, but it does suggest that substance abuse directly (through injection and possibly through other routes) and indirectly (by altering immune function over time) plays larger roles than does sexual activity itself.

HIV: the ever-lengthening incubation

In the earlier years AIDS — defined substantially more narrowly than now — survival was measured in months to a few years. By the time HIV antibody test kits were available, the time between alleged infection by HIV and the onset of symptoms of AIDS began a breathtaking ascent. The "incubation period" was stretched from three to five to seven years — indeed, with each passing year of AIDS and the accumulation of computer printouts from ELISA and Western Blot test kits, it became apparent that another 12 months of incubation could safely be ascribed to a virus which seemed endlessly to lie in wait (save in spectacular cases of "fast AIDS" when it seemed to kill within a matter of a few months to years after exposure).

By the end of the 1980s, the ever-lengthening incubation period was not only fortifying the position of Duesberg and others that HIV, at least by itself, might not be the cause, but was provoking grumbling even from the informed public. By the 1990s, it was becoming established doctrine that HIV might incubate for anywhere from 10 to 15 years before striking — if it ever struck at all. A review of AIDS patient "cohorts" led to the conclusion that at least some AIDS-prone people might be "HIV-positive" for the whole of their lives and escape "full-blown" AIDS.[68]

And, a general pre-AIDS syndrome loosely called "AIDS-related complex" (ARC) had been added to the picture: in many cases, long before any of the (was it two dozen, 30, 32, 34?) "opportunistic diseases" and "forms" of cancer appeared, allegedly due to HIV-induced immune depression, there might be long periods of non-fatal general malaise, joint and bone pains, headaches, respiratory distress, extreme fatigue, swollen glands, rashes, gastrointestinal disturbances, nightsweats, spiking fevers, some diarrhea and weight loss.

Without HIV antibodies such a profile could be described as mononucleosis, secondary syphilis, endocrine imbalance and a dozen other things. But should the patient "test positive" for HIV it automatically became "AIDS-related" and the patient was informed he — or she — would be counting the weeks, months or years until "full-blown" AIDS took over, at which time 100 percent fatality was predicted.

The pattern slowly emerged that, as HIV took longer and longer to wend its evil way, more and more conditions could be lumped together as ARC, or pre-AIDS. This pattern was developing just as the "standard literature" was beginning to take note of AIDS-like cases in HIV-negative people and the press was reporting on more and more seemingly healthy people known to have had HIV antibodies for years who had failed to develop AIDS.

There was, as I noted whenever possible, the possible scenario of a virus in search of a disease. Just as, in the early times of Western medicine when it had been faced with "the great imitator," it was easy to dismiss all otherwise inexplicable symptoms as syphilis, and as, in later times, to attribute many of them to mononucleosis, it now became equally easy to blame everything on HIV/AIDS. Even forgetfulness and occasional mood swings on the part of a carrier of HIV antibodies became not simply empty-headedness but "AIDS dementia complex" (ADC) — and, yes, it could be demonstrated that HIV was present in the central nervous system, as it was everywhere else.

But arithmetic was beginning to mount inexorably against

the key AIDS concepts: estimates of the people in the world said to be carrying HIV ranged into the millions, while actual definable AIDS cases remained, until the mid-1990s, essentially in the thousands. The CDC several times redefined what AIDS was, automatically adding diseases to the syndrome, just as some diseases seemed ready to be leaving the standard definition (old standbys PCP and KS among them).

(So convinced were some researchers and physicians that HIV not only was not the cause of AIDS or anything else that they offered to drink or inject themselves with HIV. At least one American, Robert Willner MD PhD, did so very publicly in Spain in 1993, in the USA in 1994, and wrote an impassioned attack on the basic AIDS premises.[69])

In defense of orthodox research into HIV, which also raises fundamental questions, it may be said that if HIV is as tricky as it has seemed to be — "hiding out" in the central nervous system (CNS), lymphoid and other tissue without showing itself in the blood, and also present in virtually every tissue or organ, then everything it does or does not do can be excused on its uniqueness.

One can hardly blame Nobel Laureate Dr. Kary Mullis for observing [see lead-in statement, this chapter] that "the mystery of that damn virus has been generated by the $2 billion they spend on it. You take any other virus, and you spend $2 billion, and you can make up some great mysteries about it too."

So, in AIDS, the HIV virus has been the villain who was either there or not there, directly or indirectly present, responsible if not visible, the culprit or presumed co-culprit, in virtually everything related to AIDS. A very tall order indeed.

HHV-6: riddle within an enigma

So, "co-factors" inexorably began to catch up with AIDS Inc., which was never any more likely to admit basic error than Cancer Inc. — with which it is so intimately interlocked — has been.

In what was an astounding change of gears, yet not originally presented this way — the original comments coming not in American but British journals — the key American AIDS explicator, Robert Gallo, who had for so long promoted the HIV-only theory, added his name to some new research. It found that, at the very least — above and beyond other possible "co-factor" viruses and the Montagnier/Lo mycoplasmas — yet *another* virus, HHV-6 (human herpesvirus number six), might be a "co-factor." [70,71,72]

The virus was conveniently said to have been isolated in Gallo's National Cancer Institute (NCI) laboratory and, shortly after its delineation, was found to be infecting very broad sectors of the human family without, in most carriers, seeming to "cause" anything. But it also became apparent that HHV-6 had at least two "strains" and one of them might be truly lethal to man.

The AIDS research community was "officially" informed (though some dissidents were previously theorizing the connection) that HHV-6 contributed to "the striking depletion of CD4 cells seen in patients with AIDS" and that HHV-6 was found to be active in autopsy studies of dead AIDS patients — that is, it was detected in all lung, lymph node, spleen, liver and kidney tissues "obtained at necropsy."[73] The infection rate was far higher than for CMV, a "co-factor" virus which, in or out of AIDS, can be the most damaging of all human viruses — and of course far more active than HIV, which often is not found in dying AIDS patients at all.

As the middle of the decade approached, the stream of research implicating HHV-6 — be it variant A or B or combinations thereof — as playing an ever-greater role in multiple AIDS pathology was growing yet received scant attention from AIDS Inc.

New information came in 1996 from Medical College of Wisconsin pathologist Konstance Knox, whose research implicated HHV-6 *variant A* as a probable co-factor. She told a gay-oriented New York newspaper:

> *"HHV-6 is present very early in HIV infection . . . We're finding HHV-6 in the lymph nodes early*

[indicating] active infection; this virus is replicating. This is unheard-of for any other opportunistic infection, even TB."[74,75]

In fact, somewhat like Mary and the little lamb, everywhere that HIV went, HHV-6 was sure to follow. Or, possibly, vice-versa.

With HHV-6 known to be infecting natural killer cells — considered to be key in the immune response to cancer — the apparently higher rates of certain "forms" of cancer in patients classed as AIDS (and Chronic Fatigue Syndrome) could be (allopathically) explained. One of AIDS Inc.'s ever-trickier explanations for HIV latency in seemingly healthy people has been the supposition that the virus is "hiding" in lymph tissue. But no sooner had this research approach settled in than Italian research indicated that HHV-6 is "hiding" there too — and that "variant A" HHV-6 has a high frequency of occurrence in cases of Kaposi's sarcoma, a role earlier attributed to HIV.[76]

Research has also linked HHV-6 with such potentially lethal complications of bone marrow transplants as pneumonitis (a severe lung disease) and the immunological disorder called GVHD — graft-versus-host-disease.[77]

And, perhaps even more intriguingly, German research found that HHV-6 could be detected in the blood of blood donors — a conceivably chilling reality which could mean that HHV-6 is as easily transmissible by blood as HIV allegedly is — and that blood supplies are at risk.[78] As of 1997, the US was not screening the blood supply for HHV-6.

Too, HHV-6 is known to activate Epstein-Barr, CMV[78a] virus and the human papilloma virus.

And Belgian research in 1997 linked HHV-6 antibodies to the development of multiple sclerosis.[78b]

Most ominously, "the most reliable source" of HHV-6 is saliva.[78b]

The AIDS Inc. research establishment was not saying, by mid-decade, that HHV-6 was the *real* AIDS virus, since such a

180-degree angle turn might paralyze the whole scientific effort and conceivably imperil billions of dollars in research. The admission, however, that a seemingly "new" virus was so strongly present in AIDS patients (and in *many others*) that it was *the* likely "co-factor," opened the door to possible abandonment of the HIV-only theory and an industrially acceptable gradual transfer of research tools and test kits to a whole new dimension of thought still slavishly in keeping with the precepts of allopathy.

The NCI could and did take credit for the discovery of HHV-6 (and HHV-7), originally dubbed HBLV — for human B-cell lymphotropic virus — but it could not easily answer the questions of from whence these viruses sprang and why hadn't the world known of them before.

The very least that can be said of the startling emergence of HHV-6 as a major factor in AIDS is that part of the hype, hoopla and outright scamming that has gone on in the ranks of AIDS Inc. has been devastatingly wrong: if HHV-6 or any virus or anything other than HIV is shown to be the major "cause" (or possibly, *any* cause) of AIDS, then billions of dollars of research funds have been wasted, and lives lost, due to a wrong theory (including those individuals who committed suicide upon learning that they were "positive" for HIV antibodies).

By the mid-1990s AIDS Inc. had painted itself into an ever dwindling corner with allegiance to allopathy, to single viruses, and to HIV. All the while, it had denigrated, blocked, thwarted or remained oblivious to other ideas and approaches — an intellectual crime of far-reaching dimensions.

Along with the possibility that the Allopathic Industrial Complex (AIC), AIDS Inc. subdivision, may have missed the boat about the real single cause — if there is one — of the ever-changing, multifactorial syndrome that is AIDS, its mad race to embrace AZT and other "anti-nucleosides," followed by the "non-nucleoside reverse transcriptase inhibitors" and "protease inhibitors" as "drugs of choice" in attempting to stop HIV, may be an even greater disaster.

(Such an embrace enhanced the coffers of Bristol-Myers Squibb, Hoffman-LaRoche and Glaxo/Wellcome, all members in good standing of the global pharmaceutical cartel [*see VIII*]).

Indeed, the all-encompassing notions of the "single cause" and the "single cure" are the flaws of allopathic thinking which, as applied to AIDS, have helped account for the so far total failure of Western medical orthodoxy to curb the killer. They constitute allopathy's twilight of the gods, a global death throe of an outmoded thought system for which the world population has paid and continues to pay an awful price.

Yet, it was to be expected:

If the AIDS Inc. research establishment — so overlapped with Cancer Inc. — had suddenly found the "cause" of the new killer syndrome, then it was only a matter of months before it would announce at least the first optimistic therapeutic approach.

The sorry saga of AZT

And, of course, this first optimistic therapeutic approach came from the Cancer Inc. apparatus. It was Burroughs Wellcome's AZT (Retrovir, zidovudine, azidothymidine), an old (1964), highly toxic (and highly dangerous) cancer chemotherapeutic drug which had been shelved years before because of both its overt toxicity and lack of efficacy in cancer.

The story of how AZT was literally rushed to market in terms of a truncated "clinical trial" has been gone into great detail elsewhere,[79] and there is no part of that story which does not vibrate between the murky, the greedy, and the dubious.

It can be synthesized that AZT was found to kill some of the target cells that "the AIDS virus" ostensibly infects. As time wore on, it became clear that AZT and the whole family of nucleoside drugs killed more than HIV-infected cells — they set into play a chain reaction to devastate cells in general since they strike at the very essence of cell reproduction (DNA chains) itself. Like most chemotherapeutic agents, AZT and its similars were/are immune suppressing themselves and capable of doing widespread damage to the host.

But because an early study seemed to show that AZT slowed down the course of AIDS — while never "curing" it — the AIC swiftly announced that the resurrected failed cancer agent should be immediately legalized for use in the new syndrome.

In 1993, ABC's "Day One" television program interviewed Dr. Itzhak Brook, a member of the 11-scientist FDA panel which approved AZT. As a scientist who had disagreed with the use of AZT from the beginning, Dr. Brook said the committee had never had a way of scrutinizing the data properly and that the drug had been rushed to capture the market quickly. He was also quoted as saying, "I felt we compromised science and compromised safety."[(80)]

Even Burroughs Wellcome (later merged with drug giant Glaxo) would later concede that "the drug has been studied for limited periods of time and long-term safety and efficacy are not known."[(81)]

So AZT was literally sped to public acceptance based primarily on research largely paid for, and later defended by, the company. It was also evidence of the FDA's yielding, as usual, not only to the drug interests which essentially control the agency, but to organized gay activism, which politically clamored for the government to "do something."

In fact, the well-intentioned efforts of gay activists to pressure the federal research octopus into "doing something" often was nothing more than a playing into the hands of the AIC. The international drug trust was all too happy to see speedier approval for experimental toxic compounds from which millions could be gleaned.

When it was re-introduced for AIDS, AZT was for a time the most expensive drug ever marketed. It was, also, as such dissenters as California's Bruce Halstead MD[(82)] and Peter Duesberg PhD would keep pointing out, also among the most dangerous. By the 1990s AZT was fetching $400 million in annual profits.

The outrageous costs of AZT — as well as of several older

drugs "approved" for the treatment of PCP and other "opportunistic diseases" said to be part of the syndrome (see *VIII*) — led to congressional surveillance, public outcries, and the "compassionate" dropping of prices by drug companies to meet the propaganda challenge. AZT, and later the workalikes ddI and ddC (some others having failed to make it even through the FDA's "fast track" approval system designed exclusively for AIDS and at the behest of AIDS activists) were held to be signs that the American medical/pharmaceutical research complex was truly "doing something."

At first, it seemed that at least in some cases AZT could "slow down" AIDS infections. But it was also becoming apparent that many patients, up to a third, could not tolerate the drug in *any* dose. There were some suggestions, mostly muted, but occasionally very vocal (Duesberg) that the AZT assault on host defense actually *caused* AIDS — particularly when given to individuals who were essentially free of symptoms but bore the tell-tale markers of HIV antibodies and/or inverted T4/T8 ratios.

As years passed, a troubling question arose: was AZT more often helping or hurting AIDS-prone patients?

Some celebrated AIDS patients — Florida co-ed Kimberly Bergalis, who went through the rapid stages of alleged HIV infection to ARC level to full-blown AIDS to death all within three years; tennis player Arthur Ashe, who had said he had wanted to give up AZT but didn't want to offend his doctors; and ballet star Rudolph Nureyev — were all AIDS victims but they also may have been AZT victims, since their rapid descent seemed to follow the beginning of their use of the drug.[83]

Frighteningly, AIDS orthodoxy began to argue that AZT should be prescribed as early as possible — and even prophylactically! If there were antibodies to HIV and a sign of immune system disturbance let alone any of the 27 to 34 clinical designations of overt pathology, it was argued, AZT should be given right away — though perhaps at more tolerable lower doses. The widely disseminated use of a toxic agent to prevent a disease remains, as we have seen in cancer, a centerpiece of allopathic thought, and is utterly logical if one cedes the premise.

By mid-decade AZT experienced a rollercoaster of public-relations ups and downs.

The first nosedive came primarily in preliminary results, and then final results, of a large three-year clinical trial in the United Kingdom, France and Ireland called the Concorde Study — in which Great Britain-based Wellcome PLC, the parent of Burroughs Wellcome, took no part.

The early results were bad enough since, among other things, a spinoff was that reliance on the CD4/T4 "helper" cell count as a guide as to when to initiate antiretroviral therapy was found to be misleading.

The key result, however, was that AZT did not slow down the advance of AIDS in asymptomatic people infected with HIV. The authors concluded: "The results of Concorde do not encourage the early use of zidovudine in symptom-free HIV-infected adults."[84]

In the midst of the two Concorde reports, a 1994 Harvard School of Public Health study of 1,338 HIV-infected people likewise found that whatever "slight benefits" there might be from taking AZT were often cancelled by the drug's side effects.[85]

All that could be said for switching patients from AZT to either ddI or ddC, the other common "nucleoside analogues," was that when tolerance for one developed, a physician might try another — but evidence was lacking that the AZT workalikes were any more efficacious than AZT and sometimes they caused just as many, if not more, side effects.[86]

A month after the Concorde trial was published, two other key studies weighed in to put further nails not only into the coffin of AZT but into the whole area of retroviral therapy with nucleoside analogue drugs:

First, an AIDS in Europe Study group analysis of 4,484 patients at 51 treatment centers in 17 European countries showed that "when initiated after the time of AIDS diagnosis," AZT was "associated with improved prognosis but for no more than two years after starting therapy." And, worse, "for patients surviving more than two years since starting [AZT], the death rate was greater than for *untreated* [*emphasis mine*] patients who had developed AIDS at the same time." This was at least a statistical suggestion that AZT had worsened the condition of treated patients.[87]

Second, a nine-year followup of 761 "HIV-positive homosexual and bisexual men" in San Francisco found that there had been a one-year increase in survival times for patients classified as AIDS by the 1987 CDC definition thereof — but the small increase was due more to increased "prophylaxis" (prevention of initial or secondary PCP attacks) than to "antiretroviral therapy."[88]

This was clear evidence that some of the antibiotic therapies aimed at PCP were "working" at least for awhile (perhaps the single ray of good news in "AIDS" treatments) — but there was no evidence that the "antiretroviral drugs" were associated with increased survival.

A last-minute reprieve for AZT also came in 1994 with the ongoing "Pediatric AIDS Clinical Trials Group Protocol 076 Study Group" in the US — and it of course raised more questions than answers.

In a study of infants born live to 477 women, with HIV infection status known in 363 births, it was found that in "women with mildly symptomatic HIV disease" and no prior treatment with antiretroviral drugs during pregnancy, AZT administered before and during birth and to newborns for six weeks reduced the risk of maternal-infant HIV transmissions "by approximately two thirds."[89] This study offset neither data suggesting that mother-to-infant transmission of HIV occurs a minority of the time nor an Asian study on AZT-linked birth defects.[90]

While the pediatric news gave a lift to Burroughs Wellcome following the battery of devastating earlier research, Centers for Disease Control and Prevention (CDC) physicians editorially noted that "the long-term effects on both mother and infant are unknown" from using a drug as toxic as AZT. Too, "zidovudine-resistant virus might emerge during a short course of zidovudine during pregnancy and might affect the mother's subsequent response to zidovudine therapy."[91]

On the "up" side, some research continued to show effectiveness of AZT and related drugs in seeming to mitigate central nervous system (CNS) conditions linked to AIDS, particularly in combination.[92]

Another nosedive occurred in August 1995 when virtually the same US research team associated with the governmental AIDS Clinical Trials Group (ACTG) which had originally suggested AZT should be used in "early intervention" in HIV-infected persons did a complete reversal:

Paul Volberding *et al.* concluded that, after all, giving AZT to symptom-free HIV positives did not slow down progression to AIDS, essentially confirming the Concorde study.[93]

If it did not slow down disease progression, one wondered, why give it at all? The failure of AZT and similar drugs opened the doors for other compounds said to be able to reduce HIV's "viral load."

Other research showed that combination drug therapy was more effective than single-drug treatments — even though no combination of such toxic compounds could "cure" AIDS and all had side effects.[94,95]

Hence, AZT's rash of upsets had, by 1995, or just on the eve of announcement of the use of drugs said to work "better" than AZT and the nucleosides, severely dented its reputation as *the* "drug of choice" against "HIV infection."

So, in the 14th year of the Plague, and despite a multi-billion-dollar research investment precariously balanced on two rickety pillars (the HIV theory of AIDS and the launching of AZT and similar drugs to attack "the AIDS virus"), AIDS Inc. had mostly come up a loser.

All of which, even by 1993, had led the non-profit, Los Angeles-based Project AIDS International (PAI) to submit to the

United Nations Commission on Human Rights in Geneva a request for an international review both of the HIV theory of AIDS causation and the continued use of AZT against the syndrome. It asked for action to ban AZT and all "non-selective analogue-DNA- chain terminating drugs."[96]

In an often startling review of data PAI had gleaned from various sources, the organization pointedly claimed that — in distinct contrast to AIDS Inc.'s general view — the "normal range" of CD4 "helper" cells in humans is far wider than usually thought — 237 to 1,817 — and that

> *[I]n tests completed on US Olympic athletes in 1984, the average range of CD4 helper cells was between 400 to 600. Certainly, the US athletes were not considered to be unhealthy; yet these are markers used to instill fear and manipulate HIV-positive persons into taking toxic chemo-therapy when they are not otherwise unhealthy.*[97]

Even AIDS researchers began noting that T-cell counts could "go up, down and sideways" due to many factors over long periods of time — and that five different T-cell tests done from the same patient at five different laboratories on five different days could produce five different widely varying results.

PAI also claimed that although by then there were over two thousand cases of HIV-free AIDS known to the CDC such "information was (and is) embargoed" (!) and that, even so, by Dec. 31, 1992, the CDC admitted to knowledge of 97 such (American) cases.

It also quoted a statement by two London microbiologists in 1990:

> *"It would be irresponsible to produce guidelines on AIDS until an infectious organism is identified and the means by which it causes disease are understood.*
>
> *"It is only now becoming obvious that infection with HIV does not usually give rise to AIDS."*[98]

AIDS theory: failing on all fronts

So by the mid-1990s, AIDS Inc. had either failed in or considerably modified virtually all of its premises.

The American public, American science, the Western world, the world in general had been sold a bill of goods which, for whatever reasons, turned out to be questionable at best.

Clearly, new thought was called for.

From the beginning, a number of innovative physicians were willing to try creative approaches to AIDS, and usually but not always these were the same kinds of men and women who, at however great a risk to their careers and professional standing, tried novel therapies against cancer and other "incurable" disorders.

With AIDS, both doctors and patients had a clearer certainty of the correctness of opting for "alternative" treatments: AIDS had no known effective treatment, no known cure and allegedly was always fatal.

AIDS medical innovators were faced by the same stone walls which faced cancer and cardiovascular innovators: how could they quantify their results, particularly if they were multifactorial, and who would publish them? Most knowledge of "alternatives" in AIDS therapy arose in the mostly-gay "AIDS underground" and in journals and publications in no way connected with the Allopathic Industrial Complex.

Just as breakthroughs in American cancer alternatives had often had to be found in such girlie magazines as *Penthouse*, such magazines and counter-culture publications also became clearing-houses for the latest ideas in AIDS treatments.

By the end of the 1980s, although American AIDS patients constituted a much smaller population than American cancer patients, a much higher percentage of them, though still in the minority, were willing to try "alternatives." This was primarily because the cancer "cure" rate in advanced disease, depending on the definition of "cure," was at least 8 to 10 percent, however discouraging such a number. But this was in contrast to 0 percent in AIDS.

Hope from the unortho-docs

Hence, increasing numbers of doctors, some as much informed by their patients as anyone, struck out on their own. On both coasts, primarily, a handful of physicians began implementing ideas of holism — detoxify the body, promote overall host defense, change diets, encourage healthy lifestyles, experiment with regimens of vitamins, minerals, enzymes, amino acids, essential fatty acids, herbs, "unapproved" but promising drugs, oxidative therapies, attitude-changing exercises.

(Included among "alternatively" treated patients was the small group which our research/medical team began seeing on a limited and intermittent basis beginning in 1983 — those who had the funds to seek out a foreign clinic. Following them through therapies and results allowed us to develop some early conclusions: just as in any other allegedly "terminal," multifactorial disorder of a chronic or acute nature, it made more sense to work with diet and natural factors, occasionally blending them with standard modalities, than to pursue allopathic approaches alone.

(This, of course, is a nod to the concept of holism — applied to AIDS, it means that it is more vital to shore up the natural defense of the host than to be obsessed with the "load" of a pathogenic virus, particularly given the fact that most viruses have never been known to be completely eradicable in any human.)

Going into the 1990s, it could be said of "unorthodox" approaches in general that long-term AIDS survivors — that is, persons either with diagnosed full-blown disease or ARC-level symptoms or even early-stage asymptomatics — had the following things in common:

— First, they had either abandoned, or never were involved in, standard therapies at all.

— Second, they were using one or several "alternative"

approaches (in which diet and supplements played central roles); and/or they occasionally blended "standard" therapies with such "alternatives." And

— Third, there was something different about their mental outlook: most of these patients saw themselves as "living with AIDS" rather than "dying from" it. Some had made victory over it a challenge which they faced exuberantly, and sometimes even joyously. They simply did not expect to die from the syndrome.

It also became statistically apparent that there was another cluster of patients difficult to quantify: those with no known treatments who were surviving in good condition for no known reason. These mainly involved early asymptomatics and their presence usually strengthened the idea that HIV antibody positivity did not necessarily mean the acquisition of an AIDS-related illness.

It is essential to note that, on the eve of AIDS Inc.'s announcement to the world of the "breakthroughs" of the new "protease inhibitor" drugs, that the public-private AIDS Research Program Evaluation Working Group, a 114-member advisory panel, had called both for a "midcourse correction" in how AIDS research was being conducted, and for a serious look at "alternative" treatments.

The Working Group in spring 1996 noted that funding methods had not kept up with "research advances" during AIDS' 15 years and that new ideas were needed.

Among them was the imperative to evaluate the various dietary/vitamin/mineral/enzyme/herbal regimens to which many HIV-infected and AIDS patients were turning, usually in desperation. Also included for evaluation were ozone and similar oxidative treatments, meditation and other holistic approaches. The panel also stressed the need to enhance research on ways to boost the human immune system and to refocus basic research from rodent-based to human-based.[98a]

Yet such a call received scant publicity and was literally muted by the "protease inhibitor"/"viral load" publicity.

It is true that in AIDS, as in cancer, there has been a field day for charlatans as well: "magic bullet" cures of all kinds have flourished in the AIDS world. But many of these approaches have at least some rationale empirically or in biological theory.

The experience has been that, whatever temporarily exciting results an herb tea, or any herb, or a vitamin, or a serum of some kind, or a machine, or anything else, may have had, there is no single "magic bullet" against a syndrome of multifactorial causality. Rather, AIDS, perhaps even more dramatically than cancer, has presented an archetypal condition in which individualized, integrated protocols alone offer hope.

The unorganized, poorly reported, anecdotal but gathering information on "alternatives" in AIDS led to various realizations:

That suppressing HIV, or any other virus, did not effect a "cure" and that a vast array of substances (mostly natural and from the plant and mineral kingdoms primarily) could play roles in both immune system modulation and stimulation, even though such factors did not absolutely "cure" AIDS.

Long-term survivors continued to be reported, and the better known of them continued either to have no "orthodox" therapy or to have long since abandoned it. It is also true that this multitude of "unorthodox" approaches had often simply lengthened the lives and reduced the suffering of AIDS patients so that they eventually succumbed to some complication of the syndrome — yet the months and years of unexpected, against-the-odds survival were precious to them and their families and slowly, but firmly, made the case for nutrition-based, individualized therapies based not on demolishing pathogens but on enhancing overall health.

Aside from surveys of our patients in Mexico, other practitioners went public with their theories, approaches and results.[99,100,101]

More affluent AIDS patients would try anything anywhere — they might gravitate between intravenous megadose Vitamin C therapy to treatments of the blood by ozone, from gobbling Japanese mushrooms and copious amounts of antioxidant-containing pills and foods to taking injections of live embryonic cells. What worked for one might or might not work for another — but, in sum, the multitude of mostly-natural approaches was proving that disease progression and suffering could be reduced, slowed, mitigated, if not stopped.

Interestingly enough, even establishment research was backing up at least some of the "unorthodox" findings by 1993.

In September of that year, a Johns Hopkins University study showed that some 15 percent of drug-using HIV infectees developed Vitamin A deficiency and that such a lack of a key nutrient might shave a year of life expectancy off infected individuals, of particular importance in "full-blown" cases.(102)

More impressively, none other than the National Institutes of Health (NIH) announced in 1993 that antioxidants "might" help keep HIV-infected patients from getting sicker.(103) Mentioned in this regard were Vitamins A, C and E. While it had taken cancer decades before US orthodoxy would admit the slightest possibility that vitamins, particularly antioxidants, might somehow help out against malignancy, it had taken AIDS only 12 years before orthodoxy got the picture.

In 1994, University of Georgia research added another bit of news pleasing to metabolic therapists — that depletion of the mineral selenium might be playing a crucial role in the progression of AIDS.

The U of G study, whose authors admitted that they did not know what the mechanism might be, suggested that somehow HIV causes selenium deficiency by producing proteins which consume the body's supply of the mineral — which is often depleted in the American diet anyway.

The Associated Press quoted University of Georgia College of Pharmacy's Dr. Will Taylor:

"*. . . the length of time it took to deplete the body's store of selenium could help account for HIV's latency period, which can last for years . . . If this is true, then selenium biochemistry may be the key to understanding the control of the life cycle of HIV and* *perhaps some of the pathology of AIDS . . . Many AIDS patients lack selenium and have taken supplements on their own. For several years, some researchers and doctors have recommended selenium as part of the patient's dietary supplements.*"[104]

In 1996, sports nutritionist and researcher William Brink assembled data from "peer-reviewed" literature which found that such antioxidants as glutathione, its precursor N-acetyl-cysteine (NAC), and Vitamins C and E greatly help AIDS-depressed immune systems.[104a]

The glutathione connection received a big boost from Stanford University School of Medicine research reported in 1997[104b], which drew attention to life extension.

And Johns Hopkins University research showed that HIV-infected men progress to overt AIDS more quickly if they are deficient in Vitamin B12.[104c]

The growing connections between antioxidant vitamins, minerals and enzymes speak to the revolution in *oxidology* (*see XVI*), which has added a new dimension to medicine and in which the research entities (Bradford Research Institute/ American Biologics) with which I have been involved have played some pivotal roles.

Earlier, Australian researchers had argued that "oxidative stress" — in essence, more reactive oxygen toxic species (ROTS) and "free radicals" (toxic oxygen breakdown products) than the body knows what to do with — induced by AIDS "risk factors" might be the primary cause of the syndrome!

Among the "risk factors" described as "potent oxidizing agents" were the inhalant nitrate drugs ("poppers"), Factor VIII (the multi-donor concentrated blood product used by hemophiliacs) — and sperm.[105,106]

I recalled that the first reported cases of AIDS in the US were of five gay men, *all* of whom used "inhalant drugs."[107]

Despite information available parallel to the outbreak of the AIDS pandemic that elements *other than* viruses might have a great deal to do with the syndrome, the AIC and its rapidly developing AIDS Inc. subdivision were not about to turn loose of the HIV theory of causation, whatever other lines of research begged to be looked at.

A syphilis connection ?

One such line of research, although it did not originate with him, was pursued by a heroic Manhattan physician with a high caseload of AIDS patients and who himself was infected with HIV — the late Stephen Caiazza MD, who in the midst of his investigation became a friend of mine.

Following up on German leads, Dr. Caiazza, and a small collaborating group around him, had found (as had investigators Joan McKenna and Harris Coulter[(108)]) that the parallels and overlaps between AIDS and late-stage syphilis were far too vast in number to be coincidental. Such probers found that the protean symptomatology of AIDS had a nearly equal similarity to the vast symptomatology of syphilis in an earlier era. Indeed, Dr. Moritz Kaposi, for whom Kaposi's sarcoma was named, had been a syphilologist.

Scattered European research suggested that a good deal of what was being called AIDS (including the purplish lesions of KS and various pulmonary calamities being attributed to PCP and other microbes) were really manifestations of advanced syphilis that had invaded the central nervous system — that is, *neurosyphilis*. The same research argued that because late-stage syphilis, let alone neurosyphilis, was not ordinarily seen in young people, and had rarely been clinically seen in the Western world (since earlier in this century anyway), younger physicians who had not been trained in the multiple sequelae of "the great imitator" were simply unaware that they were often looking at syphilis.

Moreover, research suggested that the syphilitic treponeme plays numerous tricks on human immune systems — and that positivity for syphilis on a standard syphilis blood test (particularly the VDRL, as favored in the USA) could obscure HIV infection while positivity for HIV could obscure syphilis. This reality led to a strange meeting at the Centers for Disease Control (CDC) in Atlanta in 1988.

A two-day conference of experts agreed that both disease states altered each other's outcomes (a nightmare for patients "co-infected" with syphilis and the "AIDS virus"), that confirmatory blood tests for either could in effect be "thrown off" by the other, that co-infection seemed to help both conditions advance, that sexually active syphilitics should be screened for HIV, that HIV patients infected through sexual intercourse or IV drug abuse should be treated for syphilis, that neurosyphilis should be considered in the diagnosis of neurological diseases being ascribed to AIDS, and that the standard treatment of choice for early syphilis, benzathine penicillin, should not be used in the treatment of neurosyphilis in either symptomatic or asymptomatic HIV-infected individuals. Rather, old-time (and patent-expired) crystalline or aqueous penicillin or procaine penicillin should be used.[(109)]

While it should also be noted that the AIDS-syphilis link never received much orthodox attention, that even the CDC's meeting on the same failed to capture much publicity and that other scattered research was said not to confirm the most stunning possibility of all (perhaps AIDS *is* syphilis), a handful of doctors who used crystalline penicillin as a drug of choice were reporting some promising results.

Dr. Caiazza had used himself as his own guinea pig: already infected with the alleged "AIDS virus" but essentially healthy, he inoculated himself with enough syphilis to make sure he became massively infected, as he recounted in his own little-known book.[(110)] He described advancing from a mildly symptomatic stage to fully advanced, near-terminal conditions in a matter of days, and how using mega-infusions of aqueous penicillin restored him to mostly good health in a short period of time.

Believing he had a tiger by the tail, Dr. Caiazza began treating more and more patients with crystalline penicillin and followup antibiotics, reporting on some spectacular successes, at least over the short term. He instantly fell under attack by New York state medical authorities, and was under investigation when, several years later, he died — allegedly of complications of his disease.

Dr. Caiazza had never believed in nutritional or other supplements as a necessary part of an AIDS protocol and, good allopath that he was, wanted to prove his point with single-shot modalities — antibiotics in general, and old-time penicillin in particular, could manage AIDS, he believed.

(Since much of AIDS is indeed bacterial, and also because mycoplasmas, though not viruses, are open to attack by antibiotics, there is an implied role for the limited use of antibiotics in an integrative, mostly-natural protocol).

Parallel to his work was that of others, who claimed that administration of the typhoid vaccine could "unmask" previously "hidden" syphilis and that aqueous penicillin could then reduce the syphilis load by crossing the blood-brain barrier. The underlying assumptions, never sharply challenged by orthodoxy, were that the standard VDRL test is not a reliable screen for neurosyphilis (that is, a negative result will occur from screening the blood but this does not mean treponemes have not already invaded the central nervous system) and that the common benzathine penicillin used in early syphilis is mostly useless in neurosyphilis.

But Dr. Caiazza had other things to report to me intermittently. The most chilling was the warning he received while in Germany that he should be less vocal about his theories since he was in a country which was a major headquarters of world pharmaceutical interests — and two apparent attempts on his life, one in an automobile near-accident and the other in a beating by thugs in which nothing was stolen.

It dawned on Dr. Caiazza over time that he, and indeed all proponents of the syphilis connection to AIDS, were playing with fire: syphilis is an altogether "curable" bacterial disease and a primary agent in "curing" it is an essentially inexpensive form of penicillin without patent protection.

Our own medical group saw several dramatic cases in which megadoses of crystalline penicillin, accompanied by hefty infusions of Vitamin C and an oxidative agent (Dioxychlor), produced relatively rapid and spectacular decreases in several

AIDS "opportunistic infections." But the syphilis-AIDS link remained heretical and, by the mid-1990s, had not seriously been followed up on.

Positivity in negativity?

Other novel magic-bullet AIDS approaches were anecdotally reported but supportive data were hard to come by. One reason was the confusing nature of the AIDS definition itself — if blood "turned negative" for HIV, did this mean that both antigens and antibodies were gone (virologically not necessarily a desired outcome) or simply that HIV was no longer active? If HIV were not causing anything, what difference did disappearance of its antigens or antibodies make? If "helper" cells were elevated and the patient remained free of disease, having never had any, did this mean he was "cured" of the syndrome? If a potentially lethal "form" of cancer associated with AIDS (as in one of our group's more celebrated cases — an HIV-positive Scandinavian) was eradicated by unorthodox therapies, had the man been "cured" of cancer, or of AIDS? (In this case, a major Southern California hospital pronounced the patient "cured" — their term — of immunoblastic sarcoma. But he remained HIV-positive. He lived in ordinarily good health for several years, dying of an indirectly related malady. Since he was still HIV-positive, had he "died of AIDS"?)

Promoters of ozone gas infusions and ozone machines spoke in glowing terms of "cures" of AIDS in the US underground and in Europe. At one point I was told that "hundreds" had been "cured," though was not provided supporting evidence. Yet research does confirm that *any* oxidative agent will, at least for a time, clear the *serum* of cell wall-deficient structures and anaerobic organisms, including virtually all viruses, retroviruses, some bacteria, mycoplasmas and yeast forms. Is clean serum evidence of a "cure"? The same had been said of the primary natural endogenous oxidative agent of all, hydrogen peroxide, and the Bradford research group's Dioxychlor and similar oxidative compounds. All have been useful and all have sprung from research relegated to the shadows of medicine in decades past primarily because they collided with the vested interests of the synthetic drug empire.

The use of "frequency machines" (see *XVII*) also generated claims of cures. The officially harassed anti-cancer products "CanCell" (said to be a synthetic of several compounds which somehow balance energy in the body) and Essiac (an herbal tea combination a half-century old in Canada) have been among "magic bullets" said to be useful in, even "curative" of, AIDS.

Highly optimistic results against, HIV/AIDS have also been reported through the use of Dr. Helmut Keller's *Carnivora* products developed from the Venus flytrap.[111] Indeed, herbs of all kinds have been reported useful against the syndrome.

By 1996/1997 SPV-30, an extract of boxwood evergreen, was among naturally derived products being looked at by "official" US research even though financial backing for such projects remained difficult and spotty.[111a]

Pharmaceutical giants were ever more turning to natural sources for AIDS drugs, not overlooking the fact that patented extracts therefrom could be great money-makers. But the fact that they were headed in the natural direction was a plus for the "holistic" side.

In 1992, Merck reportedly spent $1 million "prospecting" for both anti-cancer and anti-AIDS drugs in the Costa Rican rain forest even though by 1996 a company spokesman claimed that only "strong synthetic drugs" had shown any real effect in eliminating "traces" of HIV.[116]

But what we came to call AIDS Inc. essentially was not looking at non-drug approaches to AIDS or following up on promising leads developed outside the AIC, as I saw time and again.

Should an "outsider" — outside the AIC — appear with a promising product for AIDS (as antiviral, immune modulator, specific against a disease, etc.) — he was run through very expensive hoops.

A case in point has been Solutein, the modern-era incarnation of earlier work involving the use of immune boosters made of snake venoms (and anecdotally found useful against polio and MS at an earlier time.)

A small but enterprising Utah company attempted to show Solutein useful against AIDS — that is, in helping stabilize numbers of T4 cells, hastening HIV antigen negativity or modulating the immune system and specific disease states in a multiplicity of ways. The company wished to do things "the American way" by going through the ponderous, progress-blocking minutiae of the FDA.

Before the Utah company began reaching the conclusion that the federal government seemed to have only tepid interest, if that, in Solutein — which already was checking out well in animal trials and was "anecdotally" being used in HIV cases treated in Mexico — it had spent, its chief executive told me, at least in the "high six figures" in attempts to comply with FDA procedures.

Since the hospital with which I have been affiliated in Mexico was the site of much, but by no means all, of the Solutein use in human HIV cases, I am aware that in at least several cases (and, outside the hospital, in many more) of some truly impressive results with the product. European research continued to be positive for it.[112]

By the time this was written, and following a full-dress hearing in Washington by the FDA's "fast track" approval committee, Solutein was still not a "legal" drug in the USA.

And this, despite an authentic effort by the company to attempt to comply with the entire FDA inanity of various animal trials followed by various stages of human ones. And the company — as a non-member of the AIC — did not have millions of dollars to invest while the FDA took its time. The matter was not over at this writing, but constitutes one more frustrating reason why so much promising American research has had to be conducted outside of the USA, despite whatever utility it truly has.

While US medical orthodoxy remains devoted to the

allopathic paradigm and the HIV theory, "goods" continue to seep out of the accumulation of statistical debris.

Among them is the likelihood that more and more HIV infectees can live a very long time without developing AIDS (the so-called "non-" or "slow progressors.")

References

1. Reuters, March 7, 1994.
2. Gullick, RM, *et al.*, "Potent and sustained antiretroviral activity of indinavir, zidovudine, and lamivudine." XI Intl. Conf. on AIDS, (abstr. Th. B. 931) Vancouver, BC, Canada, July 7-12, 1996.
3. Voelker, Rebecca, "Can researchers use new drugs to push HIV envelope to extinction?" *J. Am. Med. Assn.* 276:6, Aug. 14, 1996.

3a. Nicolosi, Michelle, "AIDS fights back against drugs." *Orange County (CA) Register,* March 2, 1997.

4. The Associated Press, July 8, 1996. Also, *AIDS Clinical Care,* October 1996.
5. *The Economist* (Great Britain), in the *San Diego Union,* July 4, 1996.

5a. National Inst. of Allergy and Infectious Disease (NIAID), Washington DC, Oct. 1996.

5b. World Health Organization (WHO), cited in *J. Am. Med. Assn.,* Dec. 11, 1996.

5c. World Health Organization (WHO), July 4, 1997.

5d. Reuters, July 5, 1997.

6. The Associated Press, March 11, 1994.
7. Dept. of Health and Human Services, January 1994. Also Gary Null, WBAI Radio, New York, Sept. 23, 1996.
8. "Pneumocystis pneumonia — Los Angeles." Centers for Disease Control (MMWR), June 4, 1981.

8a. "Bad blood." "Sixty Minutes," CBS-TV, Oct. 13, 1996.

9. Culbert, ML, AIDS: *Hope, Hoax and Hoopla.* Chula Vista CA: Bradford Foundation: 1989, 1990.
10. Eighth National AIDS Update Conference, San Francisco CA, March 1996.
11. "Identification of HIV-1 Group 0 infection — 1996." *J. Am. Med. Assn.* 276: 7, Aug. 21, 1996.
12. "TB deaths reach all-time high." *J. Am. Med. Assn.,* 276: 12, Sept. 25, 1996.
13. Ho, DD, *et al.*, "Rapid turnover of plasma virions and CD4 lymphocytes in HIV-1 infection." *Nature* 373, Jan. 12, 1995.
14. Wain-Hobson, Simon, "Virological mayhem." *Nature* 373, Jan. 12, 1995.
15. Moskowitz, LB, *et al.*, "Frequency and anatomic distribution of lymphadenopathic Kaposi's sarcoma in the acquired immunodeficiency syndrome: an autopsy series." *Hum. Path.* 16, 1995.
16. Chang, Yuan, *et al.*, "Identification of herpesvirus-like sequences in AIDS-associated Kaposi's sarcoma." *Science,* Dec. 16, 1994.
17. *Lancet,* May 29, 1995.

17a. Foreman, KE, "Propagation of a human herpesvirus from AIDS-associated Kaposi's sarcoma." *New Eng. J. Med.,* 336: 3, Jan. 16, 1997.

17b. Mocarski, ES, "Propagating Kaposi's sarcoma-associated herpesvirus." *New Eng. J. Med.,* 336: 3, Jan. 16, 1997.

17c. Harrington, W., *et al.*, "Activation of HHV-8 by HIV-1 tat." *Lancet,* 349, March 15, 1997.

18. Sepkovitz, KA, *J. Am. Med. Assn.,* Feb. 12, 1992.

19. Papadopoulos-Eleopulos, E, *et al.*, "Is a positive Western blot proof of HIV infection?" *Bio/Technology* 11, June 11, 1993.
20. Kashala, Oscar, *et al.*, "Infection with human immunodeficiency virus type 1 (HIV-1) and human T cell lymphotropic viruses among leprosy patients and contacts: correlation between HIV-1 cross-reactivity antibodies to lipoarabinomanan." *J. Infect. Dis.* 169, 1994.
20a. Null, Gary, "AIDS special report." WBAI Radio, New York, Sept. 25, 1996.
21. Clerici, Mario, *et al.*, "HIV-specific T-helper activity in seronegative health care workers exposed to contaminated blood." *J. Am. Med. Assn.*, Jan. 5, 1994.
22. Kremer, H, *et al.*, "AIDS: death by prescription." *Continuum* (Great Britain), August 1996.
22a. Levy, JA, editorial, "Surrogate markers in AIDS research: is there truth in numbers?" *J. Am. Med. Assn.* July 10, 1996.
23. Feinberg, MB, "Changing the natural history of HIV disease." *Lancet* 348, July 27, 1996.
24. Culbert, ML, *op. cit.*
25. Levy, JA, "Human immunodeficiency viruses and the pathogenesis of AIDS." *J. Am. Med. Assn.*, May 26, 1989.
26. Horton, Richard, "'Renegade' HIV immunity hypothesis gains momentum." *Lancet* 342, Dec. 18/25, 1993.
27. Kurth, Richard, *et al.*, *Nature*, December 1995.
28. *Science*, Dec. 15, 1995.
29. Livingstone, WJ, *et al.*, "Frequent infection of peripheral blood CD8-positive T-lymphocytes with HIV-1." *Lancet* 348, Sept. 7, 1996.
29a. Belott, David, "Media complicity in the AIDS fraud." And Fumento, Michael, "The 'epidemic' that confounds the 'experts.'" Anaheim CA: *Orange County Register,* May 6, 1996.
30. Haney, DQ, The Associated Press, Jan. 30, 1994.
31. *Brit. Med. J.* and Reuters, March 25, 1994.
32. Peter Duesberg interview, *Spin* magazine, September 1993.
33. Duesberg, PH, "Human immunodeficiency virus and acquired immunodeficiency syndrome: correlation but not causation." *Proc. Natl. Acad. Sci.*: 86, February 1989.
34. Duesberg, PH, *Inventing the AIDS Virus*. New York: Regnery, 1996.
35. Duesberg, PH, "HIV is not the cause of AIDS." *Science* 241, July 20, 1988.
36. Miller, Jeff, "AIDS heresy." *Discover*. June 1988.
37. Root-Bernstein, Robert, *Rethinking AIDS: The Tragic Cost of Premature Consensus.* New York: The Free Press, 1993.
37a. Hodgkinson, Neville, *AIDS: The Failure of Contemporary Science*. London: Fourth Estate, 1996.
38. Culbert, ML, *AIDS: Terror, Truth, Triumph*. Chula Vista CA: Bradford Foundation, 1986.
39. Culbert, ML: *AIDS: Hope. . . . . op cit.*
40. Sonnabend, JA, *et al.*, "A multifactorial model for the development of AIDS in homosexual men." *Ann. NY Acad. Sci.* V, 1984.
41. Lo, S-C, *et al.*, "Identification of mycoplasma incognitus infection in patients with AIDS: an immunohistochemical, in situ hybridization and ultrastructural study." *Am. J. Trop. Med. Hyg.*, November 1989.
42. Lo, S-C, *et al.*, "Fatal infection of silvered leaf monkeys with a virus-like infectious agent (VLIA) derived from a patient with AIDS." *Am. T. Trop. Med. Hyg.*, April 1989.
43. Barnett, SW, *et al.*, "An AIDS-like condition induced in baboons by HIV-2." *Science*, Oct. 28, 1994.
44. "Baboons with AIDS spur hopes for tests." (Reuters). *San Diego Union*. Oct. 28, 1994.
45. Lipsky, JJ, "Antiretroviral drugs for AIDS." *Lancet* 348, Sept. 21, 1996.
46. Voelker, Rebecca, "New HIV drugs cast in supporting roles." *J. Am. Med. Assn.*, 276: 8, Aug. 28, 1996.
47. Gorman, Christine, "The exorcists." *Time*, Fall 1996.

48. Altman, LK, New York Times News Service, July 12, 1996.
49. *USA Today*, cited in *The Choice*, XX: 2-3, 1994.
50. Konotey-Ahulu, FJ. "AIDS in Africa: misinformation and disinformation." *Lancet*. July 24, 1987.
51. Garrett, Laurie. *The Coming Plague*. New York: Penguin, 1994.
52. Lauritsen, John, *The AIDS War: Propaganda, Profiteering and Genocide from the Medical-Industrial Complex*. New York: Pagan Press, 1993.
53. Dondero, TJ, and JW Curran, "Excess deaths in Africa from HIV: confirmed and quantified." *Lancet*, April 23, 1994.
54. Mulder, DW, *et al.*, "Two-year HIV-1-associated mortality in a Ugandan rural population." *Lancet*, April 23, 1994.
55. Vigniel, Corinne, Reuters, Dec. 12, 1994.
56. Kashala, *op. cit.*
57. Papadopoulos-Eleopolus, *op. cit.*
58. *Discover*, April 1996.
59. Purvis, Andrew, "Cursed, yet blessed." *Time*, Dec. 6, 1993.
59a. Fowke, KR, *et al.*, "Resistance to HIV-1 infections among persistently seronegative prostitutes in Nairobi, Kenya." *Lancet*, Nov. 16, 1996.
60. Rowland-Jones, Sarah, *et al.*, *Nature Medicine*, January 1995.
61. O'Brien, Stephen, *et al.*,*Science*, Sept. 27, 1996.
62. Parmentier, Marc, *et al.*, *Nature*, Aug. 22, 1996.
63. Landau, Nathaniel, *et al.*, *Cell*, Aug. 9, 1996.
63a. O'Brien, Stephen, *Science*, Aug. 15, 1997.
64. *Philippines Star*, Feb. 23, 1994.
65. "AIDS: the third wave." *Lancet*, Jan. 22, 1994.
66. Cohen, Jon, "The epidemic in Thailand." *Science*, Dec. 9, 1994.
67. *Manila Bulletin*, Feb. 21, 1994, and author interviews with Philippine health officials.
67a. Philippine Dept. of Health Figures cited by Manalad, AC., in *What's On/Expat*, Manila, Aug. 10, 1997.
68. Culbert, *AIDS: Hope, . . ., op. cit.*
69. Willner, RE, *Deadly Deception*. Peltec Publishing, 1994.
70. Lusso, Paolo, *et al.*, "Infection of natural killer cells by human herpesvirus 6." *Nature*, April 1, 1993.
71. Corbellino, Mario, *et al.*, "Disseminated human herpesvirus 6 infection in AIDS." *Lancet* Nov. 13, 1993.
72. Lusso, Paolo, and Robert Gallo, "Human herpesvirus 6 in AIDS." *Lancet*, March 5, 1994.
73. Knox, KK, and DR Carigan, "Disseminated active HHV-6 infection in patients with AIDS." *Lancet*, March 5, 1994.
74. Knox, Konstance, *J. AIDS and Human Retrovir.*, April 1, 1996.
75. Cited in *The Choice* XXII: 2, 1996.
76. Ostrom, Neenyah, "More on the virus the AIDS establishment is covering up." *New York Native*, Sept. 26, 1994.
77. *Ibid.*
78. Wilborn, F, *et al.*, "Detection of herpesvirus type 6 by polymerase chain reaction in blood donors: random tests and prospective longitudinal studies." *Brit. J. Haem.* 88, 1994.
78a. Levy, JA, "Three new human herpesviruses (HHV6,7 and 8)." *The Lancet* 349, Feb. 22, 1997.
78b. "MS cause said found, sparking vaccine hope." *Orange County Register*. Anaheim CA, March 1997.
78c. Levy, "Three . . ." *op. cit.*
79. Lauritsen, John, *Poison by Prescription*. New York, 1990.
80. Quoted by Charles L. Ortleb, *New York Native*, Nov. 1, 1993.

81. Bethell, Tom, "The cure that failed." *National Review*, May 10, 1993.
82. Halstead, Bruce, introduction, in Culbert, ML, *AIDS: Hope, op. cit.*
83. Bethell, *op. cit.*
84. Concorde Coordinating Committee, "Concorde: MRS/ANRS randomised double-blind controlled trial of immediate and deferred zidovudine in symptom-free HIV infection." *Lancet*, April 19, 1994.
85. Lenderking, WR, *et al.*, "Evaluation of the quality of life associated with zidovudine treatment in asymptomatic human immunodeficiency virus infection." *New Eng. J. Med.*, March 17, 1994.
86. Abrams, DI, *et al.*, "A comparative trial of didanosine or zalcitabine after treatment with zidovudine in patients with human immunodeficiency virus infection." *New Eng. J. Med.*, March 10, 1994.
87. Lundgren, JD, *et al.*, "Comparison of long-term prognosis of patients with AIDS treated and not treated with zidovudine." *J. Am. Med. Assn.*, April 13, 1994.
88. Osmond, Dennis, *et al.*, "Changes in AIDS survival time in two San Francisco cohorts of homosexual men, 1983 to 1993." *J. Am. Med., Assn.*, April 13, 1994.
89. Connor, EM, *et al.*, "Reduction of maternal-infant transmission of human immunodeficiency virus type 1 with zidovudine treatment." *New Eng. J. Med.*, Nov. 3, 1994.
90. Kumar, RM, *et al.*, "Zidovudine use in pregnancy: a report on 104 cases and occurrences of birth defects." *J. AIDS* 7, July 1994.
91. Rogers, MF, and HW Jaffe, "Reducing the risk of maternal-infant transmission of HIV: a door is opened." *New Eng. J. Med.*, Nov. 3, 1994.
92. Portegies, Peter, "HIV-1, the brain, and combination therapy." *Lancet*, Nov. 11, 1995.
93. Volberding, PA, *et al.*, "A comparison of immediate with deferred zidovudine therapy for asymptomatic HIV-infected adults with CD4 cell counts of 500 or more per cubic millimeter." *New Eng. J. Med.*, Aug. 17, 1995.
94. Cheo, Vivien, "Combination superior to zidovudine in Delta trial." *Lancet*, Sept. 20, 1995.
95. Eron, JJ, *et al.*, "Treatment with lamivudine, zidovudine, or both in HIV-positive patients with 200 to 500 CD4+ cells per cubic millimiter." *New Eng. J. Med.*, Dec. 21, 1995.
96. "An urgent appeal for action." Project AIDS International, March 25, 1993.
97. *Ibid.*
98. *Ibid.*
98a. *The Choice*, XXII: 2, 1996.
99. Badgley, Lawrence, *Healing AIDS Naturally*,. San Bruno CA: Human Energy Press, 1986.
100. Chaitow, Leon, and Simon Martin, *A World Without AIDS*. Great Britain: Thorsons Ltd., 1988.
101. Cichoke, AJ, "AIDS update: there is hope on the horizon." *Townsend Letter for Doctors*, Feb./March 1995.
102. *The Choice* XIX: 3-4, 1993.
103. *Ibid.*
104. The Associated Press, Aug. 21, 1994.
104a. Brink, WD, "Reexamining AIDS/potential non-toxic protocols." *Townsend Letter for Doctors and Patients*. December 1996.
104b. Herzenberg, Leonore and Leonard, to American Assn. of Immunologists annual meeting, San Francisco, February 1997.
104c. Tang, AM, *J. Nutr.*, Feb. 1997, reported by the *New York Times*, Feb. 1, 1997.
105. Eleopolus, EP, "Reappraisal of AIDS — is the oxidation induced by the risk factors the primary cause?" *Med. Hypoth.* 25, 1988.
106. Eleopolus, EP, *et al.*, "Oxidative stress, HIV and AIDS." *Res. Immunol.* (Institut Pasteur) 143, 1992.
107. "*Pneumocystis* pneumonia," *loc. cit.*
108. Coulter, Harris, *AIDS and Syphilis: the Hidden Link*. Richmond CA: North Atlantic Books,

1987.
109. Centers for Disease Control, Atlanta GA: *Morbid. Mort. Weekly Rep.*, Oct. 7, 1988.
110. Caiazza, Stephen. *AIDS: One Doctor's Personal Struggle*. Highland Park NJ, 1989.
111. Walker, Morton, "The carnivora cure for cancer, AIDS and other pathologies." *Townsend Letter for Doctors*, June 1991, May 1992.
111a. Dodds, Paisley, The Associated Press, Dec. 1, 1996.
111b. *Ibid.*
112. Haney, Jeffrey, "Snake venom may take bite out of AIDS." Ogden UT *Standard Examiner*, Dec. 10, 1995.
113. Munos, Alvaro, *et al.*, *J. AIDS and Human Retrovirol.*, May 1995, cited in *New York Native*, Nov. 20, 1995.
114. *Brit. Med. J.*, April 25, 1997.
115. Food and Drug Administration, June 11, 1997.

NOTE

Data presented to the American Society of Microbiology in 1997 found that in large groups of patients on experimental antiviral "cocktails" HIV had returned to "detectable levels" in a half or more of cases in a year's time. A spokesman for the University of California-San Francisco, styling the first year of the "cocktails" as "a honeymoon period," added that "all of our 'failures' are clinically feeling very well. It's very important to understand we have no idea of the prognosis of people who have resistant virus."[1]

Such a statement could be interpreted to mean that HIV viral loads do not mean much, or that HIV alone is not the sole cause of AIDS.

(1) "Promising AIDs therapy starting to fail." Haney, DQ, The Associated Press, in the *San Diego Union-Tribune*, Sept. 30, 1997.

XIV
CHRONIC FATIGUE, GULF WAR SYNDROME, 'EMERGING VIRUSES' AND THE NEW THREATS TO CIVILIZATION:
Biological warfare, nature's revenge — or both?

"[T]he speculation that AIDS jumped species naturally to initially infect people, virtually simultaneously, on two far removed continents, and more oddly, in the two exact regions wherein the suspected AIDS-like virus and vaccine experiments took place, must be seriously questioned. Moreover, based on the mass of evidence compiled herein, scientists (including those at the NCI and CDC) who advocated such farfetched notions of the origin of AIDS, in contrast to their knowledge of the NCI's Special Virus Cancer Program and recombinant viral vaccine experiments, have obviously incriminated themselves."

— **Dr. Leonard G. Horowitz, *Emerging Viruses: AIDS and Ebola — Nature, Accident or Intentional?* 1996**

"The mycoplasma that we have found in Desert Storm vets has very *unusual retroviral DNA sequences; thus in all probability it was 'engineered' and did not evolve naturally. The possible origin and illegal testing, sale and transfer of this microorganism to the Iraqi Atomic Energy Commission is the subject of one of the articles written by my wife . . . We have possibly uncovered one of the messiest controversies and coverups since Watergate and this one makes Watergate seem like a tea party . . . There is a huge coverup of immense proportions . . . a lot of people are not happy about this getting out."*

— **Cancer researcher/investigator Garth L. Nicolson PhD, 1995**

"Apparently, individuals in the US National Institute(s) of Health and National Cancer Institute have combined with the United Nation's World Health Organization to attack the United States with bio-weapons . . . The intentional introduction of disease began in Africa where sibships were inoculated by the WHO's International Agency for Research on Cancer (IARC) with diseases obtained from the [NIH's] New Bolton Center (NBC) cell lines or diseases previously inoculated were mixed by IARC's unsterile procedures. Other diseases were probably inoculated from other available cell cultures at other locations. In American homosexuals the virus may have been engineered to reproduce faster and for specific attack."

— **Robert Strecker MD, and Ted Strecker, Esq., in *This is a Bio-Attack Alert,* 1986**

Enter CFS, the Crippler

While the world was learning about the horrors of AIDS, the Killer, yet another parallel disorder, the Crippler, was silently but relentlessly spreading beyond the huge shadow cast by AIDS until, finally, its presence could no longer be denied.

The disorder, and its seeming incurability in so many cases, have added a whole new dimension to the menace of "emerging new diseases" which may in fact be man-made or at least man-influenced — and stimulated new medical approaches which must be mounted to meet the challenges of our species' very survival.

AIDS was several years old when Western medical journals began reporting cases of individuals who seemed to have AIDS-*like* conditions, but not full-blown disease. Such patients were instantly assumed to be in no way associated with AIDS because they were not, in the main, from the "AIDS risk groups" — that is, they essentially were not promiscuous male homosexuals, intravenous drug users, hemophiliacs or receivers of tainted blood products, or the sexual partners of any of the above, and were not HIV-positive.

Yet they were "presenting with" a mind-boggling constellation of symptoms (up to 60 separate ones) redolent of what came to be called the ARC stage of AIDS — swollen glands, nightsweats, spiking fevers, muscular, bone and neurological complaints, gastrointestinal and respiratory stress, sensitivity to light, occasional weight loss, sore throats, earaches, headaches, mood swings, short-term memory disturbances, personality changes, and, almost always, yeast infection and long periods of debilitating, extreme fatigue. The latter could last days to months — and even, in some cases, years.

But standard blood and other tests failed to reveal anything particularly wrong with these patients. Since the first cluster of them was reported in the resort area of Lake Tahoe/Incline Village, on the Nevada-California border, they were called sufferers of the "Lake Tahoe Syndrome." Since other clusters broke out among younger, more affluent and usually Caucasian people, they were also called victims of the "yuppie flu." The mild ridiculing of them in the media and even in the first few reports of their malady in the "literature" was excused by the fact that whatever was going on seemed to be transitory and nobody died.

Yet, the syndrome or something like it had been noted even earlier in other areas of the English-speaking world, where the countries in question equally had had a difficult time finding a phrase to define what surely was yet another syndrome. But this one, if anything, seemed more associated with *activated* than *depressed* immune systems. And in all areas it seemed to be more prevalent among women than men — a reason, some feminists argued, among several to explain why it received so little attention.

Even by the time (1988) the US officially took note of this combination of symptoms and baptized them Chronic Fatigue Syndrome (CFS; an unofficial earlier title was CFIDS, for "chronic fatigue/immune dysfunction syndrome") a significant number of clinicians and researchers were of the opinion this was essentially an all-in-your head version of schoolgirl panic attack among adults, a kind of "in" hypochondria.

At the very worst, it seemed that it might be an extreme form of yeast infection, since the general syndrome provoked by the human cohabitating yeast *Candida albicans* was also coming into its own as a pathology about whose parameters medical orthodoxy did not agree.

It also had to be distinguished from mononucleosis, thyroid disorders, general endocrine imbalances, influenza infections, occasionally secondary syphilis, hypoglycemia, the closely associated fibromyalgia, and premenstrual syndrome (PMS). All of these, along with the ARC stage of AIDS, produced a similar clinical pattern.

But AIDS was already distinguishable from any such presentation of confusing and conflicting symptoms thanks to the HIV antibody test and the standard helper/suppressor immune cell inversions — though CFS patients occasionally had some of the latter.

For a time, since blood tests to determine activity for new or reactivated Epstein-Barr Virus (EBV) were often positive in such patients, and the patients also had diagnosable yeast infection, some physicians thought they were seeing a recurring mononucleosis infection in adults, in which the yeast problem and other signs were secondary events.

But as numbers of cases came to be reported in Western medical journals, primarily though not exclusively among North Americans, inhabitants of the British Isles, Iceland, northwest Europe, Japan, Australia and New Zealand, it become evident that for numerous patients there were no elevated "titers" of EBV, even though yeast infection remained a virtual constant. This naturally gave rise to an allopathic medical industry already obsessed with the viral connection to AIDS to look for one in CFS.

By the early 1990s, CFS had ceased to be a laughing matter: its numbers anecdotally growing much faster than AIDS, some patients seemed to be permanently disabled, and some were forced to stay in bed for *years* at a time.

Yet by mid-decade it was difficult to get an "official" feel for real numbers of CFS patients, if only because the multiplicity of symptoms could so easily be confused with so many other things.

Earlier, the Centers for Disease Control and Prevention (CDC) had estimated that only 20,000 Americans fit the CFS "case description." But after a thorough review of data, CDC by 1995 had conservatively upped the estimates of carriers of CFS illnesses to between 118,000 and 520,000 — and added the syndrome to its "Priority-1 New and Emerging Infectious Diseases" list.[1]

One of CFS' medical discoverers, Paul Cheney MD, estimated in 1996 that at least 1 percent of the US population — or well over 2,600,000 — was afflicted with the syndrome even though he thought its numbers might have "peaked."[2]

The mental aspects of CFS often were as devastating as the physical symptoms: memories failed, personalities were altered, behavior patterns would swing violently, concentration diminished, IQ levels dipped, victims variously describing themselves as "unfocused," "un-wired," "coming apart." CFS caseloads and numbers grew, expanding from their younger (and even much younger) to older age brackets, and all economic levels.

The fact that the syndrome often occurred in clusters (classrooms, bands, orchestras, athletic teams, groups of doctors and nurses, any close-quarters arrangement) strongly suggested contagion, yet sexual contagion was unlikely: it became as common, if not more common, to find a mother and daughter showing symptoms as a husband and wife.

There also developed the strong possibility that CFS, whatever it was, was linked to an increased risk of some "forms" of cancer even though the syndrome itself did not at first seem to be killing anyone and a certain group of patients seemed to fully recover on their own while others went through frustrating, unpredictable periods of being healthy and restored or terribly ill and unable to study, hold a job or even think straight. Several physicians and patient support groups demanded to know what was going on, but it was difficult to hear their cries for help over the din caused by AIDS, held to be the great plague which had a 100 percent fatal outcome.

CFS became so variable in symptoms that it was not easy to distinguish it particularly from fibromyalgia syndrome, and in fact the one could be part of the other. Later, as Lyme Disease broke out (a potentially devastating infection ostensibly spread by a treponemal bacterium carried by ticks), it became equally difficult to separate Lyme cases from CFS ones.[3]

Numerous physicians thought they were seeing AIDS-like conditions in an ever-growing number of people, yet conventional wisdom was that this could not be because such patients were negative for HIV antibodies and were not from the AIDS "risk groups." For many, AIDS was a "dirty," CFS a "clean" — the one was a killer, the other a crippler, and they had no real points of similarity.

Or did they?

AIDS, CFS: parts of one syndrome?

In a 1993 book,[4] based primarily on research from the first 10 years and 2,200 patients (whom we originally called "no-name disease" victims) from our Mexican hospital, and at an international seminar our group presented in 1992, I outlined 14 large groups of symptoms (hematological, viral, bacterial, endocrinological, clinical) which pre-AIDS and CFS patients seemed to share. I asked a rhetorical final question: "*Are* these different kinds of patients?"

They could only be so on the basis of the absence of HIV in the CFS patients and the fact that pre-AIDS patients often (but by no means always) advanced into full-blown AIDS (though a few advanced CFS patients have exhibited some aspects of full-blown AIDS as well). Research from various quarters turned up some interesting items: there increasingly were thought to be aspects of "immune excitation" or "autoimmunity" in AIDS patients — and there were aspects of "immune depression" in CFS sufferers.

Our research group (Bradford Research Institute) thus proposed[5] a new model:

A Syndrome of Immune Dysregulation (SID), which covered a broad span of *immune dysregulation,* ranging from the takeover of the host by parasites, yeasts, fungi, bacteria, mycoplasmas, viruses and cancer, as was being seen in immune-depressed AIDS patients, to the over-excited immune responses of what some were calling "universal reactor syndrome" (URS). This is a condition in which the body is engaged in so many antigen-antibody immune responses and has so many confused signals it is now turning upon itself and the patient allergically reacts to everything — from all manner of food and drink to heat, cold, dryness, dampness, hair sprays, perfumes, industrial chemicals, natural and unnatural environmental allergens of all kinds, and even to the clothes on his back and bedsheets.

We reasoned that URS — and/or "environmental illness" or

so-called "multiple chemical sensitivity/environmental illness" — is a possible endpoint for unresolved CFS and that numerous "autoimmune" diseases, occurring mostly in the civilized Western world by the century's end, were stops along a general curve of SID.

While it seemed highly unlikely that a single factor was capable of causing the full spectrum of immune dysregulation — along whose pathological curve could be found many often new, mostly-Western "autoimmune diseases" (multiple sclerosis, scleroderma, various forms of lupus, Sjogren's syndrome, rheumatoid arthritis, possibly *all* arthritis, and various strange disorders simply never seen, or at least never adequately reported on, before this century) — it became more reasonable that a combination of ingredients was necessary in setting up a "substrate," a matrix on which a catalyst, or catalysts, might build.

(Such a matrix would contain the following elements [in no particular order of importance]: our chemically and hormonally altered food supply, particularly involving the overabundance of essentially nutritionless refined carbohydrates, known excesses/deficiencies in certain vitamins, minerals, enzymes and essential fatty acids, overuse of antibiotics and synthetic hormones [steroids], immunizations/vaccinations, overexposure to continual low-level radiation poisoning and/or low-level electromagnetic frequencies, fluoridated/chlorinated water, industrial and agricultural chemicals, "recreational drugs" — and mercury amalgam dental fillings and even root canals.

(The relevance of the latter two elements was particularly brought home to me in 1993/1994 as guest speaker at meetings of patients of alleged "fibromyalgia" — and/or CFS — in Missoula and Billings, Montana, where large groups of CFS-like conditions had broken out. In both meetings, of about 200 patients each, when I asked who had had a significant amount of mercury amalgam fillings prior to the onset of symptoms, 90 percent of hands went up. In Billings, when I asked who had had a root canal prior to the onset of symptoms, virtually *every* hand went up.

(All of the above elements constitute a possible witch's brew of conceivably immune-altering substances, yet they almost certainly need, whatever their numbers or combinations, one or more "triggers" or catalysts to begin the domino-like advance to pathology.)

If catalysts were involved, and if one stood out more than any other, it was a reasonable speculation it might be found among species-jumping, easily-mutating viruses from the animal kingdom (for viral inhabitants of humankind, involving dozens of varieties, have long coexisted in man without, in the main, causing significant pathology), if not from biological warfare.

HHV-6, of whatever origin, seemed to some a particularly strong candidate as a key virus in initiating a series of immune dysregulating events, particularly in a vast spectrum of individuals already "immunologically compromised." The widespread presence of HHV-6 in AIDS and CFS and its affinity for some of the same key components of immunity as targeted by HIV as well as its ability to activate other herpesviruses plus its affinity for "forms" of cancer made it a high-profile suspect.[5a]

There remained other viral suspects as well. In 1994 University of Southern California pathologist W. John Martin added a "stealth" virus, which apparently caused CFS symptoms in laboratory animals, to an ever-growing list of agents listed as possible "causes."[6]

It was observed that immunological disorders in humans are often accompanied by those in house pets or even other animals in close proximity. I pointed to the well-known statistical unusuality in which former President and Mrs. George Bush reportedly shared a single "autoimmune" disorder, Grave's disease, while their famous pet dog, Millie, reportedly had canine lupus. In 1993 I also pointed to the high prevalence of sheep (Visna virus?) in the countries which from earliest times had reported what many were calling myalgic encephalomyelitis (the equivalent of CFS in the United States) — particularly Iceland, whose outbreaks of "Icelandic disease" cases dated back to the 1940s.

HHV-6: the AIDS-KS-CFS link?

Throughout their parallel histories, US medical orthodoxy has absolutely not wanted to see connections between AIDS and CFS, even though they everywhere abound.

We have already indicated the widespread (and widening) presence of HHV-6 (human herpesvirus number 6, variants A and B) in both syndromes and have reported that some investigators find HHV-6 to be "the" likely "co-factor" to HIV — and, perhaps, far more important *than* HIV — in AIDS (*XIII*).

By 1995, the National Institutes of Health (NIH) had belatedly pumped more than $23 million into CFS research while the CDC was spending about $6 million a year to track it.[(7)]

As numbers of people fully or mostly disabled for up to years at a time continued to surface (with the strong likelihood that cases of CFS might eventually fill more hospital beds than cancer and AIDS combined), some investigators still clung to the notion CFS was mostly a psychiatric disorder.

(Unless it is unusually psychosomatic and capable of producing numerous physical symptoms, this analysis seems destined for extinction.)

With CFS estimated to be three to seven times more likely among women than men, there conceivably may be hormonal or genetic involvements, none likely to be singly definitive.[(8)]

In 1996 two landmark events occurred in the short history of CFS:

First, journalist Hillary Johnson published a 720-page roundup of nine years of investigating CFS which contained detailed information not only on the misuse of government research funds but also the systematic denial by the government that CFS is, in fact, a *communicable* disease and hence a threat to public health.[(9)]

And a New York congressman, Jerrold Nadler, was beginning a probe into the possibility that CFS research by the NIH and CDC had not been properly conducted. He also sought a full-scale General Accounting Office (GAO) investigation.

Research links between CFS and AIDS, primarily through HHV-6 (variant A), have continued to grow, not diminish, and sometimes have taken odd twists:

CFS delineator Paul Cheney told our groups' international symposium (1996) that among the characteristic signs of CFS (as also reported by other investigators) are "purple crescents" in the throat (other common signs: lymphatic swelling on the left side, deteriorating fingertips).[11]

Such crescents have also been correlated to HHV-6 infection, oral cancer and Kaposi's sarcoma, the most common "cancer" in AIDS cases, and which not all researchers agree should always be considered cancer.[12,13,14,15]

Indeed, whether Kaposi's sarcoma is actually "caused" by what has been called either KSHV (Kaposi's sarcoma-associated herpesvirus) or HHV-8 (human herpesvirus 8) raises the same problem as HIV in AIDS: is presence (correlation) construable as causation?

The small band of researchers following HHV-6 (variants A and B) see this particular virus as a likely catalyst (if in fact there is a single catalyst) in Kaposi's sarcoma (particularly the "inflammatory" variety which has turned out to be far more widespread than previously thought and able to take many forms, whether in the presence of HIV or not) as well as CFS and AIDS.

If this virus (particularly its more lethal variant A) is found to be a primary catalyst for all three or even a major contributor to all three, then serious questions are raised:

— What is HHV-6 and where did it come from?

— Since it seems to be highly communicable (saliva,[16] blood), is it or is it not a public health threat?

— If it is the major link between CFS, AIDS and possibly KS (Kaposi's sarcoma), what does this do to the HIV theory?

— If there is a contagious immune system-altering virus "out there" and government researchers are aware of it, why aren't we being told?

— And if, as some research suggests, the relatively new antiviral drug Ampligen, and a long-available extract of pig liver (Kutapressin), have anti-HHV-6 properties,[17] why aren't they in general use?

And, just as AIDS and CFS were raising such as-yet unanswered questions, quite another medical nightmare arose.

Gulf War Illness/Syndrome — the making of a scandal

In 1991, as chairman of the Committee for Freedom of Choice in Medicine Inc., I received a call from Saudi Arabia. The caller identified himself as a soldier (deployed to the Middle East during the troop buildup for what would become the Persian Gulf War) and as a former member of the Committee for Freedom of Choice in Cancer Therapy Inc., the predecessor of the current organization.

He told me he and other troops were being asked to take "vaccinations" against possible biological warfare agents and he wondered what his rights were if he refused. I was not particularly concerned about the call or the problem at the time. I should have been.

The Gulf War came and went, a quick-kill for American-led troops against America's one-time ally, Saddam Hussein of Iraq. For a brief moment, America revelled in a rapid military triumph which had seemingly caused few American casualties (while inflicting enormous damage on the civilian, let alone the military, population of Iraq.)

So hundreds of thousands of troops returned home from the Middle East in phases. Then the rumors started.

Our own medical and advocacy groups, as well as others, began hearing strange complaints from either returning veterans or members of their families — all kinds of symptoms were occurring which had all the multiple symptomatic trappings of the "ARC" stage of AIDS and the rapidly developing CFS. As time went by, females who had served in the Gulf or who were married to Gulf War soldiers complained of bringing defective babies into the world.

We started hearing about odd rashes, "burning" semen, devastating fatigue, a vast array of neurological disorders, swollen glands, states of extreme mental confusion, respiratory, ophthalmological, auditory, musculoskeletal and other sensory problems . . . that is, a syndrome.

We began hearing stories from Gulf War vets and their families that had the oddly familiar ring of the early days of CFS and even of AIDS:

The returnees went from one doctor to another to another, none of whom could adequately identify the condition (but might identify a symptom or two), and the more persistent, who spoke of ruined emotional lives, loss of jobs, extreme anxiety, were finally dispatched to the psychiatrist with the ultimate medical put-down: "It's all in your head."

It was of course, not all in anybody's head except for the damage being done to the brain.

Just as US medical orthodoxy took a long time to admit that CFS existed and might be contagious, US medical orthodoxy *and* the Pentagon took an inordinate amount of time realizing that there really was such a thing as Gulf War Syndrome or Illness (GWI), (GWS) and, even at this writing (1997), seemed distressed to find that at least some of it is *highly contagious.*

In fact, some medical professionals who treated GWS patients revealed they, too, had developed GWS symptoms.[70,70a]

Part of the problem was, of course, political and economic: should all the vets reporting Gulf War Syndrome be eligible for disability benefits? And if they were, would this not add billions to defense costs? (In an interesting development, in 1993 Veteran Affairs Secretary Jesse Brown announced that veterans who were diagnosed with CFS — an illness belatedly but "officially" recognized by the US government — could collect disability.)

It was unofficially estimated that within just a few years of returning from the Gulf at least *six thousand* US military personnel and family members had died of strange symptoms. It was reported that hundreds of thousands, perhaps millions, of residents in the Gulf War theater of operations were desperately ill with a range of symptoms sounding suspiciously like GWS.[18] (1997 estimates set the US death toll at 20,000,[18a] or higher.[18b])

As if to quiet such concerns, two studies of Gulf War veteran deaths and hospitalizations published in 1996 claimed not to find such unusual incidences at least in the first two post-war years, with a medical editorialist noting that "only careful epidemiologic studies can identify whether there is, in fact, any excess disease."[66]

By late 1993 several researchers, including those at Walter Reed Army Medical Center, had acknowledged that GWS was in fact "a chronic fatigue (CFS/CFIDS) -like syndrome."[19]

But the Pentagon and Department of Defense steadfastly insisted there was no such syndrome, and that the various complaints returning veterans had experienced could be explained in several mundane ways.

But the complaints kept right on coming. Veterans formed support groups both to counsel their ever sicker comrades and to lobby the Pentagon and Congress for a peek into what was going on. An army nurse told me in 1996 that not only she but her "entire unit" were now ill with a myriad of symptoms.

At an American Public Health Association annual meeting in 1995, Centers for Disease Control and Prevention (CDC) scientists reported "hallmark symptoms of CFS" in sick Gulf War veterans.[20] By then, some 43,000 Gulf War veterans had registered with the Department of Defense and Veterans Affairs as having developed health problems following the war.

By 1996, the information dam was beginning to burst:

First, the Pentagon began admitting that there just might be a Gulf War Syndrome, but that the numbers of afflicted individuals were small. Duke University research indicated that the overuse of chemicals used to protect troops from insects and nerve gas might account for some of the cases.[21] Another study pointed to stress as a central cause.

In the meantime, a well-credentialed Texas cancer researcher had been able to get to the public an alarming observation based on research and personal interest — that a biological warfare-derived microbe engineered in the United States and made available to Iraq had been used against US troops and that it was showing up in the blood of many vets (*see next section*).

By fall 1996 the Pentagon was accepting the validity of the GWS syndrome — but was claiming that the vast amount of cases had to do with exposure of US troops to the deadly nerve gases sarin and cyclo-sarin just *after* the war when "chemical warfare rockets" were blown up by US combat engineers in two attacks in March 1991.

An initial Pentagon study found that 5,000 troops "might have been exposed" to a nerve gas-containing cloud arising after the first detonation at the Khamisiyah military complex in southern Iraq. A few weeks later, and reporting on a second detonation, it said 15,000 might have been exposed and that exposure figures might go much higher — even to 100,000 and beyond.

The "Iraqi chemical weapons depot" story reached new levels of strangeness which it surfaced in 1997 that the CIA had known by the mid-1980s that there was such a depot.

But for some troops, who began noticing symptoms well before any attacks on Khamisiyah were carried out, the idea that one or more toxic clouds emanating from one site might explain tens of thousands of chronic symptoms seemed much too convenient.

A putatively independent presidential panel in November 1996 condemned the Pentagon's own investigation into whether or not American troops had been exposed to Iraqi chemical weapons, claiming the official probe had "lacked vigor, fallen short on investigative grounds and stretched credibility."[67]

A month earlier, the CIA and Pentagon were at great pains to dismiss the findings by two former CIA intelligence analysts who had claimed that Americans "might have been exposed" to such weapons.[68]

By the end of 1996, another governmental entity — the Centers for Disease Control and Prevention (CDC) — reported that 4,000 Air Force veterans in the Gulf War in fact were three times more likely to suffer memory loss, joint and muscle pain and other ills than people who had served elsewhere during the same period.[69]

In 1997, two official GWS boards were told of Texas research which indicated there might be six separate — though often overlapping — Gulf War Syndromes![70,71]

The same Texas researcher who made the claim of biological warfare noted how many symptoms seemed to be shared between GWS and CFS patients. I heard this correlation expressed, with bewilderment, by other doctors across the country.

The same rage which had characterized CFS patients in clamoring for their malady at least to be recognized was occuring among GWS victims. There was no blood test, no single confirmatory diagnosis of the new syndrome, and the victims, who *knew* they were sick, were mightily offended by the oft-expressed medical opinion that they were hypochondriacs or simply mentally unstable.

An extensive 1997 study claimed not to find an unusual risk of birth defects among children of Gulf War veterans. But it admitted to "certain limitations" and that "not all congenital defects are evident at birth — and thus cannot be included in a study limited to birth records."[72]

In mid-1997, a General Accounting Office (GAO) report found "substantial evidence" of a link between GWS, nerve gas and chemical weapons. It added that the Defense Department should not "rule out" the possibility of "biological weapons."[73]

As congressional investigators began demanding some answers and the Gulf War veterans community and their families continued to grow, some alarming questions were raised:

Is it possible that aspects of AIDS, CFS and GWS reflect a single pathology?

It is possible that one or more viruses, or other microbes, contribute, as catalysts, to these conditions?

Is it possible that at least some of these viruses are actually man-made and that coverups involving AIDS, CFS and GWS have been conducted to obscure or deflect this reality?

It is possible there are many other man-made viruses out there, all far more contagious than blood-borne HIV, and may be "out of control" — hence the need for the global population to be conditioned into expecting "coming plagues"?

Biological warfare — the gathering evidence

From the beginning of the AIDS pandemic conspiracy theories as to its origin and that of its presumed etiological agent abounded. While some of the ideas have hardly been worth considering, others beg to be elucidated.

Were AIDS the single new calamity facing civilization, conspiracy theories as to its nature and origin, while important, might have less impact.

But it isn't. And, as we shall see, some relatively solid new research has raised serious questions which must be answered, and suggests scandals of far-reaching magnitude.

I have detailed the conspiracy theories as they relate to AIDS elsewhere.(23) Synthesizing them:

— Information developed by Glendale CA gastroenterologist Robert Strecker MD and his late attorney brother Ted (a "suspicious" suicide) suggested that "the AIDS virus" is a man-made splice-together of two bovine viruses — *Visna maedi* virus (VMV) in sheep and the bovine leukemia virus (BLV) in cattle — "evolved upward" in humans, and that World Health Organization (WHO) and other documents can be interpreted as "calling for" creation of just such an experimental virus with which to suppress the human immune system(s).

— Information developed by British venereologist John Seale that HIV is a tampered-with version of the Visna virus that has been available as a biological warfare weapon among the superpowers for years.

(The Strecker thesis held that the "man-made virus" probably was a product of Soviet biological warfare aimed at the United States. Seale was variously quoted saying that both the

Americans and Soviets developed the virus for biological warfare.)

— An intriguing claim by a former US army engineer that the former Soviet Union used "scalar electromagnetic" methods to "beam in" the "AIDS virus" to the US (*see XVII*).

— The vaccine theories. These hold that man-made experimental viruses were "tested" on Africans and on male homosexuals by inoculating both populations with vaccines — the smallpox vaccine in central Africa, a special hepatitis B vaccine in New York. They are paralleled by the idea that a mutated simian virus causing human AIDS was spread through an earlier form of the injectable polio vaccine. Various sub-theories hold that these inoculation programs were either purposeful experiments, laboratory mistakes, or one or more parts of a coordinated conspiracy to reduce the human population. (Dr. Alan Cantwell's *AIDS and the Doctors of Death* and *Queer Blood* make interesting cases.)

While officially pooh-poohed, a case can be made for them all to some extent:

That there has been international research into immune-suppressing viruses is a fact. This in itself need not be sinister (a primary problem in the failure of organ transplants, for example, has long been how to overcome the human immune system attack on foreign tissue). That the superpowers, despite signing anti-biological warfare treaties, engage in and have engaged in biological warfare for decades is an essentially open secret. That many countries have the technological knowhow to manipulate, alter, splice together or seemingly create "new" viruses is also true.

These realities may encompass both human conspiracy (what better weapon than a virus which wipes out an immune system and is thus killing millions of people before its presence is even detected?) as well as human foibles (errors in high-tech gene research, gene-splicing and viral manipulation have been widely reported. In an era of petri-dish "immortal cell lines" and the exchange of active viral strains between laboratories and scientists, an "Andromeda strain"-like disaster is waiting to occur at any time).

The timeframes for the seemingly sudden appearance of AIDS in Africa and among male homosexuals in the United States neatly coalesce with the smallpox and hepatitis B vaccine theories, each of which has some other intriguing twists and turns which could either lead to chilling new revelations or go nowhere. The widespread appearance of AIDS in "third world" countries also comfortably dovetails with polio inoculations.

An African swine fever connection?

Another theory, part of which may — or may not — fall into what international spy network participants class as "disinformation," holds that "AIDS" is really what arrived in the United States in lieu of "swine flu" — an alleged epidemic warned about during the Gerald Ford presidency (1970s) and for which a vaccine was developed which killed several people and sickened others while no epidemic appeared.

Indirectly connected with this theory is that African Swine Fever Virus (ASFV), an extremely lethal structure which can wipe out entire pig populations and antibodies to which have been found in human AIDS patients (among others), has long been an American biological warfare research item and was in fact deployed against Cuba to wreck the island's pork production. Part of the theory also holds that ASFV, man-mutated for human inoculation, became the true "AIDS virus."

There should be more than passing interest in the latter statement.

As I noted in 1986, researcher Jane Teas originally proposed[24,25] that ASFV might be the real "cause" of AIDS — that is, the catalyst virus. Later, researcher John Beldekas argued that ASFV is in reality HHV-6, and that the virus was pirated by the NCI, which provided its present name and description.[26]

The AIDS Inc. orthodoxy denied any connection between ASFV and HHV-6, yet some of that very orthodoxy at this writing was yielding to the rising importance of HHV-6 in AIDS, as well as CFS.

In 1994, Michigan Senator Donald Riegle's Senate Committee on Banking, Housing, and Urban Affairs probe into Gulf War Syndrome uncovered the fact that between 1984-1989 the United States had shipped numerous biological warfare agents to Iraq. Staff researchers made the "disturbing proposal" that some of these agents had been used *against* American troops in the Gulf War.[27]

When a reporter asked a US Department of Agriculture official: "Can M1-AL Abrams tanks or Bradley fighting vehicles carry hoof-and-mouth disease, African swine fever, or the anthrax bacteria?" the answer was yes.[28] Did US troops return from the Middle East suffering from the effects of biological warfare weapons which had originated in the USA?

Or even from experimental vaccines provided US troops upon the outbreak of the Gulf War?

Karl Grossman, a reporter for a Long Island newspaper, wrote about what he called "the mystery-shrouded island" — Plum Island, at the east end of Long Island, New York — as a long-time center of closely-guarded biological warfare (described by the military establishment as "defensive") research and at which, he and others asserted, African swine fever virus (ASFV) was actively studied for years.[29]

Grossman quoted *Newsday* in 1993 (*Newsday* having already reported in the 1970s on an alleged CIA plot to weaken Cuban pig herds through ASFV inoculations):

> "*A 1950s military plan to cripple the Soviet economy by killing horses, cattle and swine called for making the biological weapons out of exotic animal diseases at a Plum Island laboratory, now-declassified Army records reveal . . . Documents and interviews disclose for the first time what officials have denied for years: that the mysterious and closely guarded animal lab . . . was originally designed to conduct top-secret research into replicating animal viruses that could be used to destroy animal livestock*

. . . While officials say any such research was short-lived and ceased when the lab was turned over to the Agriculture Department in 1954, two of the diseases targeted by the military — hoof-and-mouth disease and African swine fever — remain top-priority research projects on Plum Island today."[30]

Supposing, for a moment, that Teas, Beldekas and some others are right, that African swine fever virus is somehow a "cause" of AIDS let alone a major catalyst virus in immune dysregulation in general, what do we know about ASFV?

Interestingly, in its natural state it seems to be as tricky and evasive as AIDS orthodoxy says HIV is.

In a 1987 textbook on the subject, researcher Eladio Vinuela noted:

The presence in African swine virus DNA of several multigene families, a finding not reported for any other virus, may be related to the ability of African swine fever virus to evade the immune system . . . The virus . . . changes easily and different virus isolates produce diseases with different clinical symptoms or no disease at all.[31]

The Nicolsons speak out

It was in 1995 through a CFS patient treated at the Mexican hospital with which I have been affiliated that I learned, in a roundabout way, of the startling discoveries and work of Garth L. Nicolson PhD and his scientist wife Nancy.

Nicolson, an impeccably credentialed Texas cancer researcher (at the time professor and chairman of the Department of Tumor Biology at the University of Texas M.D. Anderson Cancer Center, about as orthodox a medical institution as exists in the USA), proposed the following:

— There are numerous symptomatic connections between Gulf War Syndrome (GWS) and Chronic Fatigue Syndrome (CFS).

— At least some of these symptoms were directly caused by a biological warfare-derived microbe which a US company had provided to Iraq.

— The new microbe, an otherwise harmless mycoplasma called *Mycoplasma fermentans incognitus,* into which the "envelope gene" of the HIV virus had been inserted, was detectable in the blood of a third or more of GWS patients through a "gene tracking" test he and his wife devised.

(This was the same mycoplasma which US scientist S-C Lo had found to "cause" AIDS symptoms in animals (*see XIII*). Dr. Lo has questioned the notion it is involved in GWS.[72])

— The first experiments with the microbe were carried out on the Texas prison inmate population.

— Treatment with doxycycline and other antibiotics had restored numerous patients to good health.[32]

While Dr. Nicolson had written a letter to a medical journal[33] on the utility of doxycycline against the illness virtually no one had taken his revelations seriously.

Checking with him in detail (and impressed by his courage) I made certain that *The Choice*, the publication of the Committee for Freedom of Choice in Medicine, Inc., published his general theory.

I sent copies of the article to the "straight" media as well as the "tabloid press." Only the latter originally responded. At any rate, the story got out, and the Nicolsons left the M.D. Anderson Cancer Center under pressure.

By 1997, more and more people were aware of the Nicolson claims even while the Pentagon and DoD ignored or denied them.[33a,33b,33c] (***See Addendum, Page 631***).

Among investigative journalists who did much to bring the Nicolson work to public attention was Gary Null, a New York journalist/health activist whose daily radio program has a huge following.

In 1996, Null provided more than four hours of radio time to what he called an extensive investigation of several years and hundreds of interviews and document searches looking into the Gulf War Syndrome.[34]

Based on extensive interviews, he found that US personnel had been repeatedly exposed to biological weapons and (as in the case of the strange telephone call made to me in 1991) vaccines. Part of the problem might have had to do with various inoculations the troops were provided with, ostensibly as protection *against* such weapons.

He found — as did the Nicolsons — that troops from all the nations that participated in the Desert Storm coalition against Iraq, save one, had come down with strange symptoms that they associated with experimental vaccines.[35] He said that troops from France, which had opted not to use the same, had avoided the symptoms. The Nicolsons reported huge casualty rates in Middle East countries.[35a]

Worse, whatever was happening to veterans was not only contagious but *extremely* contagious, they reported: even clothing and part of uniforms sent home were able to contaminate whole families with strange symptoms. *Majorities* of spouses and children swiftly developed symptoms.

At the same time Gary Null was involved with his in-depth probe into GWS, another investigator was ferreting out even more sinister information.

The manufacture and deployment of AIDS ?

The Strecker brothers referred to earlier were the first American professionals (Robert, the gastroenterologist; Ted, the attorney and investigator) to gather documents from "official" US and global (World Health Organization) sources — particularly one document[36] — which at the very least strongly suggested that certain research efforts were underway in the early 1970s to find ways in which viruses could affect human immune functions.

By linking much data together they reached the conclusion that HIV, the "AIDS virus," was a manufactured splice-together of two animal viruses designed to be mutated "upward" in man. In

1986 they put this information into a bundle of papers under the title *This is a Bio-Attack Alert,* which was sent to various and scientific personalities and publications in the US. Our Committee for Freedom of Choice in Medicine was one of the recipients.

Later, Robert Strecker MD made a commercially available videotape, *The Strecker Memorandum*, which outlined his findings.

Among interested parties who paid attention to information from Dr. Strecker was Leonard G. Horowitz DMD, a Harvard public-health graduate and medical investigator whose exposé of the Florida dental AIDS tragedy, *Deadly Innocence,* was at the time the major of his 10 books.

It was when he learned in 1993 of a Strecker-produced document — congressional hearing testimony detailing a Department of Defense appropriations request for $10 million for the development of "AIDS-like" viruses[(37)] — that he set forth to try to unravel the HIV/AIDS mystery and check out Strecker point by point.

This led, he told me,[(38)] to a review of more than 2,500 pertinent scientific papers and governmental documents during which "I learned that there was no direct evidence for the natural evolution of HIV-1 from monkey to man. On the contrary, a scientific assessment raised the distinct possibility that HIV-1 and its relatives, HIV-2 and the simian immunodeficiency viruses (SIVs), more likely evolved as a result of laboratory cancer virus experiments." And this may also have been true for such terrible viruses as Ebola and Marburg, he argued.

The upshot of his tenacious pursuit of one lead after another resulted in a 565-page blockbuster exposé called *Emerging Viruses: AIDS and Ebola — Nature, Accident or Intentional?*[(39)] — which he virtually had to promote and market on his own.

The Horowitz findings, while calling into question ethics and morality at the highest levels, paint a detailed picture of coverup, deceit and trickery involving major governmental and research figures, the Department of Defense, CIA, major defense contractors, noted AIDS research figures, and the National Cancer

Institute (NCI).

In synthesis:

> *The evidence shows that a channel through which experimental (mutant) viruses, viral vaccines, other reagents and drugs flowed between the NCI and affiliated testing laboratories at Litton Bionetics and Fort Detrick, to MSD (Merck, Sharp & Dohme) and its related research labs in New York and Central Africa, was the Drug Development Branch of the NCI. Through this channel, or another, the CIA, or a saboteur, may have delivered a single roller bottle containing AIDS viruses to experimental vaccine producers or directly to Merck's hepatitis B (and perhaps other multicomponent) vaccines — the vaccines that appear to have played a principal role in infecting scores of human subjects in the early 1970s in New York City, Central Africa, and other regions of the world hardest hit by AIDS.*[40]

If his composite research is anywhere near the mark, it helps clear up several mysteries, such as:

— Why, even in the face of continuing failure to provide much of a connection between the viral theory and human cancer, the NCI, in the 70s in particular, continued to receive huge federal grants to pursue such research.

— Why the first AIDS cases (and those linked to other viruses as well) broke out when and where they did.

— Why HIV is so "different" from "natural" viruses. If in fact it has been genetically engineered as a "viral hybrid," as the Horowitz research indicates, many of the mysteries of HIV vanish — by this thinking HIV can't be compared to any normal or natural virus *because it isn't one.*

His extensive data collection incriminates the government of the US and many of its collaborating political, military and scientific figures with violations of international anti-biological warfare treaties and even of genocide by the testing of experimental viruses on selected populations at home and abroad.

The general pattern he paints is this:

• America's Cold War preoccupation with worldwide communism led elements of the government to undertake biological warfare experiments under the belief or knowledge that some other nations were doing the same. American oncology's interest in the viral theory of cancer and research into anti-cancer vaccines was a useful cover for the acquisition of funds to be earmarked for more sinister purposes. In essence, the NCI to a large extent became a conduit for biological warfare research.

• America's major biological weapons testing center (at Fort Detrick MD)was transmuted into the Frederick Cancer Research Facility of the NCI in 1971 which was to become a showcase for President Nixon's "Conquest of Cancer" program.

Just years before, Nixon's security chief, Henry Kissinger (with Rockefeller and globalist credentials [*see VI*]), had ordered a reassessment of this nation's chemical/biological weapons capabilities "from which the option to develop immune-system-destroying viruses was selected." Kissinger also ordered the CIA (whose scientists developed and stockpiled numerous deadly viruses for Project MKNAOMI [code for the CIA biological weapons program]) "to conduct covert military operations in the Zaire/Angola area — the region of Africa hardest hit by the AIDS and Ebola epidemics."[42]

The Defense Department and NCI paid biological weapons contractors "millions of dollars during the 1960s and early 1970s to produce immune-system-depleting and cancer-causing viruses. These would include the viruses with the pathological effects of the HIV and the hemorrhagic fever viruses, Ebola and Marburg."[42]

• The CIA obtained "dozens of biological weapons, including deadly viruses, and illegally maintained them in storage facilities on the grounds of Fort Detrick as late as 1975. Thereafter [it] possibly retained private firms for such purposes despite all such actions being illegal."[43]

• "The CIA conducted dozens of biological warfare experiments on hundreds of thousands of unsuspecting human subjects both domestically and in foreign lands" while Defense Department contractors "conducted numerous AIDS-like virus and vaccine experiments during the 1960s and early 1970s simultaneously in New York City and/or Central Africa — the two areas hardest hit by the AIDS epidemic."[44]

Horowitz conceded that it is "highly plausible" that the earliest AIDS, Ebola and Reston virus outbreaks were accidental even though the mishaps were incidental to biological weapons research and that "government and industry standards disregarded simian virus contaminants" in the vaccines, beginning but not limited to the polio vaccines developed in the 1950s. He noted:

> *Contamination of experimental and production vaccines . . . occurred routinely, very likely giving rise to viral recombinants that might have crossed species barriers as, in many cases, they had been engineered to do through human tissue culturing. All told, such methods and materials used by NCI researchers could have easily created AIDS-virus progenitors including . . . HIV-2"* (the second "AIDS virus," which this line of inquiry suggests came first.)[45]

He added that "it is reasonable to propose that HIV-1, HIV-2, or other progenitors . . . were accidentally transmitted to . . . experimental vaccines that were then tested on retarded children, gay volunteers, and others in New York City as early as 1970."[46]

In accord with other research and suggestions, Horowitz found that, although the theory of contaminated polio vaccines as the chief vectors of AIDS is still plausible, "the unique epidemiology, and concurrent outbreaks of AIDS in New York City and Central Africa, appear to coincide more closely with the administration of the experimental hepatitis B vaccines . . . "[47]

Even so, there is the possibility that what was first called HTLV-III evolved in mentally retarded children at the Willowbrook State School [New York] or male homosexuals as a result of viral recombination — that is, first the polio, then the hepatitis B vaccines.[48]

Utilizing available documents, Horowitz found how US researchers were able to "make" viruses — an issue separate from just why they would be made:

— Synthetic RNA cat leukemia viral components were combined with human "type C" viruses (associated with lymph tissue cancer) to create genetically engineered "viral hybrids" to increase the rate of cellular DNA (master replicatory template) as many as 30 times — structures able to "cause" leukemia, lymphoma and sarcoma.[49]

— "NCI scientists elaborated the specific enzymes and other biochemical processes needed to induce immune system collapse."[50]

— Scientists "commonly modified monkey viruses enabling them to induce immunosuppression, cancer wasting and death in monkeys, humans, and lower animals."[51]

It is the "monkey vectors" through which so many hybrid viruses may have spread, he pointed out. While the "company line" has long been that somehow an African green monkey bit an African and transmitted a virus which evolved into HTLV-III (HIV-1), the painstaking Horowitz and related research suggests that, if anything, mankind infected the monkeys!

"Thus, all it might have taken was one monkey, infected with an AIDS-like virus . . . to have caused the AIDS pandemic," he wrote. "Alternatively, all it might have taken was one mad person, with access to . . . hepatitis B vaccine lots, to have initiated a 'population control' experiment."[52]

None of the above research specifically proves the intent to mass-murder anyone. It *does* highly suggest the use of human guinea pigs (Africans, gays, retarded children, prison inmates) in experiments at least some of which were guided by biological warfare concerns, whatever else some of the scientists may have had in mind.

There is naturally a visceral reaction among Americans to

disbelieve that our government or its scientists, for any reason, would use other Americans — let alone other humans anywhere — as guinea pigs.

But the fact that such has been going on is not new — even though it may be something most people do not like to think about.

Aside from 1996 disclosures in the Gary Null "white paper" on Gulf War Syndrome (which detailed some documented modern-era outrages in which various groups of Americans were either intentionally or accidentally experimented upon, including cases in which military bacteriological weapons simply "got out of control" and poisoned humans and animals alike[53]), the government record of human experimentation is relatively open:

— Between 1932 and 1972 in an experiment conducted by the US Public Health service, 400 poor black syphilitics were never told they had the disease and were allowed to develop its symptoms and remain untreated, simply to see what would happen.[54]

— A shocking tome (*A Higher Form of Killing*) described in detail how the CIA conducted drug experiments on unwilling, unsuspecting American citizens in New York, San Francisco, and elsewhere.[55]

— In the 1950s and 1960s the US Army "bio-attacked" unsuspecting US citizens and civilians, the most famous being a six-day "germ fog" experiment in San Francisco.[56]

— US government experimental "biowarfare" attacks took place in subways, on highways and at airports in the USA as well as at US military bases.[57]

— The US Army admitted in 1977 to at least 239 instances since 1949 in which unsuspecting civilians and military personnel were the subjects — that is, test animals — for germ warfare experiments involving bacteria, fungi and chemicals. These, and nerve gas experiments at Dugway Proving Ground, have now been described in detail.[58,58a]

"Biological testing involving human subjects by the Department of Defense," a US Senate hearing in 1977, detailed much of the above.[58b]

So did a shocking Senate Committee on Veterans Affairs report in 1994.[58c]

In many talks I had with him, Dr. Strecker (semi-retired as this was written) had not sought to define the politics of "who did what to whom and why" — that was left up to the conspiracy buffs, for whose theories his work (which simply showed how certain it was that US and global research had in fact manufactured "the AIDS virus") has served as useful fodder.

The "suspicious suicide" of Ted Strecker[59] and the alleged drug overdose-related death of Illinois State Rep. Douglas Huff, said to be a champion of getting the Strecker information before the Illinois Legislature[60], could only fuel such speculations.

As head of the advocacy group Committee for Freedom of Choice in Medicine Inc. for years, I heard just about every possible theory — Communists doing it to the West, the West doing it to the Communists, Arabs doing it to Israel, Israel to the Arabs, anti-gay "homophobes" plotting the destruction of all homosexuals, white racists (prodded by Nazi doctors brought to this country after World War II) exterminating racial "minorities," extraterrestrials eradicating the hybrid humans they had had a hand in creating anyway. And so forth.

One theory, though, seems to have a shade more credibility in the area of *intentional* genocide through biological warfare (rather than possible *accidental* genocide as an unfortunate consequence *of* biological warfare): the planned general reduction of the human population, given the technological reality that massive warfare is no longer a "viable option" to achieve the same.

What cries out — from the Strecker, Horowitz, Nicolson and related research — is the utter need for an airing of all aspects of the possible biological warfare components involved in the creation of new diseases and an exposé of just how far an American "secret government" — perhaps begun with the best of patriotic interests as a counter to a worldwide foe whose passage through this century left so many millions dead or brutalized — has become so entrenched, so greedy and so powerful that it is no longer accountable to anyone.

More diseases of civilization

While AIDS, CFS and "universal reactor syndrome" or URS represent huge groupings of cases in which immune dysregulation of some kind is going on, the Western world is also beleaguered by a raft of new disorders and conditions, some of which have no official names, and all of which involve some degree of immune-system derangement.

While it is not certain they should all be lumped under what we have suggested may be called the Syndrome of Immune Dysregulation (SID), certainly they should be called disorders of civilization in that they are so far essentially limited to the Western world. They include but are not limited to:

— The general constellation of conditions generally classed as "environmental illness" or "multiple chemical sensitivity" and strongly linked to exposure to organophosphates, pesticides, insecticides and an ever-lengthening list of industrial and mostly petrochemicals.

— Attention-deficit disorder (ADD), afflicting untold thousands, perhaps millions, of children — and even adults — and the true extent of which is far from known.

— Silicone-induced immune disorder (among other names) — in which women, particularly in the United States, have reported an impressive series of immunological and other disturbances seemingly linked directly or indirectly to silicone breast implants, over which billions of dollars in lawsuits have occurred, and about which scientific research has at best been confusing.

— Agent Orange Syndrome, a constellation of symptoms strongly correlated to exposure to this Vietnam War defoliant, and which, like CFS and GWS, the government long denied existed.

— Sick Building Syndrome — a galaxy of symptoms which seem to occur in clusters among workers in particular buildings, apparently associated with exposure to various chemicals involved in construction materials and air conditioning.

— Acute disturbances in behavior, including depressive disorders and sudden acts of violence, which seem to relate to any number of synthetic chemicals both in the environment and food supply.

Diametrically opposed suppositions suggest reasons and causes. All may be involved:

The first is that man has so overchemicalized his environment that the accumulated effects of industrial molecules are now beginning to manifest themselves in a vast variety of physical and mental conditions. They are grossly akin to earlier known disasters of civilization: mercury poisoning among "mad" hatters and the long-term slow poisoning of whole populations by lead — from lead pipes, for instance, a probable contributor to the gradual deterioration of the Roman Empire.

The second is the possible immune system-altering effects of the depletion of earth's ozone layer, a kind of shield through which the sun's ultraviolet radiation is diffused. A considerable school of thought believes this depletion (the extent of which remains controversial[61] since partial depletion may indeed be transitory and normal to earth's atmosphere) is more connected with immune alteration than any other single factor.

The third, and now more historic, holds that radiation (both known and unknown, or "occult"), disturbances in electromagnetic fields and related phenomena are primary suspects in immune dysregulation, since such energy alterations at the subcellular level (*XVII*) are subtle and probably cumulative.

Since the vast amount of severe immune dysregulation occurs in more civilized nations — yet the ozone depletion effect should be planet-wide — it would seem that the chemical toxicity/radiation views are more consistent for most expressions of immune damage among humans. Chemicalization as well as presumptive damage from ozone depletion may also account for increased evidence in the 1990s of immunological disturbances among animals, some of whose species are indeed threatened by the expansion of human civilization.

As we note in *XV*, depletion from soils of vital minerals is playing an undoubted role in mineral-deficient states in Western countries. The composite effects of reduced oxygen concentration (by some estimates down from 38 percent to 22 percent in the atmosphere since the 1940s and even lower in urban complexes[(62)]) are difficult to estimate, but oxygen deprivation theoretically should favor the existence of *anaerobic* life — as in cancer.

Certain medical mavericks, such as Canada's embattled Dr. Charles Reich, suggest that dietary deficiencies in calcium and Vitamin D, exacerbated by body coverings of people in cold climates (clothing as a block to already-diminished sunlight) may be major contributors to establishing a foundation for chronic disease.[(63)]

Whatever the root causes, mankind in general and Western man in particular may truly be reaching the end of their ecological/biological tether — unless they act responsibly and intelligently, and the sooner the better.

Sentinels of calamity

This writer was not particularly popular in Iceland when, in 1993, examining the spiralling rates of cancer, CFS and general immune dysregulation in a tiny population $^{1}/_{10}$th of 1 percent that of the United States — rates which are roughly the same as those in the USA, with its far greater population cushion — he warned that Western civilization faces extinction at the hands of civilization itself.[(64)]

In fact, civilized Iceland, far to the north; and civilized New Zealand, far to the south, with a larger but still small population; and, to some extent Australia, may be considered "sentinel countries" for the extinction or survival of the Western gene pool — and, by implication, of mankind itself.

In all Western countries, rates of chronic, metabolic disorders and immunological dysregulations match and occasionally bypass those of the United States and represent a palpable threat to the population. Complexing this situation with the rapid development of antibiotic-resistant bacteria and the presence of "new" viruses, both worldwide phenomena, the threat becomes one of possible human extinction.

In a grim kind of way, I was intellectually satisfied to realize, following my 1993 appearances in Iceland and in Canada and New Zealand in 1996 warning of imminent catastrophe, that I was a Johnny-come-lately.

In 1982, the aforementioned Canadian physician/researcher Carl Reich MD, upon whom medical authorities there have not always looked kindly, wrote prophetically in an Australian "alternative medicine" magazine:

> *Two hundred years ago, while the human knew starvation and infection, the human organism was exposed to no pollution (or) drugs but the smoke of wood fires and the rare use of tranquilizing or hallucinating drugs. In contrast, in recent decades, the human has been veritably steeped in an environment which contains thousands of synthesized chemical substances . . . Most of these . . . were never present in the world prior to this decade . . . (and) are entirely foreign to the human organism.*
>
> *That the human organism has survived so well in the face of this chemical onslaught is testimony to the tremendous adaptive potential inherent in an organism that has slowly evolved over a long period of time . . . There must be a limit to this adaptive potential of the human organism, however, and I regret to suggest that the human race may soon be approaching such a limit of its adaptive potential. Once this adaptive potential of the human organism has been exceeded, one may expect that various of these adaptive physiological mechanisms may break down.*
>
> *Adaptive mechanisms, which may now be proceeding asymptomatically but which are being taxed, may therefore break down at some future date* to create disease states which are currently unknown to the human body.(Emphasis mine.)

For reason of this hazard of chemical agents, I warn the public that they not only take a new look at their chemically laden environment and chemically laden diet but that they also take a new look at the modern [medical] profession, the aim of which is to provide them with health largely by chemical means.[65]

These musings by a fiercely independent medical thinker, it must be stressed, were printed only one year into the AIDS epidemic and well before the elucidation of most of the SID-connected calamities now plaguing the Western world. Dr. Reich learned, as have so many pioneers who dared to go against the grain, that a prophet is without honor in his own country.

The holistic challenge

For the holistically inclined, it is unlikely that there is a single cause of CFS, AIDS or the full spectrum of a Syndrome of Immune Dysregulation, but even if there is, the challenge to research is the same: determining why some individuals remain essentially healthy, while others become gravely ill or even die. This holistic concern supersedes allopathic obsessions with single causes, however much viruses (new or old, man-made or natural), uncontrolled parasites, bacteria, mycoplasmas and other elements may be involved.

The restored holistic paradigm for the 21st century is focused less on causes than on the elaboration of individualized, multifactorial treatment regimens (protocols) which already have become the only rational, workable approaches to AIDS, CFS and what lies between.

The challenge of immune dysregulation is that of human survival itself: SID is evidence of the imbalances man has largely brought about within himself and on his planet. Enmeshed with the devastation of cancer, SID represents what may be the final physiological challenge to the survival of the species itself.

In the spirit of dualism, the cancer-SID menace — threatening, as it does, the whole of the human species — represents at the same time challenge and opportunity.

References

1. Holzschlag, Molly, "Congressional testimony smashes CFS myths." *Healthwatch* (CFIDS Buyers Club), Summer 1995.
2. "Eighth International Symposium in Mallorca." *The Choice,* XXII:2, 1996.
3. Steere, AC, *et al.,* "The overdiagnosing of Lyme disease." *J. Am. Med. Assn.,* April 14, 1993.
4. Culbert, ML, *CFS: Conquering the Crippler.* San Diego: C and C Communications, 1993. German ed.: *CFS, Das Chronische Mudigkeitssyndrom.* Ritterhude: Waldhausen, 1993.
5. Culbert, ML *Toward a Unified Theory of Immune Dysfunction and its Management.* Chula Vista CA: Bradford Research Institute, 1992.

5a. Levy, JA, "Three new human herpesviruses (HHV-6,7, and 8)." *Lancet* 349, Feb. 22, 1997.

6. Martin, WJ, *Am. J. Path.,* August 1994.
7. "CFSwatch." *The Choice,* XXII:2, 1996.
8. *Ibid.*
9. Johnson, Hillary, *Osler's Web: Inside the Labyrinth of the Chronic Fatigue Syndrome Epidemic.* New York: Crown, 1996.
10. Ostrom, Neenyah, "Jerry Nadler's mission." *New York Native,* June 24, 1996.
11. "Eighth International . . .," *loc. cit.*
12. Yadav, M, *et al.,* "Frequent detection of human herpesvirus 6 in oral carcinoma." *J. Natl. Ca. Inst.* 86, Dec. 7, 1994.
13. Bovenzi, P, *et al.,* "Human herpesvirus 6 (variant A) in Kaposi's sarcoma." *Lancet* 341, May 14, 1993.
14. Cunha, BA, "Crimson crescents — a possible association with the chronic fatigue syndrome." *Ann. Int. Med.* 116, February 1992.
15. Marchesani, RB, "Crimson crescents facilitate CFS diagnosis." *Infec. Dis. News* 5 (11): 1, November 1992.
16. Kruger, GRF, *et al.,* "Clinical correlates of infection with human herpesvirus-6." *In vivo* 8, 1994.
17. *Ibid.*
18. Null, Gary, "The Gulf War Syndrome — a second opinion." Radio station WBA1, New York, Aug. 5-9, 1996.

18a. Riley, Joyce, RN, Gulf War Veterans Assn., to CFS/Fibromyalgia Support Group, La Jolla CA, July 20, 1997.

18b. Interview, Garth L. Nicolson PhD, *ICHF Newsletter* I: 3-4, 1997.

19. Ostrom, Neenyah, "The three faces of 'AIDS.'" *New York Native,* Nov. 20, 1993.
20. "Deny everything." *The Choice*, XXII: 1, 1996.
21. "Veterans' battle continues." *The Choice*, XXII: 1, 1996.
22. Walters, Nolan, Knight-Ridder News Service, Oct. 2, 1996.
23. Culbert, ML, *AIDS: Hope, Hoax and Hoopla.* Chula Vista CA: The Bradford Foundation, 1989, 1990.
24. Teas, Jane, "Could AIDS agent be a new variant of African swine fever virus?" *Lancet*, April 23, 1983.
25. Teas, Jane, "African swine fever virus and AIDS." *Lancet*, March 8, 1986.
26. Ostrom, Neenyah, "Did Gallo and Downing steal credit for discovering ASFV in humans from Teas and Beldekas?" *New York Native*, Feb. 28, 1994.
27. *United States Dual-Use Exports to Iraq and their Impact on the Health of the Persian Gulf War Veterans.* Senate Committee on Banking, Housing and Urban Affairs, May 25, 1994. Washington: US Government Printing Office, 1994. Also, *New York Native*, Feb. 28, 1994.
28. *New York Times*, March 20, 1991.

29. Ostrom, Neenyah, "The coming desert storm." *New York Native*. Feb. 7, 1994.
30. McDonald, John, *Newsday*, Nov. 21, 1993.
31. Vinuela, Eladio, "Molecular biology of African swine fever virus," in Becker, Yechiel (ed.), *African Swine Fever*. Boston: Nijoff, 1987.
32. Culbert, ML, "GWS-CFS: the 'coverup' and the 'cure.'" *The Choice*, XXI: 2, 1995.
33. Nicolson, GL, *J. Am. Med. Assn.* 273, 1995.
33a. Nicolson, Garth, and Nicolson, Nancy L, written testimony, House Committee on Government Reform and Oversight, June 26, 1997.
33b. "Mycoplasmal infections — diagnoses and treatment in GWS/CFIDS patients." Nicolson, Garth L, and Nicolson, Nancy L, *CFIDS Chronicle*, Summer 1996.
33c. Nicolson, Garth L, and Nicolson, Nancy L, "The Eight Myths of Operation 'Desert Storm' and Gulf War Syndrome." *Medicine, Conflict and Survival*. (UK), 13: 140-146, 1997.
34. Null, Gary, *loc.cit.*
35. *Ibid.*
35a. *Newsletter* of the Intl. Council for Health Freedom (ICHF), I: 3-4, 1997.
36. Bulletin of the WHO, Vol. 47, pp. 257-274, 1972.
37. *Department of Defense Appropriations for 1970: Hearings before a Subcommittee of the Committee on Appropriations, House of Representatives, 91st Congress, First Session, HB 15090, Part 5, Research, Development, Test and Evaluation, Dept. of the Army*. Washington: US Government Printing Office, 1969.
38. Horowitz, LG, "New evidence on manmade origin of AIDS." Abstract released to Committee for Freedom of Choice in Medicine Inc. and International Council for Health Freedom, Fall 1996.
39. Horowitz, LG, *Emerging Viruses: AIDS and Ebola — Nature, Accident or Intentional?* Rockport MA: Tetrahedron Inc., 1996.
40. *Ibid.*
41. *Ibid.*
42. *Ibid.*
43. *Ibid.*
44. *Ibid.*
45. *Ibid.*
46. *Ibid.*
47. *Ibid.*
48. *Ibid.*
49. Horowitz, "New Evidence," *op cit.*
50. *Ibid.*
51. *Ibid.*
52. *Ibid.*
53. Null, Gary, *loc. cit.*
54. Jones, JH, *Bad Blood: the Tuskegee Syphilis Experiments*. New York: Free Press, 1981.
55. Harris, Robert, and Jeremy Paxman, *A Higher Form of Killing*. New York: Hill and Wang, 1972.
56. "Army germ fog blanketed SF for 6 days in '50 test." *Los Angeles Times*, Sept. 17, 1979.
57. "Army used live bacteria in tests on US civilians." *Los Angeles Times*, March 9, 1977.
58. Cole, LA, *The Eleventh Plague: the Politics of Biological and Chemical Weapons*. New York: Freeman, 1997.
58a. Cole, LA, *Clouds of Secrecy: The Army's Germ Warfare Tests over Populated Areas*. Savage MD: Littlefield, Adams, 1990.
58b. *Biological Testing Involving Human Subjects by the Department of Defense, 1977*. Hearings, Senate Subcommittee on Health and Scientific Research. March 8, May 23, 1977. Washington: US Government Printing Office, 1977.
58c. *Is Military Research Hazardous to Veterans' Health? Lessons Spanning Half a Century*. US

Senate Committee on Veterans Affairs, Dec. 8, 1994.
59. Personal communication.
60. The Strecker Group, cited by Horowitz, L, *Emerging Viruses, op. cit.*
61. Lee, RW, "The global warming freeze." *The New American,* March 21, 1994.
62. Charles McWilliams MD to Consumer Health Organization of Canada, April 3, 1993.
63. Personal communications, 1993-1994.
64. *The Choice*, XIX: 3-4, 1993.
65. Reich, CJ, "Pseudo-scientific medicine." *Health and Healing* (Australia), April-June, 1982.
66. Campion, EW, "Disease and suspicion after the Persian Gulf War." *New Eng. J. Med.,* Nov. 14, 1996.
67. Shenon, Philip, New York Times News Service, Nov. 8, 1996.
68. Reuters, Oct. 31, 1996.
69. The Associated Press, Nov. 11, 1996.
70. Moehringer, JR, "Gulf War ailment called contagious." *Los Angeles Times,* March 9, 1997.
70a. Testimony, CFS/Fibromyalgia Support Group, La Jolla CA, July 20, 1997.
71. Haley, RW, *et al.*, "Is there a Gulf War Syndrome?" *J. Am. Med. Assn.,* Jan. 15, 1997.
72. Cowan, DN, *et al.*, "The risk of birth defects among children of Persian Gulf War veterans." *New Eng. J. Med.* 336: 23, June 5, 1997.
73. Shenon, Philip, New York Times News Service, June 16, 1997.

ADDENDUM

The *Mycoplasma fermentans incognitus* (MFI) controversy was reaching alarming dimensions in 1997 as it became clear that the microbe is transmitted casually and might be making its way into the civilian population. The Nicolsons and other researchers found the altered microbe in growing numbers of CFS and Gulf War Illness (GWI) patients even while US medical orthodoxy denied it could be found in the former and that, even when found in the latter, was not dangerous. Government physicians have questioned the Nicolsons' research and conclusions.[1]

By 1997, several mysteries were escalating the GWI controversy: the "shot charts" (immunization records) of the bulk of upwards of 700,000 US participants in the Gulf War were said to be "missing," the nature of experimental vaccinations provided Gulf-bound troops remained "classified," and squalene (used in the elaboration of potential HIV vaccines) had appeared in the blood of numerous veterans.[2]

From international contacts, the Nicolsons estimated that huge numbers of military and civilians alike in the Gulf War area had died or had become sick from the use by Iraq of biological/chemical/biological weapons provided by the US, United Kingdom, Japan and former USSR.[3]

Testimony by patients and doctors themselves meeting at the Scripps medical complex in La Jolla CA in 1997 emphasized the apparent ease of transmission of MFI, which was found in their blood by the Nicolsons' "gene-tracking" and PCR tests. It was not clear, however, for what other microbes their blood might be positive. In their own research, the Nicolsons found increasing numbers of patients they described as suffering from "GWI/FM/CFS"

(Gulf War Illness/fibromylagia/chronic fatigue syndrome) positive for MFI as opposed to low numbers in the "non-deployed" healthy adult population.[4]

The Nicolsons and others believe there are multiple causes of the GWI/FM/CFS constellation but that a substantial portion have conditions caused by mycoplasmic and bacterial infections which are susceptible to antibiotic treatments.[5]

In addtition to a five-antibiotic drug regimen (doxycycline, ciprofloxacin, azithromycin, clarithromycin, and minocycline), the Nicolsons and other investigators have added sublingual B-complex vitamins, Vitamins C and E, co-enzyme Q10, zinc, chromium, magnesium, selenium and dietary recommendations to suggested protocols.

Cases in which the primary causative agent may be MFI apparently have good prospects of recovery. However, deaths and intermittent illness continue to plague thousands of individuals in the GWI/FM/CFS category, the precipitating causes for which may be other than MFI.

A San Diego husband/wife research team (he allegedly infected simply by proximity to Marines shopping at a store; the wife infected by the husband) established a mycoplasma "tracking" registry which, among other things by 1997 found links between MFI and military/civilian personnel at or around US military ordnance depots.[6]

1. Kenneth W, Kiser, US Dept. of Health Undersecretary for Health, Symposium, "Is the government taking the right approach toward Gulf War Illness?" *Insight*, Jan. 27, 1997.
2. *Newsletter* of the International Council for Health Freedom (ICHF), I: 3-4, Fall-Winter 1997.
3. *Ibid.*
4. Nicolson, Garth L; Nicolson, Nancy L.; Narsalla, Marwan, "Mycoplasmal infections and fibromyalgia/chronic fatigue illness (Gulf War Illness) associated with deployment to Desert Storm." *Int. J. Med.* 1997 (in press).
5. Nicolson, Garth L., and Nicolson, Nancy L., written testimony to the House Committee on Government Reform and Oversight, Subcommittee on Human Resource and Intergovernmental Relations, June 26, 1997.
6. Presentation, Sean and Leslie Dudley, CFS/Fibromyalgia Support Group, La Jolla CA, July 20, 1997.

XV
SIEGE OF THE SOIL, TERROR AT THE TAP:
The revolution in food, water, diet and supplements

"Whoever pays no attention to these things, or paying attention, does not comprehend them, how can he understand the diseases which befall a man? Wherefore, it appears to me, necessary for every physician to be skilled in nature and to strive to know what man is in relation to the articles of food and drink and what are the effects of each of them to everyone."

— **Hippocrates**

"The doctor of the future will give no medicine but will interest his patients in the care of the human frame, in diet, and in the cause and prevention of disease."

— **Thomas Alva Edison**

"The greatest derangement of the mind is to believe in something because one wishes it to be so."

— **Louis Pasteur**

"He is less remote from the truth who believes nothing, than he who believes what is wrong."

— **Thomas Jefferson**

". . . Perhaps the most notorious adherents to the false notion that the diet has any specific influence on the origin or progress of cancer are the food faddists . . . There is no scientific evidence whatsoever to indicate that modifications in the dietary intake of food or other nutritional essentials are of any specific value in the control of cancer."

— **AMA Council on Pharmacy and Chemistry,**
Journal of the American Medical Assn. **(1949)**

"In its biggest shift of gears in a decade, the American Cancer Society (ACS) . . . has begun a mammoth survey of middle-aged Americans' dietary habits to find substances which may cause or inhibit the disease. The project began this fall just as the National Cancer Institute (NCI) released results of a survey of 156 studies linking cancer with diet. The survey found 'extraordinarily consistent scientific evidence' of just such a connection."

— ***The Choice*****, Fall 1992**

A conceptual revolution

As the millennium comes to a close, a conceptual dichotomy nags at the Allopathic Industrial Complex (AIC) as the revolution in new medical thought everywhere abounds:

From the standpoint of pure science — and we mean here biochemistry — the debate is essentially over: what we eat, and drink, and what goes into what we eat and drink, is of profound importance in health and disease.

Yet this reality is only slowly seeping through the layers of vested interests of the Complex because of the enormous economic implications of the reality:

• Food reform, water reform, lifestyle reform mean the prevention of a great deal of chronic disease and the promotion of health, which medically will be the guidepost of the 21st century.

• But enormous economic/political interests are involved in the treatment of disease by the drug empire and the utilization of a veritable "chemical soup" in the mass production of foodstuffs for the Western world — which, in turn, feeds much of the planet.

Nutrition and all it means are of extreme importance to medicine, but even by the 1990s organized (allopathic) medicine was only belatedly taking an interest in this central truth.

It has been the cancer pandemic which, more than any other aspect of disease, has so strongly riveted global scientific attention on the areas of nutrition and diet, even though elements of both had long been discussed in relationship to the complex of pathologies described as "heart disease" (*X*).

As late as 1949, the American Medical Assn.'s Council on Pharmacy and Chemistry had set the AIC party line as to diet and cancer (and, by implication, chronic disease in general):

> *There is no scientific evidence whatsoever to indicate that modifications in the dietary intake of food or other nutritional essentials are of any specific value in the control of cancer.*[1]

This was an early statement of Divine Law as presented by the AIC through the primary "learned journal" of American allopathic medicine. Even then there were enough vitamin pills and "food faddists" around to pose a threat, however distant, to the developing allopathic medicine/pharmaceutical empire in the United States.

But in the final decade of this millennium, a surge of research from the very bowels of orthodoxy and enshrined in orthodoxy has knocked the earlier, paleolithic view into a cocked hat:

• In 1992, the National Cancer Institute (NCI) released results of a survey of 156 studies from standard, peer-reviewed "literature" which linked a vast range of dietary aspects with cancer. Gladys Block, University of California-Berkeley School of Public Health, the lead author, found "extraordinarily consistent scientific evidence" of the connection.[(2)]

• In 1993, the health freedoms-oriented group Citizens for Health unearthed a suppressed US Department of Agriculture study which had been done in *1971* which had made strong connections between diet, chronic disease and cancer. It was charged that this extensive $30 million federal study had been suppressed at the behest of the food-processing industry.[(3)]

• The same year, 1993, results of a massive five-year trial by Chinese and American scientists found that vitamin/mineral supplementation had reduced the risk of cancer by 13 percent among residents of north-central China aged 40 to 89.[(4)] China was the subject of various nutritional studies involving chronic disease due to the size of its population, the variations of that population in terms of geography and the fact that Chinese society, by being far less mobile that the American one, provided long-term observations of relatively fixed subgroups.

• In 1994, the American Association for the Advancement of Science (AAAS) was told that of 172 studies in the orthodox medical archives on the role of fruits and vegetables in the prevention of cancer, 129 had shown a "significant protective effect."[(5)]

• In 1995, the American Institute for Cancer Research

learned that studies of the links between cancer and dietary factors, very much including the more recently described *phytochemicals*, actually had begun as early as 1933 and in 62 years had included 200 studies. These had turned up, according to cancer research scientist John Potter MD, "fairly consistent epidemiological data."[6]

As this was happening, more and more research reported in standard allopathic journals was reporting the usefulness of various nutrients and diets against "heart disease."[7] (*See also X*) It was already a given that more exercise and a reduction in dietary fats and fewer carbohydrates seemed to relate to less heart/circulatory problems, although such information — if it reached the patient at all — was usually within a treatment scheme still emphasizing cholesterol-lowering or hypertension-lowering drugs, vasodilators and/or other "heart disease" medications.

Lessons from Hawaii and Arizona

The negative effect of the Western or appropriately named SAD (standard American diet) on indigenous populations within the Western world has been among contributory elements in a greater understanding of food, health and disease and how racial/cultural differences may influence them — or vice-versa.

Cases in point are Hawaii and Arizona.

While Hawaii has long had among the best longevity rates in the USA its native Hawaiian population has had among the worst mortality rates of cancer, heart disease and diabetes and a majority of Hawaiians are obese.

But then came Dr. Terry Shintani and his belief that when native Hawaiians switched from a diet based on taro root, seaweed, sweet potatoes, greens, fruits and small amounts of fish to Spam (a Hawaiian "staple" as late as this decade, largely thanks to the US military presence in the islands) and refined carbohydrate "junk foods" they were metabolically shocked.

He hence developed the three-week native food immersion plan called the Wai'anae Diet (or Hawaiian Diet).

Startling effects were reported in 1993 — and again in 1997 — in which huge reductions in weight, lowering of "bad" cholesterol and other blood fats and the ability of some patients to go off diabetes and hypertension drugs were reported. Governor Ben Cayetano went public with his own dramatic response to the program in 1997.[87,88]

At the same time, the Tucson AZ-based Native Seeds/ SEARCH program, dedicated to saving traditional desert food plants, began accumulating evidence to show that Arizona's native Pima Indians might be "genetically adapted" to the foods which once grew in abundance around them. The research came none too soon: the Pimas' diabetes rate (half of all adults over 35) was reportedly the highest in the world.

The native Hawaiian and Pima diets emphasize low fat and high natural fiber, elements Western orthodoxy now associates with less chronic disease in general and which are components of the "poor people's diet" in Third World countries which increasingly is associated with far less chronic disease than in the West.

They also help substantiate the low-fat diet (combined with meditation and exercise) championed by California's Dr. Dean Ornish, which some insurers were beginning to cover in this decade.[89]

The squelching of nutrition

As I learned from the late Dean Burk PhD, a founder and long-time cytochemistry division chief of the National Cancer Institute (NCI) — he was the single proponent of laetrile within the federal research entity (*XII*) — NCI scientists had "breathed nutrition" in the early days of the NCI, and numerous NCI scientists were fully aware of dietary connections to cancer. But their voices were not heard, or at least not heard at the front office. For the drug industry was already in effective control of American medicine and American medical research and the search for viruses as causes of diseases was underway.

With the counterculturalism and dietary reform movements in full swing by the 1970s, an editorial in the *Journal of the American Medical Assn. (JAMA)* abstracted what was for the *JAMA* an alarming new trend:

> *There is evidence that certain vitamins can cause acute toxicity but little attention has been given it because no one thought the day would come when public figures would promote something as outlandish as megavitamin therapy.*[8]

The same editorial was arguing that the then-current efforts to limit Food and Drug Administration (FDA) authority over vitamin and mineral supplements would lead to "pharmaceutical lunacy."

It should be noted that by even that date the "recommended daily allowances" for nutrients, as established by government bodies largely beholden to the food and drug industries, were awesomely low.

It was held throughout the 1970s, by Cancer Inc., that "the first sign of a cancer quack" was any attempt to connect diet with cancer.

But no such observations by medical orthodoxy could keep Americans away from a growing array of nutritional supplements and the readership of popular books on diet and nutrition. This is not to say that opportunists of every hue were not present at every stage to promote worthless nostrums, silly diets and unprovable theories — the very actions which occasionally sustained arguments of the need *for* a stronger FDA and *for* coordinated actions against "health fraud." What comprised the latter, however, often ranged from truly bogus cures for any number of diseases to simple dissidence from the basic concepts of allopathic medicine. It was something of a replay of the Church in the Middle Ages: both the village rapist and the village Protestant might equally face death at the stake, the one for a crime of commission, the other for a crime of free thought.

The medical esoterics

More than any other element in the assembling of a new paradigm, the laetrile revolution flushed into the open increasing numbers of physicians (mostly MDs, but also MD-DOs and DCs) who not only espoused laetrile against cancer but who came to call themselves nutritional doctors, practitioners of "megavitamin therapy," or even "metabolic physicians," persons who began sounding like modern-day Eastern esoterics: they were not treating diseases but rather were treating people.

In the main, they were advancing a *holistic* concept of health and disease. They were often mavericks and antiestablishmentarians by nature, as eager to demonstrate "unproven" EDTA chelation therapy against heart disease (*X*) as the use of megavitamins and nutrition against disease in general. They talked of "bolstering the immune system" and "enhancing host defense," and, eventually, of "multifactorial therapies" as opposed to the one-drug-at-a-time "monopharmacy" of the allopathic majority. They were recapturing the ancient medical reality that *attitude*, even the demeanor of the healer, is as important in healing (and in inducing disease) as any physical remedy. They were, thus, flirting perilously with what the AIC would describe, depending on its mood, as "unconventional," "unproven," "unscientific," "dubious" therapy — or even "quackery," the worst pejorative of all.

The metabolic virus had largely been let loose by the laetrile movement, and it spread rapidly even while the AIC orthodoxy belatedly responded to the laetrile "menace" by developing the largest combined research/judicial/statutory attack in the history of American medicine (*XII*). Practitioners of preventive medicine, of megavitamin therapy, of holistic treatments, of nutritional healing were now largely accepting the appellation of "alternative" or "complementary" to define their practice (while the Europeans originally preferred "biological"). As this shift was occurring in a small but vocal group of allopaths, homeopathy began experiencing a renaissance in the United States which continues today, and naturopathy began battling (again) for sanction at every level.

Worldwide communication and cooperation played roles in helping the new paradigm along: the utility of acupuncture and acupressure in Eastern (particularly Chinese) medicine could not be hidden from Western view. But to accept its techniques without its corresponding philosophical bedrock (cosmic dualism, concepts of *yin* and *yang*, holism in man and nature) was a thorny problem, one still unresolved. Nor could the American public be denied the reality of the explosion of "alternative" treatments in Europe and the fact that the vast majority of Earth's population remained — and remains — in the hands of village-level lay practitioners, medicine men, *brujos* and *curanderos* as "primary-care physicians," most wielding herbs (as well as incantations and other attitude-altering gimmicks) in their medical practices, and among whose patients there are very low numbers of the "diseases of civilization."

And, of course, there were free thinkers (of the cut of the Canadian Shute brothers, who single-handedly did so much to advance the core concept of Vitamin E as a highly useful vitamin,[(9)] an idea that would take decades to be borne out; and of the late Roger Williams MD) within American and North American science who, running the risk of peer rejection and even legal jeopardy, brought new ideas to the fore. Popular writers (such as the late Adelle Davis, from whom "you are what you eat" became the faulty, if widely-coined, defining utterance) continually drummed in the twin realities that there are dietary connections to health and disease and that the American — indeed the "civilized" — food supply had been, was being, contaminated by many thousands of chemical compounds.

Siege of the soil

Increasingly, researchers turned to another aspect of the food problem: aside from chemical alteration and the American predilection for refined carbohydrates and animal proteins, there lurked the long-reported and also long-understated problem of nutrient depletion of soils. Oddly, veterinarians had known of this long before mainstream physicians did — and nutrient administration for animals presumed to be living off foods grown in nutrient-depleted soils was a common practice. Indeed, veterinarians had made the links between diet, health and disease in farm animals long before doctors arrived at any such conclusions about humans.

For instance, former American Naturopathic Medical Assn. (ANMA) President Joel Wallach, trained in veterinary medicine and agriculture as well as naturopathy, has strongly made the case that there is a dramatic link between the sudden deaths or cripplings of young American athletes and the runaway death rates of young people in Keshan Province, China. In a majority of cases, the deaths were attributed to cardiomyopathy — muscular dystrophy of the heart.[9]

It is known that the soil of Keshan Province is almost totally devoid of selenium — and it is increasingly apparent that much of the agriculture-producing soil of North America is also deficient in this mineral, leading to its presumed decrease in the standard diet. Researchers such as Dr. Wallach argue that simple administration of selenium as a supplement would not only save lives of young American athletes who otherwise drop dead on the basketball court but would be good for Americans overall, since the deficiency of this mineral has been associated in research to cancer, heart disease and immune problems all by itself.

Dr. Wallach has also noted how simple mineral deficiencies — recognized as such decades ago — led to metabolic disorders in farm animals which mimic or are symptomatically similar to those in humans (e.g., "stargazing rooster" syndrome correlates to human Alzheimer's), but that informed farmers and veterinarians moved to curb such deficiencies. It remained astonishing, for Dr. Wallach and others, why it took so long for human-oriented physicians to make the connection between mineral deficiencies and chronic disease.

(An avid reader of obituaries, the iconoclastic Dr. Wallach has also claimed that the longevity rates of AMA physicians are, on average, about 20 years below that of the population at large [a point some physicians are eager to dispute], and that "what's really scary" is that cardiologists — those who will train heart specialists and who have some presumed knowledge of heart health themselves — are among those physicians who often drop dead in early middle age while jogging or otherwise over-exerting themselves.[10])

Terror at the tap

It was known by the US government decades ago that there were serious mineral deficiencies in the nation's topsoil, but this information rarely received top billing in the media.

The topsoil deficiency problem is parallel to that of the overuse on crops grown in such soil of herbicides, pesticides, fungicides, insecticides and artificial fertilizers which in turn is directly linked to perhaps the most ominous single end-of-century environmental/nutritional problem: industrial pollution of the water supply.

All these elements — nutrient depletion from soils, cumulative chemicalization of agriculture (and farm animals), contamination of even subsurface water let alone of surface water into which tons of synthetic chemicals have been dumped, leached or which has migrated from farming areas — involve complicated interplays between corporate needs, governmental oversight, politics and social perceptions. Legislation passed in 1996 represented a modest effort at compromise.

The water problem — in the West in particular, the United States in general — became notorious in the 1980s. The enormity of surface runoff and underground seepage from chemically treated fields began to make it difficult to find any truly "healthy" water anywhere, including allegedly pristine mountain streams and underground wells far removed from urban centers.

In 1991, officials of the Soil Conservation Service, US Department of Agriculture, found "terrible groundwater problems" related to agricultural chemicals, and the Environmental Protection Agency (EPA) had categorized 46 different pesticides in drinking water as directly attributable to agricultural use.[12]

The private advocacy organization Environmental Working Group of Physicians for Social Responsibility released two shocking reports in 1994 and 1995 which signaled a long-delayed wakeup call for those concerned with the herbicide/pesticides problem:

In *Tap Water Blues,* a study the Working Group circulated in 1994, it was reported that 14 million Americans were drinking tap water "contaminated with cancer-causing herbicides" every year and that no small part of the problem was the fact that there were weaker standards for such contaminants in water than for those in food.(13)

A year later, the Environmental Working Group claimed that the number of Americans drinking herbicide-contaminated water had risen to between 20 to 25 million and that tap water in the Corn Belt was the most seriously laced with agricultural weed-killers.(14)

Adding a dangerous new global dimension to the problem, an Indiana University study within months of the Working Group report found, in an analysis of tree bark, that insecticides and fungicides had spread throughout the world, often thousands of miles from where they were used, and that some chemicals sprayed decades before were still affecting the environment.(15)

The Indiana research on tree bark from 90 sites, ranging from the tropics to the chilled latitudes, revealed that after decades there were still traces of chemicals related to DDT, lindane, chlordane, aldrin and 18 other pesticides and fungicides. Some traces occurred in such remote regions as the rain forests of South America.

Tap Water Blues, which was essentially funded by private foundations (though not the major ones we cite in *VI* as in lockstep with the Allopathic Industrial Complex), largely bore on the triazine family of compounds, with some 150 million pounds of these (atrazine, cyanazine, simazine, alachlor and metolachlor) reportedly applied every spring by farmers in the Corn Belt on corn and soybean fields.

Among those constantly consuming such compounds were, noted the report, "an estimated 65,000 infants [who] drink these herbicides from birth via infant formula reconstituted with herbicide-contaminated tap water."[16]

Tap Water Blues noted that atrazine, introduced in 1958 by drug giant Ciba-Geigy, had been banned in Germany, Italy, Sweden, Norway "and elsewhere" yet was still the most used agricultural pesticide in the USA, with between 70 and 75 million pounds applied each year.

The triazine herbicides, noted David Rall MD PhD, of PSR's Science and Environmental Health Policy Project, "have been linked with health problems ranging from developmental abnormalities, birth defects, genetic mutations, and reproductive and other cancers." He added that children may be more susceptible to harm from such toxins because "they drink more water per pound of body weight than adults, and they're still growing, which makes them particularly vulnerable to health risks posed by these toxic substances."

In 1996, in a report immediately attacked by the pesticide industry, the Environmental Protection Agency (EPA) claimed that the use of pesticides in the US reached all-time levels in 1994/1995 — to 1.2 billion pounds of active ingredients per year in both years, or an increase of more than 100 million pounds over 1993.

Expenditures for the same reached $10.4 billion in 1995, the same year farmers used more fungicides than ever before and more insecticides than in any previous year since 1981-82, the EPA added.[17]

The herbicide/pesticide/insecticide runoff problem in tap water is simply a huge added ingredient to the already demonstrated problems of fluoridation and chlorination. As we have reported in detail elsewhere[18] connections between industrial fluorides — as byproducts of the aluminum production industry added to water supplies — to immune dysregulation and higher rates of cancer are far too great to be ignored.

Gender-bender pollutants — a new threat

A chilling new scenario involving industrial chemicals

opened up in 1996 and immediately led to a controversy splitting science as well as pitting ecologists vs. industry:

Following up on earlier studies in preceding years that "sperm counts" were dropping in the Western population (data from British, French and Danish sources[19]), crusading zoologist Theo Colburn and other researchers published the startling book *Our Stolen Future*.[20]

This immediately-assailed[21] volume strongly argued that among unexpected results from the slew of chemicals found in pesticides, industrial pollutants and plastics have been wholesale hormonal disruptions in the endocrine systems of both man and beast, leading not only to lower sperm counts but to hormone-associated cancer and all manner of developmental, behavioral and other problems in humans and animals.

In some ways it was an update and replay of Rachel Carson's ancestral warnings about industrial chemicals in the 1960s in *Silent Spring* (DDT was eventually banned.)[22]

While research in the US was said not to have confirmed lower sperm counts, at least in American males,[23] *Our Stolen Future* created enough of a fuss that a putatively independent research panel of the National Research Council, part of the also putatively independent National Academy of Sciences, was gathered to examine the problem.

In its hastily issued report[24] the panel, somewhat sidestepping the issue, argued that there is more cancer-causing danger to Americans from eating foods with too many fats and calories than there is from pesticide residues and additives found in the food.

Pro-industry groups also issued rebuttals to the work of Colburn *et al.*, but she had made enough telling points to cause great concern.

The concern was enhanced months later when a Tulane University team found that pesticides which have been associated with breast cancer and male birth defects are up to one thousand times more potent when combined.[25]

The study — called into question a year later[25a] — by John

McLachlan *et al.* focused on endosulfan, dieldrin, toxaphene and chlordane, all of which are known to "turn on" a gene which manufactures the female estrogen in animals.

The flawed finding, said a US environmental official, might lead to a "revolution" in the way the environmental effects of chemicals are measured.[26]

This was additional fodder for many researchers who have long known that a raft of chemicals in the air, water and food supply can both mimic estrogen and block its opposite hormonal number, the masculine androgen hormones.

It also strengthened the notions of some that modern civilization is hermaphroditizing the human race (more effeminate males, more masculine women) faster than politics can establish equal political rights among the sexes.

Topsoil terror

While the debate over industrial chemicals and their effects on humans is usually dominated by the extremes — industrial nay-sayers on the one hand, arguing that there is far more benefit to the food supply than dangers to humans after decades of pesticides, artificial fertilizers, synthetic hormones and the like; ecological terrorists on the other hand, ready to destroy civilization in order to save it and to blame all calamities faced by the human race on industry while hoping that massive government controls can somehow save the day — there can be little doubt that man has altered both his external and internal ecology to an alarming degree.

As of 1991, an estimated 46 billion pounds of synthetic fertilizers and 840 million pounds of pesticides had been applied annually on American food crops (while the multi-billion-dollar agricultural market had made a brisk rebound from a slump in the 1980s). This was happening as some 440 species of insects had developed resistance to insecticides with at least 20 of these being ineradicable by *any* known pesticide.[27]

The Natural Resources Defense Council reported in 1994

that conventional pesticide use had grown from about 540 million pounds in 1964 to almost a billion pounds by 1991. However,

> *[W]hen wood preservatives, disinfectants and sulfur are included, the actual amount of pesticides applied in 1991 was 2.2 billion pounds, approximately eight pounds for every man, woman and child in the country.*[28]

Moreover, much of the burden of toxicity fell on farmers, farm workers and children, who were said to have received up to 35 percent of an average lifetime dose of certain allegedly carcinogenic pesticides by age five.[29]

Destroying the habitat

And there is an insidious new threat in the vanishing of natural seeds by civilization's onrushing destruction of the planetary habitat and their replacement by gene-altered hybrids the patents on which are in the hands of major components of the Allopathic Industrial Complex (AIC), pharmaceutical subdivision.

Seeds of Change noted in 1994 that

> *[T]he grave reality today is that plant extinctions are running at 1,000 times the natural rate: 27,000 species a year, 75 a day, 3 an hour. When only one plant species becomes extinct, so too will the 20 to 40 animal and insect species which rely on it.*[30]

While industrial defenders of the chemicalization of the food supply tend to downplay such potential ecological disasters by painting a brave new world of better living through chemistry — as, of course, mandated by some kind of super-international governmental/corporative combine which already is germinating — they at least should pay glancing attention to Harvard biologist E.O. Wilson, who wrote:

> *Biological diversity is responsible for the maintenance of the world as we know it. This is the assembly of life that took a billion years to evolve. It has eaten the storms, folded them into its genes, and*

created the world that created us. It holds the world steady.[31]

But such steadiness is now under undoubted threat by civilization — even if such threat should properly also be seen as an opportunity for civilization to work with, rather than against, nature.

On an ominous note, the United Nations' first comprehensive report on fading planetary biodiversity — the 1,140-page Global Biodiversity Assessment, reportedly the work of 1,500 scientists from around the world — was released in 1995.

It found that 10,000 species of plants and animals (out of an estimated 13 to 14 million — only about 1.75 million species having been formally identified) were currently threatened with extinction through mankind's continuing disruption of the planetary habitat, or balance between species, numbers, climate and sustenance.

The figure was far more conservative than warned about in some circles, but was a cause for alarm by the Global Environmental Facility of the UN Environmental Program, which found that "biodiversity represents the very foundation of human existence."[32]

Destruction of the planetary habitat is, however, only one of the major problems which threaten plant-based food as we know it — the international, corporative, transnational control over the ever-more-hybridized seed industry is the other.

Kevin Watkins, in a study by the Catholic Institute of International Relations (England), observing potential profits by transnationals from "intellectual property rights" accruing through patents on genetic mutations of seeds from crop materials selected and developed for ages by native farmers (who, one might think, should have first crack at any such profits), noted:

The main beneficiaries will be the core group of less than a dozen seed and pharmaceutical companies which control over 70 percent of the world seed trade.[33]

Seeds of Change observed that:

> *In the last 20 years, more than a thousand independent seed houses have been acquired by major chemical and pharmaceutical companies such as Monsanto, Lilly, Dow, ICI, and Royal Dutch Shell. These corporations — the major players in synthetic fertilizers, pesticides and agricultural chemicals — view the seed acquisitions as vertical integration, from the gene to the bank. Today in Europe, the corporations have instituted the Common Catalog, which restricts the marketability of seeds to those that are patented or registered. As a result, three quarters of traditional European folk varieties are under threat. Biology does not favor centralization, and this corporate vector of concentration may well end in vertical disintegration of incomprehensible proportions.*[34]

So there are stark warnings concerning the chemicalized future of the food supply.

But, happily, there are countermeasures already forming to at least broaden the dialogue. They range from the industrial production of hormone-less beef to the tidal wave of organic farming in general.

Between 1991 and 1994 the amount of US farmland devoted to producing organically raised crops doubled, and the number of organic farmers rose from 2,841 to 4,060 while profits for the same were reaching almost $3 billion annually.[84]

At least a little more attention is being paid to Sir Albert Howard, pioneer of "natural farming" earlier in the 20th century, one of the first voices raised against chemically-dependent farming methods. Such farming, he said, is

> *based on a complete misconception of plant nutrition. It is superficial and fundamentally unsound. It takes no account of the life of the soil . . . Artificial manures lead inevitably to artificial nutrition,*

artificial food, artificial animals and finally to artificial men and women.[35]

By some estimates, man's ancestors derived somewhere between a fourth to a third of their nutritional minerals from the water they drank. Modern research has found that populations which consume water rich in magnesium and calcium — minerals often lacking or severely depleted in modern man's polluted and/or tampered-with supply — have lower rates of cardiovascular disease, heart attack and high blood pressure.[36]

While industrial propagandists and "quackbusters" routinely sneer at the notion of "organically" grown (that is, naturally cultivated *without* synthetic chemicals) fruits and vegetables as being somehow healthier than the chemically-altered varieties, considerable observation over time, as well as competent research such as that at the Universities of Maine and Vermont, has demonstrated the superiority of the organics. The latter research showed higher levels of beta-carotene, Vitamin C, magnesium and calcium in organically grown vegetables.[37]

Western civilization is hence increasingly confronted by interlocked problems involving food production methods: a considerable amount of water has been polluted as an offshoot of such methods, leading to decreased minerals; this depletion could be compensated for by nutrients in fruits and vegetables but they, too, are deficient due to commercial cultivation methods.

These are problems apart from the dangers to the water supply from fluoridation and chlorination and from the over-chemicalization through food processing of fruits, vegetables, fibers, grains and meats for storage, transportation and marketing.

(And they are apart from the growing controversy over "genetically-engineered" foods, concern over the long-term use of which has led to demands that such products be properly labelled.)

The connections, thus, between dietary/nutritional/food elements (deficiencies, excesses, chemicalization) and health problems have accumulated over the years.

It is scandalously clear that the US government knew early

in the 1970s about such connections — and chose to cover them up.

Uncovering a coverup

As mentioned earlier, it was not until 1993, and thanks primarily to Citizens for Health, that it could be reported that a long-suppressed US government report had found — in 1971 — that the nation's major health problems were related to diet, that the solution to illness may often be found in nutrition, and that dietary improvement may defer or modify the course of many diseases.

The document, a US Department of Agriculture publication called *Human Nutrition Report No. 2, Benefits from Human Nutrition Research*, was a referenced, 129-page report, ostensibly suppressed by then Secretary of Agriculture Earl Butz at the behest of the food-processing industry.

Said CfH's executive director, Alexander Schauss, after the organization reprinted the "one copy which mysteriously missed confiscation and recently surfaced":

> *The government has known for 21 years that such illnesses as heart disease, many types of cancers, and other serious degenerative diseases can be prevented by diet . . . It is inexcusable that they have kept this information from the public all these years.*
>
> *Had this information been made available in 1971 we would have been ten years ahead of where we are today in our knowledge of the role nutrition [plays] in the prevention and treatment of disease. The loss of lives and suffering of two generations of citizens denied this information should go down in history as one of the greatest tragedies of modern medicine . . .*[38]

Because the government destroyed copies of the 1971 document, it was not until the 1977 *Senate Select Committee on Nutrition and Human Needs, Diet Related to Killer Diseases* report that the public was made aware of the amount of supportive evidence of a role for diet in the prevention of disease.

Yet due to the destruction of the 1971 report, even the 1977 Senate committee was unaware of the wealth of evidence available from our own government agencies.

By then, more researchers were drawing links between excess chemicalized processed foods, excess animal fats and proteins, the enormous consumption of refined sugar in the USA and the Western world, and the ever-more-noticeable deficiencies in essential nutrients, ranging from Vitamin C to magnesium, selenium and other minerals.

A carbohydrate calamity

A former co-author of mine, the late Harold W. Harper MD, probably did as much as anyone to rivet national attention on the refined sugar problem, arguing that the excess of refined sugars and starches (carbohydrates) in the civilized Western diet was, above and beyond all other problems with the food supply, the fundamental basis — as the cause of glucose metabolism dysfunction (GMD) — of much chronic, metabolic disease.[(39)]

His arguments, echoed by other researchers and current investigators[(40,41,42,43,86)], were that refined carbohydrates, particularly refined sucrose, act as "metabolic thieves" in depleting the body's store of B vitamins and other nutrients. GMD led ineluctably to hypoglycemia, a condition possibly affecting a majority of Americans, and over time hypoglycemia could lead to diabetes; in turn, the connections between diabetes and cancer were strengthened year by year. GMD's contribution to atherosclerosis was an early counter to the rapidly growing "cholesterol theory of heart disease" (*X*) and was frequently overlooked in the industrial race to develop ostensibly cholesterol-lowering drugs and cholesterol-lowering foods. If the proponents of GMD as a "substrate" for chronic, metabolic diseases are anywhere near the mark, "heart disease" is far more apt to be due to too many refined carbohydrates than simply to fatty and meat-oriented diets.

Indeed, the problem of excess carbohydrates in general is increasingly being seen as *the* primary culprit in the Western food disaster and — as we shall shortly see — may be connected with oxidative processes as "the anvil and the hammer" in the onset of much disease (*XVI*).

The American obsession over weight loss has been among the factors which stimulated a number of researchers to reassess the carbohydrate problem. Losing weight while stimulating good health is the root of such low-carbohydrate (but high-protein) diets as that advocated by Robert Atkins of New York, whose approach has turned in long-term victories over chronic disease.[44,45]

Correct carbohydrate intake (as a stimulant for the hormone insulin, correct levels of which are described by the researcher as a key to good health and longevity), a proper protein-to-carbohydrate ratio and a balance between essential fatty acids leading to production of so-called "super-hormone" eicosanoids, is the root of the dietary theory proposed in *Enter The Zone*, Dr. Barry Sears' bestseller of the 1990s.[46]

That the Western diet is rampant with too many carbohydrates in general and far too many refined ones in particular has now become virtually accepted. But for many dietary researchers awareness of the refined carbohydrate problem was just the beginning:

Western scientists looked ever more closely at non-Western eating habits to find clues between chronic metabolic disorders and food, endeavors which could only be viewed as threatening to significant sectors of the food-processing industry, the chemical industry, and, ultimately, to the pharmaceutical industry. This was because of industrial group-think which rightly perceived the chain of thought: if dietary elements were central to chronic diseases, if chemicalization of the food supply were a considerable portion of the problem of chronic diseases, and if the management (rather than the prevention of) chronic diseases were the central concern of the pharmaceutical cartel, then too much probing into worldwide eating habits represented a thinly veiled economic menace.

But clues loomed everywhere:

The Los Angeles Basin might be among the most atmospherically polluted areas in North America, yet one group of residents there, not definable by race or sex, was consistently reporting lower rates of cancer, heart disease and metabolic disorders in general. Exposed to the same polluted air and water, the Seventh-Day Adventists were (are) simply healthier overall. This is not due to genes but to habits: professed SDAs are essentially vegetarians and eschew nicotine and alcohol. A similar case has been made over time for Utah's Mormons (confirmed again in 1997), but the analogy is less precise because Utah is generally healthier than the LA metropolitan complex to begin with.[(47)]

The early results of a huge collaborative study between Cornell University and mainland China on the relationship between diet and disease risk in 1990 provided more solid information. Summarized the New York Times News Service: the initial 920 pages of data, "the Grand Prix of epidemiology," in fact "paints a bold portrait of a plant-based eating plan that is more likely to promote health than disease."[(48)]

There had been many other clues, particularly in the connections between diet, cancer and longevity, with laetrile proponents (including ourselves) noting how little cancer existed in populations (Vilcabamba Indians of Ecuador, Hunzakuts of Pakistan, Arctic Circle Eskimos of an earlier era, southern and non-urban Filipinos, Abkhasians of the former Soviet Union, and others) who consumed diets very high in plants, grains, fibers, vegetables (and natural laetriles). (*See XII*)

A US Navy study of American pilots shot down and captured during the Vietnam War who underwent years of dietary privation as contrasted with pilots who were not captured and whose health/disease components were studied years later made it dramatically obvious that the mostly-meatless, essentially vegetarian, minimal-portion subsistence diet of captivity was strongly related to less chronic disease later — assuming the pilots survived at all.[49]

In 1994, Knight-Ridder News Service reported on "some of the bleakest health statistics compiled in the Western world" — those of Scotland, already known to have the highest concentration of cancer spread across its population.

In a two-year study by the Scottish government, a panel of experts found that Scots have the highest mortality rate from coronary heart disease in the world, are more likely to die before age 69 than the citizens of any other Western nation — and that 20 percent of men, 13 percent of women and nearly 20 percent of children never eat vegetables and that the sale of fruit and vegetables actually fell in the country from 1990 to 1992.

The Scottish diet has long been extremely high in fats and animal proteins but almost entirely devoid of fruits and vegetables, the latter — if apparent at all — more apt to be utilized as decorations than foods.

Part of the problem is political and economic — new Scottish eating habits took root after the disruptive era of World War II, when Britain evolved a mass food distribution system and stores became dependent on processed and packaged foods from England while local vegetable farmers were given incentives to switch to meat and dairy foods.

Even in the 1990s, reported Knight-Ridder, Scots who still were growing produce were compelled by the European Union to destroy crops to keep prices down.[50]

Indeed, the general overview from many angles of research is decisive:

Populations which consume more unrefined grains, more fruits and vegetables in as natural a state as possible, and which consume fewer or no refined carbohydrates, stimulants and drugs and less animal fat and animal protein, and by sheer dint of poverty eat smaller portions, in general have far less chronic metabolic disease than do those of the more "civilized" world, whatever other pathological problems they may have.

McGee, also citing Price, Cleave and others,[51,52,53] has pointed out how the introduction of modern refined foods (refined carbohydrate products so often leading the pack) was followed by the development of chronic, degenerative diseases — an outcome which occurred *regardless* of the fat content of native diets, other lifestyle variables, and even prior genetic dispositions.

Problem one: the food business

While this reality has been obvious, thus, to hundreds of researchers for decades, the answer to why Western populations, particularly Americans, have for so long been unaware that what we might call the primitive, poor people's diet correlates with an essential absence of major chronic metabolic diseases is to be found in politics and economics — and naturally leads the unwary straight into the vested interests of the enormous food-processing industry, quite aside from the Allopathic Industrial Complex (AIC).

For years, America's views as to what constitutes "proper diet" (and the vaunted, if changing, "food groups"), let alone the government's various efforts in establishing "recommended daily allowances" (RDAs) of nutrient supplements, have been dominated by the food-processing industry and, to a lesser extent, the drug industry.

As early as 1983, in a survey of the above problems I reported[54] that the medical/pharmaceutical/nutritional establishment — even in the face of growing evidence to the contrary at that time — continued to tell Americans we were the best-fed people on earth and that there was no need for vitamin and mineral supplementation as long as we ate a "balanced diet."

There might be some substance in this claim if the components of such a diet in themselves were either balanced or natural. But this is hardly the case. Even if an American of adequate economic means consumes the presumed proper amounts of leafy greens, fruits and vegetables and their juices, meat, eggs, and carbohydrates, he is absorbing foods the great majority of which have been tampered with in some way. This would include the thousands of chemicals (estimates range from 1,500 to 10,000) with which foods have been prepared, stored, treated, preserved, colored, buffered, and so forth.

A century ago, Americans were consuming wheat with a protein count of up to 20 percent, untampered-with meat and organically grown fruits and vegetables. The balancing of that diet was in fact something worth defending. But even by 1983, American bread was 9 to 12 percent protein, meats were often artificially colored and came essentially from artificially fattened and hormone-and-antibiotic-laden cattle, hogs, and poultry, and rare indeed was the table set with natural fruits and vegetables.

Americans were already brainwashed by the US Department of Agriculture and the FDA into believing that the MDRs (minimum daily requirements) and RDAs on nutrients were sufficient. I pointed out in 1983 the lack of logic: surely the allowable amounts of certain nutrients vary greatly between a Swedish longshoreman, an African pygmy, a ninety-pound octogenarian retiree and a 19-year-old fullback. Indeed, such recommended amounts had been based by the official Food and Nutrition Board on what it called the "reference man and woman," described as being of "normal" height and weight, living in a temperate zone, and being 22 years old!

It was Senator William Proxmire who did most to take on the notion of the RDAs and the food industry's influence on government, as he warned that

> *[A]t best the RDAs are only a "recommended" allowance at antediluvian levels designed to prevent terrible disease. At worst, they are based on conflicts of interest and self-serving views of certain parts of the industry . . .*
>
> *The* [Food and Nutrition Board of the National Research Council] *is both the creature of the food industry and heavily influenced by the food industry.*
>
> *. . . The RDA standard is established by the Food*

and Nutrition Board of the National Research Council, which is influenced, dominated and financed in part by the food industry. It represents one of the most scandalous conflicts of interest in the Federal Government.[55]

It should be realized he made these remarks in Congressional testimony in 1976. Even then, of course, total profit-taking from the totality of industries and companies comprising the food industry constituted the number-one stock investment in America, with the drug companies in number-two position. (By 1993, the total food industry was estimated at about $280 billion per year.[56])

I reported in 1983 that at the time

> *Most loyal AMA physicians and dedicated readers of the* Journal of the American Medical Association *will readily admit they know little about nutrition and had no more than one or two hours of nutrition in their medical school courses.*
>
> *When they need information about nutrition, they turn to the few "A-Okay-" stamped nutritionists who are supposed to be worthy of the name, including — sometimes first and foremost — those of the Department of Nutrition at the Harvard University School of Public Health. Yet this school has accepted millions of dollars in grants from such food giants as General Foods, Kellogg, Nabisco, the Sugar Association and the International Sugar Foundation. One of the school's foremost professors of nutrition has been a consultant to the sugar and drug industries as well as a member of the Continental Can Company board of directors. It is an honest exercise to speculate about how fair and objective food science instructors can be when linked one way or another to the food industry.*[57]

As early as 1976, Congressman Benjamin S. Rosenthal brought part of the problem to light as he and a consumer group claimed that some of America's eminent nutritionists had traded independence for industry favors and that some of the nutritionists who were making public analyses of consumer products were on the boards of, or otherwise had ties to, major food companies.[58]

Rep. Rosenthal found that the Harvard Department of Nutrition had received $2 million in donations from the food industry between 1971 and 1974, some of them coming from Amstar, Beatrice Foods, Coca-Cola, Kellogg, Gerber, and Oscar Mayer. Harvard vehemently denied, of course, that much contributions in any way influenced research.

Things have changed only slightly since then, although more physicians receive slightly more education in nutrition than before.

In the meantime, parallel to the organized "quackbuster" attack on nutritional therapy, metabolic treatments, holistic medicine, etc., a coordinated campaign has developed over several years around the co-opting of the term "dietitian" — only individuals said to be board-certified or otherwise sanctioned are to be allowed even to *discuss* nutrition and health with the public. This AIC state-by-state tactic, which ran into increased opposition by the 1990s, was a way, among other things, to stop proprietors and employees of healthfood stores and/or other informed laymen from even making nutritional supplement suggestions to consumers.

Yet the past decades have only served to shore up the connections between diet and health, nutrition and disease. They constitute belated conceptual victories for such progressive thinkers as the National Cancer Institute's Dr. Gio B. Gori, who ran into severe institutional opposition after he testified in 1976 that:

> *Until recently, many eyebrows would have been raised by suggesting that an imbalance of normal dietary components could lead to cancer and cardiovascular disease. Today, the accumulation of epidemiologic and laboratory evidence in man and animals makes this notion not only possible but*

certain.[59]

But at that time, as even in its earliest days, the industry-dominated NCI was not ready to shift much interest into the food-cancer connection. Perhaps that was because it had its propaganda hands full at the time staving off the Laetrile Revolution, which was making precisely such a connection.

Making the dietary connection

The relentless rise in cancer incidence and mortality, suddenly accompanied by exponential increases in AIDS — almost a quarter of which is, by definition, cancer — has caused many researchers to look elsewhere for answers, very much including dietary/nutritional links.

As the AIDS crisis grew, more research funds were dumped into studies of immunology during the plague's first decade than in all prior years combined. Areas of research tying nutritional factors to immune depression, about which we have gone into some detail in other publications,[60,61] included these:

• Deficiencies in zinc leading to PEM, or protein-energy malnutrition, an immune system-altering condition well-known in the impoverished Third World but unexpectedly cropping up in the "civilized" Western world as well.

• The introduction of "plastic fats" into the American diet, primarily through margarine, refined vegetable oils and many products developed thereafter. The alteration of essential fatty acids (EFAs) by a food processing technique called hydrogenation caused the addition of abnormal EFA variants or *isomers* to the food chain. Scattered but growing research has implicated deficient or altered EFAs in the imbalance of the hormone-like substances called prostaglandins, at least one variety of which is strongly implicated in immune function.

(While some maverick medics and researchers had warned about the addition of industrially produced *trans* fats into margarine and certain vegetable oils decades before they were, as usual, ignored by the AIC.

(Yet, in 1994, in what The Associated Press called a "startling new report," Harvard University nutritionists found that diets high in margarine and similar foods could double the risk of heart attack and lead to as many as 30,000 of the nation's annual heart disease deaths.[62]

(At the root of the controversy is — as metabolic doctors had argued for decades, usually preaching only to the choir — the hydrogenation process for the solidifying of liquid oils. Hydrogenated or partially hydrogenated vegetable oils are used to make margarine, shortening and a wide range of cookies, crackers, chips and other processed foods — i.e., elements abounding in "civilization" while mostly unknown among primitive peoples.)

• Vitamin C deficiency. While the late two-time Nobel Laureate Linus Pauling PhD did yeoman research in elevating ascorbic acid to a prominent role against the common cold, cancer and disease in general, important research had gone on earlier by Vitamin C's delineator, Albert Szent-Gyorgyi, and the indefatigable Irwin Stone. The latter argued that man's inability to produce his own ascorbate, when accompanied by a lack of sufficient Vitamin C from the food chain, produced a state of "chronic, subclinical scurvy" which underlay much of disease. Early efforts using Vitamin C against AIDS produced considerable reduction in symptoms and seemed to correlate with longer survivals of AIDS patients.

Pauling, who died in 1994, and Hamburg cardiovascular specialist Matthias Rath MD added greatly to knowledge of how Vitamin C helps in overall heart/circulatory health and how Vitamins C and E, together with the amino acids proline and lysine, help prevent or reverse atherosclerosis. Rath has pointed out how a broad range of nutrients can successfully treat heart conditions in general[63] [*X*].

By 1992, a compilation of major research from around the world proved[64] once and for all that nutritional aspects (deficiencies and excesses) are strongly linked to the body's innate defense system, so that immunological disturbance could have as much to do with these factors as anything else. But there was also the very understated problem of nutritional deficiencies induced by standard allopathic (that is, drug-based) medicine — medications and drugs of all kinds given for reasons of all kinds could, whatever else they might be doing of a therapeutic nature, cause wholesale deficiencies of all manner of nutrients, a situation which could worsen an organism which was already nutrient-depleted due to the nature of (and the alterations in) the food being consumed daily (*immunotoxicology*).[(65)]

Perhaps the biggest boost of all for nutrients has come as part and parcel of the breakthrough concept of *oxidology* in health and disease (*see XVI*), which has added a whole new dimension to medicine.

That many long-used nutrients are in fact "scavengers" of toxic oxygen breakdown products — or *antioxidants* — and that such substances play central roles in health and disease is a bridgehead reality joining the so-called "orthodox" and "unorthodox" medical camps in the developing new health paradigm.

State-of-the-art research has also suggested correlations between foods, health and blood types, which point to long-term patterns of inheritance among population groups. Blood-type correlations may provide part of the answer as to why there is no single one-diet-fits-all for good health.[(90)]

The Club co-opts

It is instructive to note that even as both public and private research exploded in the 1980s and 1990s tracing the connections between dietary factors and nutrients to health and disease, the hard core of the AIC had a significant problem in how to integrate the rapidly onrushing new information with the established medical model and the pharmaceutical hydra which suckled it.

For, as Dean Burk PhD had observed in the matter of laetrile, once a chink in the armor of orthodoxy had appeared, it would widen: the aphorism that "that which prevents, also cures" would not be lost on rank-and-file physicians facing a tidal wave of chronic, systemic, metabolic dysfunctions and immune challenges for which the allopathic armamentarium offered little in the way of cures. The specter of *disease prevention* through nutritional changes (and lifestyle alterations) loomed, and with it the implied threat to the need for a gigantic AIC and the international drug cartel which nourished and sustained it. How work the new knowledge into the old system?

The AIC turned to co-optation and semantical manipulation, its long-time *modus operandi* in dealing with inexorable forces.

Bowing to the growing evidence that nutritional supplements and nutrients themselves might indeed play a role in thwarting disease, yet not wanting to turn loose of the medical lexicon which protected old ideas, the AIC or Club concocted the word "chemoprevention" — as hilarious a co-optation as we have seen in decades of doctor-watching. "Chemo" retains the *chemical* nature of medicine (as in toxic *chemo*therapy, a rapidly failing cancer therapeutic approach) but adds on "prevention" — so that the subliminal phrase "chemicals used to prevent" might flourish in the psyche.[(66)]

As we noted, the drug industry, whose $65-$100 billion gravy train (as of 1994) was substantially threatened by the surging industry in food supplements ($14 billion by 1997), swiftly sought to accommodate unwanted new information while grabbing a share of a swiftly developing pie — so that major drug companies, by the late 1980s, increased their line of vitamin/mineral supplements, basing the same on random establishment research on animals which seemed to "suggest" that such supplements could, for example, positively impact on immunity.

This was, of course, rank heresy to the allopathic thinking of recent decades, but did underscore the genius of the marketplace: despite "quackbuster" attacks on vitamin pills, the people were going to have their pills, so why should the drug giants be left off the bandwagon even while running a distant risk that adequate supplementation might ultimately hinder the need for many, if not most, of the expensive medications in which the pharmaceutical market was awash?

The research establishment, still allopathic in tone, almost always accompanied every new disclosure of a nutrient being found successful against a disease or a condition with a "cautionary note," usually from an appropriately allopathic medical school researcher at a major university or within the federal research community, warning against "pill-popping" or simply taking supplements on a routine basis.

The pill-popping medics

But by the early 1990s, even this ploy was beginning to fail — many doctors, some of them originally anti-vitamin, were gobbling vitamin pills and admitting it.

Even by 1990, a survey showed[(67)] that an amazing 87 percent of family practitioners were recommending or prescribing vitamin and mineral supplements to some 25 percent of their patients, and that 28 percent of the medics were taking the food supplements themselves. And, as a "quackbuster" journal reported,[(68)] citing the American Dietetic Association, of a group of cancer patients studied, 92 percent of the women and 63 percent of the men admitted that, whatever other therapy they were on, they were taking vitamin supplements.

In 1993, the *Wall Street Journal* quoted an octogenarian nutrition expert and professor emeritus of the University of St. Louis School of Medicine, who was said to regularly rail about "the over-feeding of vitamins" to Americans but who was taking Vitamin E himself: "I'm ashamed to do it because of my attitude toward taking vitamins," he said, as he honestly admitted the explosion of studies on the vitamin's positive effects could no longer be overlooked.[(69)]

Two major studies in the *New England Journal of Medicine (NEJM)* in May 1993 made the case for a significant reduction in the risk of coronary heart disease with Vitamin E (Shute brothers vindicated at long last), yet the reports were coupled with the usual admonition that the general public should not start dosing themselves with Vitamin E pills.[70] Angry doctors balked.

Wrote Dr. James O'Keefe, Kansas City MO:

> *A substantial number of physicians . . . are sufficiently convinced of the potential benefits and nontoxic nature of Vitamin E to supplement their own diets with it. If Vitamin E is good enough for doctors, should it not be good enough for our patients?*[71]

In 1993 *USA Today* reported galloping increases in profits from the sales of Vitamins E, C and beta-carotene — antioxidants all and the subjects of intense public/private investigation — and it noted that Dr. Walter Willett, Harvard School of Public Health, was taking one multivitamin tablet and one Vitamin E capsule a day, while relying on food for Vitamin C and beta-carotene.

It quoted antioxidant expert Jeffrey Blumberg of Tufts:

> *"We're at an admittedly frustrating stage, where I think one well-informed, rational person would decide to take a supplement, and the other could decide not to."*[72]

This was a hedging-of-all-bets assessment made in the midst of the continuing outpouring of new information, and certainly an honest viewpoint.

A 1997 assessment was that in 1996 the US public swallowed more than *10 billion* multivitamin tablets at a cost of $700 million — walkaround change compared to drug industry profits.[85]

Cancer Inc. does an about-face

By 1992, in what was the biggest shift of its gears in a decade or more, the American Cancer Society (ACS), for prior decades an impassioned foe of the notion that diet had much to do, if anything, with cancer, announced the start of a mammoth survey of middle-aged American dietary habits. It was launched just as the governmental National Cancer Institute (NCI) released the aforementioned results of *156* studies which linked cancer with diet — a sweeping review which forever ended any debate about whether nutritional factors have at least a role in the malignant process[73] [*XI*].

Virtually all the 156 studies confirmed the connection between eating more fruits and vegetables and lower cancer rates.

Peter Greenwald, chief of the NCI's cancer prevention and control branch, said the findings constituted part of the basis for the agency's recent recommendation that everyone eat five servings a day of fruits or vegetables.[74]

The survey was "so compelling," said analysts, that it meant that even cigarette smokers who also ate large amounts of fruits and vegetables derived major anti-lung cancer benefits.

The same year, the largest and most detailed study ever carried out to measure the effects of Vitamin C and death rates concluded[75] that the vitamin helps both sexes live longer — but only if taken in amounts far above those recommended by the federal government.

Among findings, reported Dr. James E. Enstrom:

Men whose Vitamin C intake was the highest — the equivalent of two oranges plus a 150-milligram Vitamin C tablet per day — had a 42 percent lower risk of death from heart disease and a 35 percent lower risk of death from any cause than the population of white men as a whole.

In continuing mixed-results research in 1993, a *New England Journal of Medicine (NEJM)* study of 89,494 nurses tracked over a nine-year period beginning in 1980 showed[76] that the consumption of foods rich in Vitamin A (particularly spinach and carrots) seemed to reduce the risk of breast cancer.

It was only one of many studies trying to get to grips with a pandemic which even by that year was killing 46,000 women per year and affecting 1 out of 9. Scattered research was indicating connections between breast cancer and a high-fat diet — though it should be noted that in the "unitarian" theory of cancer (it is a single disease) connections between excess fats and excess animal proteins in *general* seem to correlate with cancer as a whole.

Victory for the concept that the better-known vitamins and

minerals might after all be truly connected with health and disease opened the door to the examination of many other food factors (as indoles, flavones, and phenols in cancer) and, much to the consternation of the "quackbuster" elite, to a reexamination of the role of herbs and their components.

The dam bursts

What was largely the province of folk medicine and alleged unabashed quackery in North America increasingly came under scientifically acceptable scrutiny: useful ingredients were found in garlic and chaparral, among many others, which vindicated the empiricism of the use of these herbs over centuries. The rediscovery by the West of ancient Chinese herbalism, and the plodding efforts of America's embattled naturopaths, brought to the fore some "scientifically" acceptable rationales for everything from spirulina, blue-green algae and wheat grass to aloe vera, herbal teas of all kinds, and such folkloric herbal war-horses as echinacea and goldenseal.

As late as 1985, after all, the World Health Organization (WHO) had estimated that 80 percent of the world's population (4 billion) used herbal medicine for some aspect of "primary health care."[77]

By the mid-1990s, research with and interest in herbs and their multitudinous compounds — called both "non-nutritive food factors" and "phytochemicals" — was growing as fast as the concepts of oxidology and multivitamin therapy. A dam had burst whose floodwaters would not be stanched by the AIC, whose major concern going into the end of the century is how to co-opt the research and provide synthetic look-alikes of natural products in order to enhance profits. Mimicry is, after all, the highest form of flattery.

By 1994, mass-market sales of medicinal herbs in US drugstores and supermarkets grew by 35 percent, worth some $106.7 million in sales, garlic and ginseng topping the list. Worldwide sales were estimated at $12.4 billion.[78]

And, as of 1995, total US sales of "natural products" increased by a whopping 22.6% — to more than $9 billion. The herbal component of this in the USA had jumped to $560 million.[79]

The US herb market itself grew 300% between 1992 and 1995[80]. US retail sales of homeopathic medicines increased 25% in 1994 over 1993 — to $165 million.[81]

As the plague of AIDS reached terrifying dimensions in the 1990s, and as other immunological disturbances became apparent, it was part of the standard allopathic "line" that while a healthy immune system was the best defense against such modern killers and cripplers, there was no known way to "enhance" immunity other than through the mixed results and often dangerous administration of synthetic interferons and interleukins.

Yet "metabolic" or "holistic" medical practitioners had long argued that overall host defense — including all aspects of what is meant by the misleading general term "immune system" — could indeed be increased or modulated through nutrition and dietary supplements, however "quackish" such an idea seemed to the AIC.

And, as we have seen, as late as 1988 even the *Harvard Medical School Health Letter* was deriding the claim that nutritional factors could bolster immunity as "simply not supportable" and that

> *[T]he use of herbs or nutrition to stimulate or strengthen the immune system is a nonsense claim . . . and to the extent that people wind up believing such claims, we can say that their brains are damaged.*[82]

This typically arrogant AIC point of view came acropper in 1992, though, when *The Lancet* reported research by Dr. Rajit K. Chandra, School of Hygiene and Public Health, Johns Hopkins, on the "effect of vitamin and trace-element supplementation on immune response and infection in elderly subjects."

In this study, it became obvious that even "modest" vitamin and trace-element supplementation positively affected the "immune systems" of the elderly and that the herb ginkgo biloba (extract from the leaf of the maidenhair tree) positively helped in cases of "mild to moderate symptoms of cerebral insufficiency."

Results were said to be "impressive" in immune enhancement even with admittedly "modest" doses of Vitamin A, beta-carotene, thiamine, riboflavin, niacin, Vitamins B6 and B12, Vitamin C, Vitamin D, iron, zinc, copper, selenium, iodine, calcium and magnesium.

Conclusion: "Supplementation with a modest physiological amount of micronutrients improves immunity and decreases the risk of infection in old age."[(83)] Followup research in 1997 confirmed the 1992 conclusions and added a strong immune-boosting role for Vitamin E.

By that time, of course, thousands of AIDS and pre-AIDS patients, often supported in their efforts by well-meaning, if incredulous, MDs, were finding that supplementation with a huge array of vitamins, minerals, enzymes, amino acids, herbs and other substances conclusively or suggestively linked to "non-specific immune enhancement" were seeing immune system improvements and life extension.

While attention was now given to many other factors of civilization and how they might be aiding or abetting the end-of-century plagues of cancer, AIDS and immune dysregulation (*see XI, XIII, XIV*), the killer diseases, by emphasizing the reality of dietary connections to health and disease, had helped correct medicine's major error, abandonment of the holistic concept.

More than any other maladies, cancer and AIDS — examples of near to total disaster on the part of the AIC — have provoked new thought and a paradigm shift to the holistic concept. And within this framework, eating habits and dietary elements play the primary *physical* roles.

And these may be *lesser* roles (*see XVII*).

The popular revolt against orthodoxy and pressure for paradigm shift *within* orthodoxy also point to a probable fail-safe mechanism within the human makeup: since survival of the species is the first and primary genetic mandate of its existence, the species will creatively find ways to survive despite the challenges before it — and despite the entrenched bureaucracies and economic/ego vested interests which are in the way.

References

1. Statement of Council on Pharmacy and Chemistry, *J. Am. Med. Assn.*, Jan. 8, 1949.
2. Block, Gladys, *et al.*, "Fruit, vegetables and cancer prevention: a review of the epidemiological evidence." *Nutrition and Cancer 18*, 1992.
3. *Human Nutrition, Report No. 2, Benefits from Human Nutrition Research.* Washington DC: US Dept. of Agriculture, 1971. And *The Choice* XIX: 1, 1993.
4. *J. Natl. Can. Inst.*, September 1993.
5. *The Choice*, XX: 1, 1994.
6. "Supplements of the future." *The Choice*, XXII: 1, 1996.
7. "There's something fishy here." *The Choice*, XXII: 1, 1996.
8. *The Choice*, II: 1, 1976.
9. Shute, WE, *Wilfrid Shute's Complete Updated Vitamin E Book.* New Canaan CT: Keats, 1975.
10. Wallach, JD, "The NBA: an endangered species?" Private publication; also printed in *The Choice*, XIX: 3-4, 1993.
11. Wallach, JD, address to annual convention, American Naturopathic Medical Assn. (ANMA), Albuquerque NM, 1993.
12. "Hard facts about chemically dependent farming." *Health Foods Business,* July 1991.
13. Wiles, Richard, *et al.*, *Tap Water Blues: Herbicides in Drinking Water.* Washington DC: Environmental Working Group/Physicians for Social Responsibility, 1994.
14. *The Choice*, XXII: 1, 1996.
15. Wites, RA, and SL Simonich, *Science*, November 1995.
16. Wiles, *op. cit.*
17. "Use of pesticides in US on rise, EPA claims." *The Washington Post,* May 29, 1996.
18. Culbert, ML, *AIDS: Hope, Hoax and Hoopla.* Chula Vista CA: The Bradford Foundation, 1990.
19. Lemonick, MD, "What's wrong with our sperm?" *Time*, March 18, 1996.
20. Colburn, Theo, *et al.*, *Our Stolen Future.* New York: Dutton, Penguin, 1996.
21. Bailey, Ronald, "Hormones and humbug." *The Washington Post.* March 31, 1996.
22. Carson, Rachel, *Silent Spring.* Boston: Houghton Mifflin, 1962.
23. Waldholz, Michael, *The Wall Street Journal,* March 10, 1996.
24. *Carcinogens and Anticarcinogens in the Human Diet.* Washington DC: National Research Council, National Academy of Sciences, February 1996.
25. McLachlan, John, *et al.*, *Science*, June 7, 1996.

25a. "Tulane yanks study on pesticides and some cancer." *USA Today*, Aug. 25, 1997.

26. Recer, Paul, The Associated Press, June 7, 1996.
27. "Hard facts . . ." *op. cit.*
28. "After Silent Spring," Natural Resources Defense Council, June 1993.
29. Goldin, Greg, "Cancerous Growth." *LA Weekly*, May 6, 1994.
30. "The theft of the ark." *Seeds of Change* Catalogue, 1994.
31. *Ibid.*
32. Associated Press, Nov. 14, 1995.
33. "The theft of the ark," *loc. sit.*
34. *Ibid.*

35. "Hard facts . . ." *op. cit.*
36. Kesteloot, Hugo, in *J. Cardiol. and Pharm.* 6, 1984.
37. *J. Food Quality* 9: 1987.
38. *The Choice*, XIX:1, 1993.
39. Harper, H, and M Culbert, *How You Can Beat the Killer Diseases*. New Rochelle NY: Arlington House, 1977.
40. Brennan, RO, *Nutrigenetics*. New York: M. Evans, 1975.
41. McGee, CT, *Heart Frauds*. Coeur d'Alene ID: MediPress, 1993.
42. Fredericks, Carlton, *Low Blood Sugar and You*. New York: Constellation International, 1974.
43. Yudkin, John, *Sweet and Dangerous*. New York: Bantam, 1972.
44. Atkins, Robert, *Dr. Atkins' Health Revolution*. Boston: Houghton Mifflin, 1988.
45. Atkins, Robert, at Eighth International Symposium (American Biologics), Mallorca, Spain, June 28-30, 1996.
46. Sears, Barry, *Enter The Zone*. New York: HarperCollins, 1995.
47. Culbert, ML, *What the Medical Establishment Won't Tell You that Could Save Your Life*. Norfolk VA: Donning, 1983.
48. Cited in *The Choice*, XVI:2,3, 1990.
49. Culbert, *What the, op. cit.*
50. Palma, Dick, Knight-Ridder News Service, June 18, 1994.
51. McGee, *op. cit.*
52. Price, Weston, *Nutrition and Physical Degeneration*. Santa Monica CA: Price Pottenger Foundation, 1945.
53. Cleave, TL, *The Saccharine Disease*. New Canaan CT: Keats, 1974.
54. Culbert, *What the, op. cit.*
55. *Ibid.*
56. McGee, *op. cit.*
57. Culbert, *What the, op. cit.*
58. *Feeding at the Company Trough*. Washington DC: Center for Science in the Public Interest, 1976.
59. Culbert, *What the, op. cit.*
60. Culbert ML: *AIDS: op. cit.*
61. Culbert, ML: *CFS: op. cit.*
62. The Associated Press, May 16, 1994.
63. Rath, Matthias, *Eradicating Heart Disease*. San Francisco CA: Health Now, 1993.
64. Beisel, WR, "The history of nutritional immunology." *J. Nutr. Immun.*, I:1, 1992.
65. Roe, DA, *Drug-Induced Nutritional Deficiencies*. Westport CT: Avi Publishing, 1996.
66. *Science*, August 1991.
67. *The Choice*, XVI: 4, 1993.
68. Cited in *The Choice*, XVI: 4, 1991.
69. Cited in *The Choice*, XIX: 2, 1993.
70. *Ibid.*
71. McVicar, Nancy, "Vitamins against aging, disease." *Orange County Register* (CA), Mar. 22, 1994.
72. *USA Today*. June 2, 1993.
73. *The Choice*, XVIII: 3, 1992.
74. *Ibid.*
75. Enstrom, JE, *Epidemiology*, May 1992.
76. *The Choice*, XIX: 2, 1993.
77. *Alternative Medicine: Expanding Medical Horizons*. Rockville MD: National Institutes of Health, 1994.
78. "The proof is in the market." *Alt. Med. Dig.* #9, 1995.

79. *Natural Foods Merchandiser* cited in *Alt. Med. Digest.* # 13, 1996.
80. *HerbalGram*, cited in *Alt. Med. Digest.* # 13, 1996.
81. *Alt. Med. Digest* # 13, 1996.
82. Cited in *The Choice*, XV: 1,2, 1989.
83. Chandra, RK, "Effect of vitamin and trace-element supplementation on immune response and infection in elderly subjects." *Lancet*, Nov. 7, 1992.
84. *Nutrition Report* 7, July 19, 1996; *Nutrition Week* 25:28, July 28, 1995, cited in *Alt. Med. Digest*, 17, 1997.
85. Andrade, Bill, Las Vegas NV *Sun*, Feb. 24, 1997.
86. Salmeron, MD. *et al.*, "Dietary fiber, glycemic load, and risk of non-insulin-dependent diabetes mellitus in women." *J. Am. Med. Assn.*, 277: 6, Feb. 12, 1997.
87. Shapiro, Laura, "Do our genes determine which foods we should eat?" *Newsweek*, Aug. 9, 1993.
88. "Governor shares results of Hawaii diet." Press release, Office of the Governor, Honolulu HI, Jan. 28, 1997.
89. Shapiro, *loc. cit.*
90. D'Adamo, Peter, *The Individual Diet Solution to Staying Healthy, Living Longer and Achieving Your Ideal Weight.* New York: Putnam's, 1996.
91. *New York Times*, June 16, 1997.

XVI
OXIDOLOGY:
The coming of a revolution

"What places (Dr. Donald) Malins in the minority . . . is his contention that cancers are primarily the result of free radical damage. He's even more in the minority . . . in arguing that metastatic cancers result because tumors eventually produce massive amounts of these free radicals."

— ***Seattle Post Intelligencer*** **(1996)**

"All diseases are caused by oxidative stress . . . Insight: spontaneity of oxidation in Nature is the root cause of aging in humans and the root of all diseases. Increased oxidant stress on human biology is caused by factors in our internal and external environments. Chronic disease results from impairments of antioxidant defenses — related to poor nutrition — or excessive oxidant stress brought about by allergy, chemical sensitivity, environmental toxins, lifestyle stress and poor physical fitness."

— **Majid Ali MD, in *RDA: Rats, Drugs and Assumptions* (1995)**

"Free oxygen radicals, like sparks that are generated by a blazing log fire, are ephemeral and exist for the merest fraction of a second. The damage that they do is roughly equivalent to the spark spreading the fire by igniting dry grass and hence the forest . . . The extraordinary number of substances that act as antioxidants may be analogically compared with a wire screen over a fire which catches or quenches the sparks."

— **Editorial, *Journal of Advancement in Medicine* 4:2 (1991)**

"We found that we could produce an enormous inactivation of [the HIV] virus, reducing it down from a million virions to no viruses at all at about four micrograms of ozone; and twice that dose had no adverse effect on the healthy white blood cells."

— **Michael Carpendale MD (1988)**

The anvil and the hammer

I alluded earlier to an "anvil and hammer" concept of the development of much chronic disease.

If we style the problem of excess carbohydrates (particularly refined carbohydrates) as a central dietary contributor to chronic disease (the hammer) we may add that the way the disease is processed or mediated — i.e., forged — is through the oxidation process (the anvil).

For an increasing body of researchers from both conceptual sides of the medical aisle it is apparent that the body's incapacity to compensate for excess toxic oxygen breakdown products is *the* central feature not only of chronic diseases in general but a major contributor to the aging process itself.

Rapidly developing research into anti-aging elements, including the reduction over time of human growth hormone (HGH) and other endocrinological factors, plus genetic factors must also be considered.

The brilliant integrative physician and pathologist/author Majid Ali MD has made the oxidative process a main theme in his medical innovation series and he assesses at one point that "spontaneity of oxidation in nature is the true cause of aging in humans and the root cause of all disease."[(1)]

Stated another way, the oxidative process "is nature's way of making sure nothing lives forever."[(2)]

Accelerated oxidative injury to human enzyme systems is thus seen as the cause of all disease processes, one which leads to disruptions of the bowel, blood and "other body organ ecosystems," he has stressed.

It is perhaps the central irony of human biochemistry that the way in which the body utilizes (metabolizes) oxygen — without which it cannot survive much beyond five minutes — is of decisive importance in the induction, prevention and management of disease.

Only belatedly, of course, is the oxygen connection being made, thanks primarily to a handful of visionaries from whom the notions of so-called "free radical pathology" and "antioxidant treatment" in relationship to chronic disease and longevity essentially developed in the latter part of this century.

While it had been known that oxygen is involved in the process by which the body converts food into energy, it took years for the implication of oxygen metabolism in preventing, managing and treating disease to become clear.

Toxic oxygen breakdown products are also produced by such external factors as radiation and cigarette smoke and also occur in immune cell activity, inflammation and other body processes. Since up to 5 percent of the oxygen we breathe survives the antioxidant system,[3] at all times there is the possibility of "free radical attack" going on internally.

Such attack over the years has been implicated in everything from cataracts to the modern-day killer conditions of cancer, AIDS, cardiovascular disease and brain dysfunctions.

The body's metabolism of oxygen, the relevance of "free-radical scavengers" — antioxidants — in therapy, the importance of toxic oxygen breakdown products in health and disease, and the use of oxygen-releasing compounds as treatments eventually seemed to be a whole new subdivision of medicine.

The Bradford Research Institute (BRI), looking into this area since the the early 1980s, became aware that there was no word to define such an important medical subspecialty, so we coined one: *oxidology* — the study of oxygen breakdown products (metabolites) in both health and disease.[4]

By the late 1970s only a handful of scientists in the world were obsessed with the importance of what usually were being called "free radicals" or more precisely "oxygen free radicals" as inducers or enhancers of disease processes. The Bradford group looked at the broader field of "reactive oxygen toxic species" (ROTS) — or, as the AIC began to co-opt, reactive oxygen species (ROS) — of which free radicals are the more prominent members in ongoing efforts to correlate ROTS with both disease *and* health.

The research establishment began widening its interest in

"antioxidant" substances — that is, compounds which had the capacity of "scavenging" or inhibiting ROTS and free radicals. To the seeming chagrin of some allopathic thinkers, it turned out that some of the commonest vitamins, flavonoids and other nutrients — beta-carotene ("precursor" of Vitamin A), Vitamins C and E, certain B vitamins, enzymes and minerals, particularly selenium and zinc — were "antioxidants," or were involved in antioxidant reactions. And, as it became increasingly clear that a good deal of chronic disease — the modern "killer diseases" of the Western world — was intimately linked to free radicals, the role of antioxidant substances took on a research life of its own.

The relationship between cancer's ability to spread (metastasize) and the production of the "ROTS/free radical cascade" became a research effort worthy of its own study — and it opened the door to the use of antioxidants against the malignant process.

Some 1994 research indicated that "free radical" mechanisms could be key in the transformation of cells from normal to cancerous.[5]

A Seattle biochemist in 1996 reported that — as the genetic theory remained the new obsession in cancer research (*XI*) — the reason for cancer-related genetic dysfunction is primarily hydroxyl radicals, "worst" of the ROTS.[5a] The work by Dr. Donald Malins suggested that it is not dysfunctional genes but rather the attack on them by free radicals that "causes" cancer. Even the damned "quackery" drug laetrile turned out to be, whatever else, an antioxidant and "scavenger" of hydroxyl radical (*XII*).

Dr. Malins' contention that the cancer metastatic process is largely due to such radicals sustains observations by such innovative investigative groups as the BRI.

That "oxidative stress" is a major role-player in AIDS (*see XIII*) has been strengthened by various lines of research.

Under oxidological theory, much of the decline in the immune systems of AIDS patients is brought about by oxidative stress, factors in which include anally deposited semen from multiple partners, impure Factor VIII concentrate, endless rounds of antibiotics used against sexually transmitted diseases, habitual use of recreational and medical drugs and the oxidizing effects of such viruses as CMV and EBV together producing a "repeated toxic and microbial assault" on defense systems.[5b]

The basic oxidology concepts are that when more toxic oxygen byproducts (ROTS, ROS, free radicals) are produced than can be compensated for by the internal defense system, or when that internal system is impaired or lacking and there is no compensatory backup system (i.e., correct nutrition) then the processes of aging and disease are enhanced.

Internal antioxidant defenses primarily consist of the enzymes superoxide dismutase (dependent on zinc, copper and manganese), catalase and glutathione peroxidase (dependent upon selenium), certain proteins and uric acid. The body must also maintain adequate levels of the antioxidant Vitamins A, C, E and beta-carotene for its internal defense system. Since the body may use toxic free radicals/ROTS in a useful oxidative therapeutic way (as in destruction of foreign microbes by immune system cells which utilize a "respiratory burst" of hydrogen peroxide and free radicals) it must balance such an assault with useful antioxidants such as Vitamin C.

Understanding the generation of ROTS/free radicals involves a detailed study of aspects of both chemistry and physics beyond the scope of this section. In synthesis, free radicals are molecules with odd numbers of electrons which seek to "match up" with other molecules, gaining or losing electrons in an effort to attain stability and in so doing being capable of damaging virtually every tissue in the body.

The typical "free radical cascade" involves the body's own hydrogen peroxide, technically not a free radical, superoxide, peroxy radical and hydroxyl radical, the most toxic of the oxygen free radicals.

In terms of subcellular damage, particularly of the basic template of all cell reproduction, DNA, researcher Bruce Ames *et al.* estimated that the latter is oxidatively "hit" by free radicals/ROTS at least 10,000 times a day even in presumably healthy humans, a continuing contributor to the aging process.[6]

The basic hypothesis in most free-radical research is that the body's internal defenses against excess free radical/ROTS (glutathione peroxidase, superoxide dismutase, catalase) are depleted or "used up" just before the onset of middle age, perhaps earlier in a man, later in a woman — which some have called "Mother Nature's dirty little secret."

If the depletion is not compensated for by antioxidants from food — as it essentially is not in the Western diet — then the slow (or even accelerated) process of chronic disease and aging is guaranteed.

'Fooling Mother Nature'

In this philosophical model, the oxidation process is the great equalizer of nature — biologically, it means that developing species are equipped with a tremendous oxidative defense system to help meet both the endogenous and exogenous challenges of physical existence, at least through that period of time necessary for the species to reproduce itself ("life will find a way").

When the internal defense system begins to recede, there is still a safety belt available — the "second" or "backup" team of natural antioxidants from food, *as long as such food is essentially "natural."*

The biological observation that the internal antioxidant defense system (primarily enzymes) begins to diminish by the early middle years (sooner in men, later in women) speaks to the logic of Mother Nature: for species reproduction, it is necessary for the mother to maintain an internal defense system for a longer period of time if only to nurture the blastula, then the fetus, then the early life of the infant.

The human obsession with seeking the fountain of youth or endless longevity, which received virtually cultic dimensions by the 1970s, helped stimulate a good deal of interest in "free radicals."

The addition of antioxidants in supplement form or by consuming natural and untampered-with foods is not the single key to longevity — but it is a way of slowing the deteriorating characteristics of the aging process which, more than any other single factor (even though genetic predispositions and a decrease in key hormones play fundamental roles), is the body's increasing inability to compensate for excess toxic oxygen breakdown products provoked by both internal and external elements.

In this model, Mother Nature is perceived as biologically ruthless in the sense that her single preoccupation is *reproduction of the species,* not the health of those physical entities surviving beyond the period of time necessary for such reproduction to occur. Indeed, from the strict view of biology (balance/conservation of energy) the animal/plant model present in all of nature demonstrates a raw planetary logic in which the drive for life to reproduce itself is the primary genetic mandate.

It is because *Homo sapiens*, of whatever origin, alone among the planetary species, presumably is equipped with the mental facilities allowing for abstract thought and survival-based logic, that we are interested in "fooling Mother Nature" by staying alive far longer than *biologically necessary for reproduction of the species,* and that we contemplate life extension both in terms of quantity and quality along with the profound philosophical implication that in terms of the universe there are things more important than the reproduction of Earth-based living species.

A revolution in motion

The oxidology revolution was breaking full force by the 1990s — and it was developing this way:

— The biochemical processes leading to chronic disease increasingly were seen to be a result of, or influenced by, or strongly related to, the inability of the body to compensate for excess reactive oxygen toxic species ("free radicals" and others). Free-radical damage — an aspect of the oxidation process — was as surely linked to the buildup of plaque in arteries as was the excess amount of carbohydrates which might comprise the bedrock on which serum fats and toxic metals could accumulate. (In fact, the "oxidation theory of arterial disease," backed by consistent research over the last decades,[7,8,9,10,11] holds that if cholesterol is truly implicated in arterial blockage, it is *not* the "reduced" form found in *natural* foods and fats that is the culprit, but "oxidized" — literally rusted — blood fats which are a result of civilization's tampering with the food chain.)

— Free-radical mechanisms are implicit in radiation sickness, chemical toxicity, in the capacity of cancer to spread (metastasize), in the general overall aging process, and probably in immune dysregulation ("self" attacking "self" may involve free radical attack). "Free radical pathology" came to be a general term defining a pathological process leading to various diseases and conditions in which toxic oxygen breakdown products were held to be catalysts or important contributors.

— British research in 1994 made the case for the contribution of increased free-radical production or defects in antioxidant defenses in amyotrophic lateral sclerosis (ALS — Lou Gehrig Disease), via superoxide dismutase (SOD) deficits, and in Parkinson's Disease, via glutathione deficits. Indeed, noted P. Jenner, such antioxidant defense problems "may be central to the neurodegenerative process."[12] US research the same year tied oxidology to inflammatory bowel disease[13] and, in 1996, to diabetes.[14] Vitamin E's ability to inhibit oxidation of brain cells was cited in 1997 as a reason the vitamin might slow progression in Alzheimer's.[14a] Indeed, dietary antioxidant deficits may be broadly involved in dementia in general.[14b]

— The antioxidant (that is, the free radical-or-ROTS-scavenging) capability of various nutrients was more and more held to be the primary utility of such important substances as Vitamins C and E, beta-carotene, and a host of minerals and enzymes. There hence was a developing reason *for* the therapeutic use of such substances, even by the medical orthodoxy, against the killer/crippler "diseases of civilization" (diabetes, cardiovascular diseases, Alzheimer's, immunological disorders, cancer), and virtually always at levels far above those officially recommended by food-and drug-industry-controlled government oversight boards. Such realities led in some quarters to the concept of "nutraceuticals" — nutrients used in certain doses against deficiency states (beriberi, pellagra, scurvy, ricketts, for example) and/or higher doses which might help "control" a condition.

— Oxidology can explain, to no small extent, just why certain primitive peoples may have high-fat diets and yet have no heart disease, diabetes or hypertension — first, their blood fats are not oxidized; second, the other aspects of their diets (grains, fruits, vegetables) provide them with enormous amounts of antioxidants, that is, substances which "sop up" or inhibit excess ROTS or free radicals. Western diets are laden with "oxidized" fats and inadequate amounts of antioxidants.

— The implication that oxidative mechanisms are involved throughout the full spectrum of disease has become stronger each passing year. The Bradford Research Institute (BRI) did ground-breaking research in this area, establishing the "ROTS theory of health and disease" as well as developing a specialized test and microscopy system to examine metabolic products in coagulated blood to detect oxidative stresses and reactions in the body.[15]

— The "mitochondrial/free radical theory of aging" — at the subcellular level — has continued to garner attention.[16]

— There is increased interest in the use of *oxidative agents* (that is, purveyors of atomic oxygen, such as hydrogen peroxide, ozone, Dioxychlor and similar products) and even hyperbaric oxygenation, as acting *similarly* to free radicals as a way to assault key elements of the infective process: cell wall-deficient or anaerobic microscopic and submicroscopic structures (viruses, retroviruses, some bacteria, mycoplasmas, yeasts and parasites). The rediscovery of the effective use of oxidative agents against a broad spectrum of pathogens has led both to new therapeutics and new controversies, particularly over the utility and/or overuse of hydrogen peroxide.[17]

By mid-decade, the usefulness of many of the common supplements in their roles as antioxidants was too overwhelming to be debated by serious people:

A non-profit public-interest group called the Alliance for Aging Research called for both FDA and Congressional action to speed the approval process for nutritional health claims and urged Americans to add antioxidants to their diets at levels far above those recommended by the government.

The media noted that the recommendations were based on information from more than 200 studies over the prior 20 years.

Said Jeffrey Blumberg, professor of nutrition and associate director of the USDA Human Nutrition Research Center on Aging, Tufts University:

> *We don't have the kind of definitive, unequivocal evidence that some people are calling for, namely the medical evidence required for the approval of new drugs. But is that the right standard when we're talking about vitamins that we have decades and decades of information on? These are not some new chemical(s) that the body has never seen before. These are things that have been in the diet since prehistoric man.*[18]

He was essentially talking about Vitamins C, E and beta-carotene — which the surge of new information was already considering, along with (interestingly enough) aspirin, as blockers of "heart disease," stroke and cancer.

The call for governmental approval of higher levels of natural antioxidants was accompanied by research on fruit flies reported in *Science* which stressed (as earlier studies had suggested) that free radicals are prime causes of the aging process and that neutralizing excess free radicals or ROTS prolongs life.

Drs. Rajindar Sohal and William Orr claimed that by providing fruit flies extra copies of genes which protect against free radicals the flies' lives were extended by 30 percent.[19]

The fruit fly studies (and laboratory tests on sub-mammalian species always need to be viewed with a touch of skepticism as to relevance) were simply more precise definitions of research conducted in large (human) population-based studies which, as it was abstracted in 1994, "reported reductions as high as 40 percent in coronary artery disease among people taking antioxidants, and some clinical studies have produced similar results."[19a]

CARET and shtick?

The antioxidant champions were set back in 1994 and 1996 with three trials involving beta-carotene, Vitamin A and Vitamin A derivatives[20,21,22] which showed no protection against cancer and heart disease. And two of them, a study of smokers in Finland and the puckishly termed CARET (Beta Carotene and Retinol Efficacy Trial), actually found increased lung cancer among groups supplemented with the Vitamin A-connected products.

These were the first studies of any consequence mounted by orthodoxy which helped stanch the otherwise abundant flow of information on the usefulness of natural food elements against chronic disease. While too little too late, it gave the harder heads in the AIC and its "quackbuster" phalanx at least a winning round in an otherwise losing 15-round match.

The nutritional supplements industry, primarily in the US, was quick to point out that in the CARET study some 75,000 daily international units of Vitamin A-related supplements had been used (that is, a dose recognized as toxic). Moreover, it was argued, all such studies really show is that high-risk cigarette smokers who have puffed one, two or more packs a day for years will not prevent cancer by beginning a supplementary program of Vitamin A-derived products alone.

Even so, *The New England Journal of Medicine* was moved to make some interesting conceptual leaps by noting that it might be too shallow to look upon single dietary supplements against specific diseases.

(In the same *NEJM* where the above research was reported, another study linked lower heart disease mortality with "relatively high" Vitamin E intake[23] and yet another 1996 study tied Vitamin E to a reduction in the incidence of heart attack.[24])

Reprising years of information connecting antioxidant supplements and dietary factors against chronic disease, Drs. E. Robert Greenberg and Michael B. Sporn editorialized in the *NEJM*:

> *[N]o one should discount the importance of the findings of epidemiologic studies of diet and chronic diseases. In most such studies, persons who ate a relatively large quantity of vegetables, fruits, and grains were found to have a profoundly lower risk of death, particularly from cardiovascular disease and cancer. Antioxidant vitamins may not account for all . . . of the benefits associated with this dietary pattern, and the myriad other substances in plants should be examined for possible preventive properties . . . For now, while we await a better understanding of these mechanisms, consumption of more vegetables and fruits . . . seems a prudent preventive strategy.*[25]

This was an open-minded assessment which called for more, not less, research into natural elements (dare one suggest laetrile let alone multifactoriality?) in plants which are protective against chronic disease.

The discovery of this or that antioxidant from Mother Nature's vast treasure trove became almost faddish in the 1990s, and researchers began learning that certain antioxidants might have specific functions: beta-carotene and Vitamin A as surveillant over membranes; Vitamin C working antioxidatively in general; selenium and Vitamin E quenching ROTS in fats; zinc standing antioxidant guard over the prostate and endocrine systems; cysteine helping protect the bladder, lungs and eyes.

The discovery of super-potent antioxidants called proanthocyanidins added new fuel to the unfolding global antioxidant research, and supplement companies were quick to develop combinations of antioxidants for an increasingly health-conscious, largely Western consumer market of people facing the dilemma of extended life paralleled by increased amounts of chronic disease — as mediated through the Anvil and the Hammer.

Oxidative agents: the fight for legitimacy

The current medical era has witnessed what seems to be a "new" concept — the use of oxygen-based products (hydrogen peroxide, the endogenous oxidative agent par excellence; ozone gas; intermediate oxygen structures) as useful against disease primarily because of their ability to release atomic oxygen which in turn attacks cell wall-deficient or anaerobic microscopic and sub-microscopic structures and thus constitutes a seemingly natural weapon against a host of viruses and microbes.

Claims for hydrogen peroxide and ozone have, like all other outside-the-pale procedures, varied from the sublime to the ridiculous, yet the persistence of what orthodoxy dismisses as "anecdotal evidence" for their use is so strong as not to be happenstance.

Yet there is little that is actually new here: as Elizabeth Baker has described[(26)] in a history of oxygen treatments, since the 1920s H2O2 (hydrogen peroxide) and ozone put into remission many a disease. The aforementioned Dr. William Koch, with his controversial Glyoxylide (*XII*), was a pioneer in the oxidative area, as was Nikola Tesla, pioneer of — among so many things — ozone therapy.

On the flip side of the antioxidant/oxidative agent equation, the most intense work on purveyors of oxygen has focused on "medical ozone," which literally has saved the lives or enhanced the health of millions of Europeans while remaining essentially cold-shouldered by America's AIC.

It is also true that ozone administration via ozone generators has been hyped as magic-bulletry, just as the overuse of hydrogen peroxide has been linked to premature aging and pathological conditions through the generation of free radicals.

More recent reviews of ozone have found[(27,28)] that this

energized form of oxygen has been used with various degrees of success over the last three or more decades in the treatment of conditions ranging from gangrene to AIDS and cancer. A 1980 German study claimed more than a thousand therapists had given more than five million ozone treatments, with 90 percent of these found to be effective.[29]

Recent research has found ozone useful in reducing cholesterol — and, as an "oxidizer," stimulating *antioxidant* protection.[29a,29b]

With purveyors of nascent atomic oxygen obviously useful in demolishing viruses (as part of a general attack on cell wall-deficient or anaerobic structures), AIDS became a target for ozone therapy at home and abroad. I am aware of an enormous body of anecdotes linking positive AIDS responses to ozone, although controlled studies on the same have been hard to come by.

Some 3,300 cities across the world, most of them in Europe, routinely ozonate their water supplies.

Oxidative agents function as antiseptics and purifiers. In the United States, industrial chlorine oxides are used as potent antiseptics for everything from fish tanks to swimming pools.

One industrially developed product, Dioxychlor, refined for human use, was literally "rescued" for utility as a broad-spectrum antiviral, antifungal, antibacterial agent. A related compound, chlorozone, added to the water supply of a Greek village, dramatically reduced an epidemic of infectious hepatitis and was successfully used in Vietnam in the treatment of civilian war casualties. Yet, neither chlorozone nor similar compounds were granted patents for medical uses in the United States.[30,31]

Due to cancer's well-known aversion to oxygen, there is a rationale for the use of oxidative agents against the malignant process — but only insofar as such utilization does not lead to the generation of ROTS or free radicals, part of cancer's ability to metastasize, or spread.

The use of oxidative agents against cancer received a major step up in 1988 when the peer-reviewed journal *Science* published laboratory evidence showing that ozone selectively inhibited the growth of cancer cells[32] — not news to south-of-the-border "alternative" clinics where ozone infusion into accessible primary tumors is a relatively common practice.

The discovery — or actually re-discovery — that oxidative agents may be among the least expensive, least dangerous and most effective antiviral agents has great relevance in the Age of AIDS. And, indeed, astonishing claims (some undoubtedly hyped beyond reason) attribute to such products some major achievements.

With the world now threatened by an increasing variety of *bacteria* resistant to antibiotics, quite aside from viruses new and old for which antibiotics are useless anyway, there has been opened a window of opportunity for the use of oxidative agents. Such modalities represent a cost-effective rescue since they are effective against anaerobic bacteria, some parasites and other microbes as well as mycoplasmas and viruses.

As this book was readied for press, impressive anecdotal evidence was mounting for the use of "cold plasma" electrostatically-generated ozone along the lines of research pioneered a century ago by inventor and genius Nikola Tesla (*see also XVII*), though, as so often is the case with "underground" treatments, hard data and followup were lacking.

It is true that claims for oxidative agents may not always hold up — and that such medical approaches have often been more commercialized than scientifically established. Yet the abundance of evidence in favor of their utilization far outweighs any argument about why such methods have not been pursued, particularly when viral diseases, by their nature, are inherently "incurable."

And, overzealous use of several agents as oxidative "magic bullets" carries with it the downside of either red blood cell damage or the generation of the "free radical cascade," in which harmful oxygen metabolic byproducts can do as much harm to the body as may be done by the very microbes the oxidative agents are deployed to attack. Yet the possibility of danger by overuse has never been used by the AIC as an excuse not to develop toxic drugs.

The utilization of either a natural substance or a portion of the atmosphere against disease swiftly ran into trouble: who could turn much of a profit using such unpatentable things? The sulfa drugs were in the wings, then came penicillin, then came other antibiotic wonder drugs, and interest in oxidative therapies was buried under a blizzard of negative propaganda.

The "trouble" with oxidative agents — as anti-cancer, anti-AIDS, anti-viral, anti-bacterial, anti-fungal compounds — is of course due to three factors:

— Their essentially inexpensive nature

— Their ubiquity

— The fact they mostly cannot be patented as drugs

The oxidative agents hence pose an awesome market challenge for antibiotics, expensive antivirals and even chemotherapeutic agents. They have been vigorously opposed in one form or another since earlier in this century for just such reasons.

Their rediscovery and amplified use constitute major contributions to the medicine of the 21st century.

Being clean from the inside out

Thanks to oxidological research, it is now clearer than ever that the key to healthy human survival in an ever-more-toxic world boils down to two prime mandates:

Enhancement of all aspects of host defense, particularly of the multiple "immune systems"; and

Enhancement of the antioxidant internal defense system, which impinges on the former.

From the point of conception to the transition of birth and throughout all of life the species is exposed to a veritable microbial toxic soup of natural substances and life forms which at any given moment can do it in. Facing this reality, the "immune systems" are in place.

Yet the species is now threatened equally, and perhaps

moreso, by a world of man-made calamities (chemically polluted air, water, food, toxic waste dumps, radiation great and small, for starters) against which the antioxidant defense system is the only real fortress.

In physical terms, then, the best bulwark against all such challenges is "to be clean from the inside out" — by enhancing the internal antioxidant system.

Up to now, our interest has been in all those natural elements which help to promote health at the physical level. Nutritional science, immunology and now oxidology have played key roles in continually developing this information.

But — in the spirit of the ancient holism which now philosophically underpins the coming medicine of the 21st century — it is increasingly understood that the physical aspect of health, however vital, is only part of the reality.

The non-physical aspect will increasingly demand the species' attention.

REFERENCES

1. Ali, Majid, *RDA: Rats, Drugs and Assumptions.* Denville NJ: Life Span Press, 1995.
2. Ali, Majid, at Eighth International Symposium (American Biologics), Mallorca, Spain, June 28-30, 1996.
3. Reiter, RJ, *et al.*, "A review of the evidence supporting melatonin's role as an oxidant." *J. Pineal Res.* 18 (1), 1995.
4. Bradford, RW, *et al., Oxidology: The Study of Reactive Oxygen Toxic Species (ROTS) and Their Metabolism in Health and Disease.* Los Angeles CA: The Bradford Foundation, 1985. (Updated, 1997.)
5. Cerutti, PA, "Oxy-radicals and cancer." *Lancet*, Sept. 24, 1994.
5a. Malins, Donald, *Proc. Natl. Aca. Sci.*, Nov. 26, 1996.
5b. Hodgkinson, Neville, *AIDS: The Failure of Contemporary Science.* (United Kingdom: Fourth Estate, 1996.) Rev. by Alex Russell, *Continuum* [UK], 4: 2, 1996.
6. Ames, BN, *et al.*, "Oxidants, antioxidants and the degenerative diseases of aging." *Proc. Natl. Aca. Sci. USA* 90, 1993.
7. McGee, CT, *Heart Frauds.* Coeur d'Alene ID: Medi Press, 1993.
8. Cathcart, RK, *et al.*, *J. Leukocyte Biol.* 38, 1985.
9. Witztum, JL, "The oxidation hypothesis of atherosclerosis." *Lancet*, Sept. 17, 1994.
10. Verschuen, WMM, *et al.*, *J. Am. Med. Assn.*, July 17, 1995.
11. Jha, P, *et al.*, "The antioxidant vitamins and cardiovascular disease: a critical review of epidemiologic and clinical trial data." *Ann. Intern. Med.* 123, 1995.
12. Jenner, P. "Oxidative damage in neurodegenerative disease." *Lancet*, Sept. 17, 1994.
13. Grisham, MB, "Oxidants and free radicals in inflammatory bowel disease." *Lancet*, Sept. 24, 1994.

14. Dandona, P, *et al.*, "Oxidative damage to DNA in diabetes mellitus." *Lancet*, Feb. 17, 1996.
14a. Thal, Leon, *et al.*, *New Eng. J. Med.*, April 24, 1997.
14b. Lethem, R, and M Orrell, "Antioxidants and dementia." *Lancet* 349, April 26, 1997.
15. Bradford, *op. cit.*
16. "A theory of aging." *Scientific American*, January 1996.
17. Bradford, RW, *Hydrogen Peroxide: The Misunderstood Oxidant.* Chula Vista CA: Bradford Research Institute, 1987
18. McVicar, Nancy, "Vitamins against aging, disease." *Orange County Register*, Mar. 22, 1994.
19. Sohal, Rajindar, *et al.*, *Science*, Feb. 25, 1994.
19a. McVicar, *loc. cit.*
20. The Alpha-Tocopherol, Beta Carotene Cancer Prevention Study Group, "The effect of vitamin E and beta carotene on the incidence of lung cancer and other cancers in male smokers." *New Eng. J. Med.* 330, 1994.
21. Hennekens, CH, *et al.*, "Lack of effect of long-term supplementation with beta carotene on the incidence of malignant neoplasms and cardiovascular disease." *New Eng. J. Med.* 334, 1996.
22. Omenns, GS, *et al.*, "Effects of a combination of beta carotene and vitamin A on lung cancer and cardiovascular disease." *New Eng. J. Med.* 334, 1996.
23. Kushi, LH, *et al.*, "Dietary antioxidant vitamins and death from coronary heart disease in postmenopausal women." *New Eng. J. Med.* 334, 1996.
24. Stephens, NG, *et al.*, "Randomised controlled trial of vitamin E in patients with coronary disease: Cambridge Heart Antioxidant Study (CHAOS)." *Lancet*, 374, 1996.
25. Greenberg, ER, and MB Sporn, "Antioxidant vitamins, cancer, and cardiovascular disease." *New Eng. J. Med.* 334, 1996.
26. Baker, Elizabeth, *The UnMedical Miracle — Oxygen.* Indianola WA: Delaware Communications, 1992.
27. Viebahn, Renate, *The Use of Ozone in Medicine*. Heidelberg, Germany: Karl F. Haug, 1994.
28. Altman, Nathaniel, *Oxygen Healing Therapies.* Rochester VT: Healing Arts Press, 1995.
29. Klein, JW, "Cancer, HIV succumb to medical ozone." *Well Being Journal,* Sept./Oct. 1996.
29a. Hernandez, F, *et al.*, "Decrease of blood cholesterol and stimulation of antioxidative response in cardiopathy patients treated with endovenous ozone therapy." *Free Radic. Biol. Med.* 19 (1), July 1995.
29b. Bocci, V, "Does ozone therapy normalize the cellular redox balance? Implications for therapy of human immunodeficiency virus infection and several other diseases." *Med. Hypoth.* 46 (2), February 1996.
30. Bradford, RW, *et al.*, *Exogenous Oxidative Mechanisms in Combating Infectious Diseases.* Chula Vista CA: The Bradford Foundation, 1986.
31. Brown, RK, *Cancer, AIDS and the Medical Establishment.* New York: Speller, 1986.
32. Cited in Klein, *loc. cit.*

XVII
TOWARD THE MEDICINE OF THE 21ST CENTURY:
A new paradigm in healing emerges

"All healing is magic. The Indian healer and the western healer have a common denominator — the trust and confidence of both the patient and the healer. They must both believe in the magic or it doesn't work. Western doctors make secret markings on paper and instruct the patient to give it to the oracle in the drug store [and] make an offering in return for which they will receive a magic potion."

— Irving Oyle DO

"I don't know what you learned from books, but the most important thing I learned from my grandfathers was that there is a part of the mind that we don't really know about and that it is that part that is most important in whether we become sick or remain well."

— Navajo medicine man Thomas Largewhiskers
(in *Imagery and Healing*)

". . . Psychoimmunology . . . will become a vitally important clinical field — perhaps the most important field in the 21st century — supplanting our present emphasis on oncology and cardiology. Healthy thinking may eventually become an integral aspect of treatment for everything from allergies to liver transplants. What all this means is that our present concept of medicine will disappear . . . Medicine will change its focus from treatment to enhancement, from repair to improvement, from diminished sickness to increased performance."

— Michael Crichton MD

". . . Regular medicine . . . likes to call itself scientific and imagines that its exclusive attention to the physical reality of bodily mechanisms is in the best spirit of twentieth-century science. What most medical doctors do not know is that the scientific model of reality has changed radically since 1900 and no longer views the universe as an orderly mechanism independent of the consciousness viewing it."

— Andrew Weil MD (in *Health and Healing*)

"If we took what we know about laughter and bottled it, it would require FDA approval."

— Dr. Lee Berk, Loma Linda University

New Medicine — or extinction

Hurtling toward the end of the century, the Allopathic Industrial Complex (AIC), educationally and philosophically enshrined in the AMA, is faced with its gravest of challenges: apparent inability to stave off the looming extinction of the human species.

Reminiscent of Hitler hallucinating in the bunker toward the end of World War II and still imagining that new weapons breakthroughs and nonexistent troops would somehow rescue the Third Reich at the last minute, the AIC is counting on biotechnology to save the day.

Perhaps it will — and certainly genetics and all it implies will be part of the medicine of the future — but at the present time there is little of merit in hoping the AIC will fend off the combination plagues of new and old — cancer, AIDS, immune dysregulation in the West; environmental poisoning, dangerous new viruses, infections and parasites in the Third World (and man-made germs and antibiotic-resistant bacteria everywhere).

But because the prime directive of human biology seems to be one and one only — survival — and because *Homo sapiens* is nothing if not supremely clever when faced with extinction, as it now is, there logically is room for optimism.

Part of our species' survival is intimately involved with the rise of a new paradigm in healing — the New Medicine — which is developing as a collective mandate as the old structure dies, however brontosaurian its death throes may be.

Thomas Alva Edison was, as usual, ahead of his time with the prophetic and oft-quoted observation that "the doctor of the future will give no medicine but will interest his patients in the cure of the human frame, in diet, and in the cause and prevention of disease."

He was, after all, paraphrasing the ancients and, to some extent, Paracelsus.

His view foreshadowed by a century the disaster of the standard medical model which is now evident.

The primary medical concept of the 21st century must be promotive health, rather — even — than preventive medicine. For the promotion of health relegates medicine to a secondary position and implies that the individual rather than the physician or the state will take upon himself the primary responsibility for what many now call "wellness."

Yet, assuming a role for medicine as long as the species exists, the new medical paradigm must be holistic and integrative — a return to the original mind/body/spirit concept of the ancients accompanied by the technological advances of our times.

The New Medicine should be a union of the composite experience of the past fused with the technology of the present — it should take from the best of all worlds (allopathy, homeopathy, naturopathy, meditation, energy medicine, etc.)

True, an integrative holistic model is revolutionary and necessarily will ruffle many feathers — those who believe that all that is natural is good and all that is man-made or synthetic bad, that there are no good drugs of any kind and that all invasive procedures are violations of the temple always to be avoided, will not enjoy making common cause with allopaths; and diehard allopaths, long trained to perceive the back-to-nature musings of the opposition as quaint at best, charlatanry of a high order at worst, will be loath to join forces with those who believe natural therapies and even attitude changes are superior to drugs and surgery.

Yet both extremes will be missing the point: it is what "works" that counts, what is best for healing to occur. No single school of medical thought has a monopoly on this.

Such integrative models are already developing. They were referred to at the precedent-setting meetings in 1992 which led to the formation of the Office of Alternative Medicine (OAM) within the allopathy-enshrining National Institutes of Health (NIH) and in which I was pleased to play a modest role.

Among attention-getting comments then were those which came from Dr. Majid Ali, a Columbia pathologist who also uses nutrition and fitness programs in environmental therapy (*see XVI*).

Tackling the question of how the outmoded standard or allopathic model could possibly be used to evaluate multifactorial therapies against the modern disease calamities, particularly when individualized for the patient, the gifted practitioner/author said:

> *We are incarcerated in the double-blind, crossover model. It is not appropriate for holistic therapy, in which there are many variables and neither the practitioner nor the patient can be blinded to the treatment.*[1]

In these impressive gatherings of proponents of all forms of medicine, ranging from diehard allopaths to Indian tribal medicine men, from promoters of Ayurvedic medicine to chiropractors, from homeopaths to naturopaths, and including well-credentialed researchers who dabbled in all medical areas, several were in agreement about the need for a new evaluative medical parameter to be able to measure the efficacy of multi-variable therapies:

End results — i.e., "outcomes."

The only real way to assess the efficacy or lack thereof of multifactorial treatment models (protocols) is indeed the final result — how long did the patient live and in what state of health? That is, after all, the true stuff of medicine, not a workout in "science".

Establishment of a new evaluative model is a primary challenge for the New Medicine, and it will surely be met.

Genetics as a last gasp

The allopathic paradigm (treatments by contraries, single causes of disease states) is still in power and is the dominant philosophical force behind medicine's high technology. It still is producing a last, dramatic gasp.

Just as, in centuries past, the allopathic mindset placed emphasis on surgery, bleedings, purgings, and intoxications; and, in generations past, it relied upon the microbial theory of disease causation, leading to its brightest moments; and, within the past decades, it refined the latter down to the viral theory of disease as the seeming end-all of therapeutic experience, it has come up with its final card:

Genetics.

If in fact, after all, burning or poisoning out the bad humours was mostly in error and even if defining much of disease as the work of devilishly clever, invisible, not-really-alive particles (viruses) has turned up few real advances, then genes — "smaller," even, "more invisible" than, viruses — must hold the clue.

The American commitment to high technology — carrying with it an almost myopic embrace of not only not seeing the forest for the trees but actually being blinded by leaves and stems — will be part of the medicine of the Twenty-First Century and will provide useful areas of human understanding.

Most medical universalists, eclecticists and integrationists would no more deny the possible gains of genetic knowledge and its application to a new medical model than would an athlete question that performance is enhanced with a better athletic shoe.

But the reliance on genes as the over-arching, all-encompassing solution to medical problems is fraught with the same perils that have haunted all prior efforts at unilateral, linear thought: the snag is in the details and the exceptions.

By the mid-1990s, a veritable flurry of discoveries had produced evidence of possible genetic "causes" for a growing number of diseases, including various "forms" of cancer (*see XI*). The deeper scientists probed into the stuff and nature of biology the more they dredged up those wonderful replicatory particles, genes, whose alteration or absence seemed to equate with diseases and to explain why some conditions seem to "run in families."

The road to medical Nirvana will not be paved with genes — but high tech's increasing interest in the invisible will ultimately force it into new understandings of reality which transcend medicine and biology.

The rediscovery that food (and the many elements of food) have something to do with health and disease — an idea as ancient as the holistic paradigm itself — has been the first major chink in the armor of the AIC. In less than two decades, medical practitioners who once obediently followed the AIC propaganda notion that what we eat has little to do with health and disease now agree that food is important — perhaps vital. The old medical aphorism which states that that which prevents also cures inexorably led to the idea that various nutritive factors not only prevent disease but can be used to manage and treat them. We have assigned a Marine Corps-like role to laetrile ("Vitamin B17") in helping stimulate this shift in concepts (*XII*).

As the new paradigm develops, simply at the physical level, certain approaches to health and disease quietly abandoned before or blatantly and at times ruthlessly suppressed are being looked at in a whole new light.

One of these, used even against cancer and AIDS, as we have seen (*XVI*), is oxygen therapy (or, more properly, oxidative therapy), whose resurgence has paralleled the gradual embrace by medical/pharmaceutical orthodoxy of its flip side — antioxidant (or "free radical") therapy. Both are pillars of what one research group has styled *oxidology,*[(2,3,4)] a major component of the New Medicine.

Co-opting live cell therapy

In the area of rediscovered medical approaches it became almost humorous to longtime observers how the AIC in the 1990s was attempting to co-opt a form of therapy American medicine had derided as ineffective at best, dangerously quackish at worst. But it provided another glimpse at the AIC's boundless capacity to alter semantics.

The therapy in question is what the Europeans have long called "live cell" or "cellular" therapy — the subcutaneous or intramuscular injection of cellular suspensions of living birth-related tissue (embryonic, fetal, placental), usually but not always of the endocrine glands, from animals.

While the pedigree of live cell therapy is ancient (consumption of animal organs for reasons of health and vitality are referred to in most ancient medical systems), it became particularly known in the 20th century through the long-time work of Paul Niehans MD of Switzerland.[5]

The late Dr. Niehans and a group of otherwise allopathically trained physicians and researchers demonstrated that suspensions of cells of birth-related tissues (birth-related so that immune responses from the host would not be triggered) could be used not only against problems of infertility, impotence and sterility, but to enhance vitality, lengthen lives, balance the endocrine system in general and, in many cases, revitalize or repair damaged organs and tissues.

While there is extensive research data in languages mostly other than English, live cell therapy in the United States has long been treated as a gimmick whereby elderly males hoped to restore sexual vitality. And while just such effects have often been reported, it was not the intention of Niehans or his followers to set up sexual-potency clinics but to demonstrate, along Paracelsian terms, that in fact "like cures like" — that injections of embryonic heart tissue from a sheep, for example, did in fact somehow stimulate or improve a flagging human heart (and vice-versa.)

Even though radioactive tagging of the material could "prove" what doctors had long empirically observed, just how this could be happening escaped full understanding, and American-led Western medicine mostly derided cellular injections. Even so, famous Americans from politics, entertainment and literature joined famous citizens of other countries in trekking to Paul Niehans' chateau/clinic for just such therapy.

In the early 1980s, live cell therapy made its appearance in Mexico and elsewhere in the Americas, usually as part of an "eclectic" or "metabolic" treatment program, and began turning in some exciting "anecdotes" which could not help but catch the eye of honest American scientists.

What was exciting to independent minds, of course, was the implicit concept of the universality of birth-related proteins in the mammalian and viviparous species — and possibly of all species.

If animal embryonic heart and lung cellular material could really improve the function of damaged human hearts and lungs, then here was an inexhaustible source of a potentially inexpensive, and possibly highly effective, therapy.[6]

During the 1980s, several lines of research among "qualified experts" (a code for allopathic investigators) began demonstrating that *human* embryonic — and other — tissue seemed to be useful in treating such human pathologies as muscular dystrophy and Parkinson's disease. The ethical problem loomed: how to secure embryonic tissue other than through the use of aborted fetuses? While other research suggested successful trans-species use of birth-related tissues (animal to animal and human to animal), the US establishment still did not take seriously the notion of animal-to-human cellular implants. The political/social debate over abortion blunted real research along these lines for more than a decade.

With the advent of the Clinton Administration (1992) a ban on the possible use of human embryonic/fetal research was lifted. But how could the medical/pharmaceutical establishment, which had long damned the Niehans and related approaches as unproven or quackery, now espouse a similar approach without calling it by the right name?

Voila — the development of "fetal cell transplantation therapy" and/or "tissue transplantation therapy" as clever semantical artifices to avoid saying "live cell" or "cellular" therapy.

True, the American orthodoxy seemed determined to make this investigative therapy all the more complicated and potentially dangerous: usually, as in Parkinson's, adrenal tissue either from the patient himself or from aborted human fetuses was injected directly into the brain.

To classical live cell therapists this was both risky and unnecessary:

Under the standard European model, the cellular suspensions (usually in saline solution) are injected into the fatty tissue of the buttocks. And, as our own research group long argued, there not only is no reason to use human tissue whatsoever but it may be more dangerous to do so.

Even so, the attempted co-optation of live cell therapy by the US medical establishment as "fetal cell transplantation therapy" was another landmark on the way to a new paradigm.

For, implicit in any consideration of cellular therapy is the underlying suggestion that, whatever else the cellular suspensions are doing, they clearly seem to work on — and possibly balance — the endocrine system, the complex of "ductless glands" whose secretions, the hormones, constitute the bridge between the physical and the non-physical.

At American Biologics-Mexico SA Medical Center and the Kuhnau Center, in Tijuana, live cell or cellular therapy has been used successfully in aspects of cancer, AIDS, impotence, and sterility as well as in:

All forms of arthritis, lupus, multiple sclerosis, Sjogren's syndrome, epilepsy, childhood learning, behavioral and cognition problems, including autism and Down's syndrome, Alzheimer's, Parkinson's, macular degeneration, ankylotic spondylosis, Klinefelter's Syndrome, ulcerative colitis, tuberous sclerosis, and hyperthyroidism. It even took one man, brain-damaged after a fall from a horse, out of a coma.[78,79]

While in most of the above cellular suspensions could not be described as "cures," they certainly played an important role in multifactorial natural therapies in securing dramatic results over the short term.

1996 brought more proof for cellular therapy:

• In India, a 32-year-old patient blind from retinitis pigmentosa (RT) underwent "varying degrees" of restoration of vision through the use of implants of retina cells taken from aborted human fetuses, and four other RT patients also showed improvement. US orthodoxy remained "guardedly optimistic."[80]

• Memorial Sloan-Kettering Cancer Center researchers showed that transferring tumor-related proteins from one species to another may trigger an immune attack on cancer. Involved were human melanoma cells and "cancer-ridden" mice.[81]

While the precise methodology of how the cellular suspensions work remains to be elucidated, the research group with which I have been affiliated has made important contributions thereto.[7] And one of them involves a homeopathic principle — it may be that all that is needed to incite a chain reaction of organ or tissue regeneration or stimulation is a *single molecule* of the foreign protein.[8]

Whatever the final determination is as to the mechanics of cellular therapy, it indicates protein universality and a linkage between the species. It will play a role in 21st century medicine.

And so may — incredibly — urine therapy, since modern research is helping vindicate the ancient (and in some societies, still current) practice of healing practically everything with one's own "perfect medicine."[10a,10b]

Can we live forever?

The resurgence of live cell or cellular therapy, together with rapidly developing information on the role of hormones in health, disease and longevity, and these together with onrushing research into how nutrients and diet affect the same, has led to an end-of-millennium fascination with a single question:

Can human beings live forever? (Aside from the more cosmic inquiry: *Should* they live forever?)

Or, at the very least, can the aging clock be slowed down and life — with good health — extended far beyond the current parameters, which are even now in the West somewhat ahead of "threescore and ten?"

A growing group of physicians and researchers has begun to look upon aging as a disease condition itself — very much involving the oxidation process (*see XVI*), the environment and genetic inheritance. For these thinkers, the multiple exogenous and endogenous challenges to humankind, so threatening at this time as to suggest the extinction of the species (*see Introduction*), may all be overcome.

There is of course a certain cultural obscenity going on:

As most of the world's human population faces the grim prospect of starvation, a dwindling food supply and an ever more difficult ability to eke out a subsistence existence in primitive conditions, the Western world — captained by the USA — seems more concerned about losing excess pounds, looking and feeling forever young, and extending the median lifespan.

The reality that life-threatening chronic metabolic conditions are manageable, even curable, has fueled interest in the concept of physical immortality or at the very least considerable life extension.

In the present decade, controversies over and the mass-marketing of three hormones in particular (human growth hormone [HGH] from the pituitary gland, DHEA [dihydroepiandrosterone] from the adrenals, and melatonin [from the pineal]), together with global research on pre-existing drugs and nutrients which might aid in cognitive or brain repair and overall life extension while helping thwart chronic disease, have brought the concept of extending the lifespan in a state of good health to the fore.

Extensive research has been done on the three hormones, the most controversial of which is HGH, which may also provide the greatest spectrum of anti-chronic disease, systemic rejuvenation and life extension of them all.[82,83]

To these may be added male and female hormones which are now provided as "hormone replacement therapy" for numerous conditions.

Because all of the above are hormones, and because a central feature of live cell or cellular therapy *is* the balancing of hormones, the use of this therapy for life extension, as theorized decades ago by Niehans, takes on a whole new meaning.

As does the administration of the hormones themselves and/or those substances, natural or unnatural, which may be regarded as precursors of the same.

A cautionary note usually accompanies news about the latest hormonal breakthrough, and with good reason: tampering with the delicate balance of the body's intricate system of messenger cells (hormones and hormone-like cells), however spectacular some short-term results may be, may run the risk of imbalances later. Research on long-term effects is wanting.

Even so, the attention accorded HGH, DHEA and melatonin helps make the case for injections of living embryonic endocrine tissues, since pituitary and adrenal solutions (in particular) are among the most commonly used cellular injections.

Whether through endocrine balancing accomplished by the cellular therapy route or through monohormonal administration the use of such substances in overcoming chronic disease and almost certainly slowing down the aging process makes them elements of the New Medicine.

Rise of the 'X factor'

The breakthroughs of nutrition, of megavitamin therapy, of continued evidence of the importance of food in health and disease, of oxidative therapies, of hormones and live cell therapy comprise ever-more-important elements of a new understanding of the *body* part of the mind/spirit/body triad.

But for many, the totality of the physical, corporeal element within the triad is the lesser. What some, including ourselves, call the "X factor" will probably become the more important of the elements, for it speaks to *mind* and *spirit*.

Larry Dossey MD has recalled that it was a particularly well-structured (and hence, more acceptable in terms of allopathy-guided Western physicians and others asea in a world of statistics, double blinds and other aspects of quantification) 1987 study in San Francisco that changed his life.[11]

Before then, Dr. Dossey, who had practiced medicine for 20 years and had been chief of staff at a Dallas medical center, was simply a successful, if unusually insightful, physician.

What particularly struck his powers of insight was a "randomized, double-blind trial" conducted over 10 months at the University of California-San Francisco Medical School.

In this particular study, self-avowed religious volunteers, participating from outside the medical school hospital, offered prayers for about half of 393 patients in the coronary care unit.

During the course of treatment it was found that the prayed-for group had a significantly lower "severity score," with the "controls" (not prayed for) more often needing ventilatory assistance, diuretics and antibiotics.

Reported the American Medical Assn.'s weekly, *American Medical News*, investigator Randolph Byrd MD concluded that the prayers had had "a beneficial therapeutic effect."[12]

After Dossey reviewed the San Francisco study, he decided to look more closely into the effect of prayer on living organisms. He even started to pray for patients (one wonders just which statutes of which medical boards might be violated by such an effort). Explained the free thinker:

> *"I reached the conclusion that withholding prayer was the equivalent of withholding any other valid medical treatment."*

Had a known quack from south of the border or the evangelical leader of a faith-healing service said this, the medical and research communities would probably have ignored the remark.

But in fact Dr. Dossey had tapped into a vein already being exploited: the role of the mind (of spirit, of attitudes) in health and disease, and his excellent 1993 book on the subject followed earlier blockbusters by the well-credentialed Bernie Siegel MD. The latter had abandoned simple surgery for medical intervention *plus* aspects of caring, love and good humor in the treatment of patients, certain they could receive such positive energy whether they were conscious or not.[13]

And, *AMN* quoted Jeffrey S. Levin PhD, associate professor of family and community medicine at Eastern Virginia Medical School: "There is a considerable amount of scientific evidence showing that prayer is effective." He has added that to do research in connecting spirituality and healing "is no longer professional death" for scientists.[14] Dossey calculated that more than 130 "sound" studies exist in the English language alone which attest to the power of prayer.[15]

Lest the Allopathic Industrial Complex (AIC) trot out one of its favorite arguments to explain the inexplicable — the "placebo effect" — Dossey and others noted that the psychological support one might expect from prayer could indeed be explained by the fact a person knows he is being prayed for, and/or is praying himself — yet it is difficult to dismiss research suggesting that adult humans, children and *animals* who and which have been unaware they were prayed for experienced positive effects.

And Dr. Herbert Benson, president of the Mind/Body Medical Institute at Boston's Deaconess Hospital and Harvard Medical School, has observed that "most of the history of medicine is the history of the placebo effect." He has called the placebo effect "remembered wellness" and adds that "faith in the medical treatment . . . is wonderfully therapeutic, successful in treating 60 percent to 90 percent of the most common medical problems."[16]

Indeed, at a 1996 conference, Dr. Benson, author of a classic on the subject,[17] said that his years of research had convinced him that the mind can work "like a drug" particularly when people have faith in God or a higher power.[18]

As of 1996, more than 200 studies which make the case for religion in healing had been "ferreted out" — as *Time* put it — by Jeffrey Levin and David Larson, a research psychiatrist at the National Institute for Healthcare Research. They included:

• A 1995 Dartmouth-Hitchcock Medical Center study found that one of the best survival predictors among 232 heart-surgery patients was the degree to which patients said they had drawn comfort from religious faith — indeed, the death rate varied 300 percent between the faithful and the faithless.

• A survey of 30 years of research showed that churchgoers have lower blood pressure than non-churchgoers, even when adjusted to account for smoking and other risk factors.

• Factoring in smoking and socioeconomic elements, other studies show that regular churchgoers have half the risk of dying from coronary artery disease as those who rarely attend.

• A study of 30 female patients recovering from hip fractures found those who regarded God as a source of strength and comfort and who attended church services could walk farther and were less depressed than those with little faith.[19]

The same year, a Yankelovich Partners survey of 269 physicians found that a startling 99 percent believed that faith can heal.[84]

To the religious, that prayer "works" is so obvious that it needs no explanation by individuals trained in the (Western) "scientific method." For the more materialistic/agnostic segment of the Western population, quantification of the observation looms as intellectually necessary.

That "faith works wonders" was quantified before the San Francisco experiment which so affected Dr. Dossey.

Between 1954 and 1989, when the data were published, 19 out of 38 research dossiers studied by a group called the International Medical Commission of Lourdes (CMIL) — which attempts an objective overview of alleged miracle cures by religious pilgrims visiting the shrine of Saint Bernadette in Lourdes, France — were essentially accepted as legitimate cures, though medically and scientifically inexplicable. The CMIL has been described as a panel of medical doctors who are "independent of interference by outside bodies."[20]

Important to the CMIL were reliability of diagnosis, precluding of "spontaneous remission" in the known natural history of the disease, and the fact that no known medical treatment could have effected the cure.

In 1977, Dr. Charles Weinstock noted, speaking of the phenomenon of "spontaneous regression" in cancer:

> *In every single case of "spontaneous" regression where the psychosocial situation is described, a favorable change in it (or the favorable psychological*

change occasionally experienced on facing death) has invariably just preceded the tumor shrinkage. Some of the former include: a sudden fortunate marriage; the experience of having one's entire order of clergy engage in intercessory prayer; sudden, lasting reconciliation with a long-hated mother; unexpected and enthusiastic praise and encouragement from an expert in one's field; and the fortunate death of a decompensated alcoholic and addicted husband who had stood in the way of a satisfying career.[21]

Substantial evidence indicates the negative effects of mental stress on human immunity (death of a spouse, divorce, separation, for example) and that difficulty in coping with mental stress may be related to allergies, autoimmune and infectious diseases, as well as cancer.[22,23,24,25,26,27]

Evidence has also accumulated that what some have called "hardiness" has had a mitigating effect on mental stress and stress-related illness (elements — sense of control, commitment and challenge), and that a "fighting spirit" has better outcomes in breast cancer.[28,29,30]

Norman Cousins' books describing long-term controls over his own condition through a seemingly perpetual sense of humor, among other positive factors, have become classics.[31,32]

In fact, by 1996 the old adage that "laughter is the best medicine" was no longer conventional wisdom but established scientific fact:

The Sixth Annual Meeting of the American Assn. for Therapeutic Humor heard that laughing lowers blood pressure, increases muscle flexion, triggers beta endorphins in the brain (causing euphoria), and raises levels of natural killer cells (active against viruses and cancer), disease-fighting gamma-interferon, antibody-producing B cells and immune system-orchestrating T cells (*Drs. Lee Berk and Stanley Tan, Loma Linda University* [California].)

Said pathologist Dr. Berk: "If we took what we know about

laughter and bottled it, it would require FDA approval." Association President Dr. Edward Dunkelblau added that "medicinal humor" is inexpensive and has no negative side effects.[75]

In 1993, California's pioneering Institute of Noetic Sciences attempted a "scientific-method" assemblage of phenomena related to "spontaneous remissions," which turned out to include 1,385 articles gleaned from 3,500 reports which appeared in 800 "standard" medical journals in 20 languages.

Of the survey, in which cancer cases represented 74 percent of the collection, investigators found widespread evidence of such "psychosocial mechanisms" as group support, hypnosis/suggestion, meditation, relaxation techniques, mental imagery, "miraculous spiritual phenomena," "faith/positive outcome expectancy," "fighting spirit," "denial," "sense of control," "sense of purpose" and "placebo effect" as correlating with many cases of remission.[33]

In 1993, the newly established Office of Alternative Medicine (OAM) began funding various projects to look into what many called "the mind-body connection." In 1994, an NIH "Reunion Task Force" actually held a "Mind-Body Interactions and Disease" symposium at which 50 researchers were gathered to address aspects of the interplay between mental states, immune function and health.

That such a symposium could be held under the aegis of federal sponsorship, let alone that the OAM could fund a tiny study at the University of New Mexico on "intercessory prayer," were — as was the establishment of the OAM itself in 1992 — landmark events.

By mid-decade, some cancer patients at Duke University Comprehensive Cancer Center, in addition to conventional therapy, were also receiving "guided imagery," meditation, biofeedback and prayer.

And Columbia Presbyterian Medical Center, New York, was offering hypnosis, reflexology, therapeutic touch ("energy field manipulation"), yoga and acupressure.[34]

All of these events represent if not a coming of age then at least a successful prepubescence for a concept which had been primarily developed in the 1980s and which had finally been given its own name (perhaps as much as anything else to keep it a pristine ideology and/or an approach susceptible at some point of coverage by insurance plans).

PNI says it all

The name for the new concept was *psychoneuroimmunology* — PNI, for short (to which some have already added *psychoneuroendocrinology*, PNE). The jawbreaking word said it all: mind to nerves to immunity. And not to be confused with *psychosomatic,* of a more general range.

The stage had been set in the 1970s primarily due to the pioneering work of psychologist Robert Ader and immunologist Nicholas Cohen at the University of Rochester. What they demonstrated, as other researchers also had suggested, was that the immune system (or, as we stress, systems) do not work independently of the brain and the emotions — but that they are somehow bound together.[35]

Pioneering work by Lawrence LeShan did much to suggest the role of attitude in cancer, a complicated pathology which, perhaps more than any other, provides the bridge between the worlds of the physical and the non-physical.[36]

In the 1980s, Dr. Lydia Temoshek, University of California-San Francisco, in reviewing the cases of long-term AIDS survivors, found that whatever the patients were doing mentally "may affect the immune system and survival."[37]

Another major PNI proponent, Dr. George Solomon, psychiatry professor at the University of California-Los Angeles, suggested that personality and emotions, particularly one's ability to cope with adversity, may help the immune system(s) respond to illness.[38]

Seemingly celebrating PNI's emergence, *Newsweek* devoted

a "cover story" on "body and soul" and the elucidation, by PNI's main proponents, of the "feedback loop" — an intricate interplay of multi-system communication in which not only does the brain seem to speak to the immune system(s), as earlier guessed by researchers, but the latter also "talk back" to the brain.[39]

The suggestion is a language of both hormones and hormone-like substances and nerve signals in which parallel systems are somehow able to converse.

By the 1990s researchers were giving increased attention to *neuropeptides*, substances which affect nerve system function and, by implication, overall host defense, including all aspects of immunity, and to where and how they are produced and their connections to attitudes and emotion.

The breakthrough linkage was achieved by the University of Alabama's J. Edwin Blalock, who discovered that an aspect of the immune system is indeed the production of neuropeptides (originally thought only to be produced by the brain).[40] Thanks to this and a groundswell of research on mind, attitudes, health, the nervous system and immunity, the ties between "mind" and immunity can be considered fully established.[41,42,43,44,45]

The PNI connection hence helps to explain, in however preliminary a way, the vital importance of attitude, belief, thoughts and emotions in both the induction and control of disease. It does not yet account for the next phase — the influence over physical events (mediated through thoughts and emotions) by unaware patients: e.g., how prayer might provide a positive effect whether the PNI "feedback loop" is involved or not.

Aside from the relatively better-known aspect of attitude in cancer (perhaps up to 20 percent of advanced cancer cases may somehow be linked to a subconscious desire of the patient to die) doctors and healers since time immemorial have known (though not in a Western scientific sense) that the mind contributes both to *ease* and *dis-ease.* This has long been an empirical observation and it is only now that rivulets of "proof" susceptible to the Western mind-set are emerging.

In 1993, the University of California-Los Angeles (UCLA) Neuropsychiatric Institute and Hospital and Johnson Comprehensive Cancer Center released results of a six-year study which examined the benefits of combining extensive psychological support with education to help melanoma cancer patients cope with their disease.[46]

This conservative but well-constructed trial of 68 patients indicated that those who learn how to "cope" may keep disease from recurring as rapidly. What remains to be demonstrated is whether teaching patients how to *reject* disease could be as successful.

Such experiments and the rise of PNI virtually demolish the "placebo" and "false hopes" arguments hurled by the AIC against practitioners of "holistic" medicine. This is because the "placebo effect" is clearly of demonstrated therapeutic benefit (that is, simple belief that a potion or a doctor visit will help stimulates the brain to release opiate-mimicking chemicals called endorphins which, whatever else they may or may not do, allow the patient to feel better — an event often of awesome importance in such pathologies as advanced cancer) and the question is now raised: "what *is* 'false hope'?"

While it is true that the charlatan preys on the ignorant by promising miracle cures, it is now clear from virtually all sides that the injection of hope in the mind of a terminal-disease patient often correlates with life extension if not outright "cure."

By far the greater ethical crime is within the current — failed — allopathic medical mindset as the continual promotion, in one hospital or clinic or doctor's office after another, of the idea that there *is* no hope. This conclusion is usually reached after a patient has tried all conceivable allopathic approaches which, having failed, allow no room for even the faintest hint that there might be a better way.

This then leads, in case after case, to the patient's being told that "you have six months to live" or some other estimate conjured up by the perhaps well-meaning practitioner who bases such a conclusion on statistical analyses and "best" — that is, allopathic — evidence. Since the patient has usually already transferred his responsibility for health or illness to the physician (symbolically equipped as the quasi-divine arbiter of life and death) the patient may be programmed by such a statement to die in six months.

The author's two-decade experience dealing with patients who flock south of the border grasping for miracles provides copious evidence of the mind/attitude connection — as a group, "terminal" patients who outright rejected the idea that another mortal on this planet can adequately predict when they are going to die tended to postpone their "terminality," often for many years; those who ceded attitudinal terrain to the physician as authority figure tended to die on schedule.

It becomes ever more evident that ideas and attitudes help induce either wellness or illness.

By 1993, it was clear that mental depression — whatever its actual source — was itself a factor so significant in American pathology that it was costing $43.7 billion a year in treatment and lost productivity.[47]

That same year, psychiatrist James Gordon, director of the Center for Mind-Body Studies in Washington and clinical professor in the departments of psychiatry and community and family medicine at Georgetown Medical School, summarized that:

> *[T]he capacity for self-regulation that once seemed unbelievable even in Indian yogis is now commonplace in our clinics. Biofeedback, relaxation and simple visual images may enable us to change our heart rate, blood flow, urine output, brain-wave patterns and even the numbers and activity of white blood cells, often with demonstrable clinical benefits . . . It has become clear too that the effect of many therapeutic interventions — conventional or alternative, Western or non-Western — may be enhanced by loving, individual attention from health care providers and group support from others with similar illnesses. This is true at every stage of life and in virtually every chronic*

illness.[48]

Holism comes West

By the 1990s, some unique societal trends had coalesced to give a boost to the Eastern concept of holism — the trinity of mind, spirit and body, the core fundamental belief of ancient and original medicine (*IV*).

First, the antiestablishmentarianism of the 1960s left, among its residue, many seedlings of conceptual change in Western minds including increased respect for Eastern religious and philosophical systems and the healing methods which sprang from them, together with reverence for ancient healing techniques among the indigenous peoples of the New World.

And the demands of world politics (America's "opening to China" among the more paramount) and the explosion of communications, through which all parts of the globe were increasingly ever more in contact with each other, caused a transfer of ideas, concepts and methods between East and West leading, as a particularly notable example, to the embrace of acupuncture by the West.

Too, the profound failures and catastrophes of Western "scientific medicine" against chronic disease led by sheer numbers to the need for an ever more open spirit of inquiry.

Within this spirit, individuals appropriately credentialed by the allopathic majority were given space to try new ideas, ranging from the sublime to the ridiculous.

Among the fusions of Eastern thought and Western methodology came aspects of using the mind against disease — for which the words "imaging" and "guided imagery" came to be descriptive. While numerous savants have entered this field, particularly solid advancement has occurred through the work of O. Carl Simonton MD[49] and psychologist Jeanne Achterberg.[50]

At meetings in which I participated which led eventually to the formation of the OAM, more than 100 proponents of various "alternative" or "complementary" therapies heard individuals with seemingly impeccable credentials refer more and more to the mind-body-spirit connection, and to emphasize the importance of attitude in healing — not only the attitude of the patient but also that of the healer.

One such presentation referred to something new to most of us: "human intention factor" (HIF) — that is, the palpable improvement of therapy administered by a clinician if his or her *intent* were to heal (rather than, for example, simply to see the 3:15 pm patient at 3:15 pm and dash off a prescription in a lackadaisical, ho-hum manner). Interest also centered on such seemingly irrelevant areas as the cheerfulness or lack of same of the doctor's office and the color of wallpaper therein. Conversations on such cosmic subjects engaged in by multiply-degreed people appearing at government-sponsored ad hoc seminars would have been unthinkable, if not impossible, a few years before.

The respect for traditions of the East had opened up primarily because of the West's meteoric interest in acupuncture (and its adjuvant approach, acupressure), some of which doubtless accompanied the political needs of accommodating mainland China with the United States. Whatever, through acupuncture a bond between Eastern and Western healing models was firmly established.

Yet the West could not absorb the physical aspects of acupuncture (obviously useful in reducing chronic pain, reducing craving in chemically addicted individuals, in altering the moods of depressed people) without taking along some of its philosophical baggage. For acupuncture, however disciplined it may seem to be at the physical level, is an expression of a philosophical/religious system: cosmic dualism, Taoism, the concepts of the equal balance of forces, of *yin* and *yang*, of harmony/disharmony.

Not only acupuncture, but many other healing systems "re-discovered" in the West in recent years, strike at the very root of the (Western) Cartesian-Newtonian postulates which, among other things, see an endless separation between mind, body and spirit. These Eastern beliefs, consonant with those of virtually the whole world before the advent of Western allopathy, hold the mind and the body to be inseparable — just as man (they would argue) is inseparable from nature and nature inseparable from the universe.

In such systems, the ideas of *ease* vs. *dis-ease* (ill health, in the Western model) are secondary to the broader concepts of balance/imblance or harmony/disharmony.

From India, the ancient systems of yoga (not itself a medical system but impinging on medicine) and Ayurvedic medicine, enjoying a rebirth in the West largely thanks to Deepak Chopra MD, have brought insights useful to the Western mind.

The "Americanization" of Eastern mind-body meditative and relaxation techniques has of course spanned the range from the eccentric and damaging (the use of psychedelic and "mind-expanding" drugs) to providing quantifiable breakthroughs in the matter of how mental gymnastics can enhance health.

Whether from faddish research from the Hippie Era, ongoing studies from Eastern occultism injected into the West (Theosophy, Rosicrucianism, certain sects of Buddhism, the Vedanta Society), or responsible quantification or results by Western-credentialed researchers (and often above and beyond the "self-actualization," "higher consciousness" and "sensitivity training" aspects which have accompanied such new thought, not without negative effects in some cases), some solid facts are beginning to emerge, particularly in the areas of "transcendental meditation" and "biofeedback."

Separating the wheat of real knowledge from the chaff of a veritable Western *melange* of *gurus, senseis, roshis, swamis* and *tulkus*, "meditation as a scientific study" has come up with important contributions to research. In this light, the works of Murphy/Donovan,[87,88,89] Benson,[90,91,92] Kabat-Zinn,[93,94] and Smith[95.-96.97] are of considerable merit, to say nothing of impressive ongoing research into yoga.[98]

Uses of the mind in pain control, muscle relaxation,

improved circulatory and respiratory function, enhanced cognitive abilities, alterations in brain waves, reductions in cholesterol levels, control of blood pressure, decreases in cortisol and some evidence of hormone balancing in general, lowering of anxiety, reductions in blood sugar levels of diabetics, positive effects in psoriasis, fibromyalgia and even cancer have been reported.

What is now excitingly underway in the Western world is the one-item-at-a-time quantification of Eastern precepts in a manner understandable to the Western "scientific method" as the new healing paradigm of the 21st century emerges.

The West, thus, is rediscovering many currents of religious and philosophical thought from the Orient and making them, in Western words, "believable."

***Of subtle energy,* prana, qi, wayqi, reiki *and* quanta**

Underlying these ancient systems is the concept of a vital, subtle, universal energy flowing through everything — the *prana* of the Indians, the *chi* or *qi* (in modern transcription) of the Chinese, the Japanese *reiki* ("boundless vital energy"), and the alterations of which (through the meridians and pressure points of acupuncture and the *chakras* of Indian holism) may bring health or disease.

Further mystifying to the Western mind is the apparent ability of "qigong masters" — that is, specialists in enhancing health and well-being through special moving and breathing exercises — to produce effects *at a distance.*

In 1988, a group of China Institute of Higher Physics and Qinghua University scientists produced solidly researched articles on the effects of "external qigong," called *wayqi.*

Abstracted in English by the Monterey Institute for the Study of Alternative Healing Arts (MISAHA), a leader in attempting to quantify Eastern energetics and healing through Western "science," "external qigong" influence could be measured at distances of as great as two thousand kilometers (!) on a number of chemical reactions.[51]

A US researcher has found that DNA, the cellular template of life itself, is sensitive both to what the Chinese call *qi* and the Western world calls an electromagnetic field.(52)

American Cleve Backster has found "evidence for primary perception at the cellular level" in plants and animals — and found "biocommunication" between humans and their white blood cells removed *in vitro* and at distances from 5 meters to 12 kilometers!(85,86)

From a Western "scientific" standpoint, the *prana, qi, wayqi* or *reiki* is "unquantifiable" and hence (cognitive dissonance!) non-existent. Subtle atoms of this energy cannot be gathered, studied, tested, reproduced, so therefore they must not truly *be*.

Yet such a concept is wholly redolent of the underlying nature of homeopathy, of 18th-century Western (German) inspiration, which evolved into an entire medical system which challenged allopathic concepts and posed the most serious threat to the vested and ideological interests thereof in the United States in the 19th century [*V*].

The same essential element in the homeopathic paradigm which eludes allopathy is exactly that element in ancient Oriental medicine which the West cannot quantify:

The notion of a subtle, cosmic energy field or vital force. Homeopathy's founder, physician Samuel Hahnemann, called it the *vis medicatrix naturae*, the vital force, the disturbance in which would lead to imbalance which would lead to disease. Because Hahnemann's method utilized infinitesimally dilute amounts of natural substances to affect the vital force, and because such substances were often so dilute as not to be palpable in and of themselves, "Western science" was both taken aback by, and never could explain (other than in elegant placebo terms), the manifest victories of homeopathics over disease.

However, I (and certainly others — by 1996 "reputable researchers" at the Menninger Clinic, Topeka KS, Stanford University and New York's Mount Sinai School of Medicine were said to be drawing a parallel between the "life force" of acupuncturists and "bioelectrical-magnetic fields that permeate the body"[76]) have argued that homeopathy, and Hahnemann, were "on to something," and that the something has to do with subtle universal energies. These energies are not now, in terms of modern physics, nearly as abstruse as they seemed in the 18th and 19th centuries — for much of physics now concerns itself with the unseen and the *presumed.*

In fact, physician Max Planck's description of *quanta* as the smallest quantity of "radiant energy" (energy as both waves *and* particles) may be construable as a Western definition of a vital force.

Indeed, homeopathy may be described as quantum mechanics applied to biology: infinitesimal disturbances in an infinitesimally dilute or subtle energy field, perhaps the very stuff of the universe itself, are the root of *dis-ease*! If the universal vital force is the wellspring of all life, all vitality, in the physical universe (cosmos), then it is the ultimate expression of a single energy — perhaps, some might argue, of a single thought.

Whether one extends this vital force to its theological conclusions, it does present science — as third-dimensionally understood by hominid mammals within our own parameters of space, mass and time — with a conceptual statement: all existence is, ultimately, a reflection of energy, and there are many states of energy. In physics it can now be stated that there are subatomic forces the ultimate limit of which — if there is one — remains unknown.

Only by perceiving the possibility of an as-yet-unquantifiable subtle energy flow do such realities that "prayer heals" mean much to the rational mind.

The concept of such a universal subtle energy force, sometimes expressible as electromagnetism, biomagnetics or some other relevant term which attempts to capture at least part of its nature, provides a possible basis for understanding of both treatment and diagnostic models which, for various reasons, have yet to be broadly accepted by mundane science.

Radionics, for example, posits that a mere part of a person as small as a lock of hair or a drop of blood emits "vibrational energies" which can be used either for diagnostics or even for healing at a distance. This approach, developed primarily in the US in the early part of this century, evolved into more modern attempts to project healing at a distance through the use of a photograph of the patient. Radionics ran afoul of the Food and Drug Administration (FDA) in the USA although various forms of the theory and practice are legal in several countries.

Homeopathy triumphant

Homeopathy, however, has surged forward on all sides and may be bringing with it a concept of ancient healing more in tune with modern physics: Hahnemann's minuscule dilutions may be operating against symptoms on the basis of *pure energy*, or at least a pure *biological* energy. That shaking (succussion) of liquids seems to enhance their potency is often observed in standard experiments — but can dilutions be literally shaken into a state of virtual pure energy to a point where no trace of the original substance is recoverable?

This of course was the core and marrow of the 1988 Benveniste experiments, which excited an international flurry of "quackbuster" activity:

French researcher Jacques Benveniste and 11 colleagues in research laboratories in France, Italy, Israel and Canada demonstrated that an antibody solution so dilute (up to 10^{120}) that not a single molecule of the substance could be present seemed to alter the chemistry and internal structure of white blood cells. The work was presented in a major British "learned journal," *Nature*, whose reviewers had been unable to find a flaw which could be used to invalidate the results. The magazine editorially expressed both "reservation" and "incredulity" — a clear conflict of cognitive dissonance: what was reported "could not be," yet the methods followed were appropriately "scientific" and the results therefore "seemed to have been," ran the logic.

But three observers soon were found (including a magician connected with America's best-known "quackbuster" group) to go over the lengthy, multi-laboratory data. In a matter of weeks they claimed to have found that the experiments had been poorly designed and constituted a "delusion." For his part, Benveniste declared the quickly-assembled and quickly-executed investigation "a mockery" and compared it to the Salem witch trials.

Also helping stir American interest was an editorial analysis by the *Washington Post* that

> *[I]f taken at face value, the research shows that the immune system's antibodies can work even when the solution they are in is so diluted that no antibody molecules are left in it. There is no known physical basis for such action. It would mean there is some bizarre way that the solution could "remember" the presence of the antibody molecules and act as if they were still there.*[53]

This, of course, would lead both a radionics proponent and a homeopath to exclaim, "Well, yes, indeed — that's the way it works."

Benveniste stood his ground despite the inability of another team to reproduce the results.

The Benveniste matter, however, was only one in a series of seeming breakthroughs for homeopathy in the modern era.

In 1986, the British journal *Lancet* published a study of homeopathy that followed what the orthodoxy described as "the rules of proper clinical research." It compared hay fever sufferers treated with a homeopathic remedy with similar patients given a dummy pill. Symptoms improved dramatically enough in the homeopathic group that by the end of the study its members had used half the antihistamines as the control group. Yet, noted *Consumer Reports*, "the remedy they had taken was so greatly diluted that none of the original material should have remained."[54]

None, a homeopath might say, except what really counted — the remedy's own "vital force."

Since these results, and later the Benveniste experiments, seemed to say that homeopathy was worth pursuing, a team of Dutch epidemiologists then began a literature search for evidence of homeopathic usefulness demonstrated through "controlled trials."

They published their results in 1991 in the *British Medical Journal:* of 105 studies with "interpretable results," 81 appeared to show that homeopathic remedies had been effective.

While numerous trials were said to be flawed in one way or another, the Dutch team pulled out 23 of those thought to be the most "scientifically" sound — and even then 15 showed positive results.

There then entered the usual dash of negative cognitive dissonance: "Based on this evidence," they wrote, "we would be ready to accept that homeopathy can be efficacious, if only the mechanism of action were more plausible." The question was implicit: *plausible to whom*? It seemed redundant at the time to note that in 1492 what Christopher Columbus seemed to have accomplished was simply not "plausible" to nautical science as then understood.

Consumer Reports, usually thought of as a bastion of disinterested rational thought, reported in 1994 how it had asked "two scientists well versed in study design" to comment on the Dutch case review, the hay fever study and two other earlier homeopathic studies involving flu and rheumatoid arthritis in which homeopathy had seemed to have a positive effect.

One of the researchers, apparently using every acceptable technique of the "rigorous scientific method," found that the flu and hay fever results had indeed been "impressive," adding that "these papers used orthodox research methods to show effectiveness, and demonstrated it soundly."[(55)]

Intriguingly, when *CR* asked him if he would prescribe these homeopathic remedies for patients with hay fever and flu he delivered a resounding no. "Ultimately, it gets to the issue of plausibility and how well it fits into your scientific view of the world," he said. "It doesn't fit."[56]

"Plausibility" and "fit" are hallmarks of paradigm capture (domination by a preheld set of beliefs) and the negative aspect of cognitive dissonance (inability or lack of interest in processing new and unwanted information). They are, as we have seen, the ideological, semantical and psychological supports of the Allopathic Industrial Complex (AIC) or The Club.

Also in 1994, as microcephalic "quackbusters" railed in ever higher decibels against the growing public awareness of homeopathy, another "scientifically" acceptable study of the healing approach appeared in a "standard" journal: J. Jacobs *et al.* reported in *Pediatrics* that homeopathic preparations had been beneficial in the management of acute diarrhea in Nicaraguan children.[57]

California pediatrician Carol D. Berkowitz, who wrote a "commentary" in *The Lancet* on this case, noted that the research was a "small but methodologically sound study." Moreover, she editorialized, in an embrace of honest objectivity:

> *Despite. . .barriers to universal acceptance of homeopathy, physicians should maintain an open mind about potential benefits. Although we have often relied on drugs such as antibiotics to manage disorders such as diarrhea, the emergence of resistant organisms may necessitate a change in strategies.*[58]

Given the rapid and ominous spread worldwide of antibiotic-resistant bacteria, this observation was an understatement.

That homeopathy could be objectively dealt with in a standard allopathic medical publication — and this observer notes that *The Lancet* seems to have taken the lead in mold-breaking medical objectivity among the allopathic "learned journals" — shows that new thought is stirring.

As did the precedent-setting decision by insurance giant Blue Cross of Washington and Alaska when, in 1994, it began a pilot project covering homeopathy, naturopathy and acupuncture for several thousand participants.

What may stand as the modern-era breakthrough thrust in

which medicine did its best to "test" homeopathy was reported December 10, 1994 — *The Lancet* again as the forum. When homeopathically inclined David Reilly *et al.*, Glasgow Royal Infirmary and University of Glasgow, published "Is evidence for homoeopathy reproducible?" the medical world was treated to a well-honed serving of truth being squeezed out through layers of "Western science" and abstracted with some of the most agonizing semantics yet mounted against a possibly unexpected reality — namely, that homeopathy "works."

Reilly *et al.* conducted a "meta-analysis" of three trials involving the use of homeopathics against asthma in 28 patients. It may be said that the analysis measured "oral homoeopathic [*British spelling*] immunotherapy" in every conceivable "rigorously scientific" way — literally, up, down and sideways.

When all was said and done, the investigators carefully noted that the results "strengthened the evidence that homoeopathy does more than placebo." The authors ended the "summary" portion of the article with a question, one possibly reflecting negative cognitive dissonance: "Is the reproducibility of evidence in favour of homoeopathy proof of its activity or proof of the clinical trial's capacity to produce false-positive results?"

In the "discussion" portion of the study, after finding the undoubted evidence that homeopathic efficacy could plainly *not* be explained by the placebo effect (i.e., it's all in your head), the authors inscribed the following historic overview, reflective of the very honest, if Western, mind attempting to explain the inexplicable:

> *For today's science . . . the main barrier to homoeopathy is the issue of serially vibrated dilutions that lack any molecules at all of the original substance. Can water or alcohol of fixed biochemical composition encode differing biological information? Using current metaphors, does the chaos-inducing vibration, central to the production of a homoeopathic dilution, encourage biophysically different fractal-like*

patterns of the diluent critically dependent upon the starting conditions? Theoretical physicists seem more at ease with such ideas [emphasis mine] *than pharmacologists, considering the possibilities of isotopic stereodiversity, clath-rates, or resonance and coherence within water as possible modes of transmission, while other workers are exploring the idea of* electromagnetic changes [emphasis mine]. *Nuclear magnetic resonance changes in homoeopathic dilutions have been reported and, if reproducible,* may be offering us a glimpse of a future territory [emphasis mine] . . . *Our results lead us to conclude that homoeopathy differs from placebo in an inexplicable but reproducible way.*[59]

Degobbledegooked, the message here actually is clear — chaos-inducing vibrations, fractal-like patterns of the diluent and isotopic stereodiversity notwithstanding — damn it, homeopathy works and we just can't explain it, but it may involve higher physics.

The resurgence of homeopathy, the delineation of PNI, even renewed interest in radionics, even the possibility that plant and animal cells can "perceive" human attitudes and emotions and react to distant stimuli,[60] speak to growing concepts of *energetic medicine* — using "vibrations," "resonances," "frequencies," various manifestations of subtle energy, both in the diagnosis and management of disease.

Everything is energy

While the field is naturally wide-open to charlatanry, the idea of subtle energies, ever more in alignment with modern physics and increasingly removed from magic and superstition, can make at least a tangential case for some of the admittedly off-the-wall techniques and therapies advanced by "New Age" thinkers and the occultists of old:

If indeed everything is energy, then manipulation of such

energy may somehow have a hand in healing — or in pathology. The therapeutic use of precious stones and quartz crystals, pillars of Western occultism and Eastern esotericism, thus may have some basis in reality: certain structures are better conductors and accumulators of energy than others. The use of colors, aromas, essences, light and even sound in therapy fall into the broad category of *energetic medicine*.

Understanding that everything is energy, and that there may be a subtle energy underlying all other expressions thereof, may explain a host of phenomena attributed to "touch" therapy and to the combination touch and visual gimmickry of the "faith healers" of the Philippines, some of whom have indeed provided some spectacular feats of apparent healing.

The same concept may bring some Western reasoning to the oft-demonstrated positive phenomena of accumulating energy in pyramidal shapes — "pyramid power" — an ancient demonstration of energy normally rejected in the West simply because it is not "plausible" under current concepts.

It is no longer necessary to be a dabbler in the occult or an exponent of an Eastern religious sect to become seriously interested in "frequency medicine," "directed energy" or "biomagnetism" — a peek at the shadows of scientific history in the West suggests that mankind has leapfrogged over some areas of science, leaving others in the darkness and forgotten or ignored, for a variety of reasons.

What some call bioelectrical therapy — the effect of energy fields on life — and/or "directed energy" (how to manipulate and direct energy for a given end above and beyond electricity and the known spectra of light and radiation) represents an aspect of healing which will play a profound role in the medicine of the 21st century.

The bridge uniting homeopathy and various forms of electromagnetism is increasingly evident in attempts to measure the frequencies and vibrations of subtle energies both for diagnostic and treatment purposes.

The therapeutic use of electromagnetic fields, electricity, bioelectricity, and magnetism is a composite new area drawing both on old-time remedies and high-tech science. Such approaches range from certain folk-medicine uses of magnets as cures to the quirky claims of radionics proponents claiming to heal at a distance and the modern technique called "heliopathic," which is a way to use magnetic energy to produce a "healing phenomenon."

Biophysics, magnets and oxidology

In the United States, some vital research has been attempted, at least anecdotally, to tie together what we have referred to as *oxidology* with magnetic-field therapy since, ultimately, the two areas are like peas in a biophysical pod.

Central to this new dimension of medicine is an understanding of the role of antioxidants and oxidative agents, the energy dynamics involved in the "catalysis" (accelerating a chemical reaction) of energy, alkaline-acid balance (pH), the seemingly universal role of calcium in metabolic functions — and manipulating negative magnetic fields by the use of magnets.

Retiring in 1990 after 40 years of medical practice, an Oklahoma researcher, physician William H. Philpott MD, set himself the task — through the Bio-Electro-Magnetic Institute — of attempting to assemble, in FDA-approved ways, sufficiently scientific data to prove his decades of empirical evidence (also gleaned by others) that:

— A static magnetic field is an energy field; a negative magnetic field exposure increases molecular oxygen in humans; a negative magnetic field is the energy activator for the enzymes that release molecular oxygen from biologically "reduced" substances; and such fields may heal inflammation, may act as antibiotics against bacteria, fungi, intestinal parasites, etc., may reduce toxins, decrease pain, normalize pH in cellular and body fluids to an alkaline state (which extensive observation from many angles equates with an absence of chronic degenerative conditions), encourage restorative sleep and in fact "govern biological healing in humans."[61]

The utilization of magnets and of magnetic beds and other devices theoretically relieves the body of having to apply such a field to one of its own damaged areas.

Dr. Philpott has described cases of seeming control of numerous conditions, including advanced cancer, simply by the proper application of negative magnetic fields mediated through industrial magnets but strongly argues that hardcore data need to be established to buttress what appears to be abundant empirical evidence. His work, with considerable nods to the "Aharonov-Bohm" effect and the work of R.O. Becker MD,[62,63] also makes a case for helping maintain an alkaline medium nutritionally for the enhancement of overall health.

Hence, as this century ends the areas of oxidology (stressing the central importance of oxygen metabolism to life and health) and of biophysics (particularly, magnetic energy applied to healing), together with renewed work in homeopathy, constitute trail-blazing events heading toward the medicine of the next century.

***Rediscovering Tesla, Reich, Rife, Priore,* et al.**

Paralleling them has been a resurgence of interest in the work and theories of Nikola Tesla, the turn-of-the-century American inventor who is best known in the electrical orthodoxy as the developer of the alternating current motor and the high-frequency coil. Tesla was seeking nothing less than "wireless transmission of energy at a distance with no losses."

Modern reviewers of Tesla's work and theories alternately call him a madman and a genius, and by the middle of this century, most of his efforts had been ignored or forgotten — or, as Teslaites claim, stamped out by the energy monopolies which perceived a threat in his ideas. (What need would there be for human social organization if, for example, all the energy and sustenance one needed to survive could literally be plucked right out of the air?)

In the current era, in a West bedazzled by scientific gadgetry, various promoters utilizing "oscillating waves" and several forms of bioelectricity claim to be able to measure the electromagnetic fields of everything from the body itself to the minutest cell, and also claim they can interfere with these fields in such a way as to promote healing. (Just as others believe pathology may be *provoked* by electrical fields.[64,65,66,67]) There may be modern names for the techniques and their champions but they are echoes of the not-too-distant past.

The names of Wilhelm Reich, Royal R. Rife and Antoine Priore loom large in this appraisal.

The scientist and mystic Wilhelm Reich, an Austrian psychoanalyst, earlier in this century claimed an understanding of energy at variance with the theories of the day, and the discovery of what he called *bions*, minute particles of energy. He developed the concept of *orgone energy* (a kind of *prana* or *qi* definable as a combination of sexual energy and cosmic life force) and believed he had described the authentic relationship between physiological and mental disturbances. He developed "orgone energy accumulators" as treatment modalities and, naturally, ran very much afoul of government authorities. While the imprisoned Reich faded from view and died, Alexander Lowen, who studied with him, though rejecting the orgone theory, developed the mind-body therapy called *bioenergetics*, now taught and practiced under various names in many countries.[68]

Royal R. Rife, a San Diego scientist, in the 1930s claimed both advanced microscopy so refined that viruses could actually be seen with the "Rife microscope," and the apparent ability to cure terminally ill cancer patients with a "ray tube" tuned to specific electronic frequencies which allegedly inhibited what he, and later others, believed to be "the cancer virus." Rife produced considerable controversy in his time, and proponents of his theories would claim, as did followers of Tesla and Reich, that vested interests were behind his harassment and the blocking of further research. But there are enough witnesses and background available for study to make the case that the inventor was doing serious work of considerable merit.[69]

(Reich's *bions* and Rife's "cancer virus" may possibly explain the visual evidence of particles of pure energy which take transitory, will-o'-the-wisp forms identifiable only in very high-resolution multi-phase microscopes, and which have haunted the fringes of both science in general and microscopy in particular for decades.

(A growing number of researchers have seen, or theorized, the presence of *pleomorphic* — that is, ostensibly and arguably, form-changing or "L-forms" — in the blood of diseased people and, allopathically, have tended to describe such now-you-see-it-now-you-don't bodies as *causes* of pathology.

(The speculated or visually inexplicable presence of tiny structures in the blood, seeming to appear and disappear, has given birth to several novel theories, aside from Wilhelm Reich's bions and Rife's "cancer virus."

(The late Dr. Virginia Livingston-Wheeler, continuing the work of several others, described a tiny particle she called *progenitor cryptocides* [ancestral hidden killer] as both the wellspring of disease and life.

(Later, Canadian biologist Gaston Naessens, also updating the work of others, elaborated the theory of *somatids* — primitive life-forms beginning with minuscule spore-like structures — describing their presumed pleomorphism as detectable through high-power microscopy and their relationship to disease. But somatids are also seemingly similar to, if not the same as, the *microzymas* described by France's Antoine Bechamp in the 19th century, and possibly the *protit*, a particle defined in this century by Germany's Guenther Enderlein.

(Involved in all such theories and research are the basic [and highly controversial] ideas of pleomorphism — even to the point of viruses and bacteria seemingly switching back and forth, with intermediate stops — and/or visual reflections of what some might call vibrational energy. They have had to be detected in powerful microscopes whose magnification/resolution powers are beyond the normal range — *incredibly* beyond them, skeptics would say — of most research microscopes.

(The American Biologics/Bradford research group also pioneered a high-resolution multiple-phase microscopy system which, particularly in darkfield, has visually, and at times transitorily, captured all manner of ill-defined and inexplicable bodies aswarm in the blood of diseased peopie. To a somatidist such structures are somatids; to followers of the "cancer microbe" theory they may be *progenitors* — who knows? Yet they are there, or at least are there part of the time. Understanding that a general rule in the development of radical scientific notions is that more often than not the genius is usually right, but for the wrong reason — and comes acropper because of theory when in fact it is *application*, as in medicine, which is important — the final explanation of what these minute forms are and what they are doing remains to be elucidated.)

In the 1960s, Antoine Priore, an Italian-born electrical genius who worked in France, demonstrated that he could overcome cancer with the "Priore ray," which allegedly altered magnetic fields.

The history of the harassment and persecution of Reich, Rife and Priore as well as the attacks on Tesla's theories is a lengthy, sad and at times disgusting accumulation of jealousy, perverted science and vested interests — of *scientism* hurled at unpopular proponents of unpopular beliefs under the guise of *science*, as occurred, on a lesser scale, with Immanuel Velikovsky (*IV*).

If Reich, Rife and Priore in general may have something in common besides a threat to vested energy interests and the politics which devolve therefrom, it would seem to be in their demonstration of the real nature of all matter: that it may be understood in electromagnetic terms; that all energy is, or ultimately is bound up in, electromagnetism; that both disease induction and healing may be understood from such a concept.

At the extreme end of this chain of thought is the obvious implication: if everything is energy and each individual could learn to harness it then there is suddenly an answer to problems of both energy in general and medicine in particular. Were even a small part of this true, then enormous industrial cartels — and dependence on government — would collapse.

All of which explains institutional hostility to any number of "free-energy" or "over-unity energy" theories and devices which seem to violate known laws of physics and electrodynamics.

"Perpetual-motion" machines, "cold fusion," "tachyon waves" are among unwelcome interlopers which are left unresolved or unaccessbile and whose proponents may be harassed, bought off — or worse.[77]

But while Reich, Rife and Priore have been consigned to history's museum of interesting relics by the would-be rationalists of today's AIC, interest in electromagnetic fields and how they relate to health and healing keeps growing and flourishing.

Persons claiming to have "Rife instruments" and other "frequency machines" have peddled many a product to both the wary and unwary, and some of them, at least in some cases, and within a sea of hype and occasional outright charlatanry, seem to have "worked."

Interest in subtle energies and energy fields has also rekindled interest in applications of the known energies and hence reopened old debates.

In this vein there is renewed interest in the work of E. K. Knott, the probable father of ultraviolet irradiation of the blood.

In a provocative tome on a "trizoid" look at the American medical monolith, physician and cancer researcher Raymond K. Brown noted that Knott's UV approach, beginning in the 1920s, was demonstrated to be useful against viral and bacterial infections and inflammatory processes.

Wrote Brown:

> *For approximately twenty-five years, observations and results from several thousand patients were summarized and presented at medical meetings and in major medical journals; blood irradiation as a*

part of medical practice gradually died out when antibiotics and other products of modern technology appeared. Despite the formation of the Foundation for Irradiation, established by patients whose lives had been saved by the process and the physicians who had used it, irradiation of blood completely faded from the medical scene by the 1970s. At this time, the FDA was given the power to control all medical equipment and devices, so the possibility of a revival of blood irradiation in this country dissolved.[70]

Yet the AIDS plague has helped resuscitate it, and scattered evidence suggests that UV treatment of blood is a useful way to rid it of pathogenic factors.

On both a terrifying yet scientifically absorbing scale, nuclear engineer and retired Army Lt. Col. Thomas E. Bearden claimed that AIDS at the point of origin was actually a man-made disease "beamed into" the USA by Soviet scientists who, advancing the theories of Antoine Priore and others, had developed "phase conjugate, time-reversed scalar electromagnetic" weapons.[71]

Bearden, who updated the Priore work and similar research, in a 1993 open letter to the leaders of the American Foundation for AIDS Research made both the astounding claim that by utilizing technological advances involving a new understanding of bioelectrical theory "the technical development of an AIDS cure should be possible in no more than three years" and that the former Soviets had used "microwave radiation" of US Embassy personnel in Moscow simply to see whether the Americans knew about Russian advances in the development of such weapons.

He also reprised the work in the former USSR of Vlail Kaznacheyev and associates who in 17,000 laboratory experiments were said to have shown that "essentially any kind of cellular death or disease pattern could be transmitted between cell cultures 'electromagnetically.'"

Wrote Bearden, whose 20-year Army career included

specialization in air defense systems, tactical and technical intelligence, nuclear weapons, and research and development of Army missile systems:

> *The point here is that, from a fundamental physics viewpoint, it's just about all electromagnetics anyway, at the most fundamental level. But the quantum physicists are unaware of the earlier research work, and so are totally unaware that the physical structure, genetics, biochemistry, etc. of the living cell can in fact be directly engineered with the strange "new" kind of electromagnetics.*[72]

What is involved is a "'new', internal, hidden electromagnetics . . . (a) fundamental extension to normal 'classical' electromagnetics that is of extraordinary importance to cellular healing," he wrote.

In his writings, Bearden relayed the hitherto hidden history of competing theories of energy and the nature of matter, originating in the 19th century, indicating that many useful theories and approaches (particularly Priore's) were simply left unresolved or were squelched by establishment science.

If there is a "new, hidden electromagnetics" capable of uses far beyond the current understanding of physics, is the human mind closer to finding *prana* or *qi* in a demonstrable way? And, if so, are we nearing a "scientific breakthrough" which can explain the power of prayer and the capacity of healing through thought?

Bearden is not the only scientist associated directly or indirectly with the space program who has made contributions to a deeper understanding of energy and matter.

In 1968, Adrian V. Clark, a researcher associated with the Saturn V Moon Vehicle project of the National Aeronautics and Space Administration (NASA), adduced that the ultimate capability of man may be the controlling of matter through the energy of thought — that is, the "intellectual control of molecular motion."[73]

Clark was enamored of the suggestions of new concepts of

energy and existence posed — as some investigators would have it — by the seemingly inexplicable phenomena attributed to unidentified flying objects (UFOs), perhaps the greatest unresolved scientific conundrum of the century, as well as by clues in the Bible as to the nature of energy and the universe.

Bearden, Clark and others are modern-era thinkers with credible backgrounds who understand energy and nature-of-matter concepts at variance with the scientific orthodoxy of our day — one, as we know from even recent history, susceptible of 180-degree turns and causing profound befuddlement. Cosmological concepts in general and quantum mechanics in particular are racing well ahead of Western rationalist science and have opened new vistas as to what may be the very nature of existence.

Toward the final link

In areas that seem less threatening and more comfortable to the ensconced orthodoxy, many scientific thinkers increasingly are describing the human body as a closed electrical system. There is, as some put it, truly a "body electric" or an "electro-vibratory body" which defines the physical aspect of the human and which, by definition, at some point impinges upon the subtle energies which in turn may be universal in nature.[(74)]

The link between body, mind, bioelectricity and subtle energy will eventually be sufficiently "quantified" to satisfy the proof requirements of the West while accommodating the intuitive truths of the East.

As this occurs, not only will the power of prayer be set forth in a comprehensible manner but it will become clear why meditation and simply thinking good thoughts — and the healing capacity of human touch — "work" in medicine.

The wheel will have come around full circle — the holistic paradigm which guided ancient medicine will have been restored in a new era. Mind-body-spirit will be seen as interdependent parts of a greater reality.

Perhaps by then it will be said that man better understands his relationship with God.

References

1. *The Choice*, XVIII: 2, 1992.
2. Baker, Elizabeth, *The UnMedical Miracle — Oxygen*. Indianola WA: Delwood Communications, 1992.
3. Bradford, RW, *et al.*, *Exogenous Oxidative Mechanisms in Combating Infectious Diseases*. Chula Vista CA: The Bradford Foundation, 1986.
4. Culbert, ML, *AIDS: Hope, Hoax and Hoopla*, Chula Vista CA: The Bradford Foundation, 1990.
5. Kuhnau, WW, *Live Cell Therapy: My Life with a Medical Breakthrough*. Tijuana, Mexico: Artes Graficas, 1983.
6. Culbert, ML, *Live Cell Therapy for the 21st Century*. Chula Vista CA: The Bradford Foundation, 1994.
7. Bradford, RW, *et al.*, *The Biochemical Basis of Live Cell Therapy*. Chula Vista CA: The Bradford Foundation, 1986.
8. Culbert, ML, *Live Cell, op. cit.*
9. Christy, Martha M., *Your Own Perfect Medicine*. Scottsdale AZ: Future Med Inc., 1994.
10. Armstrong, JW, *The Water of Life*. United Kingdom: Health Science Press, 1971.
10a. Barnett, Beatrice, *Urine Therapy*. Botsford CT: Water of Life Publishing, 1989.
10b. Thakkar, *Wonders of Urotherapy*. Athens: 16th World Congress of Complementary Medicines, 1989.
11. Dossey, Larry, *Healing Words: The Power of Prayer and the Practice of Medicine*. New York: Harper, 1993.
12. Greengard, Samuel, "Doctor says prayer can be an essential part of cure." *American Medical News*, Dec. 20, 1993.
13. Siegel, Bernie, *Love, Medicine and Miracles*. New York: Harper and Row, 1986.
14. Wallis, Claudia, "Faith and Healing." *Time*, June 24, 1996.
15. Greengard, *op. cit.*
16. Wallis, *op. cit.*
17. Benson, Herbert, *Timeless Healing*. New York: Scribner, 1996.
18. Cited in *Townsend Letter for Doctors & Patients*, April 1996
19. Wallis, *op. cit.*
20. Kent, Jaylene, *et al.*, "Unexpected recoveries: spontaneous remission and immune functioning." *Advances* (Institute for the Advancement of Health), VI:2, 1989.
21. Weinstock, Charles, "Recent progress in cancer psychobiology and psychiatry." *J. Am. Soc. Psychosom. Dent. & Med.* 24, 1977.
22. Chen, CC, *et al.*, "Adverse life events and breast cancer: case control study." *Brit. Med. J.*, Dec. 9, 1995.
23. Mittleman, M, "American Heart Assn. Conference on Cardiovascular Disease and Epidemiology, 1996" Harvard Medical School: *Fam. Pract. News*, April 15, 1996.
24. Rogers, MP, *et al.*, "The influence of the psyche and the brain on immunity and disease susceptibility: a critical review." *Psychosom. Med.*41, 1979.
25. Holmes, TH, *et al.*, "Psychosocial and physiological studies of tuberculosis." *Psychosom. Med.* 19, 1957.
26. Dohrenwend, BS, and BP Dohrenwend, eds., *Stressful Life Events; Their Nature and Effects*. New York: Wiley, 1974.
27. Minter, RE, and CP Kimball, "Life events and illness onset: a review." *Psychosomatics* 19, 1978.
28. Kobasa, SC, "Stressful life events, personality and health: an inquiry into hardiness." *J. Pers. & Soc. Psychol.* 37, 1979.
29. Greer, S, and KW Pettingale, "Psychological response to breast cancer: effect on outcome." *Lancet* 11, 1979.
30. Levy, SM, *Behavior and Cancer*. San Francisco: Jossey-Bass, 1985.
31. Cousins, Norman, *Anatomy of an Illness*. New York: Norton, 1979.
32. Cousins, Norman, *The Healing Heart*. New York: Norton, 1983.
33. Regan, B, and C Hershberg, *Spontaneous Remission: An Annotated Biography*, Sausalito CA: Institute of Noetic Sciences, 1993.
34. "A new age of healing hands." *US News & World Report*, Feb. 5, 1996.
35. *Powers of Healing*. Alexandria VA: Time-Life Books, 1989.
36. Leshan, Lawrence, *You Can Fight for Your Life: Emotional Factors in the Causation of Cancer*. New York: Evans, 1977.
37. Grady, Denise, "AIDS survivors." *American Health*, September 1988.
38. Solomon, GE, *Psychoneuroimmunology*. New York: Academic Press, 1987.
39. Gelman, David, and Mary Hager, "Body and Soul." *Newsweek*, Nov. 7, 1988.
40. Cited in Culbert, *AIDS, op. cit.*
41. Vollhardt, LT, "Psychoneuroimmunology: a literature review." *Am. J. Orthopsychiatry* 61, Jan. 1991.
42. Baban, A, "Psychoneuroimmunology." *Rev. Roum. Physiol.* 29, January-June, 1992.
43. Kook, AI, *et al.*, "Depression and immunity: the biochemical interrelationship between the central nervous system and the immune system." *Biol. Psychiatry*, June 1, 1995.
44. Kiecolt-Glaser, JK, and R Glasser, "Psychoneuroimmunology and health consequences: data and shared mechanisms." *Psychosom. Med.*, May-June 1995.
45. O'Leary, A. "Stress, emotion, and human immune function." *Psychol. Bull.*, November 1990.
46. *The Choice*, XIX: 3,4, 1993.
47. *Orange County Register*, in *The Choice*, XX:1, 1994.
48. Gordon, JS, "Healing with feeling." *The Washington Post*, August 29, 1993.
49. Simonton, Carl, *et al.*, *Getting Well Again*. New York: Bantam, 1986.
50. Achterberg, Jeanne, *Imagery in Healing: Shamanism and Modern Medicine*. Boston: New Science Library, 1985.
51. "Studies of *wayqi* — external *qigong* in China." Monterey CA: Monterey Inst. for the Study of Alt. Healing Arts. *Newsletter*, April-June, 1996.
52. *Ibid.*
53. Cited in *The Choice*, XIV: 3, 1988.
54. "Homeopathy: much ado about nothing?" *Consumer Reports*, March 1994.
55. *Ibid.*
56. *Ibid.*

57. Jacobs, J, *et al.*, "Treatment of acute childhood diarrhea with homeopathic medicine: a randomized clinical trial in Nicaragua." *Pediatrics* 93, 1994
58. Berkowitz, CD, "Homoeopathy: keeping an open mind." *Lancet*, Sept. 10, 1994.
59. Reilly, David, *et al.*, "Is evidence for homoeopathy reproducible?" *Lancet*, Dec. 10, 1994.
60. Stone, RB, "Cells caught in the act of communication." Monterey CA: Monterey Inst. for the Study of Alt. Healing Arts. *Newsletter*, Oct.-Dec. 1995.
61. Philpott, WH, *Cancer: the Magnetic Oxygen Answer*. Choctaw OK, 1994.
62. Aharonov, Y, and D Bohm, "Significance of electromagnetic potentials in quantum theory." Cited in Philpott, *op. cit.*
63. Becker, RO, and G Seldon, *The Body Electric: Electro-Magnetism and the Foundation of Life*. New York: Morrow Co., 1986.
64. Becker, Robert O., *Cross Currents: The Perils of Electropollution, The Promise of Electromedicine*. New York: Tarcher, 1990.
65. Brodeur, Paul, *Currents of Death: Powerlines, Computer Terminals, and the Attempt to Cover Up Their Threat to Your Health*. New York: Simon and Schuster, 1989.
66. Smith, Cyril W., and Simon Best, *Electromagnetic Man: Health and Hazard in the Electrical Environment*. New York: St. Martin's Press, 1989.
67. Sugarman, Ellen, *Warning: the Electricity Around You May be Hazardous to Your Health*, New York: Simon and Schuster, 1992.
68. *Powers of Healing*, *op. cit.*
69. Lynes, Barry, *The Cancer Cure that Worked!* Toronto: Marcus Books, 1987.
70. Brown, RK, *AIDS, Cancer and the Medical Establishment*. New York: Speller, 1986.
71. Bearden, TE, *AIDS: Biological Warfare*. Greenville TX: Tesla Book Co. 1988. Also, Bearden, TE, "Soviet phase conjugate weapons (weapons that use time-reversed electromagnetic waves)." *Bulletin of the Committee to Restore the Constitution*, January 1988. Cited in Culbert, *AIDS, op. cit.*
72. Bearden, TE. Open letter to Elizabeth Taylor and Dr. Mathilde Krim. *Bulletin of the Committee to Restore the Constitution*. September 1993.
73. Clark, AV, *Cosmic Mysteries of the Universe*. West Nyack NY: Parker, 1968.
74. Beasley, Victor, *Your Electro-Vibratory Body*. Boulder Creek CO: University of the Trees Press, 1978.
75. Ricks, Delthia, *Orlando Sentinel*, cited in *San Diego Union*, Nov. 10, 1996.
76. Langene, John, "Challenging the mainstream." *Time*. Special Issue (148:14), Fall 1996.
77. Masen, Erik, "Suppressed energy." *Perceptions*, Oct./Nov. 1996.
78. Culbert, ML, *Live Cell. . . op. cit.*
79. *ICHF Newsletter*, Spring 1997.
80. "Surgery helps blind man in India." *San Diego Union*, Nov. 19, 1996.
81. Paul Recer, Associated Press, Dec. 11, 1996.
82. Klatz, Ronald, *Grow Young with HGH*. New York: HarperCollins, 1997.
83. Klatz, Ronald, and Robert Goldman, *Stopping the Clock*. New Canaan CT: Keats, 1996.
84. *Parade*, Dec. 1, 1996.
85. Backster, Cleve, "Evidence for a primary perception at the cellular level in plant and animal life." Am. Assn. for Advancement in Science (AAAS) annual meeting, 1975.
86. Backster, Cleve, "Biocommunications capability: human donors and *in vitro* leukocytes." *Int. J. Biosoc. Res.* 7(2), 1985.
87. Murphy, M, *The Future of the Body: Explorations into the Evolution of Human Nature*. Los Angeles: Tarcher, 1992.
88. Murphy, M, and S Donovan, "A bibliography of meditation research 1931-1983." *Transpers. Psych.* 15:2, 1988.
89. Murphy, M, and S Donovan, *The Physical and Psychological Effects of Meditation*. Sausalito CA: Institute of Noetic Sciences, 1997.
90. Benson, Herbert, *The Relaxation Response*. New York: Morrow, 1975.
91. Benson, Herbert, *Beyond the Relaxation Response*. New York: Times Books, 1984.
92. Benson, H, and W Proctor, *Your Maximum Mind*. New York: Avon, 1987.
93. Kabat-Zinn, J, *Full-Catastrophe Living: Using the Wisdom of Your Body and Mind to Face Stress, Pain, and Illness*. New York: DeLaCorte Press, 1990.
94. Kabat-Zinn, J, *Wherever You Go, There You Are: Mindfulness Meditation in Everyday Life*. New York: Hyperion, 1994.
95. Smith, JC, *Meditation: A Sensible Guide to a Timeless Discipline*. Champaign IL: Research Press, 1986.
96. Smith, JC, *Relaxation Dynamics: Nine World Approaches to Self-relaxation*. Champaign IL: Research Press, 1985.
97. Smith, JC, *Understanding Stress and Coping*. New York: Macmillan, 1993.
98. Monro, R, *et al.*, *Yoga Research Bibliography: Scientific Studies on Yoga and Meditation*. Cambridge MA: Biomedical Trust, 1989.

APPENDICES

APPENDIX A

SOLVING THE HEALTHCARE CRISIS WHILE

RESCUING LIBERTY

An American challenge

In the final decade of this century, it is evident that the healthcare system of the United States is failing on various fronts:

— Despite its earlier success against infectious disease and the development of the most advanced biomedical high technology in the world, it seems utterly unable to curb the exponential growth of chronic diseases and multifactorial disorders, most of them the results of civilization. Such disorders now pose a threat to the survival of the species itself.

— Because of its mechanical successes in increasing overall life extension (if maintenance of one or more viable life systems is itself the extension of "life" rather than the prolongation of death) it has helped increase the numbers of people most apt to be affected by the chronic disorders of civilization.

— It is unable to evaluate new medical techniques and approaches because it is conceptually held hostage to an essentially unworkable paradigm — allopathic medicine — in which monotherapy, single causes, treatment by opposites and linear thought are the philosophical anchors. And the paradigm is, in turn, held hostage to vested economic interests.

— Increasing numbers of the population simply cannot afford the system even if they wish to utilize it.

Any number of politicians and social critics would have us believe that the answer is in the social distribution of the system, *not* in the philosophical essence of the system itself.

They hence have attempted to narrow the debate to being one of "universal healthcare" (socialized medicine) vs. private healthcare.

While this study has explained that what the United States currently has is a hybrid most classifiable as *fascist* medicine, it should be clear that the political issue of how healthcare is to be made available is separate and apart from the *nature* of medicine:

While it is certainly true that most civilized countries have a form of socialized medicine (though many, such as Germany, allow freedom of choice for other medical models not "covered" by the state), there is no correlation between the method of healthcare delivery and the implied goal of any system: delivery of good health.

No greater a model for socialized medicine existed than in the prior Soviet Union (and indeed, in all socialist-bloc states) — yet the rates of chronic, systemic diseases and metabolic disorders were as bad — and at times worse — in the USSR than in any Western nation.

Do not look to Canada

Americans who look to Canada should also be aware that, whatever the successes of Canada in redistributing the cost of medicine (while hiking taxes) so that it is of universal access, increasingly Canadian medics and citizens have opted out of the system:

— In 1994, most of the 23,000 doctors in Ontario, Canada's most populous province, took a one-week "vacation" without pay because the Canadian healthcare system could not afford to pay them for a full year.(1)

— In 1993, a record number of Canadian doctors — 650 — moved to the United States, while thousands of nursing graduates were said to be "flocking south" in search of greener fields. Why not? They had taken a 2 percent pay cut and hospital staffs faced reductions across the country.(2)

— More affluent Canadians, frustrated over long lines and long waits, routinely slip across the border for therapy in the USA. The Fraser Institute reported that 177,297 Canadians were on waiting lists for surgery in 1992, and that, as in Newfoundland, there were two-month waits for patients seeking CAT scans and two-month delays for women needing "urgent" Pap smears.(3)

In 1994, it was reported that a tenth of the 40,000 hospital beds in Toronto had been closed in the past three years due to funding shortages.(4)

In 1996, doctors in British Columbia unleashed a campaign of "reduced activity days" (seeing only emergency cases) after taking a 3 percent pay cut.(5)

Do not look to the UK

As we have seen (*VII*), the United Kingdom's long-time flirtation with socialized medicine on a population base far inferior to that of the United States not only has failed to significantly curb degenerative diseases but has led to cries for reform there, including far more assent by the status quo to "complementary" therapies in that country than in ours.

By 1997, the National Health Service (NHS), regarded as the world's most tightly run socialized medicine system, was in such dire straits due to consistent funding cutbacks and ever-longer waits even for emergency services that the deputy chairman of the British Medical Assn.'s consultants' and specialists' committee described the system as "unraveling."(6)

Long waits — the Bristol Oncology Centre had some patients, expected to live for only two months, on one-month-long waiting lists for acute pain relief following funding cutbacks; *two-year* waits for magnetic resonance (MRI) scans and *four-year* waits for orthopedic consultations were reported — were among the many reasons that some 12 percent of Britons had opted for private medical insurance and "untold numbers" were paying out-of-pocket for emergency and specialized treatments.(7)

Any governmental health system (as we have seen in Medicare and Medicaid in this country) faces the same problems:

— Availability and funding at the whim of master planners and politicians. In totalitarian societies, access to "free medicine" is a political function, so that dissidents (enemies of the state) may be denied such service.

— Increased demand (much of it from hypochondriacs and the chronically ill) will *always* exceed availability with the concomitant problems of ever-increasing waiting periods and rationed medical services.

— Caregivers will be either chronically overworked or even underworked, depending on where they are, with an increase in frustration and inattentiveness.

It cannot be stressed enough that international pharmaceutical interests, the motor of the allopathic paradigm, essentially do not care *what* the medical system is politically as long as it remains drug-dependent. The drug behemoths will be paid whether the payer is the patient, an insurance company or the government.

Comparing the United States with small, homogeneous countries in the distribution of healthcare services, as frequently done by proponents of socialized medicine, is a case of mixing apples and oranges.

Centralized planning, control and distribution are easier, even more effective, in small-population countries even if, over time, the same problems giant nation-states face with centralized planning will occur.

We would strongly argue that the urge to centralize control and planning, however seemingly rational and convenient it may seem for the short-term resolution of problems of social organization, is the central flaw in collective political thought which ineluctably leads to tyranny.

Liberty vs. central planning

This is because of the historically long observed phenomenon that there can be no effective central planning without an equal portion of central compliance — and that centralized compliance is the wellspring of political tyranny. The criminal actions of this nation's Food and Drug Administration (FDA) against "alternative" healers and their patients is a stark and unforgiving manifestation of this basic truth.

There are those who would argue that, by the end of the 20th century, it is somehow too late to argue about the relevance of giant government in the management and ultimate control of our lives (including all decisions on healthcare) — that the sands of time have irreversibly blown in the direction of gigantic governments, gigantic corporations, gigantic planning.

But some of us beg to differ. It is extremely unlikely that human liberty — assuming this to be a worthwhile goal at all — can flower in a collectivistic, big-government statist environment, no matter what the excuses or pretexts for such gargantuan governance are.

The framers of the American republic — frequently dismissed in the modern era as well-meaning gentlemen agrarian aristocrats who could not foresee the eventual need for huge government to "manage" everything — were far shrewder than the historical revisionists give them credit for.

They fully understood the need not to further unleash the government and to put chains on the people but to free the people and place chains on the government. That — originally — was what this country was all about.

By the 1990s, as the nation engaged in a raging debate over the healthcare crisis, at least several of the States had taken steps to attempt to impose healthcare reform within their borders — a decentralist move in keeping with the spirit of the US Constitution.

Others were moving to protect medical practitioners who engaged in "alternative therapy" — a state-by-state effort redolent of that which in the 1970s and early 1980s had led to the "decriminalization" of laetrile in 24 states. (See *XII*)

That effort had demonstrated how a grass-roots, *decentralist* activity could rapidly outpace central planners and the central (federal) government. This constitutionally republicanist effort vindicated the wisdom of the Founding Fathers and proved to Americans that liberty in general was still rescuable.

In 1993, the Committee for Freedom of Choice in Medicine Inc. presented a conceptual program to the Clinton Administration as a model for an attempt at healthcare reform for earth's mightiest power within both the spirit and letter of the US Constitution.

The program (Appendix B) is a suggested mingling of federal and state actions to defang both governmental *and* private monopoly and to restore medical freedom of choice — with informed consent — for physician and patient, the single guiding doctrine of the Committee.

For if — in keeping with the spirit of the Constitution — the people and their healthcare practitioners (of *any* school) have access to freedom of choice in medicine the political barriers to medical reform will have ended and a free people can get about the business of a new paradigm:

The promotion of health.

References

1. Jacobson, Sherry, *The Dallas Morning News*. Feb. 27, 1994.
2. *Ibid.*
3. Lee, RW, "Should we copy Canada?" *The New American*. Nov. 1, 1993.
4. Jacobson, *op. cit.*
5. "Physicians react to budget woes." *J. Am. Med. Assn.*. Dec. 11, 1996.
6. Lyall, Sarah, "For British health system, bleak prognosis." *The New York Times*, Jan. 30, 1997.
7. *Ibid.*

APPENDIX B

THE COMMITTEE FOR FREEDOM OF CHOICE IN MEDICINE INC. PLAN FOR HEALTHCARE REFORM

(Originally Presented February 19, 1993, to the Presidential Task Force on Healthcare Reform)

Dear Chairperson Clinton:

The Committee for Freedom of Choice in Medicine, Inc. takes this opportunity to congratulate you on your appointment and to extend our best wishes as well as our ideas on the urgent need for healthcare reform in America.

You are aware of the healthcare crisis in this nation. Synthesizing our organization's views and suggestions on (a) the nature of this crisis and (b) how it may be managed and, hopefully, solved, we set forth the following:

THE PROBLEM(S): The extraordinarily high cost of medical care (to the extent that between 37 and 40 million Americans are unable to afford medical coverage) which will assume a constant-dollars total cost of $1 trillion by mid-decade and already consumes 15 percent of gross domestic product (GDP), while the existing medical structure is essentially a failure in coming to grips with the modern chronic killer diseases, now poised to destroy Western civilization.

GOALS: To solve the above while enhancing overall access by the public to achieving promotive health through the availability of options and choices within a political model which respects the virtues of Constitutional republicanism without enhancing the grasp and reach of government.

SOLUTIONS TO THE PROBLEM(S)

— Replacing the current allopathic paradigm with an integrative model in which all medical approaches are assured a level playing field.

— Decentralizing medical decision-making so that the States may assume greater burdens and their own innovations in the matter of licensure, surveillance, sanction and insurance. (President Clinton, at least rhetorically, has suggested this in terms of the diffusion of Medicare/Medicaid.)

— Dismantling the Food and Drug Administration (FDA) as currently constituted.

— Protecting consumer access to dietary and nutrient supplements as first-line preventive maintenance health options and allowing honest and accurate health claims to be made about them by producers and distributors.

— Providing tax incentives for corporate structures and companies to establish promotive-health programs and/or private group medical plans.

— Enhancing antitrust and racketeering enforcement against organizational and professional combines which seek to prevent the free interstate flow of medical information and/or to monopolize the medical marketplace for a single school of medical thought.

This endeavor implies a paradigm shift from emphasizing management of disease and the prolongation of death to encouraging promotive health. Politically, this means a vast decentralization on the federalist model, with the States assuming far more individual and creative responsibilities, the resurrection of an authentic free market of competitive medical ideas (thus an end to the Allopathic Industrial Complex/monopoly), a dismantling of the frequently corrupt Food and Drug Administration (FDA) or a rewriting of its enabling legislation to capture the original intent of establishing responsible surveillance over the purity (and labeling honesty) of foods and drugs.

Decentralizing medicine to the States and allowing States to assume many more of the functions of existing federal programs should vastly eliminate the bureaucratic paperwork gridlock at the top which is itself a significant contributor to our (currently) $900 billion healthcare tab. The overall economic goal: vast reduction in the cost of healthcare delivery.

Such a shift also implies empowering the general population (medical consumers) to make first-line or primary decisions on their health and well-being through access to a free market of medical practitioners of their choice as well as access to health-oriented products consisting of vitamins, minerals, amino acids, enzymes, herbs and/or any combination of the above, along with such parallel State-level developments as the legalization of midwifery and consumer-level nutritional counselors.

State-level legislative action (if necessary) should in effect persuade private insurers to provide fair and equal coverage of *all* forms of competitive medicine with the view in mind of vastly reducing the cost of medicine through free-market forces and hence lowering the cost of private medical insurance. Existing federal insurance schemes, however currently bloated and out of control (Medicare, Medicaid), should gradually be diffused in power, administration and authority to the States, with federal funds (matching or otherwise) available solely as safety-net operations for the most disadvantaged.

The IRS code should allow for tax incentives for companies and corporations for group private insurance plans.

Parallel to these developments, the nation's pharmaceutical industry should be congressionally investigated along the lines of domestic monopolism, restraint of trade, racketeering and, if necessary, legislatively trust-busted to allow for the competition of smaller firms involved in the research, development and distribution of medically oriented products. This investigation should look deeply into the international aspects of the major pharmaceutical companies with emphasis on monopolism, price-fixing, restraint of trade and racketeering, along with whatever conflict-of-interest relationships as may exist between pharmaceutical companies, the FDA and other federal and State governmental agencies.

Equal enforcement efforts should be mounted against any professional organization or combination of organizations, societies or individuals who or which are involved in restricting the free flow of information concerning medical products, medical theories and treatment practices for reasons of exclusion or monopoly, or who or which utilize positions of privilege to defame, malign, vilify or intimidate individuals, organizations or enterprises for reasons of exclusion or monopolism.

At the federal and State levels there should be an immediate end to the multi-agency harassment of medical practitioners and/or healthfoods and supplement companies who or which make honest claims on their products simply because the former may be practicing "non-mainstream" medicine or because the latter represent an economic threat to the Allopathic Industrial Complex.

NATURE AND CAUSES OF THE PROBLEM(S)

The generic root of the problems lies in two of the great defining elements of human nature (greed and ego, with a greater proportion of the former than the latter) which devolve into these aspects:

— The primacy of a single model of medical thought, a paradigm which has guided American and therefore Western medicine for the better part of a century. This model, *allopathy* — which is usually what the existing American medical/pharmaceutical establishment actually means when it utilizes such terms as "mainstream", "orthodox", "conventional" and even "rigorously scientific" medicine, and even by use of the exclusive term "medicine" itself (the same establishment having also co-opted the term "physician" while indirectly attempting to appropriate "doctor") — has driven from the field all competitors in the ideological and conceptual marketplace except for those which have achieved partial rescue through legal action (chiropractic) and others which survive as allopathic hybrids (osteopathy).

So sweeping and total has been the genesis and nurturing of this paradigm that the majority of American medical practices/products consumers are not aware that there are other schools of legitimate medical thought. Allopathic medicine is that which is protected by sanction and licensure, with only trained allopaths accorded full access to patients and only allopaths bearing full hospital access. The allopathic model or paradigm is sustained and buttressed by the media and so interlocked with related vested interests that what is or is not "medicine" is often obscured in the public mind.

— The use or capture of this particular model of medical thought by international pharmaceutical interests. Extensive data detail the rise of drug-based medicine in this country (and elsewhere) as parallel to the enshrining of the allopathic model as the single healing paradigm to be accorded sanction and licensure in the United States. Several historical trends converged in the first two decades of the present century to allow the profit-driven pharmaceutical combines to utilize allopathy as a channel for their products (while, to be sure, assisting in notable victories over infectious disease) and to dominate "medical" education and "medical" literature. A huge role in this effort was played by the amassed-wealth foundations of several ultrawealthy families whose profits were protected by the tax-free foundation scheme while protected funds were deflected into such educational, research and propaganda measures as would build what is today the Allopathic Industrial Complex.

This complex (of interlocking pharmaceutical houses, research centers, universities, corporations, companies, hospitals, insurance plans, medications, drugs, hospital equipment, high-technology diagnostics) is so intertwined with corporate America (transportation, publishing, utilities, department stores, energy, etc., etc.) that lines of demarcation between the Allopathic Industrial Complex itself and its overlap with this broader complex, and the multitude of interests influenced by, or dependent upon it, are often vague, which helps explain the seemingly ubiquitous presence of the allopathic medical paradigm and its seemingly wide acceptance by the consuming public.

— The American Medical Association (AMA), which actually grew out of mid-19th-century efforts to organize the "regulars" (that is, allopathic dispensers of minerals and surgery) against the "irregulars" (primarily the homeopaths, who represented both a conceptual and economic threat to the regulars), which has become the organized voice not of medicine itself but of allopathy, constituting in effect a labor union for allopathic physicians and an ongoing propaganda voice for the concept of "scientific medicine" (essentially an oxymoron, in that until this century medicine was essentially conceived of as an art rather than a science).

AMA is the education-orienting force of allopathy whose "seal of approval" on techniques, theories and products is the ever-present guiding hand of the medical establishment. Its ruthless efforts to suppress competitors only became fully public in the 1980s with the federal court victory by chiropractors against the AMA and its allies.

State medical boards, state "medical quality assurance" boards, state medical vigilance and punishment boards, are comprised in the main of AMA members. State-level AMAs constitute major political action committees (PACs) in every state and, in sum, constitute one of the major federal lobbying forces at the legislative level. It is perhaps more than symbolic that the *Journal* of the AMA is laden, cover to cover, with high-tech advertisements from the very international/pharmaceutical behemoths whose gargantuan profits depend on the primacy of the allopathic model.

— The Food and Drug Administration (FDA), an example of a good governmental idea gone woefully wrong. The "compliance" wing of this bloated federal satrapy has been used time and again in recent decades to suppress, harass, prosecute, persecute and intimidate the burgeoning healthfoods and supplements industries (which the Allopathic Industrial Complex regards as a major threat), as well as healthcare practitioners of all kinds (including progressive allopaths) who dare abandon the key elements of allopathy (surgery, radiation, toxic chemicals, invasive techniques, awesomely expensive diagnostics).

MDs, chiropractors, naturopaths, homeopaths, herbalists, Native American healers, acupuncturists, and even midwives have been among targets of the FDA and compliant State agencies involved in an ongoing conspiracy to punish medical rebels and protect the profits of the pharmaceutical industry. The attached litany of recent FDA-associated actions against individuals, companies and organizations constitutes a shameful and viciously tyrannical chapter in American history, and the most dispassionate review of FDA "compliance" behavior should indicate how far afield this bureaucracy-for-life has strayed from its original enabling legislation as a monitor of safety and purity in foods and drugs. As presently constituted, the FDA, compliance division, is little more than a police force for drug interests and, as recent history has shown, has often been corrupted.

CURRENT SITUATION

The above synthesis of the situation, and the out-of-control costs of delivering the allopathic medical product (with its attendant swollen prices in medicines, diagnostics, practices, etc.) would very likely be well tolerated by our people if in fact we were receiving value in kind. A synthesis of the current medical reality, however, discloses that we are not:

Despite the costliest medical establishment in the world, the United States has no cure for *most* of metastatic cancer, *all* of AIDS, and even much of that complex of conditions referred to as "heart disease", and is *24th* in infant mortality. It stands impuissant in the face of an ever-lengthening list of allegedly incurable maladies of the young and old: cystic fibrosis, muscular dystrophy, lupus, rheumatoid arthritis, multiple sclerosis, Parkinson's, Alzheimer's's, chronic fatigue, ALS, osteoporosis, and a veritable maze of conditions and metabolic disorders unknown earlier in this century.

Despite increases in overall life expectancy, allopathy's earlier triumphs over major infections and improvements in sophisticated diagnostic techniques, this nation does not have a health-care delivery system so much as a death-prolonging "sick business". A few extra years of physical existence achieved by electronic hookup and stultifying drugs can only vaguely be defined as "life".

It is because so many Americans are increasingly informed of the above that they are turning — in droves, as recent information now proves — to so-called "alternative" or "unconventional" therapies. They first seek these out in the United States — that is, when their practitioner is not too afraid to provide them and who may risk his/her professional and social standing and medical license by so doing. Yet because the Allopathic Industrial Complex is so vast and nationwide in scope it is difficult to find healthcare givers in *any* State who are not in some way (be it statutorily or professionally) hamstrung in their efforts to provide more choices for our ever-sicker population (one member of which dies every 60 seconds from cancer).

With the compliant media also interlocked with the Allopathic Industrial Complex and the allopathic model the only one seemingly operative at the conscious level in the minds of so many journalists, American medical consumers are often left either uninformed or ill-informed about available medical options and are, at the least, socially pressured into acceptance of the standard medical system even if it means certain death and suffering. Hence, should they be adequately informed and economically advantaged, they seek healthcare outside their home country. The Hobson's choice for an American with a life-threatening disorder who seeks "alternatives" to allopathy is simple: do without, attempt to go underground and locate a practitioner willing to place himself in jeopardy, or flee the country.

As these lines are written, no less than 30 clinics, hospitals and other operations claiming to offer "alternative medicine" and serving a clientele made up of up to 90% or more Americans now function in the area of Tijuana, Mexico, alone. This is a giant leap from a decade ago, when American medical and pharmaceutical front groups ("quackbusters") began their noisy if failing campaign to "alert" Americans to "quackery" and "quack clinics". While many of these operations are indeed suspect and some are outright frauds, in their totality they reflect the abject failure of American medicine against chronic degenerative disease. Studies continue to point out that Americans who seek "alternative" therapies either at home or abroad are, in the main, among the better-educated of our citizens.

There is no moral reason why an American citizen should have to leave this country to save his/her life! There is no *good* reason (though there are many *bad* ones) why an American with a life-threatening disease should have to face the prospect of being abandoned by this country and its medical establishment in an effort — however remote — to save his/her life.

SOLUTIONS: AN OVERVIEW

Approaches to this problem run the gamut of political theory, and it is not the Committee's position that any single individual or organization has a total solution. But we add here both suggestions and recommendations.

1. Socializing medicine (that is, establishing the federal government as a single payer) is not the solution if we are seeking promotive health for the general population. A socialist system might take the immediate sting out of medical costs for a majority of people, but history is eloquent in displaying how the costs of government in general rise when *any* presumed right is guaranteed and/or nurtured by the government. Western countries with socialist and semi-socialist systems have the same (and at times worse) rates of chronic disease as does the United States.

The role of the federal government in assuming medical care (if it be the nation's will that government should play any such role) should be, at best, what it often already is in several areas: safety net of last resort when all else fails. That is, neither the paying for nor setting forth the treatment parameters of healthcare should be mandated from top-down; rather they should rise, albeit disproportionately, from the ground up.

2. A free market in medicine is the proper goal of a republican society which also engages in competitive (rather than monopolist) capitalism. With the cancer and AIDS crises alone poised to wipe out not only American civilization but the Western gene pool itself, the times cry out not for more restrictive adherence to a set of postulates and doctrines which have plainly failed (as in allopathic medicine) but for the encouragement of the broadest possible field of options and ideas. If there is a federal role in this paradigm shift, it should be as a stated policy, not a new statute to be exercised by yet another tax-enhancing bureaucracy. In the federalist mold, that of our Constitution, the manner in which a free market is approached should be at the State level.

WHAT THE STATES CAN DO

The States might undertake legislatively several changes:

1. It may not be necessary to license physicians at all. The licensure procedure itself is prone to corrupting influences.

2. But degrees from qualified (and state-licensed) medical schools (of all concepts) should be necessary for the practice of any form of medicine.

3. State legislation . . . should protect the right of *all* qualified practitioners to engage in putatively "unorthodox" or "non-mainstream" medical practices under the following qualifications:

   a. That the condition be life-threatening (though some States might waive this qualification).

   b. That the procedure, treatment or compound *itself* not be dangerous to the patient.

   c. That the practitioner discuss all known available options with the patient.

4. Existing medical insurance plans should not discriminate in reimbursing for medical services as long as the qualified practitioner and patient have made an informed-consent decision for the service.

5. There should be freedom on the part of all qualified practitioners of all schools of medicine to advertise for their services and freely compete for consumers within the statutory and regulatory confines of an orderly profession.

6. State medical boards of oversight, compliance/ regulation, etc., should be composed of representatives of *all* forms of medicine practicing within that State.

Each State may view differently the issue of licensing midwives and allowing therapeutic abortions. The intent here is to decentralize medicine from its allopathic center to allow a broad range of options, which are both therapeutically and economically competitive. It is also assumed the States will continue to enforce statutes on the safety and purity of drugs, nutrients and medical equipment.

WHAT THE FEDERAL LEVEL CAN DO

At the federal level, real change could be accomplished swiftly in a single stroke (as suggested in 1992 at the "working group on unconventional medical practices" of the National Institutes of Health) by:

1. Removing the so-called Kefauver amendments ("efficacy clauses") of the Food, Drug and Cosmetic Act as amended in 1962. The language in the above equipped the FDA with enormous policing/compliance power, virtually all of it used *against* non-allopathic therapies and the healthfoods and supplements industries. The amendments allow the state to intervene in the doctor-patient relationship at precisely the point it should not: freedom of choice of both to reach an informed decision on therapy. Only the doctor and patient, working together, are in any real position to know what does or does not have "efficacy". In addition:

2. The food-purity aspects of the FDA might be transferred to the US Department of Agriculture.

And, however a new food and drug law is to be rewritten, it should be clear that:

3. No agency shall use the fact that a valid health claim is made on the label of a food, food supplement, nutrient, herbal or similar product as a pretext to attempt to monitor or control the same as a "drug".

4. Therapeutically high doses of vitamins, minerals, enzymes, amino acids, herbal compounds and similar products might be statutorily protected at both the federal and State levels by classifying them as "nutraceuticals", as suggested by several distinguished American researchers.

5. The primary federal research parameter for acceptance of a new drug, technique or practice should be one:

Disease-free survival time.

This does not preclude a reasonable review of foreign literature for non-American products seeking access to the American market, nor an end to limited testing on animals for toxicity of certain compounds. The reliance on animal test models and the numbing persistence of the monofactorial, randomized, placebo-controlled, double-blind cross-over approach may still have some merit in the toxicity assessments of single therapeutics but is essentially irrelevant in the development of multifactorial, natural therapies for individualized use in humans.

The presence of 17th-century "rigorously scientific" postulates for monopharmacy has been a major roadblock — together with the enormous costs of developing the same through FDA channels — in the elaboration both of new single compounds and certainly in the advent of individualized, multifactorial protocols against chronic disease.

The IRS code should be revised to allow for tax incentives for companies, corporations and other business structures and/or labor unions or any other business or professional or bureaucratic organization or combination to establish promotive-health programs for employees, members, associates or shareholders and/or to encourage such entities to provide, at least as partial payment, private-enterprise group medical coverage.

Such coverage should not discriminate on the basis of a given medical theory or school of thought and should include payment for the services of all recognized healthcare practitioners whose validity or certification may be determined by the individual States.

The IRS code should be changed, if necessary, to provide tax incentives for the elderly, the retired, or the elderly retired on fixed incomes, to seek out private medical insurance coverage (as a way to shift significant elements of the population off Medicare, Medicaid, etc.)

There should be an inducement at the federal level for insurance companies to explain billing procedures in a uniform way and to attempt as far as feasible to set fair, understandable, acceptable and provable rates for all those covered regardless of the State or Territory in which they live, notwithstanding the insurance company's conceivably legitimate explanation of why rates might have to vary from one locale to another.

The costs and administration of Medicare, Medicaid and any other similar federal program should be transferred increasingly and over time to the States on a State-by-State basis.

Coverage by Medicare, Medicaid or any other federal program should not discriminate on the basis of medical schools of thought and medical theories. Such programs should not discriminate in coverage between health practitioners as duly and separately certified, licensed or accepted based on the separate provisions of the States, Territories or the District of Columbia.

The Veterans Administration and/or any federal agency or department involved in healthcare delivery should not discriminate on the basis of medical schools of thought and medical theories.

It should be clear that the will of the nation is that no existing federal law, bureau or department has been or will be established to engage directly in the practice of medicine.

There should be a Congressional-level investigation of possible price-fixing activities and monopolism within the pharmaceutical industry, an overview of the domestic industry's links with international pharmaceutical conglomerates, and an investigation of the pharmaceutical industry's relations, particularly involving conflicts of interest and retirement policies, with federal and State governments, and of the lobbying efforts of AMA-aligned or AMA-directed State or federal level political action committees (PACs) in connection with attempts to establish, maintain or protect monopolies and/or hinder the free flow of medical information.

The federal government should not inhibit the importation into the USA from foreign sources by American patients of medicines, compounds and medical devices which may or may not be approved by federal or State statutes or regulations absent the finding that any such medicine, compound or device poses a direct, palpable danger to the patient or to society at large.

WHAT BOTH LEVELS CAN DO

Consumers (the general public) should be empowered to make medical decisions in no small part on their own and have access to nutritional therapies and products which credible scientific evidence suggests may assist them in the goal of promotive health, preventive medicine and at-home management of some disease conditions.

Insurance companies should be encouraged to provide coverage for *all* forms of medical endeavor based upon the certification, licensure or acceptance of any given school of medical thought in any State. Their guidelines at the federal level should be equally broad.

State and federal agencies should not be involved in the denial of medical options and choices either to consumers (the general public) or to healthcare providers, nor should any combination of State and federal agencies together or separately or in combination with professional and other organizations, individuals and combinations thereof seek to harass, prosecute, persecute, intimidate or undermine the legitimate interests of medical freedom of choice in options and the free market thereof or engage in any practice, tactic or endeavor which seeks to establish, empower, maintain or protect a medical monopoly for economic, ego, or any other reason.

State and federal law enforcement should investigate and prosecute any attempt by public or private agencies, bureaus, boards, professional groups or individuals who or which seek to establish, maintain or protect any form of medical-practice monopoly be it in services, techniques, equipment or products, or to slander, vilify or bring into public discredit the proponents, defenders, or owners or operators of "non-mainstream" medical centers, medical practices, medical techniques or products held not to or be part of allopathic services, techniques, equipment or products. Enforcement should be along the lines of investigating monopolism, trust-making, collusion, conspiracy, racketeering, and civil rights violations.

To the extent practicable, the practice of any form of medicine should be separate from and distinct to the provision of goods and services which might be involved in this form of medicine.

Federal and state tax codes should be revised to allow for tax incentives for companies, corporations and other business structures and/or labor unions or any other business or professional or bureaucratic organization or other combination of citizens to establish promotive-health programs for employees, members, associates or shareholders and/or encourage such entities to provide, at least as partial payment, group medical coverage. Such coverage should not discriminate on the basis of a given medical theory or school of thought and should include payment for the services of all recognized healthcare practitioners whose validity or certification may be determined by the individual States. Nor should any such coverage be mandated or enforced as a requirement for employment, membership or association.

There should be a computer-based or other reliable tracking system so that a patient might know if a practitioner of any kind has undergone loss of insurance, legal problems, disciplinary problems, etc., so that a patient, particularly one with a life-threatening disorder or who is about to give birth in a hospital setting, would know the possible "negatives" about the practitioner into whose hands one is placing his/her body or life.

We believe that attempts to reform healthcare conceptually, economically and politically along the lines described above will result in a resurrection of medical freedom of choice for all Americans, a wholesale reduction in the runaway costs of the provision of medical goods and services, eventual victory over the killer diseases of the current era through unleashing the creative energies of the unfettered human mind operating in an essentially free marketplace of ideas, goods and services and research, and a reorienting of society toward promotive health rather than the management of death and disease.

With such a goal in mind, we reiterate our congratulations and best wishes to you in overseeing the considerable task with which you have been charged, and express our support and availability to discuss with you or work with you in the furtherance of these aims and objectives.

M.L. CULBERT,DSc, *chairman emeritus*
R.W. BRADFORD,DSc, *President-founder*

APPENDIX C
MODEL STATE-LEVEL LEGISLATION for MEDICAL FREEDOM OF CHOICE

1) Neither the State of ________________ nor any agency, division, department or bureau thereof, shall interfere with the medical practices of any duly qualified practitioner of the medical arts because such practitioner engages in a form of the medical arts which may not be considered standard or orthodox practice by prevailing standard definitions *absent the finding* that any such practice represents a direct threat to the life or health of the patient.

2) Any duly qualified practitioner of the medical arts in ____________ shall, at the request of a patient, provide information on optional treatments, or allow patient access to such information, particularly in those cases in which prevailing medical opinion has determined the patient to be in a "terminal," "incurable" or "end-state" condition.

3) Neither the State of ________________ nor any agency, division, department or bureau thereof, shall interfere with the right of a duly qualified practitioner of the medical arts to receive into the state for his or her professional use any nutrient, herbal or other natural substance or combination of substances or any chemical substance or combination thereof or any device or technique which is not considered standard or orthodox practice for medical or diagnostic or evaluative use by prevailing standard definitions of orthodox medicine *absent the finding* that any such substance or combination of substances or device or technique represents a direct threat to the life or health of the patient.

4) Neither the State of ________________ nor any agency, division, department or bureau thereof, shall interfere with the right of a duly qualified practitioner of the medical arts to counsel with, or provide information to, his or her patients concerning substances, therapies, devices or techniques which may not be considered standard practice by prevailing standard definitions, *absent the finding* that such counsel or information represents a direct threat to the life or health of the patient.

APPENDIX D

RESOURCES

ORGANIZATIONS

Governmental

Office of Alternative Medicine (OAM)
National Institutes of Health
OAM Information Center
9000 Rockville Pike, Mail Stop 2182
Bethesda MD 20892
Tel. (310) 402-2466
FAX (301) 402-4741

Research, information, education, referral, advocacy, supplements industry, patient services, etc.

Academy for Guided Imagery
P.O. Box 2070
Mill Valley CA 94942
Tels. (415) 389-9324 / 1-800-726-2070
FAX (415) 389-9342

Alliance for Alternative Medicine
160 NW Widmer Place
Albany OR 97321-1589
Tel. (503) 926-1626
FAX (503) 684-9705

Alternative Therapies Health Assn.
P.O. Box 891630
Oklahoma City OK 73189-1630
Tels. (405) 634-3799 / 1-800-988-1238
FAX (405) 634-7320

American Academy of Medical Acupuncture
5820 Wilshire Blvd., Suite 500
Los Angeles CA 90036
Tel. 1-800-521-2262

American Alliance of Aromatherapy
P.O. Box 750428
Petaluma CA 94975-0428
Tel (707) 778-6762
FAX (707) 769-0860

American Assn. of Holistic Nurses
4101 Lake Boone Trail, Suite 201
Raleigh NC 27607
Tel. (919) 787-5181

American Assn. of Naturopathic Physicians (AANP)
6010 Valley St., Suite 105
Seattle WA 98109
Tel. (206) 298-0126
FAX (206) 298-0129

American Assn. of Oriental Medicine
433 Front St.
Catasauqua PA 18032-2506
Tel (610) 266-2448
FAX (610) 264-2768

American Board of Chelation Therapy
1407B N. Wells
Chicago IL 60610
Tels. (321) 787-ABCT/1-800-356-2228

American Botanical Council
P O Box 201660
Austin TX 78720-1660
Tels. 1-800-373-7105 /
(512) 331-8868
FAX (512) 331-1924

American Chiropractic Assn.
1701 Clarendon Blvd.
Arlington VA 22209
Tel. (703) 276-8800
FAX (703) 243-2593

American College for Advancement in Medicine (ACAM)
23121 Verdugo Drive, Suite 204
Laguna Hills CA 92653
Tels. (714) 583-7666 / 1-800-532-3688
FAX (714) 455-9679

American Foundation of Traditional Chinese Medicine
505 Beach St.
San Francisco CA 94133
Tel. (415) 776-0502
FAX (415) 776-9053

American Herb Association
P.O. Box 1673
Nevada City CA 95959
Tel. (916) 265-9552
FAX (916) 274-3140
(Includes information on herb schools/classes)

American Herbal Products Assn.
4733 Bethesda Ave., Suite 0585
Bethesda MD 20824-0585
Tel. (301) 951-3204
FAX (301) 951-3205

American Herbalist Guild
P O Box 746555
Arvada CO 80006
Tel. (303) 423-8800
FAX (303) 423-8828

American Holistic Health Association
P.O. Box 17400
Anaheim CA 92817-7400
Tel (714) 779-6152

American Holistic Medical Assn.
4101 Lake Boone trail, Suite 201
Raleigh NC 27607
Tel. (919) 787-5146
FAX (919) 787-4916

American Holistic Nurses Association
4101 Lake Boone Trail, Suite 201
Raleigh NC 27607
Tels. (919) 787-5181/1-800-278-2462
FAX (919) 787-4916

American Institute of Homeopathy
925 East 17th Ave.
Denver CO 80218-1407

American Massage Therapy Assn.
820 David St., Suite 100
Evanston IL 60201-4444
Tel. (847) 864-0123

American Naturopathic Medical Assn. (ANMA)
P O Box 96273
Las Vegas NV 89193
Tel. (702) 897-7053

American Preventive Medical Assn.
459 Walker Road
Great Falls VA 22066
Tels. (703) 759-0662 / 1-800-230-2762

American Reflexology Certification Board
P.O. Box 620607
Littleton CO 80162
Tel. (303) 933-6921
(Certification, information on reflexologists and reflexology schools)

American Yoga Association
513 South Orange Ave.
Sarasota FL 34236
Tels. (941) 953-5859/1-800-226-5859
FAX (941) 364-9153

Associated Bodywork and Massage Professionals
28677 Buffalo Park Rd.
Evergreen CO 80439-7347
Tels.((303) 674-8478/1-800-458-2267
FAX (303) 674-0859

Association for Applied Psychophysiology and Biofeedback
10200 W. 44th Ave #304
Wheat Ridge CO 80033-2840
Tels. (303) 422-8436/1-800-477-8892

Ayurvedic Institute
11311 Menual NE, Suite A
Albuquerque NM 87112
Tel. (505) 291-9698
FAX (505) 294-7572

Bradford Research Institute
1180 Walnut Avenue
Chula Vista CA 91911
Tels. (619) 429-8200/1-800-227-4458
FAX (619) 429-8004
(*Answers American Biologics*)

Cancer Control Society/Cancer Book House
2043 N. Berendo St.
Los Angeles CA 90027
Tel. (213) 663-7801

Cancer Support and Education
1035 Pine St.
Menlo Park CA 94025
Tel. (415) 327-6166

(The) Cancer Support Community
350 Bay Street
San Francisco CA 94133
Tel. (415) 648-9400

CANHELP
3100 Paradise Bay Road
Port Ludlow WA 98365-9771
Tel. (206) 437-2291

Center for Attitudinal Healing
33 Buchanan Drive
Sausalito CA 94965
Tel. (415) 331-6161

Center for Frontier Sciences
Temple University, Ritter Hall 003-00
Philadelphia PA 19122
FAX (215) 204-5553

Center for Mind-Body Medicine
5225 Connecticut Ave., NW, Suite 414
Washington DC 20015
Tel. (202) 966-7338
FAX (202) 966-2589

Center for Reiki Training
29209 Northwestern Highway #592
Southfield MI 48034
Tel. (810) 948-8112
FAX (810) 948-9534

Citizens for Health
P O Box 1195
Tacoma WA 98401
Tel. (206) 922-2457
FAX (206) 922-7583

Chronic Fatigue & Immune Dysfunction
Media Awarness Assn. of America
17131 Village 17
Camarillo CA 93012
Tel. (805) 383- 1043
FAX (805) 384-1077

Citizens for Health
P.O. Box 2260
Boulder CO 80306
Tel. 1-800-357-2211
FAX (303) 417-9278

Committee for Freedom of Choice in Medicine, Inc.
1180 Walnut Avenue
Chula Vista CA 91911
Tels. (619) 429-8200 and 1-800-227-4458
FAX (619) 429-8004
(Answers American Biologics)

Commonweal Cancer Help Program
P O Box 316
Bolinas CA 94924
Tel. (415) 868-0970

(The) Council for Homeopathic Certification
1709 Seabright Ave.
Santa Cruz CA 95062
Tel. (408) 421-0565

East West Academy of Healing
Arts/Qi Gong Institute
450 Sutter St., Suite 210
San Francisco, CA 94108
Tel. (415) 788-2227
FAX (415) 788-2242

Environmental Health Assn.
1800 Robertson Blvd., Suite 380
Los Angeles CA 90035
Tel. (310) 837-2048

Fetzer Institute
9292 West KL Avenue
Kalamazoo MI 49009-9398
Tel. (616) 375-2000
FAX (616) 372-2163

Foundation for Advancement in Cancer Therapy
P O Box 1242
Old Chelsea Station
New York, NY 10113
Tel. (212) 741-2790

Foundation for Homeopathic Education and Research
2124 Kittredge St.
Berkeley CA 94702
Tel. (510) 649-8930

Foundation for the Advancement of Innovative Medicine (FAIM)
2 Executive Blvd., Suite 404
Suffern NY 10901
Tel. (914) 368-9797
FAX (914) 357-8883

Health Comm, Inc.
5800 Soundview Drive, #E-102
P O Box 1729
Gig Harbor WA 98335

(The) Health Resource
564 Locust St.
Conway AR 72032
Tels. (501) 329-5272/1-800-949-0090
FAX (501) 329-9489

Heliopathic Research Institute and Academy
P.O. Box 281298
Memphis TN 38168-1298

Herb Research Foundation
1007 Pearl St #200
Boulder CO 80302
Tels. (303) 449-2265 / 1-800-748-2617
FAX (303) 449-7849

Himalayan Institute
RR1 Box 400
Honesdale PA 18431
Tel. (717) 253-5551
FAX (717) 253-9078

Holistic Dental Assn.
P.O. Box 5007
Durango CO 81301

Institute for Traditional Medicine and
Preventive Health Care
2017 SE Hawthorne
Portland OR 97214
Tels. (503) 233-4907/1-800-544-7504
FAX (503) 233-1017

Institute of Noetic Sciences (IONS)
P O Box 909 • Sausalito CA 94966-0909
Tels. 1-800-383-1586 / 1-800-383-1394
(415) 331-5650
FAX (415) 331-5677

International Academy of Nutrition and Preventive Medicine
P O Box 18433
Asheville NC 28814-0433
Tel. (704) 258-3243
FAX (704) 253-7781

International Assn. of Cancer Victors and Friends (IACVF)
7740 West Manchester Avenue # 203
Playa del Rey CA 90293
Tel. (310) 822-5032

International Bioxidative Medicine Foundation
P.O. Box 891954
Oklahoma City OK 73189
Tel. (405) 478-4266

International Chiropractic Assn.
1110 N. Glebe Rd., Suite 1000
Arlington VA 22201
Tels. (703) 528-5000/1-800-423-4690
FAX (70) 528-5023

International Council for Health Freedom
5580 La Jolla Blvd., B-429
La Jolla CA 92037
TEL/FAX (619) 581-6640

International Oxidative Medicine Assn.
P.O. Box 890910
Oklahoma City OK 73189
Tel. (405) 634-1310
FAX (405) 634-7320

International Foundation for Homeopathy
P. O. Box 7
Edmonds WA 98020
Tel. (425) 776-4147
FAX (425) 776-1499

International Society for the Study of Subtle Energies
and Energy Medicine
356 Goldco Circle
Golden CO 80401
Tel. (303) 278-2228
FAX (303) 279-3539

Life Extension Foundation
P. O. Box 229120
2490 Griffin Rd.
Ft. Lauderdale FL 33012
Tels. (305) 966-4886 / 1-800-841-LIFE

(The) Mankind Research Foundation
1315 Apple Ave.
Silver Spring MD 20910
Tel. (301) 587-8686
FAX (301) 585-8959

Monterey Institute for the Study
of Alternative Healing Arts
1216 Lawton Avenue
Pacific Grove CA 93950
Tel. (408) 646-0339
TEL./FAX (408) 646-8019

National Assn. for Holistic Aromatherapy
219 Carl St.
San Francisco CA 94117
Tel. (415) 564-6785
FAX (415) 564-6799

National Center for Homeopathy
801 N. Fairfax St., Suite 306
Alexandria VA 22314
Tel. (703) 548-7790
FAX (703) 548-7792

National Council for Improved Health (NCIH)
1555 West Seminole St.
San Marcos CA 92069
Tel. (619) 471-5090

National Health Federation
212 West Foothill Blvd.
Monrovia CA 91016
Tel. (818) 357-2181
FAX (818) 303-0642

National Wellness Institute, Inc.
1300 College Court
Stevens Point WI 54481
Tel. (715) 342-2969
FAX (715) 342-2979

New Mexican Academy of Healing Arts
P.O. Box 932
Santa Fe NM 87504
Tel. (505) 982-6271
FAX (505) 988-2621

New Mexico School of Natural Therapeutics
117 Richmond NE
Albuquerque NM 87106
Tel. (505) 268-6870
FAX (505) 268-0818

(The) New York Open Center
83 Spring St.
New York, NY 10012
Tel. (212) 219-2527
FAX (212) 219-1347

(The) North American Society of Homeopaths
10700 Old Country Rd. #15
Plymouth MN 55411
Tel. (612) 593-9458
FAX (612) 593-0097

Omega Institute for Holistic Studies
260 Lake Drive
Rhinebeck NY 12572-3212
Tel. (914) 266-4444
FAX (914) 266-4828

People Against Cancer
P O Box 10
Otho IA 50569-0010
Tel. (515) 972-4444
FAX (515) 972-4415

Peoples Medical Society
462 Walnut St.
Allentown PA 18102
Tel. (610) 770-1670

Physicians Committee for Responsible Nutrition
5100 Wisconsin Ave. NW., Ste. 404
Washington DC 20016
Tel. (202) 686-2210
FAX (202) 686-2216

Positive Alternative Therapies in Healthcare, Inc.
P O Box 651285
Miami FL 33265

Price-Pottenger Nutrition Foundation
P O Box 2614
La Mesa CA 91944-2614
Tels. 1-800-366-3748
(619) 574-7763 / (619) 582-4168
FAX (619) 574-1314

Professional Assn. of Traditional Healers
1660 Gilpin St
Denver CO 80218
Tel. (303) 333-WELL

Project Cure
16801 Addison Rd., Suite 207
Dallas TX 75246
Tel. (972) 732-7960
FAX (972) 732-7961

(The) Reiki Alliance
P.O. Box 41
Cataldo ID 83810
Tel. (208) 682-3535
FAX (208) 682-4848

Rolf Institute
205 Canyon Blvd.
Boulder CO 80302
Tel. (303) 449-5903

Rosenthal Center for Alternative/Complementary Medicine
College of Physicians and Surgeons
Columbia University
630 W 168th St
New York, NY 10032
Tel. (212) 305-4755

Sarasota School of Natural Healing Arts
8216 South Tamiami Trail
Sarasota FL 34238
Tel. 1-800-966-7117
FAX (813) 966-4414

Society for Orthomolecular Medicine
2698 Pacific Ave.
San Francisco CA 94115
(415) 922-6462
FAX (415) 346-4991

Team Victory
Bethany Community Church
6240 S. Price Road
Tempe AZ 85283-3399

Trager Institute
21 Locust Ave.
Mill Valley CA 94941
Tel. (415) 388-2688

(The) Upledger Institute
11211 Prosperity Farms Rd.
Palm Beach Gardens FL 33410
Tel. 1-800-233-5880

Wellness Referral Network
5307 East Mockingbird Lane, Ste. 404
Dallas TX 75206
Tels. (214) 827-9355/1-800-520-WELL
FAX (214) 828-4064

Wellspring Center for Life Enhancement
3 Otis St.
Watertown MA 02172
Tel. (617) 924-8515

Women for the Advancement of Alternative Medicine
P.O. Box 891630
Oklahoma City OK 73189
Tel. (405) 634-0207

World Chiropractic Alliance
2950 North Dobson Rd., Ste. 1
Chandler AZ 85224
Tel. 1-800-347-1011
FAX (602) 732-9313

World Life Research Institute
23000 Grand Terrace Ave.
Colton CA 92324
Tel. (909) 825-4773
FAX (909) 783-3472

World Research Foundation
20501 Ventura Blvd., #100
Woodland Hills CA 91364
Tel. (818) 999-5483
FAX (818) 227-6484

Collegiate (or advanced or specialized) education

Bastyr University
14500 Juanita Drive NE
Bothell WA 98011-4995
Tel. (206) 823-1300
FAX (206) 823-6222

California Institute of Integral Studies
9 Peter York Way
San Francisco CA 94109
Tel. (415) 674-5500

Capital University of Integrative Medicine
5039 Connecticut Ave. NW
Washington DC 20008
Tel. (202) 237-2446
FAX (20) 237-2448

Chiropractic institutions and programs.
Information on accredited and licensed schools of chiropractic:

- *(The) Council on Chiropractic Education*
  7975 N. Hayden Rd., Ste. A-210
  Scottsdale AZ 85258
  Tel. (602) 443-8877
  FAX (602) 483-7333

- *Federation of Chiropractic Licensing Boards*
  901 5th Ave., Ste. 101
  Greeley CO 80364
  Tel. (970) 356-3500
  FAX (970) 356-3599

Institute for Holistic Healing Studies
San Francsico State University
1600 Holloway Ave.
San Francisco CA 94132
Tel. (415) 338-1200
FAX (415) 338-0573

Maharishi International University
(Center for Health and Aging Studies)
1000 N. 4th St. DB 1028
Fairfield IA 52557-1028
Tel. (515) 472-7000
FAX (415) 472-1189

National Accreditation Commission for Schools of
Acupuncture and Oriental Medicine
8403 Colesville Rd., Ste. 370
Silver Spring MD 20910
Tel. (301) 608-9680
FAX (301) 608-9576
(*Information on accredited schools/programs of acupuncture and Oriental medicine*)

National College of Naturopathic Medicine
11231 SE Market St.
Portland OR 97216
Tel. (503) 255-4860

(The) New Center for Wholistic Health
Education and Research
6801 Jericho Turnpike
Syosset, NY 11791-4413
Tel. (516) 364-0808
FAX (516) 364-0989

North American University
13402 N. Scottsdale Rd., Suite B-150
Scottsdale AZ 85254-4056
Tel. (602) 948-3353
FAX (602) 948-8150

Southwest College of Naturopathic Medicine
and Health Sciences
6535 East Osborn Rd., Suite 703
Scottsdale AZ 85251
Tel. (602) 990-7424
FAX (602) 990-0337

SELECTED BIBLIOGRAPHY

(Recommended reading in aspects of medical history, medical politics and economics, iatrogenic medicine, metabolic and nutritional therapies, integrative treatments, medical futurism and novel theories)

Achterberg, Jeanne, *Imagery in Healing: Shamanism and Modern Medicine.* Boston: New Science Library, 1985.

Ackerknecht, E. K., *Therapeutics: From the Primitive to the 20th Century.* New York: Hafner, 1973.

Adams, Ruth, and Murray, Frank, *Megavitamin Therapy.* New York: Larchmont Books, 1975.

Airola, Paavo, *Hypoglycemia: A Better Approach.* Phoenix AZ: Health Plus, 1977.

Ali, Majid, *Healing, Miracles and the Bite of the Gray Dog.* Denville NJ: Life Span Press, 1997.

Ali, Majid, *RDA: Rats, Drugs and Assumptions* Denville NJ: Life Span Press, 1995.

Ali, Majid, *The Butterfly and Life Span Nutrition.* Bloomfield NJ: Institute of Preventive Medicine, 1992.

Ali, Majid, *The Canary and Chronic Fatigue.* Denville NJ: Life Span Press, 1994.

Ali, Majid, *The Cortical Monkey and Healing.* Bloomfield NJ: Institute of Preventive Medicine, 1990.

Allen, Gary, *The Rockefeller File.* Seal Beach CA: '76 Press, 1976.

Allenberg, Henry, *Holistic Medicine: A Meeting of East and West.* New York: Japan Publishing, 1992.

Alternative Medicine. (The Goldberg Group) Puyallup WA: Future Medicine Publishing, 1993.

Alternative Medicine: Expanding Medical Horizons. Rockville MD: National Institutes of Health, 1994.

Anders, George, *Health Against Wealth.* Boston: Houghton Miffin, 1996.

Andrews, L. B., *Deregulating Doctoring: Do Medical Licensing Laws Meet Today's Health Care Needs?* Emmaus PA: People's Medical Society, 1984.

Annis, E. R., *Code Blue — Health Care in Crisis.* Washington DC: Regnery Gateway, 1992.

Atkins, Robert, *Dr. Atkins' Health Revolution.* Boston: Houghton Mifflin, 1988.

Badgley, Lawrence, *Healing AIDS Naturally.* San Bruno CA: Human Energy Press, 1986.

Balch, James F. and Phyllis A., *Prescription for Nutritional Healing.* Garden City Park NY: Avery, 1990.

Barnett, Beatrice, *Urine Therapy.* Botsford CT: Water of Life Publishing, 1989.

Beall, Morris A., *Super Drug Story.* Washington DC: Columbia Books, 1962.

Beasley, Joseph, *The Betrayal of Health.* New York: Times Books, 1991.

Bearden, T.E., *AIDS: Biological Warfare.* Greenville TX: Tesla Book Co., 1988.

Beasley, Victor, *Your Electro-Vibratory Body.* Boulder Creek CO: University of the Trees Press, 1978.

Becker, Robert O., *Cross Currents: The Perils of Electropollution, The Promise of Electromedicine.* New York: Tarcher, 1990.

Becker, R. O., and Seldon, G., *The Body Electric: Electro-Magnetism and the Foundation of Life.* New York: Morrow, 1986.

Bellavite, Paolo, and Signorini, Andres, *Homeopathy A Frontier in Medical Science.* Berkeley CA: North Atlantic Books, 1995.

Benson, Herbert, *Timeless Healing.* New York: Scribner, 1996.

Benson, H., and Proctor, W., *Your Maximum Mind.* New York: Avon, 1987.

Bennett, J. T., and DiLorenzo, T. J., *Unhealthy Charities: Hazardous to Your Health and Wealth.* New York: Basic Books, 1994.

Berger, Stuart M., *What Your Doctor Didn't Learn in Medical School.* New York: Avon Books, 1989.

Berman, Edgar, *The Solid Gold Stethoscope.* New York: Macmillan, 1976.

Binzel, Philip E., *Alive and Well.* Westlake Village CA: American Media, 1995.

Bland, Jeffrey, *Nutraerobics.* San Francisco: Harper & Row, 1983.

Bogdanovich, Walt, *The Great White Lie: How America's Hospitals Betray Our Trust and Endanger Our Lives.* New York: Simon and Schuster, 1991.

Beik, John, *Cancer and Natural Medicine.* Princeton MN: Oregon Medical Press, 1995.

Borysenko, Joan, *Minding the Body, Mending the Mind.* New York: Warner, 1996.

Bradford, Robert W., and Culbert, M. L., *Now That You Have Cancer.* Chula Vista CA: The Bradford Foundation, 1992.

Bradford, Robert W., et *al., Oxidology: The Study of Reactive Oxygen Toxic Species (ROTS) and Their Metabolism in Health and Disease.* Los Altos CA: The Bradford Foundation, 1983. (Update, 1997.)

Bradford, Robert W., *et al., The Biochemical Basis of Live Cell Therapy.* Chula Vista CA: The Bradford Foundation, 1986.

Braverman, E. R., and Pfeiffer, C. C., *The Healing Nutrients Within.* New

Canaan CT: Keats, 1987.

Brecher, Arline and Harold, *Forty Something Forever*. Herndon VA: Health Savers Press, 1992.

Brennan, R. O., *Nutrigenetics*. New York: M. Evans, 1975.

Brodeur, Paul, *Currents of Death: Powerlines, Computer Terminals, and the Attempt to Cover Up Their Threat to Your Health.* New York: Simon and Schuster, 1989.

Brodie, Douglas, *Cancer and Common Sense.* White Bear Lake MN: Winning Publications, 1997.

Brown, R.E., *Rockefeller Medicine Men: Capitalism and Medical Care in America.* Berkeley CA: University of California Press, 1979.

Brown, R. K., *AIDS, Cancer and the Medical Establishment.* New York: Speller, 1986.

Burk, Dean, *A Brief on Foods and Vitamins*. Sausalito CA: The McNaughton Foundation, 1975.

Burns, Richard, *High Blood Pressure.* Old Noarlunga, Australia: Stirling Press, 1995.

Caiazza, Stephen, *AIDS: One Doctor's Personal Struggle*. Highland Park: NJ, 1989.

Cameron, Ewan, and Pauling, Linus, *Vitamin C and Cancer*. Menlo Park CA: Linus Pauling Institute of Science and Medicine, 1979.

Cannon, Walter B., *The Wisdom of the Body*. New York: Norton, 1960.

Cantwell, Alan, *AIDS and the Doctors of Death*. Los Angeles: Aries Rising, 1988.

Carlson, Rick, *The End of Medicine*. New York: Wiley, 1975.

Carper, Jean, *Stop Aging Now!* New York: HarperCollins, 1995.

Carse, Mary, *Herbs of the Earth*. Hinesburg VT: Upper Access Publishers, 1989.

Carson, Rachel, *Silent Spring.* Boston: Houghton Mifflin, 1962.

Carter, J. O., *Racketeering in Medicine*. Norfolk VA: Hampton Roads, 1992.

Carter, Richard, *The Doctor Business*. New York: Doubleday, 1985.

Carver, Cynthia, *Patient Beware.* Scarborough, Ontario, Prentice-Hall Canada, 1984.

Cassell, E. J., *The Healer's Art.* New York: Penguin, 1978.

Chaitow, Leon, and Martin, Simon, *A World without AIDS*. Great Britain: Thorsons Ltd., 1988.

Chang, S. T., *The Complete Book of Acupuncture*. Millbrae CA: Celestial Arts, 1976.

Chappell, Terry, *Questions from the Heart.* Norfolk VA: Hampton Roads, 1996.

Cheraskin, E., *Psychodietetics*. New York: Bantam, 1974.

Cheraskin, E., and Ringsdorf, W. M., *New Hope for Incurable Diseases*. Hicksville NY: Exposition Press, 1971.

Cheraskin, Emanuel, *et al., The Vitamin C Connection*. New York: Harper and Row, 1983.
Chopra, Deepak, *Quantum Healing*. New York, Bantam, 1990.
Chopra, Deepak, *Unconditional Life*. New York: Bantam, 1991.
Christopher, John R., *School of Natural Healing*. Provo UT: BiWorld Publishers, 1976.
Christy, Martha M., *Your Own Perfect Medicine*. Scottsdale AZ: Future Med., 1994.
Cichoke, A. J., *New Hope for AIDS*. Portland OR: Seven C's Publishing, 1993.
Clark, Adrian V., *Cosmic Mysteries of the Universe*. West Nyack NY: Parker, 1968.
Cleave, T. L., *The Saccharine Disease*. New Canaan CT: Keats, 1974.
Collins, Thomas M., *Comprehensive Health Care for Everyone*. Nevada City CA: Blue Dolphin, 1995.
Cooper, K.H., *Antioxidant Revolution*. Atlanta: Thomas Nelson, 1994.
Corea, Gena, *The Hidden Malpractice*. New York: Harper and Row, 1985.
Coulter, Harris L., *AIDS and Syphilis: the Hidden Link*. Richmond CA: North Atlantic Books, 1987.
Coulter, Harris L., *Divided Legacy: the Conflict Between Homoeopathy and the American Medical Association*. Richmond CA: North Atlantic Books, 1973.
Coulter, Harris, and Fisher, B.L., *DPT: A Shot in the Dark*. New York: Harcourt Brace Jovanovich, 1985.
Cousins, Norman, *Anatomy of an Illness*. New York: Norton, 1979.
Cousins, Norman, *The Healing Heart*. New York: Norton, 1983.
Cranton, Elmer, and Brecher, Arline, *Bypassing Bypass*. Norfolk VA: Donning, 1989.
Crook, William G., *The Yeast Connection*. Jackson TN: Professional Books, 1984.
Culbert, Michael, *AIDS; Hope, Hoax and Hoopla*. Chula Vista CA: The Bradford Foundation, 1990.
Culbert, Michael, *AIDS: Terror, Truth and Triumph*. Chula Vista CA: The Bradford Foundation, 1986.
Culbert, Michael, *CFS: Conquering the Crippler*. San Diego CA: C and C Communications, 1993.
Culbert, Michael, *Freedom from Cancer*. New York: Pocketbooks, 1977.
Culbert, Michael, *Live Cell Therapy for the 21st Century*. Chula Vista CA: The Bradford Foundation, 1993.
Culbert, Michael, and Camino, D.I., *Nutritional and Herbal Factors in the Prevention and Management of Cancer*. San Diego: C and C Communications, 1997.
Culbert, Michael, *Vitamin B17: Forbidden Weapon Against Cancer*. New Rochelle NY: Arlington House, 1974.

Culbert, Michael, *What the Medical Establishment Won't Tell You that Could Save Your Life*. Norfolk VA: Donning, 1983.
Damasio, Antonio R., *Descartes' Error:* New York: Putnam, 1994.
Davis, N. M., and Cohen, M. R., *Medication Errors: Causes and Prevention.* Philadelphia: George F. Stickley, 1981.
deGrazia, Alfred, ed., *The Velikovsky Affair (the Warfare of Science and Scientism).* Hyde Park NY: University Books, 1966.
DeMarco, Carolyn, *Take Charge of Your Body.* Canada: The Well Woman Press, 1994.
Dermer, G. B., *The Immortal Cell.* Garden City Park NY: Avery, 1994.
Diamantidis, Spiro, *Homoeopathic Medicine*. Athens: Medical Institute for Homoeopathic Research and Application, 1989.
Dienstfrey, Harris, *Where the Mind Meets the Body.* New York: Harper Collins, 1991.
Diet, Nutrition and Cancer. (National Research Council) Washington DC: National Academy Press, 1982.
Dohrenwend, B. S. and B. P., eds., *Stressful Life Events: Their Nature and Effects*. New York: Wiley, 1974.
Dossey, Larry, *Healing Words: the Power of Prayer and the Practice of Medicine*. New York: Harper, 1993.
Dossey, Larry, *Meaning and Medicine.* New York: Bantam, 1991.
Dossey, Larry, *Prayer is Good Medicine.* San Francisco: Harper, 1996.
Dossey, Larry, *Space, Time & Medicine*. Boston: Shambhala, 1982.
DuBois, J. E., *The Devil's Chemists*. Boston: Beacon, 1952.
Dubos, Rene, *The Mirage of Health.* New York: Harper, 1979.
Duffy, John, *The Healers: The Rise of the Medical Establishment.* New York: McGraw, 1976.
Dufty, William, *Sugar Blues*. Radnor PA: Chilton, 1975.
Epstein, Samuel, *The Politics of Cancer.* San Francisco: Sierra Club Books, 1978.
Fasciana, Guy, *Are Your Dental Fillings Poisoning You? The Hazards of Mercury in Your Mouth.* New Canaan CT: Keats, 1986.
Ferguson, Wilburn, *The Jivaro and His Drugs*. Quito, Ecuador: Editorial Casa de la Cultura Ecuatoriana, 1957.
Feuer, Elaine, *Innocent Casualties*. Pittsburgh: Dorrance, 1996.
Fink, John, *Third Opinion.* Garden City Park NY: Avery, 1988.
Flynn, J. T., *God's Gold: the Story of Rockefeller and His Times*. New York: Harcourt Brace, 1932.
Forman, Brenda, *B-15: The 'Miracle' Vitamin*. New York: Grosset and Dunlap, 1979.
Fox, Arnold, and Fox, Barry, *Immune for Life.* Rocklin CA: Prima, 1990.
Fredericks, Carlton, *Breast Cancer and the Nutritional Approach.* New York: Grosset and Dunlap, 1977.

Fredericks, Carlton, *Eat Well, Get Well, Stay Well.* New York: Grosset and Dunlap, 1980.
Fredericks, Carlton, *Eating Right for You.* New York: Grosset and Dunlap, 1972.
Fredericks, Carlton, *PsychoNutrition.* New York: Grosset and Dunlap, 1976.
Fredricks, Carlton, and Goodman, Herman, *Low Blood Sugar and You.* New York: Grosset and Dunlap, 1969.
Friedman, Alan, *Spider's Web.* New York: Bantam 1993.
Friedman, Steven, and Burger, Robert, *Forbidden Cures.* New York: Stein and Day, 1976.
Freese, A. S., *Managing Your Doctor.* New York: Stein and Day, 1975.
Fuchs, V. H., *Who Shall Live?* New York: Basic Books, 1974.
Garceau, Oliver, *The Political History of the American Medical Association.* Cambridge MA: Harvard University Press, 1941.
Garrett, Laurie, *The Coming Plague.* New York: Penguin, 1994.
Garrison, Omar, *The Dictocrats.* Chicago: Books for Today, 1970.
Gerson, Max, *A Cancer Therapy — Results of Fifty Cases.* New York: Whittier Books, 1958.
Gittleman, Ann Louise, *Super Nutrition for Men and the Women Who Love Them.* New York: Evans, 1996.
Gittleman, Ann Louise, *Super Nutrition for Women.* New York: Bantam, 1991.
Glasscheib, H. S., *The March of Medicine: Emergence and Triumph of Modern Medicine.* (tr. Savill) New York: Putnam, 1964.
Glassman, Judith, *The Cancer Survivors and How They Did It.* New York: Dial Press, 1981.
Gofman, J. W., and O'Connor, E., *X-rays: Health Effects of Common Exams.* San Francisco: Sierra Club Books, 1985.
Golan, Ralph, *Optimum Wellness.* New York: Ballantine, 1995.
Goulden, Joseph, *The Money Givers.* New York: Random House, 1971.
Greenberg, Kurt, ed., *Challenging Orthodoxy.* New Canaan CT: Keats, 1991.
Greenwald, Peter, ed., *Cancer, Diet and Nutrition.* Chicago: Marquis Who's Who, 1985.
Gregory, Scott, and Leonardo, Blanca, *They Conquered AIDS!* Palm Springs CA: Tree of Life Publications, 1989.
Griffin, G. E., *World without Cancer.* Westlake Village CA: American Media, 1974. (Update, 1996)
Griggs, Barbara, *Green Pharmacy.* New York: Viking Press, 1981.
Guinther, J., *The Malpractitioners.* New York: Doubleday, 1978.
Haas, Elson, *Staying Healthy with Nutrition.* Millbrae CA: Celestial Arts, 1991.
Haggard, H. W., *Mystery, Magic and Medicine: the Rise of Medicine from Superstition to Science.* Garden City NY: Doubleday, Doran, 1933.
Halstead, Bruce, *Amygdalin Therapy.* Los Altos CA: Choice Publications,

1978.
Halstead, Bruce, *Metabolic Cancer Therapy.* Colton CA: Golden Quill, 1978.
Halstead, Bruce, *The DMSO Handbook.* Colton CA: Golden Quill, 1981.
Halstead, Bruce, *The Scientific Basis of EDTA Chelation Therapy.* Colton CA: Golden Quill, 1981.
Harmer, Ruth Mulvey, *American Medical Avarice.* New York: Abelard-Schuman, 1975.
Harper, Harold, and Culbert, M. L., *How You Can Beat the Killer Diseases.* New Rochelle NY: Arlington House, 1977.
Hastings, A.C., *et al., Health for the Whole Person.* New York: Bantam, 1980.
Hausman, Patricia, *The Right Dose*. Emmaus PA: Rodale Press, 1987.
Hay, Louise, *You Can Heal Your Life, and Heal Your Body.* Santa Monica CA: Hay House, 1984.
Heiby, W.A., *The Reverse Effect.* Deerfield IL: MediScience, 1988.
Heimlich, Jane, *What Your Doctor Won't Tell You*. New York: HarperCollins, 1990.
Heinerman, John, *Double the Power of Your Immune System.* West Nyack NY: Parker, 1991.
Heinerman, John, *The Treatment of Cancer with Herbs.* Orem UT: BiWorld Publishers, 1980.
Hilfiker, David, *Healing the Wounds*. New York: Pantheon, 1985.
Hoffer, Abram, *Orthomolecular Nutrition for Physicians.* New Canaan CT: Keats, 1989.
Hoffman, W. H., *Using Energy to Heal.* (Privately published), 1979.
Hong-Yen Hsu and Preacher, W. G., *Chinese Herb Medicine and Therapy.* Nashville TN: Aurora Publishers, 1976.
Horne, Ross, *The Health Revolution*. Australia: Happy Landings Pty Ltd, 1989.
Horowitz, L.G., *Emerging Viruses: AIDS and Ebola.* Rockport MA: Tetrahedron, 1996.
Houston, Robert G., *Repression and Reform in the Evaluation of Alternative Cancer Therapies*. Washington DC: Project Cure, 1989.
Hoxsey, Harry, *You Don't Have to Die*. 1956: reprinted by Nature Heals, Chapala, Mexico, 1977.
Huard, Pierre, and Wang, Ming, *Chinese Medicine*. New York: McGraw-Hill, 1972.
Huggins, Hal, *It's all in Your Head: Diseases Caused by Silver-Mercury Amalgams.* Life Sciences Press, 1989.
Hunt, Steven B., and Allen, James, *In Failing Health.* Skokie IL: National Textbooks Co., 1977.
Hunt, Valerie, *Infinite Mind: The Study of Human Vibration.* Malibu CA: Malibu Publishing, 1995.

Hur, Robin, *Food Reform: Our Desperate Need.* Austin TX: Heidelberg, 1975.

Illich, Ivan, *Medical Nemesis*. New York: Random House, 1976.

Inlander, C. B., *et al., Medicine on Trial*. New York: Pantheon Books, 1988.

Isaacs, James, and Lamb, John C., *Complementarity in Biology*. Baltimore: Johns Hopkins Press, 1969.

Jayasuriya, Anton, *Clinical Acupuncture*, 10th ed. Sri Lanka: Medicina Alternativa, 1985.

Jayasuriya, Anton, *Clinical Homeopathy*, 4th ed. Sri Lanka: Medicina Alternativa, 1985.

Jeffreys, Toni, *The Mile-High Staircase.* London: Hodder and Stoughton, 1982.

Jensen, Bernard, *Foods that Heal*. Garden City Park NY: Avery, 1988.

Jones, Rochelle, *The Supermeds*. New York: Macmillan, 1990.

Josephson, Matthew, *The Robber Barons*. New York: Harcourt Brace, 1934.

Kanfiran, M., *Homeopathy in America: the Rise and Fall of a Medical Heresy.* Baltimore: Johns Hopkins University Press, 1971.

Kaptchuk, T. J., *The Web that Has No Weaver: Understanding Chinese Medicine*. New York: Congdon and Weed, 1983.

Kaptchuk, T. J., and Croucher, Michael, *The Healing Arts*. New York: Summit, 1978.

Kastner, Mark, and Burroughs, Hugh, *Alternative Healing: The Complete A-Z Guide to over 160 Different Alternative Therapies.* La Mesa CA: Halcyon, 1993.

Kiev, A., ed., *Magic, Faith and Healing*. New York: Macmillan, 1974.

Kittler, Glenn, D., *Laetrile — Control for Cancer*. New York: Paperback Library, 1963.

Klatz, Ronald, *Grow Young with HGH.* New York: HarperCollins, 1997.

Klatz, Ronald, and Goldman, Robert, *Stopping the Clock.* New Canaan CT: Keats, 1996.

Klaw, Spencer, *The Great American Medical Show.* New York: Penguin, 1976.

Kloss, Jethro, *Back to Eden*. Santa Barbara CA: Lifeline Books, 1974.

Koch, W. F., *The Survival Factor in Neoplastic and Viral Diseases.* Detroit: Vanderkloot Press, 1961.

Kramer, C., *The Negligent Doctor*. New York: Crown, 1968.

Kuhnau, W. W., *Live-Cell Therapy: My Life with a Medical Breakthrough.* Tijuana BC, Mexico: Artes Graficas de Baja California, 1983. Rev. ed., 1992.

Kunin, R. A., *Mega-Nutrition*. New York: McGraw-Hill, 1980.

Kunnes, Richard, *Your Money or Your Life.* New York: Dodd, Mead, 1974.

Kushi, Michio, and Blauer, Steven, *The Macrobiotic Way.* Garden City Park NY: Avery, 1985.

Lambert, E. C., *Modern Medical Mistakes.* Bloomington IN: Indiana University Press, 1978.
Lambert, Samuel, and Goodwin, G. M., *Medical Leaders from Hippocrates to Osler.* Indianapolis: Bobbs-Merrill, 1929.
Lanctot, Guylaine, *The Medical Mafia: How to Get Out of It Alive and Take Back our Health and Wealth.* (Published in Canada) Morgan VT: Here's the Key Inc., 1995.
Lander, Louise, *Defective Medicine.* New York: Farrar, Straus, Giroux, 1978.
Lauritsen, John, *Poison by Prescription.* New York: Pagan Press, 1990.
Lauritsen, John, *The AIDS War: Propaganda, Profiteering and Genocide from the Medical-Industrial Complex.* New York: Pagan Press, 1993.
Lauritsen, John, and Wilson, Hank, *Death Rush: Poppers and AIDS.* New York: Pagan Press, 1986.
Lederberg, J., *et al.,* eds., *Emerging Infections: Microbial Threats to Health in the United States.* Washington DC: National Academy Press, 1992.
Lerner, Michael, *Choices in Healing.* Cambridge MA: MIT Press, 1994.
LeShan, Lawrence, *You Can Fight for Your Life: Emotional Factors in the Causation of Cancer.* New York: Evans, 1977.
Levine, Stephen, *Healing into Life and Death.* New York: Anchor, 1987.
Levine, Stephen, and Kidd, Paris, *Antioxidant Adaptation: its Role in Free Radical Pathology.* San Leandro CA: Allergy Research Group, 1986.
Levy, S. M., *Behavior and Cancer.* San Francisco, Jossey-Bass, 1985.
Lin, David J., *Free Radicals and Disease Prevention.* New Canaan CT: Keats, 1993.
Lisa, P. J., *Are You a Target for Elimination?* Huntington Beach CA: International Institute of Natural Health Sciences, 1985.
Lisa, P. J., *The Great Medical Monopoly Wars.* Huntington Beach CA: International Institute of Natural Health Sciences, 1986.
Livingston, Virginia: *Cancer: a New Breakthrough.* San Diego: Production House, 1972.
Livingston, Virginia: *The Conquest of Cancer — Vaccines and Diet.* New York: Franklin Watts, 1984.
Longgood, William, *The Poisons in Your Food.* New York: Pyramid, 1960.
Love, Susan, *Dr. Susan Love's Hormone Book.* NY: Random House, 1997.
Lucas, Richard, *Nature's Medicines.* New York: Award Books, 1966.
Lucas, Scott, *The FDA.* Millbrae CA: Celestial Arts, 1978.
Lynes, Barry, *The Cancer Cure that Worked.* Toronto: Marcus Books, 1987.
Lynes, Barry, *The Healing of Cancer.* Toronto: Marcus Books, 1989.
Major, R. H., *A History of Medicine.* Springfield IL: Charles C. Thomas, 1954.
Manner, Harold, W., *et al., The Death of Cancer.* Evanston IL: Advanced Century, 1978.
Marti, James E., *The Alternative Health and Medicine Encyclopedia.* Detroit:

Visible Ink Press, 1995.
Martin, Rose, *Fabian Freeway.* Belmont MA: Western Islands, 1966.
Martin, Wayne, *Medical Heroes and Heretics.* Old Greenwich CT: Devin-Adair, 1977.
McCully, Kilmer S., *The Homocysteine Revolution: Medicine for the New Millennium.* New Canaan CT: Keats, 1997.
McDonagh, E. W., *Chelation Can Cure.* Kansas City MO: Platinum Pen, 1983.
McGee, Charles, T., *Heart Frauds.* Coeur d'Alene ID: MediPress, 1993.
McTaggart, Lynne, *What Doctors Don't Tell You.* San Francisco: Thomson/ HarperCollins, 1996.
Melville, A., *Cured to Death: the Effects of Prescription Drugs.* New York: Stein and Day, 1982.
Mendelsohn, Robert S., *Confessions of a Medical Heretic.* New York: Warner, 1979.
Millman, Marcia, *The Unkindest Cut.* New York: Morrow, 1977.
Mills, Simon, and Finando, Steven, *Alternatives in Healing.* New York: New American Library, 1988.
Mindell, Earl, *Earl Mindell's Vitamin Bible.* New York: Rawson, Wade, 1980.
Montgomery, E. R., *The Story Behind Great Medical Discoveries.* New York: Dodd, Mead, 1945.
Moore, M. J., and Lynda, *The Complete Handbook of Holistic Health.* Englewood Cliffs NJ: Prentice-Hall, 1983.
Moore, Thomas J., *Deadly Medicine.* New York: Simon & Schuster, 1995.
Moore, Thomas, J., *Heart Failure.* New York: Random House, 1989.
Moskowitz, Reed C., *Your Healing Mind.* New York: Avon, 1993.
Moss, Ralph, W., *Cancer Therapy: the Independent Consumer's Guide to Non-Toxic Treatment and Prevention.* New York: Equinox Press, 1992.
Moss, Ralph W., *Questioning Chemotherapy.* New York: Equinox Press, 1995.
Moss, Ralph W., *The Cancer Industry.* New York: Paragon House, 1991.
Moss, Ralph W., *The Cancer Syndrome.* New York: Grove Press, 1980.
Moyers, Bill, *Healing and the Mind.* New York: Doubleday, 1993.
Mullins, Eustace, *Murder by Injection.* Staunton VA: Council for Medical Research, 1988.
Murphy, M., and Donovan, S., *The Physical and Psychological Effects of Meditation.* Sausalito CA: Institute of Noetic Sciences, 1997.
Murray, M. T., and Pizzorno, J. F., *An Encylopedia of Natural Medicine.* Rocklin CA: Prima Publishing, 1990.
Myss, C.A., and Shealy, C.N., *The Creation of Health: Merging Traditional Medicine with Intuitive Diagnosis.* Walpole MA: Stillpoint, 1988.
Needleman, Jacob, *The Way of the Physician.* San Francisco: Harper and Row,

1985.
Nichols, Joe D., "*Please, Doctor, DO Something!*" Dallas TX: Universal Media, 1992.
Nuland, Sherwin, *How We Die: Reflections on Life's Final Chapters.* New York: Knopf, 1994.
Nuland, Sherwin, *The Wisdom of the Body.* New York: Knopf, 1997.
Null, Gary, *Healing Your Body Naturally: Alternative Treatments to Ilness.* New York: Four Walls Eight Windows, 1992.
Nutrition Almanac (Nutrition Search, Inc.) New York: McGraw-Hill, 1984.
Orient, J.M., *Your Doctor is Not In.* New York: Crown, 1994.
Ornish, Dean, *Dr. Dean Ornish's Program for Reversing Heart Disease.* New York: Random House, 1990.
Ornstein, Dolph, *Medicine Today, Healing Tomorrow.* Millbrae CA: Celestial Arts, 1976.
Ornstein, Robert, and Sobel, David, *The Healing Brain.* New York: Simon and Schuster, 1987.
Osler, Sir William, *The Evolution of Modern Medicine.* New Haven CT: Yale University Press, 1923.
Ostrom, Neenyah, *Fifty Things You Should Know About the Chronic Fatigue Syndrome Epidemic.* New York: St. Martin's Press, 1993.
Owen, Bob, *Roger's Recovery from AIDS.* Cannon Beach OR: DAVAR, 1987.
Page, M.E., and Abrams, H.L., *Your Body is Your Best Doctor.* New Canaan CT: Keats, 1972.
Passwater, Richard, *Cancer and Its Nutritional Therapies.* New Canaan CT: Keats, 1978.
Passwater, Richard, *Selenium as Food and Medicine.* New Canaan CT: Keats, 1980.
Passwater, Richard, *Supernutrition.* New York: Dial, 1975.
Passwater, Richard, *Supernutrition for Healthy Hearts.* New York: Dial, 1977.
Pauling, Linus, *How to Live Longer and Feel Better.* New York: Avon, 1987.
Pelletier, K. R., *Mind as Healer, Mind as Slayer.* New York: Delacorte Press, 1977.
Pelletier, K.R., *Sound Mind, Sound Body: A New Model for Lifelong Health.* New York: Simon and Schuster, 1994.
Peltzman, Sam, *Regulation of Pharmaceutical Innovation: the 1962 Amendments.* Washington DC: American Enterprise Institute for Policy Research, 1974.
Pfeiffer, Carl, *Mental and Elemental Nutrients.* New Canaan CT: Keats, 1975.
Philpott, W. H., *Cancer: the Magnetic/Oxygen Answer.* Choctaw OK, 1994.
Philpott, W. H., and Kalita, D. W., *Brain Allergies: the Psycho-Nutrient Connection.* New Canaan CT: Keats, 1987.
Pizzorno, Joseph, *Total Wellness.* Rocklin CA: Prima, 1996.

Powers of Healing. Alexandria VA: Life-Time Books, 1989.
Preston, Thomas, *The Clay Pedestal*. Seattle: Madrona, 1981.
Price, Weston, *Nutrition and Physical Degeneration*. Santa Monica CA: Price Pottenger Foundation, 1945.
Queen, H.L., *Chronic Mercury Toxicity: New Hope Against an Endemic Disease*. Colorado Springs CO: Queen & Co., 1988.
Rapp, Doris, *Is This Your Child?* New York: Morrow, 1991.
Rappoport, Jon, *AIDS, Inc*. San Bruno CA: Human Energy Press, 1988.
Rath, Matthias, *Eradicating Heart Disease*. San Francisco CA: Health Now, 1993.
Regan, B., and Hirshberg, C., *Spontaneous Remission: An Annotated Biography*. Sausalito CA: Institute of Noetic Sciences, 1993.
Riordan, H. D., *Medical Mavericks, vol. 1*. Wichita KS: Bio-Communications Press, 1988.
Richardson, J. A., and Griffin, P., *Laetrile Case Histories*. New York; Bantam, 1977.
Robbins, John, *Diet for a New America*. Walpole NH: Stillpoint Publishing, 1987.
Robertson, W. O., *Medical Malpractice: a Preventive Approach*: Seattle: University of Washington Press, 1985.
Roe, D. A., *Drug-Induced Nutritional Deficiencies*. Westport CT: Avi Publishing, 1976.
Rogers, E.E., *Biological Medicine*. New Westminster BC, Canada: Everwood, 1980.
Rona, Zoltan, *Childhood Illness and the Allergy Connection* Rocklin CA: Prima, 1997.
Rona, Zoltan, *Return to the Joy of Health*. Burnaby, BC, Canada: *Alive* Books, 1995.
Rona, Zoltan, *The Joy of Health*. Toronto: Hounslow Press, 1991.
Root-Bernstein, Robert, *Rethinking AIDS: the Tragic Cost of Premature Consensus*. New York: Free Press, 1993.
Rosenbaum, Michael, and Susser, Murray, *Solving the Puzzle of Chronic Fatigue Syndrome*. Tacoma: Life Sciences Press, 1992.
Rosenberg, Harold, *The Doctor's Book of Vitamin Therapy*. New York: Berkley Windhover, 1974.
Rubik, Beverly, ed., *The Interrelationship Between Mind and Matter*. Philadelphia PA: Center for Frontier Science, Temple University, 1992.
Ruesch, Hans, *Naked Empress*. Zurich: Buchverlag CIVIS, 1982.
Sarnat, Michael, *Physician, Heal Thyself*. Battleboro UT: Herbal Free Press, 1995.
Satillaro, Anthony, *Recalled by Life*. Boston: Houghton Mifflin, 1981.
Schauss, Alexander, *Diet, Crime and Delinquency*. Berkeley CA: Parker House, 1980.

Scheiber, S. C., and Doyle, B. B., *The Impaired Physician.* New York: Plenum Press, 1983.
Schlosser, Thea, *Beyond the Dark Cloud.* Santa Barbara CA: Chronic Fatigue and Immune Dysfunction Media Awareness Assn. of America, 1995.
Schneider, Robert, *When to Say No to Surgery.* Englewood Cliffs NJ: Prentice-Hall, 1982.
Schrauzer, G., *ed., Inorganic and Nutritional Aspects of Cancer.* New York: Plenum, 1978.
Scott, C. J., and Hawk, J., eds., *Heal Thyself: the Health of Health Care Professionals.* New York: Brunner/Mazel, 1986.
Sears, Barry, *Enter the Zone.* New York: HarperCollins, 1995.
Selye, Hans, *The Stress of Life.* New York: McGraw-Hill, 1956.
Sherman, Harold, *Your Power to Heal.* New York: Harper & Row, 1972.
Shilts, Randy, *And the Band Played On.* New York: St. Martin's Press, 1987.
Shute, Wilfred E., *Wilfred Shute's Complete Updated Vitamin E Book.* New Canaan CT: Keats, 1975.
Sidel, V. W. and R., *A Healthy State.* New York: Pantheon, 1983.
Siegel, Bernie, *Love, Medicine and Miracles.* New York: Harper and Row, 1986.
Siegel, Bernie. *Peace, Love and Healing.* New York: Harper and Row, 1989.
Silverman, Milton, and Lee, Philip R., *Pills, Profits and Politics.* San Francisco: University of California Press, 1974.
Simon, H.B., *Conquering Heart Disease.* New York: Little, Brown, 1994.
Simonton, Carl, *et al., Getting Well Again.* New York: Bantam, 1986.
Smith, Cyril W., and Best, Simon, *Electromagnetic Man: Health and Hazard in the Electrical Environment.* New York: St., Martin's Press, 1989.
Smith, L.H., *How to Raise a Healthy Child.* New York: Evans, 1996.
Smith, Russell, *The Cholesterol Conspiracy.* St. Louis: Green, 1991.
Solomon, G. E., *Psychoneuroimmunology.* New York: Academic Press, 1987.
Starr, Paul, *The Social Transformation of American Medicine.* New York: Basic Books, 1982.
Stefansson, Vilhjalmur, *Cancer: Disease of Civilization.* New York: Hill and Wang, 1960.
Steingraber, Sandra, *Living Downstream — An Ecologist Looks at Cancer and the Environment.* New York: Addison-Wesley, 1997.
Sugarman, Ellen, *Warning: the Electricity Around You May be Hazardous to Your Health.* New York: Simon and Schuster, 1992.
Tansley, David V., *Radionics: Interface with the Ether-Fields.* London: Health Science Press, 1975.
The New Wellness Encylopedia. Eds., University of California-Berkeley Wellness Center. Boston: Houghton-Mifflin, 1995.
Tierra, Lesley, *Herbs of Life: Health & Healing Using Western & Chinese*

Techniques. Freedom CA: Crossing Press, 1992.

Tilden, John H., *Toxemia: The Basic Cause of Disease*. Chicago: Natural Hygiene Press, 1974.

Tinney, Louise, *The Encylopedia of Natural Remedies*. Pleasant Grove UT: Woodland, 1995.

Trever, William, *In the Public Interest*. Los Angeles: Scriptures Unlimited, 1972.

Trowbridge, J. P., and Walker, Morton, *The Yeast Connection*. New York: Bantam, 1986.

Tyler, Varro E., *The Honest Herbal: A Sensible Guide to the Use of Herbs and Related Remedies*. New York: Pharmaceutical Products Press, 1993.

Venzmer, Gerhard, *Five Thousand Years of Medicine*. (tr. Koenig) New York: Taplinger, 1968.

Unconventional Cancer Therapies (H. Gelband, Project Director) Washington DC: US Congress, Office of Technology Assessment, 1990.

Vitamin A: Everyone's Basic Bodyguard. Emmaus PA: Rodale Press, 1972.

Vithoulkas, George, *Homeopathy: Medicine of the New Man*. New York: Arco Publishing, 1979.

Vithoulkas, George, *The Science of Homeopathy*. New York: Grove Press, 1980.

Vogel, Virgil J., *American Indian Medicine*. New York: Ballantine, 1973.

Wade, Carlson, *Nature's Cures*. New York: Award Books, 1972.

Wade, Carlson, *The Rejuvenation Vitamin*. New York: Award Books, 1970.

Walker, Kenneth, *The Story of Medicine*. New York: Oxford University Press, 1954.

Walker, M. J., *Dirty Medicine*. London: Slingshot Publications, 1993.

Walker, Morton, *Chelation Therapy*. Atlanta GA: '76 Press, 1980.

Walker, Morton, *DMSO: The New Healing Power*. Old Greenwich CT: Devin-Adair, 1983.

Walker, Morton, *Total Health*. New York: Everest House, 1979.

Wallach, J. D., and Ma Lan, *Let's Play Doctor!* Alexandria VA: Lifestyle Horizons, 1993.

Wallach, J. D., and Ma Lan, *Rare Earths*. Alexandria VA: Lifestyle Horizons, 1994.

Walters, Richard, *Options: The Alternative Cancer Therapy Book*. Garden City Park NY: Avery, 1993.

Weaver, Warren, *U.S. Philanthropic Organizations: Their History, Structure, Management and Record*. New York: Harper and Row, 1967.

Webster, David, *Achieve Maximum Health.* Cardiff CA: Hygeia, 1995.
Webster, James, *Vitamin C: The Protective Vitamin.* New York: Award Books, 1971.
Weil, Andrew, *Health and Healing.* Boston: Houghton Mifflin, 1983.
Weil, Andrew, *Natural Health, Natural Medicine.* Boston: Houghton Mifflin, 1990.
Weil, Andrew, *Spontaneous Healing.* New York: Knopf, 1995.
Weinberger, Stanley, *Healing Within.* Larkspur CA: Healing Within, 1993.
Weiner, Michael A., *The Herbal Bible.* San Rafael CA: Quantum Books, 1992.
Weitz, Martin, *Health Shock.* Englewood Cliffs NJ: Prentice-Hall, 1982.
Werbach, Melvyn, R., *Foundations of Nutritional Medicine.* Tarzana CA: Third Line Press, 1997.
Werbach, Melvyn R., *Healing through Nutrition.* New York: HarperCollins, 1993.
Werbach, Melvyn R., *Nutritional Influences on Illness.* Tarzana CA: Third Line Press, 1987.
Werbach, Melvyn, and Murray, Michael, *Botanical Influences on Illness.* Tarzana CA: Third Line Press, 1994.
Wheelwright, E. C., *Medical Plants and Their History.* New York: Dover Books, 1974.
Wigmore, Ann, *Be Your Own Doctor: a Positive Guide to Natural Living.* Garden City Park NY: Avery, 1982.
Wigmore, Ann, *The Hippocrates Diet and Health Program.* Garden City Park NY: Avery, 1984.
Wiles, Richard, *et al., Tap Water Blues: Herbicides in Drinking Water.* Washington DC: Environmental Working Group/Physicians for Social Responsibility, 1994.
Williams, Roger J., *Nutrition Against Disease.* New York: Bantam, 1971.
Williams, Roger J., *Physician's Handbook of Nutritional Science.* Springfield: Charles C. Thomas, 1975.
Willner, Robert E., *Deadly Deception.* Peltec Publishing, 1994.
Wohl, Stanley, *The Medical Industrial Complex.* New York: Harmony Books, 1984.
Wolfe, Sydney, *et al., Worst Pills/Best Pills II.* Washington DC: Public Citizen Health Research Group, 1993.
Wolinski, Howard, and Bruno, Tom, *The Serpent and the Staff: The Unhealthy Politics of the American Medical Association.* New York:

Tarcher, 1994.
Wood, Matthew, *The Magical Staff: the Vitalist Tradition in Western Medicine.* Berkeley CA: North Atlantic Books, 1992.
World Medicine: the East-West Guide to Healing Your Body. New York: Tarcher/Perigee, 1993.
Wright, Jonathan V., *Dr. Wright's Guide to Healing with Nutrition.* Emmaus PA: Rodale Press, 1989.
Yiamouyiannis, John, *Fluoride, the Aging Factor.* Delaware OH: Health Action Press, 1983.
Yudkin, John, *Sweet and Dangerous.* New York: Bantam, 1972.

INDEX

A

B

C

D

E

H

J

K

L

M

N

O

P

Q

T

U

V

W

X

Y

Z

American Medical Avarice
by Ruth M. Harvev

The Solid Gold Stethoscope
Dr. Edgar Bergman

The Unkindest Cut Marcia Millman

Confessions of a Medical Heretic
Dr. Rbt. Mendelsohn

Medicine On Trial

The Impaired Physician

How We Die, Dr. Sherwin Nuland

Confessions of a Medical Heretic, R. Mendelson

Solid Gold Stethoscope E. Bergman MD

In the Public Interest, Wm. Trever

Your Money Or Your Life Rich Kunnes MD

Slaughter of the Innocent
Naked Empress
Hans Ruesch